# SANDERS' STRUCTURAL FETAL ABNORMALITIES

## NOTICE

# SANDERS' STRUCTURAL FETAL ABNORMALITIES

## Third Edition


EDITOR

**W. Allen Hogge, MD, MA**
Professor and Chair, Emeritus
Department of Obstetrics, Gynecology, and Reproductive Sciences
University of Pittsburgh, Magee-Womens Hospital
Pittsburgh, Pennsylvania
Clinical Professor
Department of Obstetrics and Gynecology
Virginia Commonwealth University
Richmond, Virginia

ASSISTANT EDITORS

**Barbara Cohlan, MD**
Professor of Pediatrics
Department of Pediatrics, University of Pittsburgh
Director of the Newborn Nurseries
Magee-Womens Hospital/Children's Hospital of Pittsburgh
Pittsburgh, Pennsylvania

**Isabelle Wilkins, MD**
Professor and Vice-Chair
Department of Obstetrics, Gynecology, and Reproductive Sciences
University of Pittsburgh/Magee-Womens Hospital
Pittsburgh, Pennsylvania

**Lyndon Hill, MD**
Professor, Emeritus
Former Director, Division of Ultrasound
Department of Obstetrics, Gynecology, and Reproductive Sciences
University of Pittsburgh, Magee-Womens Hospital
Pittsburgh, Pennsylvania



Mc Graw Hill Education

New York Chicago San Francisco Athens London Madrid Mexico City
Milan New Delhi Singapore Sydney Toronto

**Sanders' Structural Fetal Abnormalities, Third Edition**



1 2 3 4 5 6 7 8 9 DSS 21 20 19 18 17 16

ISBN 978-1-25-964137-4
MHID 1-259-64137-6

This book was set in Arno Pro by Cenveo® Publisher Services.
The editors were Andrew Moyer and Regina Y. Brown
The production supervisor was Richard Ruzycka.
Project management was provided by Raghavi Khullar, Cenveo Publisher Services.
The cover designer was Dreamit, Inc.

**Library of Congress Cataloging-in-Publication Data**

Names: Hogge, W. Allen, editor. | Wilkins, Isabelle A., editor. | Cohlan, Barbara, editor. | Hill, Lyndon, editor.
Title: Sanders' Structural fetal abnormalities / editor, W. Allen Hogge ; assistant editors, Isabelle Wilkins, Barbara Cohlan, Lyndon Hill.
Description: Third edition. | New York : McGraw-Hill Education, [2016] | Preceded by Structural fetal abnormalities / editor, Roger C. Sanders ; assistant editors, Lillian R. Blackmon ... [et al.]. 2nd ed. c2002. | Includes bibliographical references and index.
Identifiers: LCCN 2016019772| ISBN 9781259641374 (pbk.) | ISBN 1259641376 (pbk.)
Subjects: | MESH: Congenital Abnormalities--ultrasonography | Fetus--abnormalities | Ultrasonography, Prenatal | Atlases
Classification: LCC RG626 | NLM QS 617 | DDC 618.3/2–dc23
LC record available at https://lccn.loc.gov/2016019772

# CONTENTS

**Timothy P. Canavan, MD, MSc.**
Associate Professor
Director, Division of Ultrasound
Department of Obstetrics, Gynecology and Reproductive Sciences
Magee-Womens Hospital/University of Pittsburgh
Pittsburgh, Pennsylvania

**Barbara Cohlan MD**
Professor of Pediatrics
Department of Pediatrics, University of Pittsburgh
Director of the Newborn Nurseries
Magee-Womens Hospital/Children's Hospital of Pittsburgh
Pittsburgh, Pennsylvania

**Stephen P. Emery, MD**
Associate Professor
Director, Center for Innovative Fetal Intervention
Department of Obstetrics, Gynecology and Reproductive Sciences
Magee-Womens Hospital/University of Pittsburgh School of Medicine
Pittsburgh, Pennsylvania

**Matthew D. Ford, MS, CCC-SLP**
Clinical Coordinator Cleft-Craniofacial Center
Children's Hospital of Pittsburgh of UPMC
Pittsburgh, Pennsylvania

**Lyndon M. Hill, MD**
Professor, Emeritus
Former Director, Division of Ultrasound
Department of Obstetrics, Gynecology, and Reproductive Sciences
University of Pittsburgh, Magee-Womens Hospital
Pittsburgh, Pennsylvania

**W. Allen Hogge, MD, MA**
Professor and Chair, Emeritus
Department of Obstetrics, Gynecology, and Reproductive Sciences
University of Pittsburgh, Magee-Womens Hospital
Pittsburgh, Pennsylvania
Clinical Professor
Department of Obstetrics and Gynecology
Virginia Commonwealth University
Richmond, Virginia

**Aviva L. Katz, MD, MA, FACS, FAAP**
Associate Professor of Surgery
University of Pittsburgh School of Medicine
Children's Hospital of Pittsburgh
Pittsburgh, Pennsylvania

**David E. Kauffman, MD**
Clinical Professor
Department of Obstetrics, Gynecology, and Reproductive Sciences
University of Pittsburgh / Magee Womens Hospital
Pittsburgh, Pennsylvania

**Michael C. Ost, MD**
Associate Professor of Urology
Division Chief, Pediatric Urology
Vice Chairman, Department of Urology
The Children's Hospital of Pittsburgh
The University of Pittsburgh Medical Center
Pittsburgh, Pennsylvania

**Devereux N. Saller, Jr., MS, MD**
Professor
Director of Clinical Genetics
Department of Obstetrics, Gynecology & Reproductive Sciences
Magee-Womens Hospital University of Pittsburgh
Pittsburgh, Pennsylvania

**Frederick S. Sherman, MD, MBA**
Professor Emeritus
Department of Pediatrics and Obstetrics, Gynecology and Reproductive Sciences
Magee-Womens Hospital/University of Pittsburgh
Pittsburgh, Pennsylvania

**Hyagriv N. Simhan, MD, MS**
Professor and Vice-Chair
Director, Division of Maternal-Fetal Medicine
Department of Obstetrics, Gynecology & Reproductive Sciences
University of Pittsburgh
Medical Director of Obstetrical Services, Magee-Womens Hospital
Pittsburgh, Pennsylvania

**Isabelle Wilkins, MD**
Professor and Vice-Chair
Department of Obstetrics, Gynecology, and Reproductive Sciences
University of Pittsburgh/Magee-Womens Hospital
Pittsburgh, Pennsylvania

# FOREWORD

It gives me great pleasure to write the foreword for the new edition of *Structural Fetal Abnormalities*. The book has an interesting history. In 1970, I joined the Johns Hopkins Department of Radiology as an instructor, on a 1-year leave of absence from my UK position at Oxford, and was put in charge of genitourinary imaging. Within a month, the hospital's woman's board announced the donation of a bistable ultrasound imaging system for use in the women's clinic. With minimal experience in ultrasound, I was asked to develop the use of the system and welcomed the opportunity to travel around the USA for training and machine selection. I started imaging fetuses, crudely assessing growth by measuring the biparietal diameter and the femur length, counting fetal number, and discovering fetal lie. I even attempted to diagnose placenta previa by imaging a fluid-filled pessary placed around the cervix after a "double setup." Fetal anomaly detection seemed a remote possibility because the images were so rudimentary. I soon became fascinated by the technique and decided to stay on when my year away from the United Kingdom was complete.

Since that time there has been steady improvement in imaging quality. Grayscale imaging became available in 1975, but the acquirement of images was tedious and technically difficult using the B-scan technique, which involved carefully dragging a transducer suspended from a gantry around the maternal abdomen. Slowly, starting with Stuart Campbell's observation of the absent cranium in anencephalus (1972) and the spinal deformity in spina bifida (1975), the ultrasonic spectrum of fetal malformations began to be revealed. It soon became apparent that a team approach, involving consultation with obstetricians, pediatric surgeons or urologists, geneticists, neonatologists, genetic counselors, and individuals in other specialties was important in pregnancy management and in discussions with anxious patients when a fetal abnormality was discovered on a sonogram. For the most part, these anomalies were an incidental finding at the time of the ultrasound study rather than the result of referral because of familial or teratogenic issues; quality sonography was the doorway into the fetal world.

Fetal anomaly management discussions, such as the one that I and colleagues started at Johns Hopkins and subsequently at the University of Maryland, became an important feature of fetal malformation management. Each week, the fetal abnormalities revealed by sonography were shown, and the representatives of the various specialties commented on the aspects of fetal care that related to their specialty. These management conferences were the stimulus for the first two editions of this book, which were developed at the University of Maryland with collaboration from authors at Johns Hopkins. I am delighted that Allen Hogge, who has been involved since the first edition, has taken on the task of editing a new edition of the book.

What is the point of these management discussions? The discovery of a fetal abnormality poses difficult ethical and management dilemmas for the sonographic examiner, the parents, and the obstetrician. What sort of difficulties with delivery, and later life, will the anomaly present? Is the anomaly lethal, or is there such a poor prognosis that cesarean section and resuscitative care are to be avoided? Has the anomaly been discovered early enough that termination is an option? This is a difficult question because termination limits vary by state. Do the parents wish to pursue in utero surgery with all the uncertainty that approach brings? Sonologists, whether radiologists or now predominantly perinatologists, and referring obstetricians are frequently faced with many questions when a possible anomaly is discovered. This book attempts to answer these questions. In addition, support staff, such as sonographers, nurses, and genetic counselors, also play a significant role in diagnosis and care, and it is hoped this book will be of help to them. This book, in a succinct and well-illustrated fashion, attempts to provide complete coverage of all the problems the affected fetus may have so that the patient is ensured a comprehensive compassionate care plan.

There are thousands of conditions and syndromes that cause fetal deformities in utero. The conditions selected for presentation in this book were chosen because they are relatively common or have distinctive features that allow definitive recognition, such as the hitchhiker thumb of diastrophic dwarfism. Some of the more common sonographic findings that sometimes indicate underlying fetal problems, such as cord cysts, are also considered. Each is presented in a standardized fashion from the viewpoint of the geneticist, sonologist (whether radiologist or perinatologist), obstetrician, neonatologist, and surgeon. A consistent format is used for each entity. Numerous high-quality ultrasound images and photographs of the fetus or infant are included. Although the book is modeled on *Smith's Recognizable Patterns of Human Malformations*, there has been no attempt to be as comprehensive. The material in this book is targeted at sonographically visible abnormalities and does not include abnormalities not discoverable by sonography. I congratulate the new team led by Allen Hogge and Lyndon Hill on the quality of the new edition.

*Roger C. Sanders*

## REFERENCES

Campbell S, Johnstone FD, Holt EM, May P: Anencephaly: early ultrasonic diagnosis and active management. Lancet 1972; 2:26-27.

Campbell S, Pryse-Davies J, Coltart TM, et al: Ultrasound in the diagnosis of spina bifida. Lancet 1975; 1:1065-1068.

# PREFACE



It has been 25 years since Dr. Roger Sanders envisioned the concept of this book. He first developed and organized a highly successful series of conferences, "Structural Fetal Abnormalities: The Total Picture." National and international experts came together not only to discuss the ultrasound diagnosis of fetal malformations but also to focus on the "total picture," from the time an ultrasound finding was visualized to the final surgical treatment of the structural abnormality. In essence, this is the information that every maternal-fetal medicine specialist, radiologist, geneticist, genetic counselor, or any professional taking care of a family whose unborn child has been diagnosed with a structural abnormality needs to know. It gives them the essential knowledge they need to provide the family counseling regarding prognosis and appropriate management. The principles of a multidisciplinary approach to a pregnancy complicated by a fetal structural malformation, which were discussed at those first conferences, provided the outline for the first edition of this book. Experts in sonography, perinatology, genetics, neonatology, and pediatric surgery were recruited to complete a comprehensive picture of the diagnosis and management of common structural fetal anomalies detected by obstetrical ultrasound. The second edition, published 10 years later, reflected the marked improvements in ultrasound technology and the growing ability to make a precise genetic diagnosis of fetal conditions.

In this third edition, much has been changed from previous editions. These changes mirror the dramatic improvements that have occurred in our ability to diagnose and treat fetal malformations. This edition includes all new images that demonstrate the new and improved ultrasound technologies, such as three-dimensional (3-D) and power Doppler. The sections on genetic etiologies of the structural malformations have required complete revision, indicating the rapid advances in genomics and molecular diagnostics that have occurred in the last decade.

The passage of 20 years also has meant that the former editor, three of four assistant editors, and a number of contributors have retired from the active practice of medicine. But, with the guidance and support of Dr. Sanders, I have assembled a new team of experts to carry on the tradition of excellence that was key to the first two editions. As in previous editions, a sonologist, Lyndon M. Hill, provides the ultrasonic findings of each anomaly, which is complemented by the perspectives of experts in genetics, maternal-fetal medicine (MFM), and neonatology. Isabelle Wilkins in MFM and Barbara Cohlan in neonatology have provided their respective expertise, and I have taken on the role of geneticist for this edition. We have been greatly aided in the endeavor by a large and diverse group of contributors who are our colleagues and collaborators from Magee-Womens Hospital and the Children's Hospital of Pittsburgh.

What has remained unchanged in this third edition is the overall format. This book has been a concise, but complete, handbook of structural fetal malformations that provides, at the reader's fingertips, the features of a condition, its differential diagnosis, how to manage the pregnancy, and what to expect in the neonatal period and beyond. The subtle changes made to the format are intended to enhance that sense of a concise but comprehensive reference. Each section has an updated bibliography of suggested readings to provide the reader a source for greater detail on each condition.

In addition to my assistant editors and contributors, others deserve my special thanks for their efforts in bringing this new edition to fruition. My wife, Joan Hogge, not only provided her encouragement and support but also served as the proofreader for the final draft. Adele Leibowitz, my administrative assistant, and Andrea Juhl, Dr. Hill's administrative assistant, were absolutely key to our ability to coordinate and organize the multiple sections of the manuscript and the many ultrasound images that are part of this book. Without the efforts of all of these people, this third edition of *Sanders' Structural Fetal Abnormalities* would not have been possible.

*W. Allen Hogge*

# CHAPTER 1

# CHROMOSOMES

# 1.1 TRIPLOIDY

## EPIDEMIOLOGY/GENETICS

**Definition** Rare, lethal chromosomal abnormality. An entire extra haploid set of chromosomes results in 69 chromosomes instead of the usual 46.

**Epidemiology** Of human conceptions, 1% to 2% are triploid, but most end in spontaneous abortion. Accounts for 20% of chromosomally abnormal spontaneous abortions. Very rare at birth, occurring in 1 in 10,000 live births.

**Embryology** A complete extra set of chromosomes results in 69 XXX (digynic) or XXY (diandric). Sixty percent result from fertilization with two sperm; 40% result from fertilization of a diploid egg. However, more recent prospective information, at the time of first-trimester screening, suggests that digynic triploidy may be more common than diandric. Central nervous system malformations include hydrocephalus, holoprosencephaly, and neural tube defects. Hypertelorism, cleft lip/cleft palate, syndactyly of the third and fourth fingers, and congenital heart defects are typical features.

**Inheritance Patterns** Sporadic

**Teratogens** None

**Screening** Serum levels of human chorionic gonadotropin and inhibin A may be extremely high in triploidy with dispermy as the cause. Very low levels of α-fetoprotein, estriol, inhibin A, and human chorionic gonadotropin (hCG) are seen in pregnancies in which fertilization of a diploid egg occurs. In the first trimester, screening, using nuchal translucency and serum markers will detect approximately 85% of fetuses with triploidy. Diandric triploids have an increased nuchal translucency, elevated hCG, and normal, or low, pregnancy-associated plasma protein A (PAPP-A). Digynic triploidy has a normal nuchal translucency, very low hCG, and very low PAPP-A. Diandric triploidy will generally look like an increased risk for trisomy 21, and digynic will generally look like a high risk for trisomy 18.

**Prognosis** Lethal antenatally or in the newborn period. Rare mosaic cases survive with moderate-to-severe mental retardation.

## SONOGRAPHY

**Findings:** Sonographic findings vary with the source of the extra chromosome.

### FREQUENT FINDINGS

- First-trimester thickened nuchal translucency
- Intrauterine growth restriction
  - Asymmetric growth restriction with large fetal head is associated with digynic triploidy
  - There is early-onset symmetrical growth restriction.
  - Some fetuses with diandric triploidy have grown normally.
- Ventriculomegaly

- Holoprosencephaly
- Micrognathia
- Low-set ears
- Single umbilical artery
- Syndactyly of third and fourth fingers
- Clubfeet
- Oligohydramnios
- Enlarged placenta with multiple cystic spaces; similar to a partial mole (diandric, XXY)
- Small placenta (digynic, XXX)
- Bilateral theca lutein cysts

### LESS FREQUENT

- Neural tube defects
- Dandy-Walker malformation
- Agenesis of the corpus callosum
- Microphthalmia
- Hypertelorism
- Cystic hygroma
- Coarctation of aorta
- Hypoplastic left ventricle
- Omphalocele
- Pyelocaliectasis
- Ambiguous genitalia
- Nonimmune hydrops
  - Pleural effusion
  - Pericardial effusion
  - Ascites
  - Anasarca

## PREGNANCY MANAGEMENT

**Investigations and Consultations** Traditional karyotyping with, or without, fluorescent in situ hybridization (FISH) analysis via amniocentesis or chorionic villi sampling (CVS) establishes the diagnosis. Once a cytogenetic diagnosis has been established, no further investigations or consultations are necessary. For patients in whom the diagnosis is made beyond the point of legal pregnancy termination or in those who decide to continue the pregnancy, a neonatologist should consult with the family about appropriate perinatal and neonatal management. The family should be offered supportive psychological care throughout the pregnancy.

**Monitoring** If pregnancy termination is not an option, monitor for preeclampsia or hyperthyroidism. Either of these complications is an indication for treatment, including immediate delivery without regard to gestational age.

**Pregnancy Course** Molar changes in the placenta predispose to hyperemesis gravidarum, early preeclampsia, theca lutein cysts, and, on occasion, hyperthyroidism. Prenatal care should be modified such that only interventions for maternal health, rather than fetal health, are offered. Intrauterine growth restriction is common, and aggressive management with fetal monitoring is inappropriate.

**Pregnancy Termination Issues** Use of suction dilatation and evacuation, or any other method of pregnancy termination, is appropriate once a cytogenetic diagnosis has been established.

**Delivery** Fetal monitoring and cesarean section are both contraindicated for the pregnancy complicated by a triploidy.

## NEONATOLOGY

**Resuscitation** Contraindicated if the diagnosis is definite because of the established lethal prognosis.

**Transport** Indicated only if diagnostic confirmation, counseling, and long-term care planning are not available locally.

**Testing and Confirmation** A peripheral blood chromosome study can confirm the chromosome abnormality.

**Nursery Management** Provision of basic supportive care—warmth, hygiene, nourishment, and comfort only— until prognosis for protracted survival is defined and long- term care decisions can be addressed with the family.

### SUGGESTED READINGS


1. Daniel A, Wu Z, Bennetts B, et al: Karyotype, phenotype, and parental origin in 19 cases of triploidy. Prenat Diagn 2001; 21:1034-1048.
2. Edwards MT, Smith WL, Hanson J, Abu Yousef M: Prenatal sonographic diagnosis of triploidy. J Ultrasound Med 1986; 5:279-281.
3. Engelbrechtsen L, Brondum-Nielsen K, Ekelund C, et al: Detection of triploidy at 11-14 weeks' gestation: a cohort study of 198,000 pregnant women. Ultrasound Obstet Gynecol 2013; 42:530-535.
4. Jauniaux E, Brown R, Rodeck C, Nicolaides KH: Prenatal diagnosis of triploidy during the second trimester of pregnancy. Obstet Gynecol 1996; 88:983-989.
5. Jauniaux E, Brown R, Snijders RJM, et al: Early prenatal diagnosis of triploidy. Am J Obstet Gynecol 1997; 176;550-554.
6. Joergensen MW, Niwmann I, Rasmussen AA, et al: Triploid pregnancies: genetic and clinical features of 158 cases. Am J Obstet Gynecol 2014; 211:370.e1-19.
7. Jones KL, Jones MC, del Campo M: Smith's Recognizable Patterns of Human Malformations. 7th ed. Philadelphia: Elsevier; 2013.
8. Kagan KO, Anderson JM, Anwandter G, et al: Screening for triploidy by the risk algorithms for trisomies 21, 18 and 13 at 11 weeks to 13 weeks and 6 days of gestation. Prenat Diagn 2008; 28:1209-1213.

9. Lockwood C, Scioscia A, Stiller R, Hobbins J: Sonographic features of the triploid fetus. Am J Obstet Gynecol 1987; 157:285-287.

10. McFadden DE, Pantzar JT: Placental pathology of triploidy. Hum Pathol 1996; 27:1018-1020.

11. Mittal TK, Vujanic GM, Morrissey BM, Jones A: Triploidy: antenatal sonographic features with post-mortem correlation. Prenat Diagn 1998; 18:1253-1262.

12. Pircon RA, Porto M, Towers CV, et al: Ultrasound findings in pregnancies complicated by fetal triploidy. J Ultrasound Med 1989; 8:507-511.

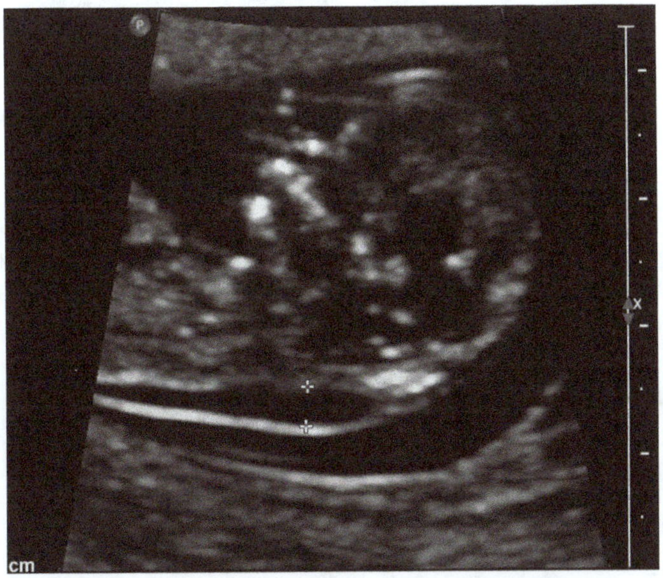

FIGURE 1.1A Triploidy—Thickened (4 mm) nuchal translucency.

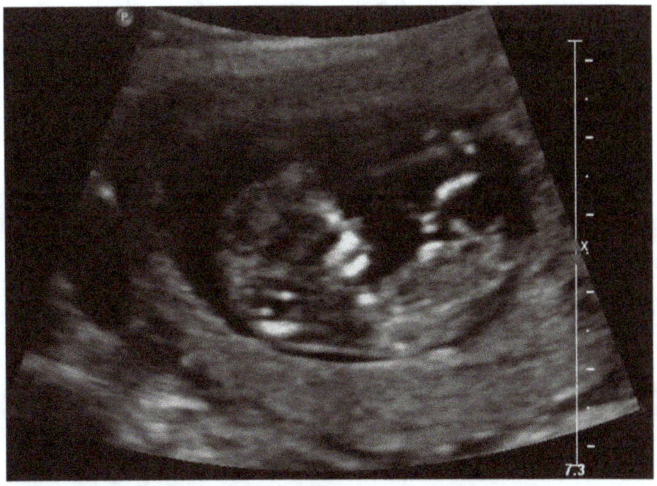

FIGURE 1.1B Digynic Triploidy—1st trimester disproportion between head and abdomen.

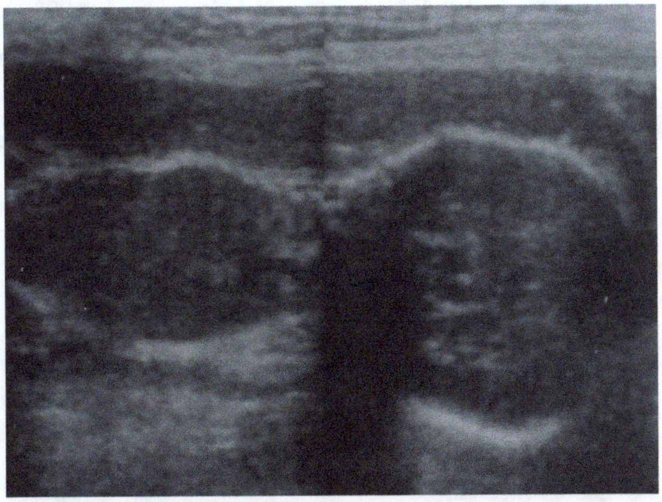

FIGURE 1.1C Digynic Triploidy—2nd trimester disproportion between head and abdomen.

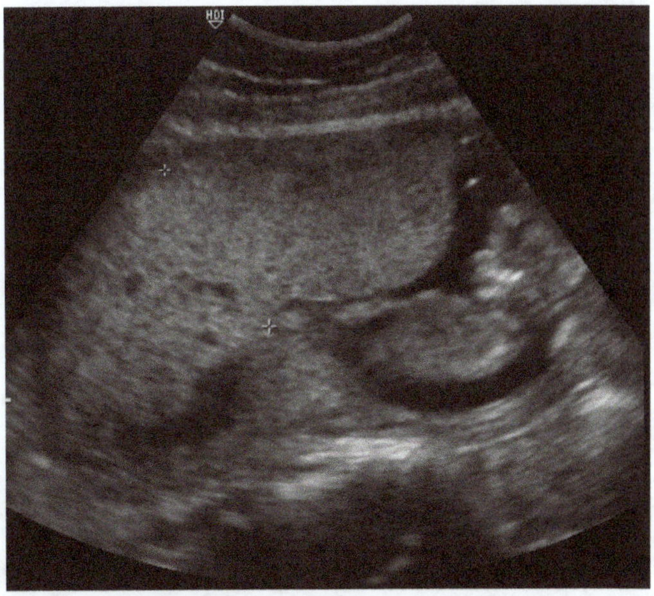

FIGURE 1.1D Diandric Triploidy—cystic placenta (+. . . +).

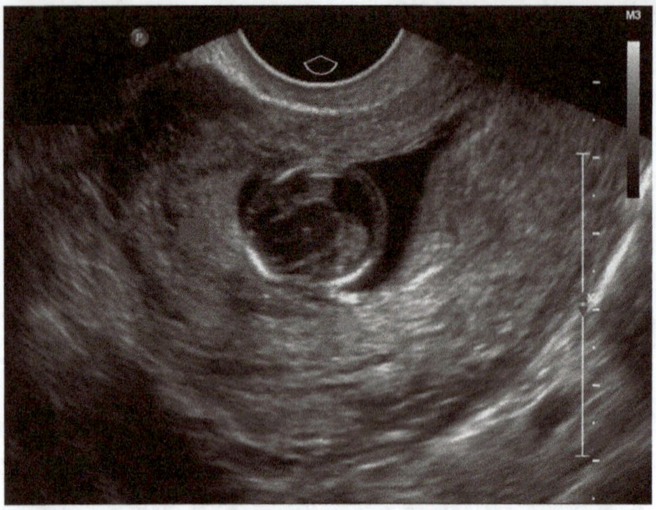

**FIGURE 1.1E** Triploidy with alobar holoprosencephaly

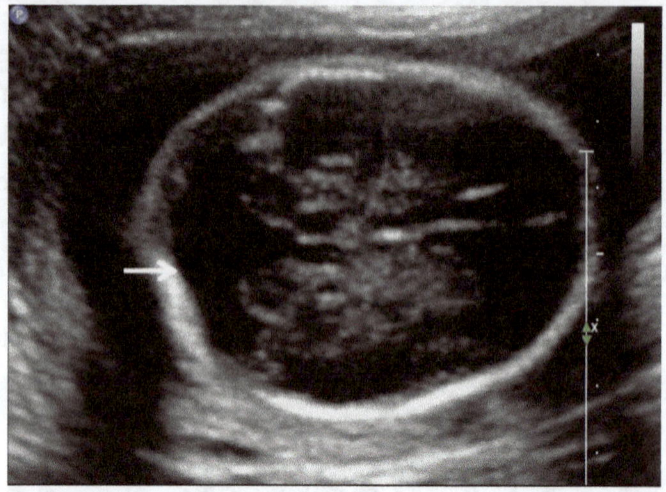

**FIGURE 1.1F** Triploidy with Dandy-Walker malformation (arrow).

# 1.2 TRISOMY 13

## EPIDEMIOLOGY/GENETICS

**Definition** Because of its higher intrauterine mortality, trisomy 13 is the least common of the major autosomal trisomies. Fetuses with trisomy 13 tend to have more craniofacial (median cleft, micro- or anophthalmia) and brain (holoprosencephaly) abnormalities. While trisomy 13 is frequently referred to as lethal, this is not always the case. The median survival is 7 days, and 90% of trisomy 13 newborns die by 1 year of age.

**Epidemiology** One in 5000 to 10,000 births

**Embryology** The phenotype is due to full trisomy 13. Increased maternal age has been documented in this disorder. Rare mosaic partial trisomy 13 syndromes (with varying phenotypes) and translocation patients have been reported. Microcephaly, holoprosencephaly, microphthalmia, polydactyly, and facial clefts are found in more than 50% of patients. Eighty percent of patients have congenital heart defects, with atrial septal defects (ASDs) and ventricular septal defects (VSDs) the most common. However, many patients have complex heart lesions. Other distinctive abnormalities include polycystic kidneys (30% of patients) and omphalocele (<50% of patients).

**Inheritance Patterns** Most cases are sporadic, with approximately a 1-in-100 risk of recurrence in future pregnancies. Rare familial translocations have a higher recurrence risk, depending on the specific translocation.

**Teratogens** None

**Screening** Second-trimester maternal serum biochemical marker screening is not helpful in detecting trisomy 13 fetuses. Some cases are diagnosed by first-trimester screening because of increased nuchal translucency and fetal malformations. Noninvasive prenatal testing (NIPT) will detect 90% to 95% of cases.

**Prognosis** This condition is lethal or has a very poor prognosis in all cases. Live births occur in 40% to 60%, but 90% die in the first year. All survivors with full trisomy 13 have profound mental retardation. In infancy, severe failure to thrive, feeding difficulties, seizures, apneic attacks, and visual and hearing deficits occur in the majority of infants, secondary to the orofacial and central nervous system defects.

## SONOGRAPHY

**Findings:** The number and severity of congenital anomalies associated with trisomy 13 are highly variable.

### FREQUENT FINDINGS

- First-trimester thickened nuchal translucency
- Holoprosencephaly
    - The presence of a cavum septum pellucidum excludes a significant forebrain abnormality.

- Microcephaly
- Central cleft lip and palate
- Enlarged cisterna magna
- Hypotelorism
- Low-set ears
- Polydactyly
- Clubfeet
- Congenital heart defect
  - Ventricular septal defect
  - Atrial septal defect
  - Hypoplastic left ventricle
  - Aortic stenosis
  - Pulmonary stenosis

### LESS FREQUENT

- First-trimester megacystis
- Agenesis of the corpus callosum
- Cerebellar hypoplasia
- Basal ganglia calcifications
- Single orbit with 2 globes, cyclops
- Microphthalmia
- Single nostril
- Proboscis
- Rocker-bottom feet
- Clubhands
- Overlapping fingers
- Echogenic enlarged kidneys containing small cysts
- Omphalocele
- Neural tube defect

## PREGNANCY MANAGEMENT

**Investigations and Consultations** Traditional karyotyping with, or without, FISH analysis via amniocentesis or CVS establishes the diagnosis. A positive result from maternal blood of cell-free circulating fetal DNA is considered a screening test and is not sufficient to establish the diagnosis. Once a cytogenetic diagnosis has been established, no further investigations or consultations are necessary. For patients in whom the diagnosis is made beyond the point of legal pregnancy termination or in those who decide to continue the pregnancy, a neonatologist should consult with the family about appropriate perinatal and neonatal management. The family should be offered supportive psychological care throughout the pregnancy.

**Monitoring** Only routine prenatal care should be performed. Monitoring for preeclampsia is appropriate, as it is more common in pregnancies complicated by trisomy 13. This complication is an indication for treatment, including immediate delivery, without regard to gestational age.

**Pregnancy Course** Prenatal care should be modified such that only interventions for maternal health, rather than fetal health, are offered. Intrauterine growth restriction is common, and aggressive management with fetal monitoring is inappropriate.

**Pregnancy Termination** Use of suction dilatation and evacuation, or any other method of pregnancy termination, is appropriate once a cytogenetic diagnosis has been established.

**Delivery** Electronic fetal monitoring and cesarean section should be avoided unless requested by the family after a thorough discussion of the prognosis for infants with trisomy 13.

## NEONATOLOGY

**Resuscitation** A decision about whether to give life support should be made prior to delivery, once the diagnosis is established. If the diagnosis is unknown prior to birth, providing life support is appropriate until a diagnosis can be established.

**Transport** Indicated only if diagnostic confirmation, counseling, and long-term care planning are not available locally.

**Testing and Confirmation** Obtain peripheral blood, or cord blood, for chromosome analysis to confirm the diagnosis.

**Nursery Management** Full life support is appropriate until the diagnosis is confirmed and the family has time for weighing options for duration and intensity of support. Care requirements will be contingent on associated organ involvement and the long-term goals of the family.

### SUGGESTED READINGS


1. Chen C-P, Chien S-C: Prenatal sonographic features of trisomy 13. J Med Ultrasound 2007; 15:58-66.
2. Hosseinzadeh K, Luo J, Borhani A, Hill L: Non-visualization of cavum septi pellucidi: implication in prenatal diagnosis? Insights Imaging 2013; 4:357-367.
3. Janvier A, Watkins A. Medical interventions for children with trisomy 13 and trisomy 18: what is the value of a short disabled life? Acta Paediatr 2013;12:1112-1117.
4. Jones KL, Jones MC, del Campo M. Smith's Recognizable Patterns of Human Malformations. 7th ed. Philadelphia: Elsevier; 2013.
5. Liao AW, Sebire NJ, Beerts L, et al: Megacystis at 10-14 weeks of gestation: chromosomal defects and outcome according to bladder length. Ultrasound Obstet Gynecol 2003; 26:338-341.
6. Loureiro T, Ferreira AFA, Ushakov F, et al: Dilated fourth ventricle in fetuses with trisomy 18, trisomy 13, and triploidy at 11-13 weeks' gestation. Fetal Diagn Ther 2012; 32:186-189.

7. Matias A, Montenegro N, Areias JC, Brandao O: Anomalous fetal venous return associated with major chromosomopathies in the late first trimester of pregnancy. Ultrasound Obstet Gynecol 1998; 11:209-213.
8. Merritt TA, Catlin A, Wool C, et al: trisomy 18 and trisomy 13. Neoreviews 2012; 13:e40-e48.
9. Quezada MS, Gil MM, Francisco C, et al: Screening for trisomies 21, 18, and 13 by cell-free DNA analysis of maternal blood at 10-11 weeks' gestation and the combined test at 11-13 weeks. Ultrasound Obstet Gynecol 2014; 20:1-6.
10. Papageroghiou AT, Avgidou K, Spencer K, et al: Sonographic screening for trisomy 13 at 11 to 13 (+6) weeks of gestation. Am J Obstet Gynecol 2006; 194:397-401.
11. Springett AL, Morris JK: Antenatal detection of Edwards (trisomy 18) and Patau (trisomy 13) syndrome: England and Wales 2005-2012. J Med Screen 2014; 21(3): 113-119.
12. Watson WJ, Miller RC, Wax JR, et al: Sonographic detection of trisomy 13 in the first and second trimesters of pregnancy. J Ultrasound Med 2007; 26:12069-1214.

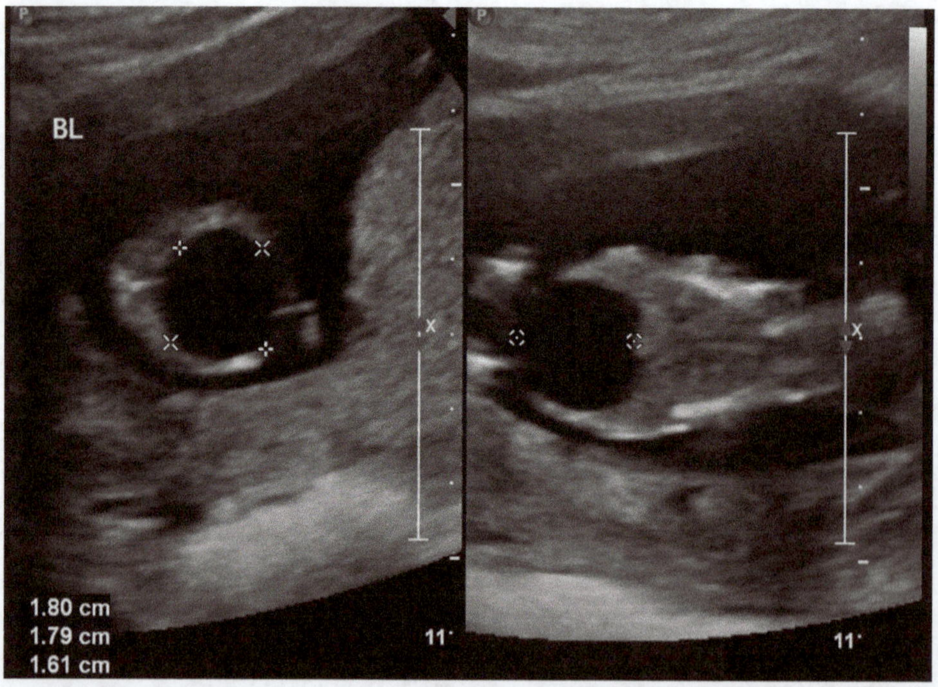


FIGURE 1.2A Trisomy 13 with 1st trimester megacystis (+. . . +).

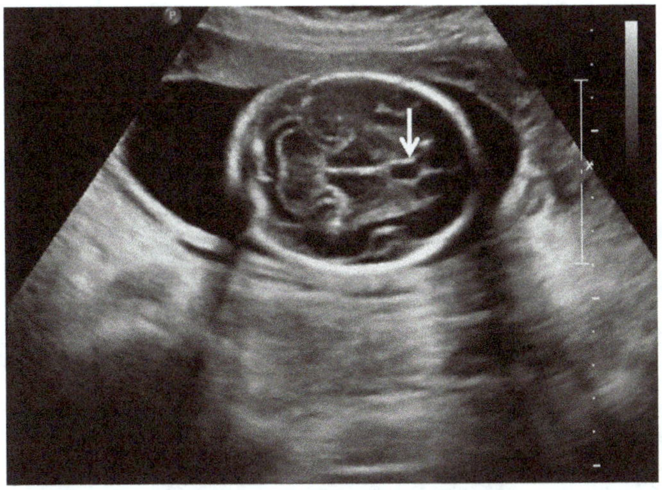

**FIGURE 1.2B** Normal cavum septum pellucidum (arrow).

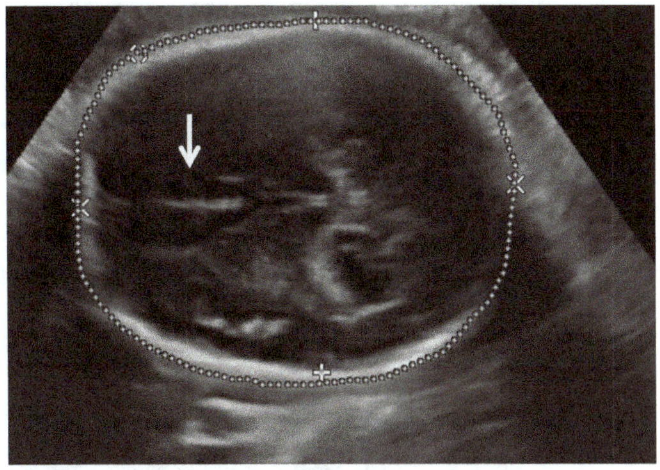

**FIGURE 1.2C** Trisomy 13 with absence of cavum septum pellucidum (arrow).

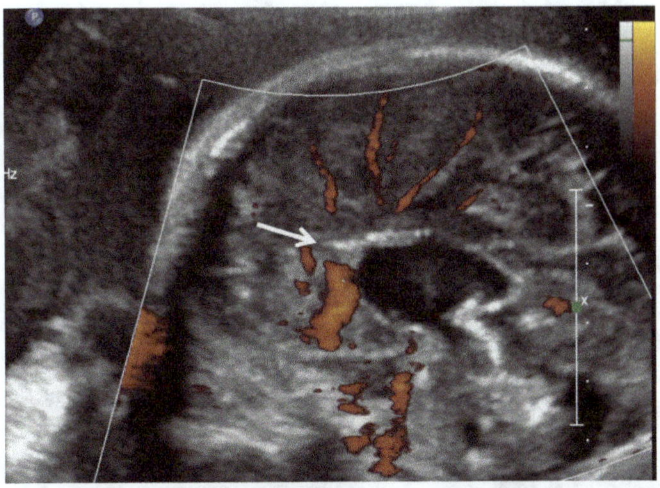

**FIGURE 1.2D** Trisomy 13 with agenesis of the corpus callosum. Note the absence of pericallosal artery and corpus callosum (arrow).

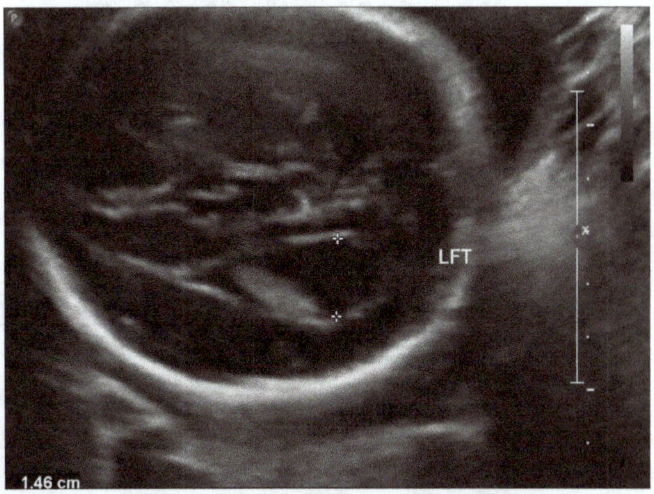


**FIGURE 1.2E** Trisomy 13 with Colpocelphaly (+. . . +) associated with agenesis of the corpus callosum.

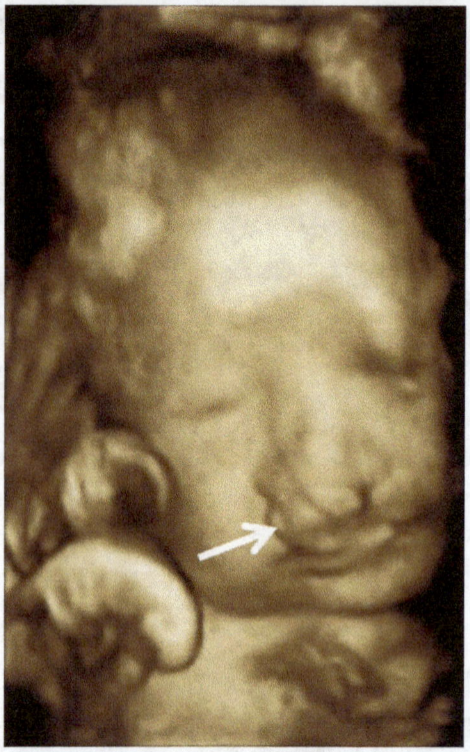

FIGURE 1.2F Trisomy 13 with pre-maxillary protuberance (arrow) indicating bilateral cleft lip and palate.

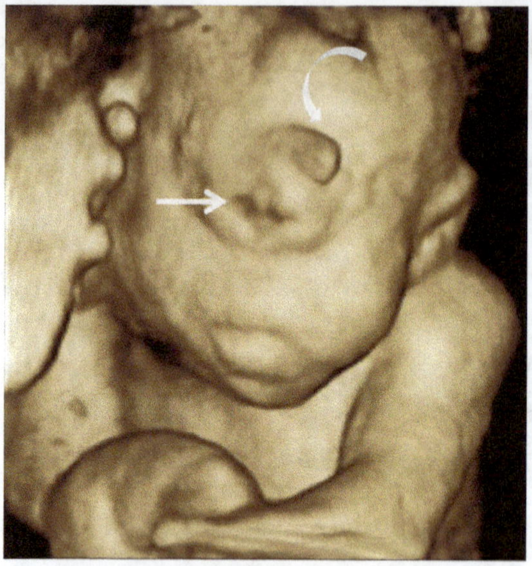

FIGURE 1.2G Trisomy 13 with cyclops—single orbit with two globes (straight arrow) and proboscis (curved arrow).

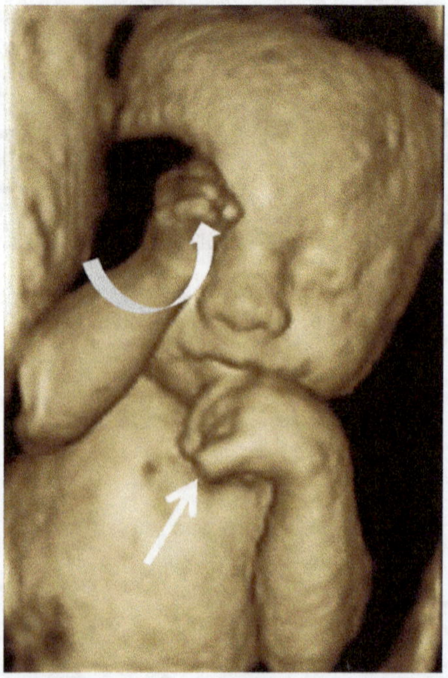

FIGURE 1.2H Trisomy 13 with club hand (straight arrow) and overlapping fingers (curved arrow).

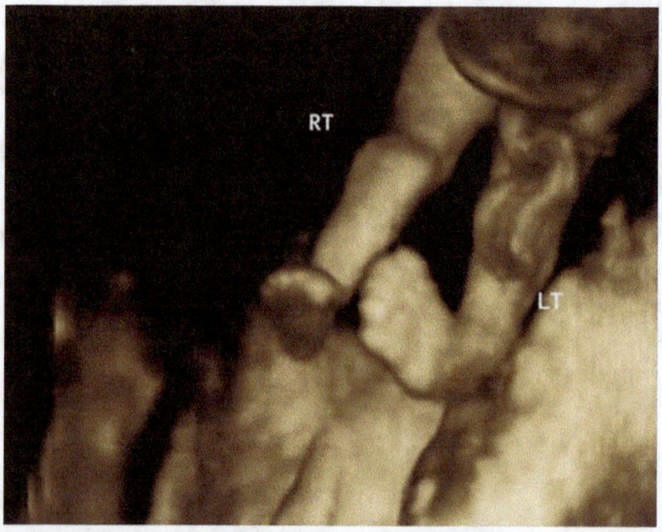


FIGURE 1.2I Trisomy 13—3D left clubbed foot.

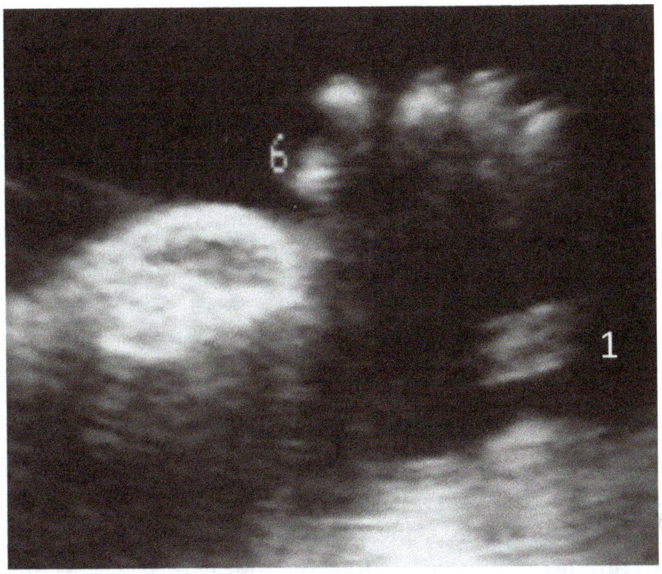


**FIGURE 1.2J** Trisomy 13 with post-axial polydactyly (6); thumb (1).

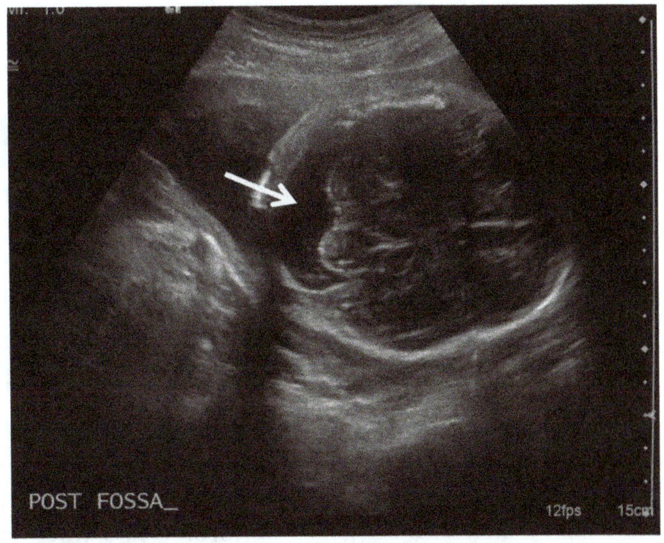


**FIGURE 1.2K** Trisomy 13 with an enlarged (> 10 mm) cisterna magna (arrow).

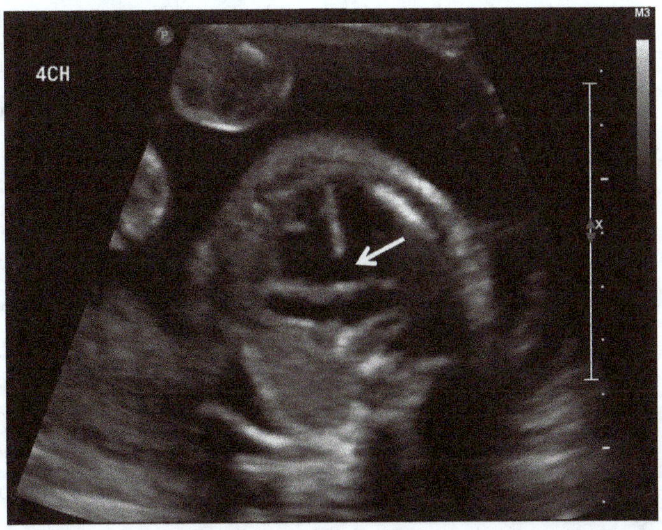


**FIGURE 1.2L** Trisomy 13 with a ventricular septal defect (arrow).

# 1.3 TRISOMY 18

## EPIDEMIOLOGY/GENETICS

**Definition** Trisomy 18 is the second most common autosomal trisomy syndrome. It presents with intrauterine growth retardation (IUGR), microcephaly, and congenital heart defects (80%).

**Epidemiology** One in 3000 to 5000 (M1:F3)

**Embryology** Most infants have full trisomy 18. Rare patients with mosaic karyotypes, partial trisomy 18 syndromes (with varying phenotypes), and translocation cases have been reported. Infants with trisomy 18 present with severe growth restriction, microdolichocephaly with a prominent occiput, malformed ears, micrognathia, clenched hands, and congenital heart defects (80%) that are characterized by complex polyvalvular abnormalities with VSDs. Malformations that occur in less than 50% of cases include cleft lip and palate, limb defects, omphalocele, and diaphragmatic hernia.

**Inheritance Patterns** Most cases are sporadic, with a 1-in-100 risk of recurrence in future pregnancies. Rare familial translocations have a higher recurrence risk, depending on the specific translocation.

**Teratogens** None

**Screening** Second-trimester maternal serum biochemical marker screening may detect as many as 80% of trisomy 18 fetuses. First-trimester screening has an equal detection rate. NIPT will detect approximately 99% of cases.

**Prognosis** Trisomy 18 is lethal or has a very poor prognosis in all cases. Of those detected prenatally, approximately 50%-60% will be either spontaneously aborted or be stillborn. Of affected infants, 50% will die in the first week of life, and 90% will die in the first year. Median survival is 14.5 days. All survivors with full trisomy 18 have profound mental retardation. Associated cardiac and gastrointestinal anomalies are usually life threatening, and definitely life limiting, if not corrected or palliated by surgery. Failure to thrive and feeding difficulties occur in all who survive the immediate neonatal period.

## SONOGRAPHY

**Findings:** More than 130 abnormalities have been reported with trisomy 18.

### FREQUENT FINDINGS

- First-trimester thickened nuchal translucency
- Thickened second-trimester nuchal fold (>6.0 mm)
- Low-set, abnormally shaped ears
- Cystic hygroma
- Ventriculomegaly
- Choroid plexus cysts (25%)
  - Only 2%-9% of choroid plexus cysts are associated with trisomy 18; therefore, an isolated choroid plexus cyst has a very low association with trisomy 18.

    - The number of choroid plexus cysts does not influence the likelihood of trisomy 18.
    - When a structural anomaly is present with a choroid plexus cyst, the likelihood of trisomy 18 is 37%.
    - A choroid plexus cyst as the sole sonographic finding with trisomy 18 is rare.
- Microcephaly
- Persistently clenched hands with overlapping of the fourth digit
- Clubfeet
- Congenital heart defect
    - Ventricular septal defect
    - Atrioseptal defect
    - Coarctation of the aorta
    - Double-outlet right ventricle
- Neural tube defect (20%)
- Omphalocele (25%)
    - Bowel containing
    - Liver containing
- Diaphragmatic hernia (10%)

### LESS FREQUENT

- Brachycephaly and a narrow frontal cranium results in the "strawberry-shaped" calvarium.
- Micrognathia
- Unilateral or bilateral cleft lip/palate
- Cerebellar hypoplasia
- Dandy-Walker malformation
- Mega cisterna magna (>10 mm)
- Rocker-bottom feet
- Radial ray defects
- Persistently extended extremities
- Preaxial upper limb reduction
- Second-trimester echogenic bowel
- First-trimester megacystis
- Cystic renal dysplasia
- Horseshoe kidneys

## PREGNANCY MANAGEMENT

**Investigations and Consultations** Traditional karyotyping, with or without FISH analysis via amniocentesis or CVS establishes the diagnosis. A positive result from maternal blood of cell-free circulating fetal DNA is considered a screening test and is not sufficient to establish the diagnosis. Once a cytogenetic diagnosis has been established, no further investigations or consultations are necessary. A neonatologist should consult with the family about appropriate perinatal and neonatal management if the diagnosis is made beyond the point of legal pregnancy termination or in those who decide to continue the pregnancy. The family should be offered supportive psychological care throughout the pregnancy.

**Monitoring** Maternal status should be monitored in standard fashion. Fetal evaluation is not appropriate because emergency intervention is not warranted.

**Pregnancy Course** Prenatal care should be modified such that only interventions for maternal health, rather than fetal health, are offered. Intrauterine growth restriction is common, and aggressive management with fetal monitoring is inappropriate.

**Pregnancy Termination** Use of suction dilatation and evacuation, or any other method of pregnancy termination, is appropriate once a cytogenetic diagnosis has been established.

**Delivery** Electronic fetal monitoring and cesarean section should be avoided, unless requested by the family, after a thorough discussion of the prognosis for infants with trisomy 18.

## NEONATOLOGY

**Resuscitation** A decision about whether to give life support should be considered prior to delivery when the diagnosis is definite. If the diagnosis is unknown prior to birth, providing life support is appropriate until the diagnosis can be established.

**Transport** Indicated only if diagnostic confirmation, counseling, and long-term care planning are not available locally.

**Testing and Confirmation** A peripheral blood chromosome study can confirm the abnormality.

**Nursery Management** Decisions regarding surgical intervention for cardiac and gastrointestinal defects are the primary concerns in the postnatal period. If the family desires no surgical intervention, care requirements are determined primarily by feeding difficulties.

### SUGGESTED READINGS


1. Ghidini A, Strobelt N, Locatelli A, et al: Isolated fetal choroid plexus cysts: role of ultrasonography in establishment of the risk of trisomy 18. Am J Obstet Gynecol 2000; 182:972-977.
2. Gratton RJ, Hogge WA, Aston CE: Choroid plexus cysts and trisomy 18: Risk modification based on maternal age and multiple marker screening. Am J Obstet Gynecol 1996; 175:1493-1497.
3. Hepper PG, Shahidullah S: Trisomy 18: behavioral and structural abnormalities. An ultrasonographic case study. Ultrasound Obstet Gynecol 1992; 2:48-50.
4. Janvier A, Watkins A: Medical interventions for children with trisomy 13 and trisomy 18: what is the value of a short disabled life? Acta Paediatr 2013; 12:1112-1117.
5. Jones KL, Jones MC, del Campo M: Smith's Recognizable Patterns of Human Malformations. 7th ed. Philadelphia: Elsevier; 2013.

6. Lam YH, Tang MHY: Sonographic features of fetal trisomy 18 at 13 and 14 weeks: four case reports. Ultrasound Obstet Gynecol 1999; 13:366-369.
7. Liao AW, Sebire NJ, Geerts L, et al: Megacystis at 10-14 weeks of gestation: chromosomal defects and outcome according to bladder length. Ultrasound Obstet Gynecol 2003; 21:338-341.
8. Liau J, Romine L, Korty LA, et al: Simplifying the ultrasound findings of the major fetal chromosomal aneuploidies. Curr Probl Diagn Radiol 2014; 43:300-316.
9. McGraw MP, Perlman JM: Attitudes of neonatologists toward delivery room management of confirmed trisomy 18: potential factors influencing a changing dynamic. Pediatrics 2008; 121:1106-1110.
10. Merritt TA, Catlin A, Wool C, et al: Trisomy 18 and trisomy 13. Neoreviews 2012; 13:e40-e48.
11. Quezada MS, Gil MM, Francisco C, et al: Screening for trisomies 21, 18, and 13 by cell-free DNA analysis of maternal blood at 10-11 weeks' gestation and the combined test at 11-13 weeks. Ultrasound Obstet Gynecol 2014; 20:1-6.
12. Sepulveda W, Treadwell MC, Fisk NM: Prenatal detection of preaxial upper limb reduction in trisomy 18. Obstet Gynecol 1995; 847-850.
13. Springett AL, Morris JK: Antenatal detection of Edwards (trisomy 18) and Patau (trisomy 13) syndrome: England and Wales 2005-2012. J Med Screen 2014; 21(3):113-119.
14. Steiger RM, Porto M, Lagrew DC, Randall R: Biometry of the fetal cisterna magna: estimates of the ability to detect trisomy 18. Ultrasound Obstet Gynecol 1995; 5:384-390.
15. Tul N, Spencer K, Noble P, et al: Screening for trisomy 18 by fetal nuchal translucency and maternal serum free β-hCG and PAPP-A at 10-14 weeks of gestation. Prenat Diagn 1999; 19:1035-1042.

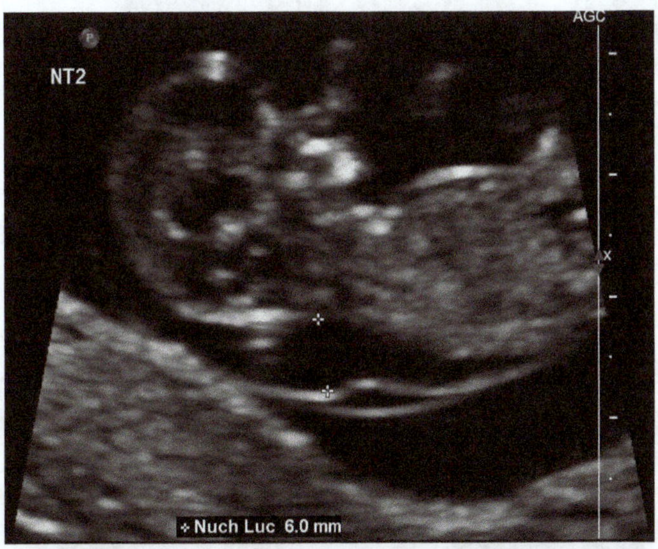


**FIGURE 1.3A** Trisomy 18. 1st trimester thickened nuchal translucency (+....+).

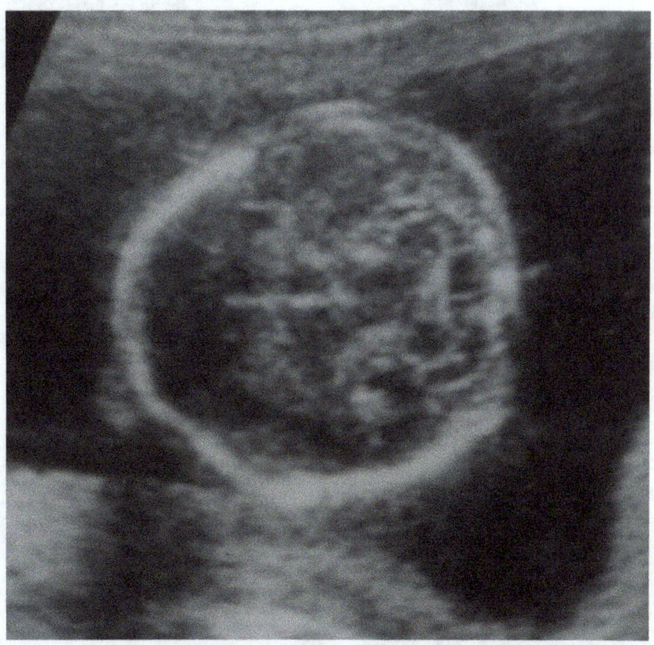

**FIGURE 1.3B** Trisomy 18 with strawberry shaped calvarium.

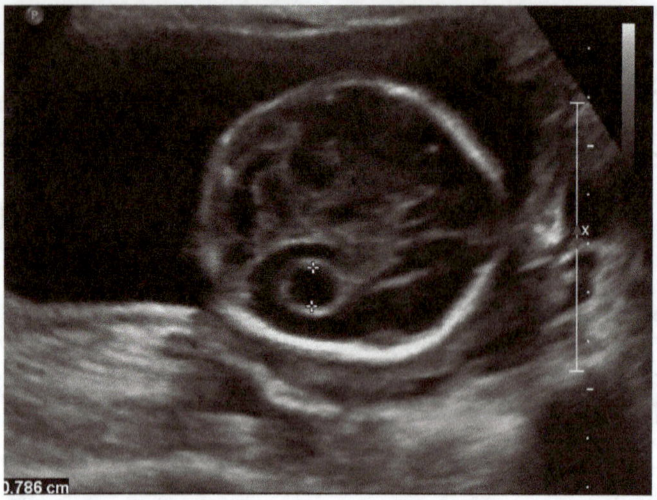

**FIGURE 1.3C** Trisomy 18 with a choroid plexus cyst (+. . .+).

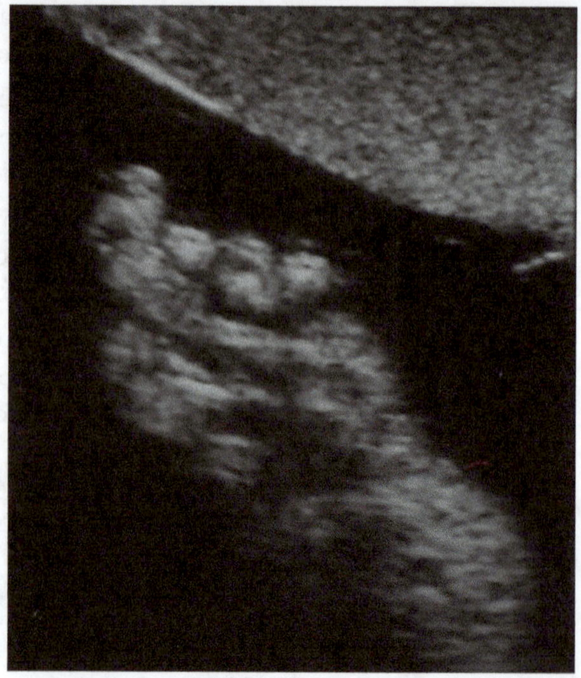

**FIGURE 1.3D** Trisomy 18 with a clenched hand.

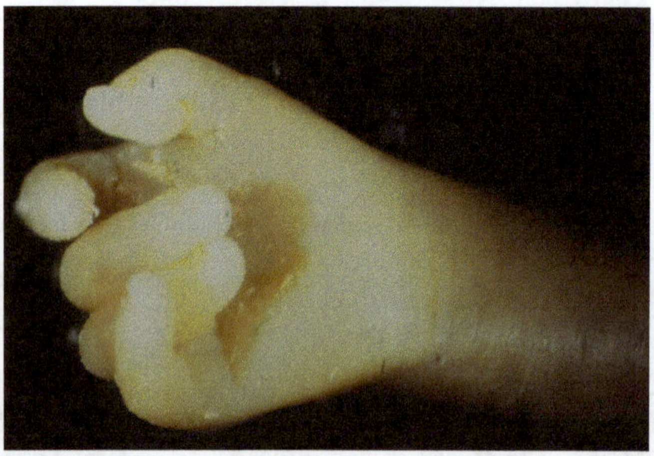

**FIGURE 1.3E** Trisomy 18 fetus with clenched hand.

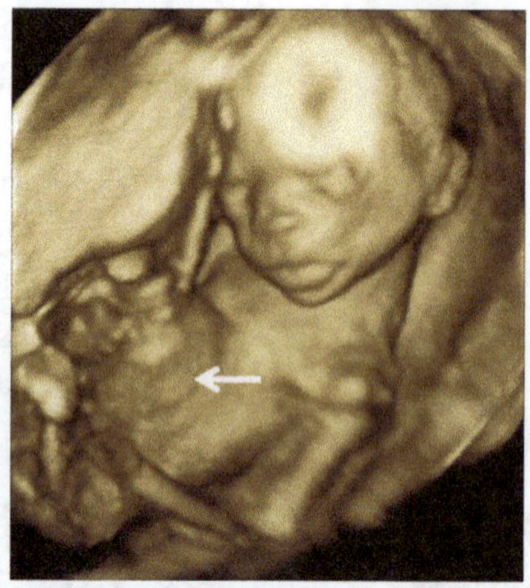

**FIGURE 1.3F** Trisomy 18 with an omphalocele (arrow).

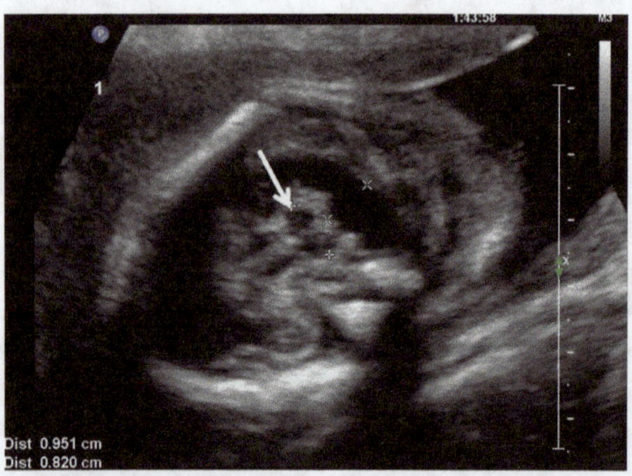

**FIGURE 1.3G** Trisomy 18 showing cerebellar hypoplasia (arrow).

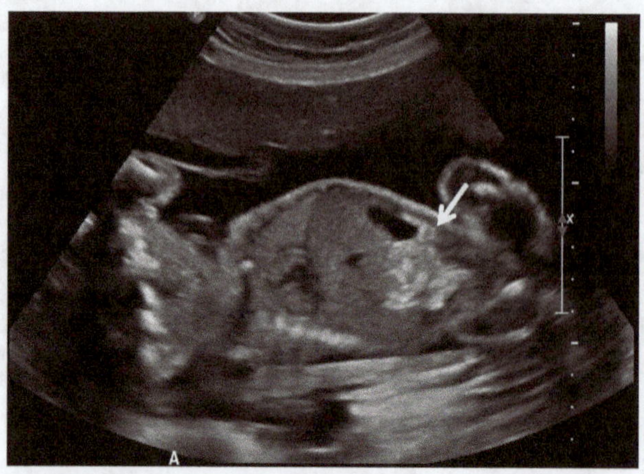

**FIGURE 1.3H** Trisomy 18 with echogenic small bowel (arrow).

# 1.4 TRISOMY 21 (DOWN SYNDROME)

## EPIDEMIOLOGY/GENETICS

**Definition** Trisomy 21 (Down syndrome) is the most common chromosomal abnormality in newborns. It results in a characteristic phenotype with major malformations, including congenital heart disease and intestinal atresias.

**Epidemiology** Occurs in 1 in 800 live births (M1:F1). No racial differences have been noted, but there is a significant increase in incidence with increasing maternal age.

**Embryology** The phenotype is due to trisomy for all or part (21q22) of chromosome 21. Of cases, 95% are due to full trisomy 21, 3% are unbalanced translocations, and 2% are mosaic. Infants with trisomy 21 have a characteristic craniofacial appearance that includes microbrachycephaly, midface hypoplasia, excess nuchal skin, and small, overfolded ears. There is generalized shortening of the limbs, with small hands, clinodactyly of the fifth fingers (50%), single palmar creases (40%), and wide spacing between the first and second toes. Approximately 40% of patients have congenital heart disease, with endocardial cushion defects and VSDs the most common lesions. Two-thirds of fetuses with endocardial cushion defects have trisomy 21. Intestinal tract defects (duodenal atresia, tracheoesophageal fistula, imperforate anus, Hirschprung disease) occur in approximately 10% of infants with trisomy 21.

**Inheritance Patterns** Most cases are sporadic, with approximately a 1-in-100 risk of recurrence in future pregnancies. Familial translocations have a higher recurrence risk, depending on the specific translocation.

**Teratogens** None

**Screening** Assuming all women would elect to have CVS or amniocentesis, the use of advanced maternal age as a risk factor would detect approximately 30% of trisomy 21 fetuses. Combining maternal age with maternal serum biochemical markers raises the detection rate to 80%. First-trimester screening has a similar detection rate. NIPT will detect approximately 99% of trisomy 21 cases.

**Prognosis** Cardiac abnormalities are the major cause of increased mortality in infancy. Mortality between infancy and the age of 40 years is not markedly increased over mortality in the general population, but there is an increase in mortality from respiratory diseases. Most patients with Down syndrome have some degree of cognitive impairment, ranging from mild (IQ of 50-75) to severe impairment (IQ of 20-35). Social performance is usually above that expected for mental age.

## SONOGRAPHY

### FREQUENT FINDINGS

- Cystic hygroma (10%)
- Mild ventriculomegaly (lateral ventricle 10-15 mm)

- Congenital heart defect
  - Ventricular septal defect
  - Atrial septal defect
    - Complete
      - Atrial septal defect
      - Large VSD
      - Common atrioventricular valve
    - Partial
      - Atrioventricular septal defect
      - Intact ventricular septum
      - Two atrioventricular valves
    - Transitional (intermediate)
      - Atrioventricular septal defect
      - Ventricular septal defect
      - Two atrioventricular valves
  - Tetralogy of Fallot
- Duodenal atresia

### LESS FREQUENT

- Macroglossia
- Shortened ear length
- Isolated pleural effusion
- Isolated fetal ascites
  - Ascites may be transient.
- Nonimmune hydrops
- Hepatosplenomegaly
- Decreased liver echogenicity
- Tracheoesophageal atresia

### KEY FINDINGS

- There are a number of subtle dysmorphic features associated with Down syndrome that can be assessed songraphically.
  - Nationally accepted standards for the dysmorphic features that should be evaluated have not been developed.
  - Gestational age, maternal body habitus, sonographer experience, and the dysmorphic features evaluated all affect the reliability of soft sonographic markers in the detection of trisomy 21.
- The most frequently assessed soft sonographic markers include
  - Thickened nuchal fold (≥6.0 mm)
  - Short femur
  - Short humerus
  - Echogenic intracardiac focus
  - Pyelectasis (≥4.0 mm)
  - Echogenic small bowel

- A hypoplastic or absent nasal bone during the 11- to 14- or 16- to 20-week ultrasound is associated with an increased likelihood of Down syndrome.
  - Racial adjustments are required when evaluating the nasal bone as a marker of Down syndrome.
- To appropriately evaluate the fetus for soft sonographic markers, all of the dysmorphic features, as well as an extended fetal anatomic survey, must be completed.
- The prevalence of multiple minor markers increases the likelihood of Down syndrome.
  - The interaction between variables selected must be evaluated with multiple logistic regression to determine which factors are significant and what their potential interaction is.
- The primary advantage of the soft markers is the risk reduction associated with an absence of all of the markers on a second-trimester ultrasound examination.

### PITFALLS

- The nuchal fold in the second trimester is difficult to measure accurately.
  - The transverse cerebellar diameter and cavum septum pellucidum should be on the transverse image of the calvarium.
  - The measurement is from the external skin line to the external edge of the occiput.
- Echogenic bowel is present with cystic fibrosis, congenital infections, intra-amniotic hemorrhage, and second-trimester growth restriction. It is most frequently a normal variant.

## PREGNANCY MANAGEMENT

**Investigations and Consultations** Traditional karyotyping with, or without, FISH analysis via amniocentesis or CVS establishes the diagnosis. A positive result from maternal blood of cell-free circulating fetal DNA is considered a screening test and is not sufficient to establish the diagnosis. For patients in whom the diagnosis is made beyond the point of legal pregnancy termination or in those who decide to continue the pregnancy, a neonatologist should consult with the family about neonatal management. The high incidence of cardiac defects requires fetal echocardiography, which also may be helpful in assessing prognosis.

**Monitoring** No alterations in prenatal care are necessary. There is a high rate of intrauterine fetal demise in trisomy 21, and whether fetal monitoring decreases the stillbirth rate is unclear. Growth restriction is more common, although it is usually mild. It is not known if fetal monitoring and aggressive management improve prognosis.

**Pregnancy Course** Duodenal atresia results in severe polyhydramnios and resultant preterm labor. Congenital heart defects may result in fetal hydrops. Follow-up ultrasounds should be scheduled to monitor for these issues, as appropriate.

**Pregnancy Termination Issues** Use of suction dilatation and evacuation, or any other method of pregnancy termination, is appropriate once a cytogenetic diagnosis has been established.

**Delivery** The fetus with Down syndrome should be managed at delivery like a fetus with normal chromosomes. Cesarean section should be performed if there are obstetric indications. If structural malformations are present, delivery should be in a tertiary center.

## NEONATOLOGY

**Resuscitation** Rarely contraindicated unless multiple complex associated anomalies have been confirmed antenatally and a prior decision has been made by family not to begin life support measures. If the diagnosis is not known prior to birth, providing life support is appropriate initially.

**Transport** Indicated if cardiac or gastrointestinal tract anomalies are suspected or if diagnostic confirmation, counseling, and long-term care planning are not available locally.

**Testing and Confirmation** Children with trisomy 21 present in the newborn period with hypotonia and a characteristic facial appearance. A peripheral blood chromosome study can confirm the chromosome abnormality.

**Nursery Management** The major objectives of care are comprehensive evaluation to identify all associated problems and the development of a postnursery plan of care to facilitate parental adaptation. The initial priorities are to determine the presence and type of cardiac defects (50%) and gastrointestinal tract anomalies, most commonly anorectal and duodenal atresia/stenosis (10%) and to plan for surgical interventions. Infants should be screened for polycythemia (65%), transient abnormal myelopoiesis (10%), hearing loss, and feeding difficulties, particularly if preterm or with concurrent cardiac or gastrointestinal anomalies. Referral to a Down syndrome center with a multidisciplinary team of specialists is recommended for long-term care.

### SUGGESTED READINGS


1. Bromley B, Benacerraf BR: The Genetic Sonogram Scoring Index. Semin Perinatol 2003; 27:124-129.
2. Bull MJ, Committee of Genetics: Clinical report—health supervision for children with Down syndrome. Pediatrics 2011; 128:393-406.
3. Hamada H, Yamada N, Watanabe H, et al: Hypoechoic hepatomegaly associated with transient abnormal myelopoiesis provides clues to trisomy 21 in the third trimester fetus. Ultrasound Obstet Gynecol 2001; 17:442-444.
4. Jones KL, Jones MC, del Campo M: Smith's Recognizable Patterns of Human Malformations. 7th ed. Philadelphia: Elsevier; 2013.
5. Morris JK, Garne E, Wellesley D, et al: Major congenital anomalies in babies born with Down syndrome: a EUROCAT population-based registry study. Am J Med Genet A 2014; 24:2979-2986.

6. Norton ME, Jelliffe-Pawlowski LL, Currier RH: Chromosome abnormalities detected by current prenatal screening and noninvasive prenatal testing. Obstet Gynecol 2014; 124:979-986.
7. Odibo AO, Ghidini A: Role of the second-trimester "genetic sonogram" for Down syndrome screen in the era of first-trimester screening and noninvasive prenatal testing. Prenat Diagn 2014; 34:511-517.
8. Paladini D, Tartaglione A, Agangi A, et al: The association between congenital heart disease and Down syndrome in prenatal life. Ultrasound Obstet Gynecol 2000; 15:104-108.
9. Penna L, Bower S: Hyperechogenic bowel in the second trimester fetus: a review. Prenat Diagn 2000; 20:909-913.
10. Roberts D, Walkinshaw SA, McCormack MJ, Ellis J: Prenatal detection of trisomy 21: combined experience of two British hospitals. Prenat Diagn 2000; 20:17-22.
11. Schlater PJ, Pritchard G: Mid-trimester sonographic findings for the prediction of Down syndrome in a sonographically screened population. Am J Obstet Gynecol 2005; 192:10-16.
12. Smith-Bindman R, Hosman W, Feldstein VA, Deeks J, et al: Second-trimester ultrasound to detect fetuses with Down syndrome. JAMA 2001; 285:1044-1055.
13. Snijders RJM, Holzgreve W, Cuckle H, Nicolaides KH: Maternal age-specific risk for trisomies at 9-14 weeks' gestation. Prenat Diagn 1994; 14:543-552.
14. Sonek JD: Nasal bone evaluation with ultrasonographic marker for fetal aneuploidy (Opinion). Ultrasound Obstet Gynecol 2003; 22:11-15.
15. Souka AP, Snijders RJM, Novakov A, et al: Defects and syndromes in chromosomally normal fetuses with increased nuchal translucency thickness at 10-14 weeks of gestation. Ultrasound Obstet Gynecol 1998; 11:391-400.

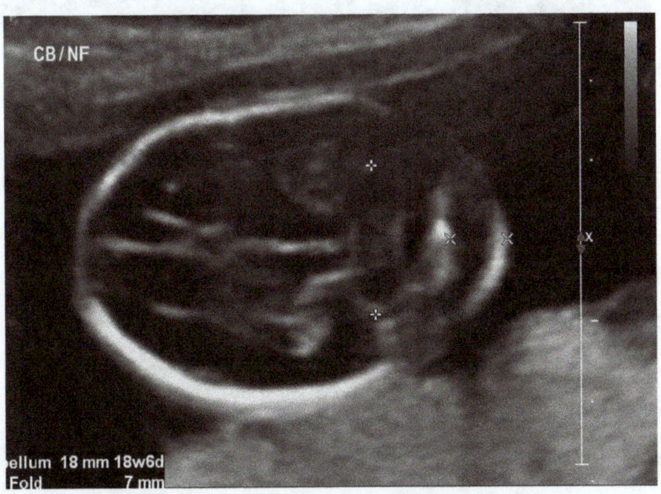


**FIGURE 1.4A** Trisomy 21. Thickened nuchal fold (x. . . x). Transverse cerebellar diameter (+. . .+).

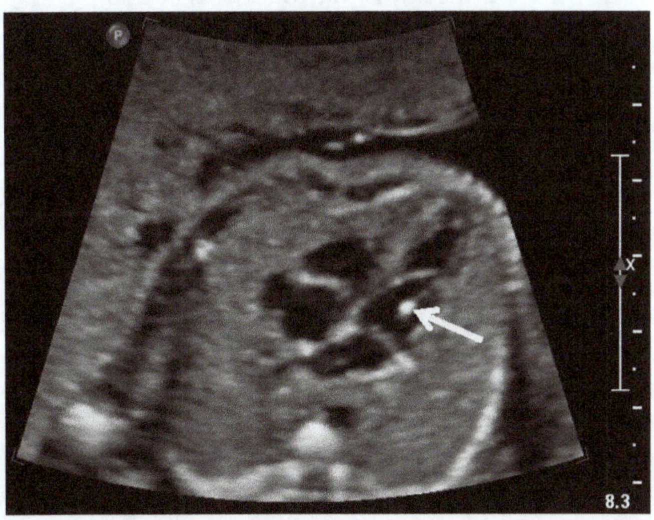


**FIGURE 1.4B** Trisomy 21 with a left echogenic intracardiac focus (arrow).

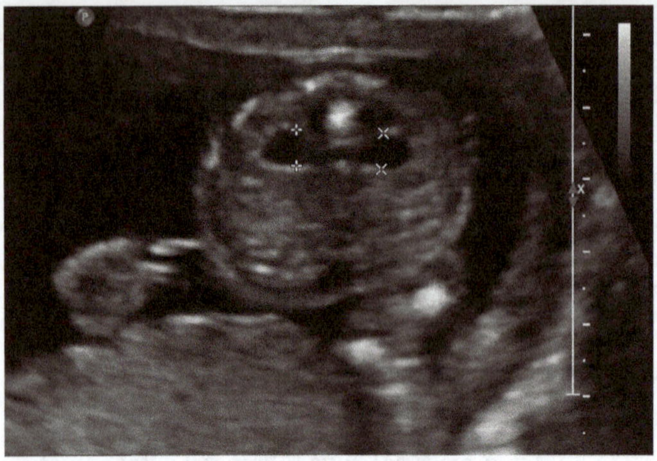

**FIGURE 1.4C** Trisomy 21 with bilateral 2nd trimester pyelectasis of 5 mm (markers).

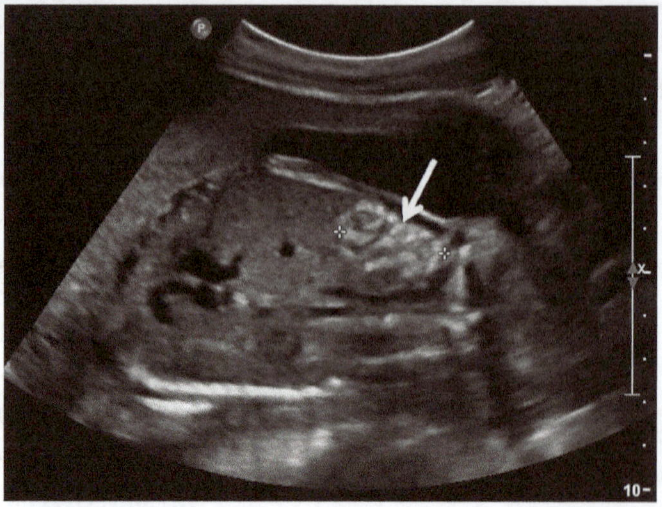

**FIGURE 1.4D** Trisomy 21 illustrating 2nd trimester echogenic fetal small bowel (arrow).

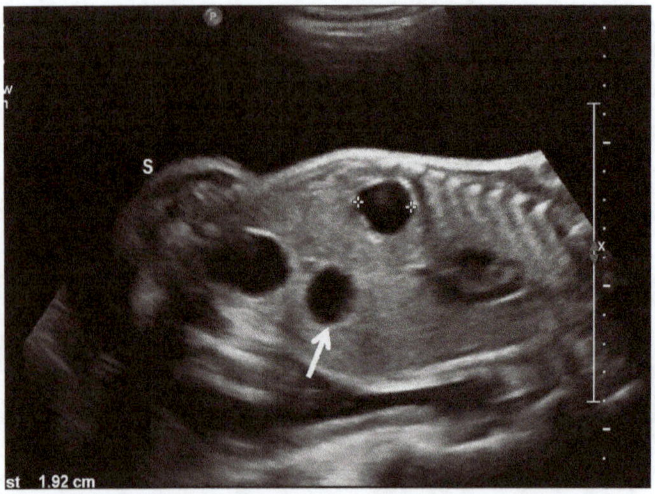


**FIGURE 1.4E** Trisomy 21 with duodenal atresia. "Double bubble" of stomach (+. . . +) and duodenum (arrow). Polyhydramnios is present.

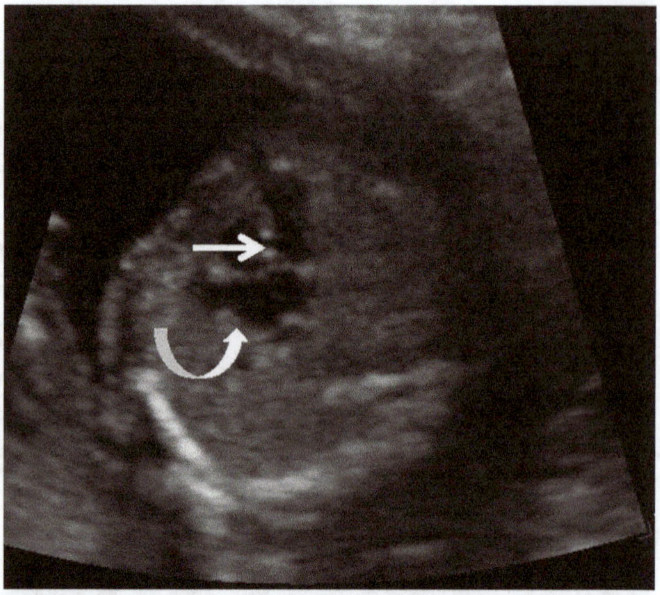

**FIGURE 1.4F** Trisomy 21 with a transitional atrioventricular septal defect. Ventricular septal defect (straight arrow) and atrial septal defect (curved arrow).

# 1.5 TURNER SYNDROME (45,X SYNDROME)

## EPIDEMIOLOGY/GENETICS

**Definition** Turner syndrome is a common sex chromosome abnormality at conception, but 90% end as a spontaneous abortion or stillbirth. It is characterized by a complete, or partial, monosomy for one X chromosome.

**Epidemiology** Occurs in 1 in 2500 births (M0:F1)

**Embryology** Turner syndrome is due in most cases to a 45,X karyotype that results from chromosomal nondisjunction. No maternal age effect has been noted. Forty percent of newborns with Turner syndrome are mosaic or have variant chromosome patterns. Characteristic cardiac abnormalities include a bicuspid aortic valve (30%) and coarctation of the aorta (10%). Horseshoe kidney or other structural renal abnormalities occur in 60% of patients. A cystic hygroma with or without hydrops is the most common antenatal presentation.

**Inheritance Patterns** Sporadic

**Teratogens** None

**Screening** Second-trimester maternal serum biochemical screening may detect cases with hydrops because the markers will suggest an increased risk for Down syndrome (low α-fetoprotein, high hCG, high inhibin A, and low estriol). First-trimester screening will detect those cases with a cystic hygroma. NIPT will detect approximately 90% of cases.

**Prognosis** If hydrops is present, fetal death occurs during pregnancy in 95% of cases. Isolated cystic hygromas, without hydrops, regress during pregnancy. Early death in infancy results from associated cardiac defects and is infrequent with current surgical and postoperative intensive care. The potential life span is normal, and those who survive early infancy usually reach adulthood. Skeletal growth restriction occurs in all, and perceptive hearing impairment occurs in 50% of cases. Absence of secondary sexual characteristics and infertility are uniformly present. Hormone replacement therapy will be necessary for maturational changes in adolescence. Most Turner syndrome women have normal, or near-normal intelligence, but the incidence of neuropsychological deficits is increased over the general population.

## SONOGRAPHY

### FREQUENT FINDINGS

- Early-onset symmetric intrauterine growth restriction
- Thickened first-trimester nuchal translucency
- Cystic hygroma
  - Multiple, internal thin septations are characteristic.
  - Of the 45,X fetuses, 60% have a cystic hygroma.
- Heart
  - Coarctation of the aorta (40%)
  - Valvular aortic stenosis

- Nonimmune hydrops: fluid within 2 areas
  - Skin edema
  - Pleural effusion
    - May be transient
  - Pericardial effusion
  - Ascites
- Short femur, humerus

### LESS FREQUENT

- First-trimester hydrops
- Horseshoe kidney
- Renal agenesis
- Ambiguous genitalia (usually seen with mosaic cases having a Y chromosome cell line)

## PREGNANCY MANAGEMENT

**Investigations and Consultations** Traditional karyotyping with, or without, FISH analysis via amniocentesis or CVS establishes the diagnosis. A positive result from maternal blood of cell-free circulating fetal DNA is considered a screening test and is not sufficient to establish the diagnosis. Once a cytogenetic diagnosis has been established, fetal echocardiography should be performed because of the high incidence of congenital heart disease. Consultations with other specialists will be dependent on the types of structural malformations seen.

**Monitoring** No alterations in prenatal care are necessary. There is a high rate of intrauterine fetal demise when a cystic hygroma and hydrops are present. Follow-up ultrasound examinations should be scheduled to monitor for hydrops and to follow any cardiac malformations, as appropriate.

**Pregnancy Course** Whereas cystic hygroma with hydrops is virtually always fatal, cystic hygroma without hydrops slowly regresses and leaves a webbed neck.

**Pregnancy Termination Issues** Should a family choose pregnancy termination, suction dilatation and evacuation or any other method of pregnancy termination is appropriate once a cytogenetic diagnosis has been established.

**Delivery** The fetus with Turner syndrome should be managed at delivery like a fetus with normal chromosomes. Cesarean section should be performed if there are obstetric indications. If congenital heart disease is present, delivery should be in a tertiary center.

## NEONATOLOGY

**Resuscitation** There is no contraindication to full resuscitation. Because coarctation of the aorta is the most frequently occurring cardiac defect, peripheral perfusion may be dependent on flow through the ductus arteriosus. Prolonged exposure to high oxygen concentrations is not advisable until the cardiac anatomy is known.

**Transport** Indicated if a cardiac malformation is suspected and counseling and long-term care planning are not available locally. If asymptomatic and no cardiac involvement is suspected, outpatient evaluation in early infancy is appropriate.

**Testing and Confirmation** Newborns present with a short webbed neck (50%) with a low hairline (80%), lymphedema of hands and feet, prominent ears (80%), and cardiac abnormalities. Patients not detected in infancy are detected in childhood with short stature and delayed puberty due to ovarian dysgenesis. Peripheral blood chromosome studies, with special attention to possible mosaicism, confirm the diagnosis.

**Nursery Management** Diagnostic evaluation should include an echocardiogram and renal sonogram, regardless of symptomatology. No intervention is usually required for lymphedema.

## SUGGESTED READINGS

1. Bronshtein M, Zimmer EZ, Blazer S: A characteristic cluster of fetal sonographic markers that are predictive of fetal Turner syndrome in early pregnancy. Am J Obstet Gynecol 2003; 188:1016-1020.
2. Chen CP, Chien SC: Prenatal sonographic features of Turner syndrome. J Med Ultrasound 2007; 15:251-257.
3. Chervenak FA, Isaacson G, Blakemore KJ, et al: Fetal cystic hygroma: cause and natural history. N Engl J Med 1983; 309:822-825.
4. Hall G, Weston MJ, Campbell DJ: Transitory pleural effusion associated with mosaic Turner syndrome. Prenat Diagn 2001; 21:421-422.
5. Jones KL, Jones MC, del Campo M: Smith's Recognizable Patterns of Human Malformations. 7th ed. Philadelphia: Elsevier; 2013.
6. Liau J, Romine L, Korty LA, et al: Simplifying the ultrasound findings of the major fetal chromosomal aneuploidies. Curr Probl Diagn Radiol 2014; 43:300-316.
7. Norton ME, Jelliffe-Pawlowski LL, Currier RH: Chromosome abnormalities detected by current prenatal screening and noninvasive prenatal testing. Obstet Gynecol 2014; 124(5):979-986.
8. Surerus E, Huggon IC, Allan LD: Turner's syndrome in fetal life. Ultrasound Obstet Gynecol 2003; 222:264-267.

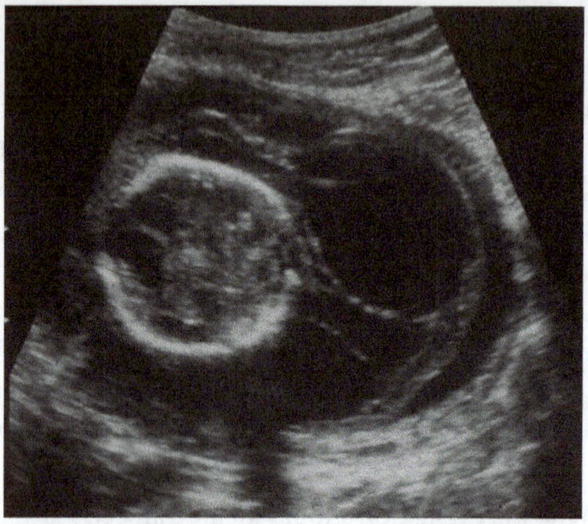

**FIGURE 1.5A** Turner Syndrome illustrating a cystic hygroma.

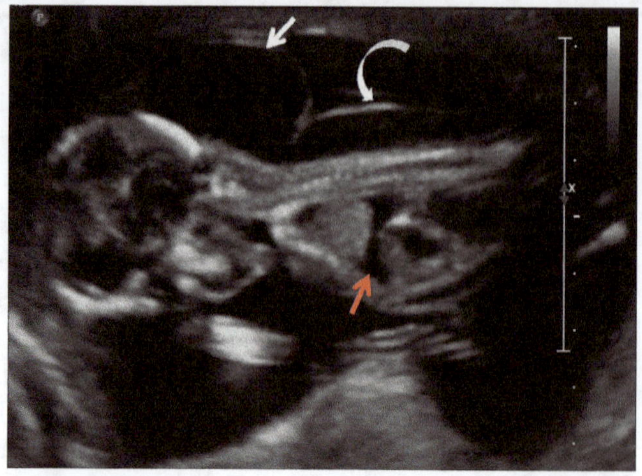

**FIGURE 1.5B** Turner Syndrome with non-immune hydrops. Note the cystic hygroma (straight arrow), anasarca (curved arrow) and pleural effusion (red arrow).

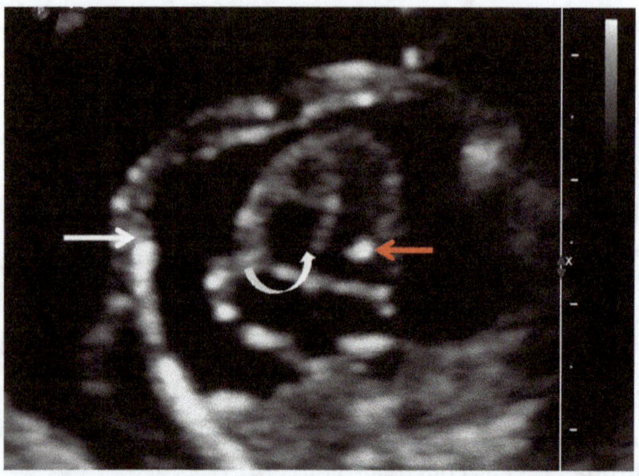

**FIGURE 1.5C** Turner Syndrome with a pericardial effusion (straight arrow), ventricular septal defect (curved arrow), and left echogenic focus (red arrow).

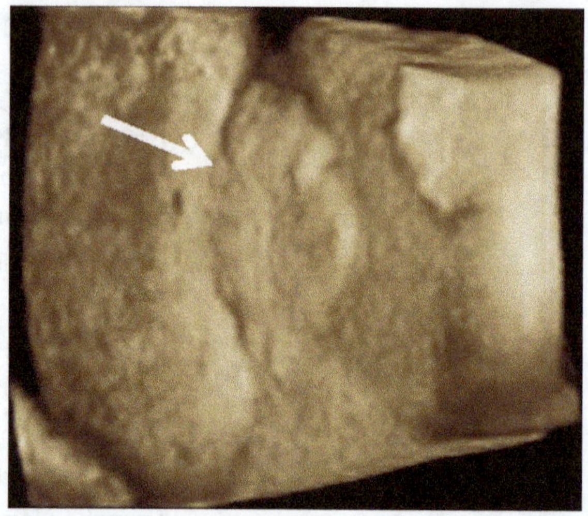

**FIGURE 1.5D** Turner Syndrome. "Tulip sign" (arrow) indicating severe hypospadias.

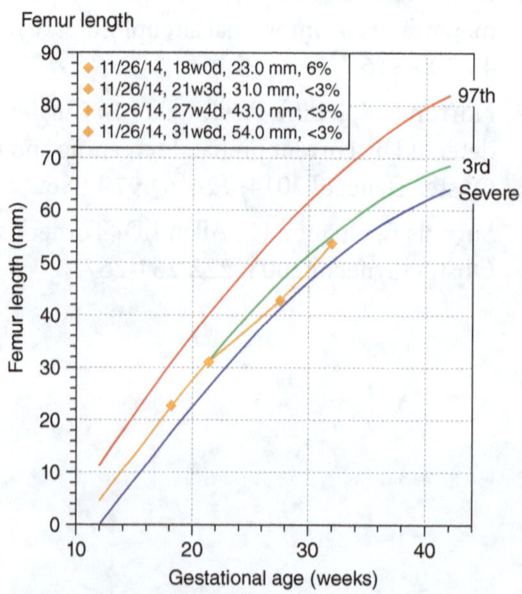


**FIGURE 1.5E** Graph of femur length measurements in Turner syndrome.

# CHAPTER 2

# CENTRAL NERVOUS SYSTEM

# 2.1 AGENESIS OF THE CORPUS CALLOSUM

## EPIDEMIOLOGY/GENETICS

**Definition** Complete or partial agenesis of the corpus callosum (ACC) is a failure of the callosal commissural fibers to cross in the midline and form the corpus callosum between the two cerebral hemispheres. Partial agenesis may also be called hypogenesis, or dysgenesis, of the corpus callosum.

**Epidemiology** Incidence may be as high as 1%, with many asymptomatic individuals.

**Embryology** The corpus callosum develops between the 12th and the 22nd week of gestation. Vascular disruption or failure of formation may cause complete or partial agenesis. Associated abnormalities include hydrocephalus, microcephaly, pachygyria, and lissencephaly. More than 80 sporadic, genetic, and chromosomal syndromes have been described with ACC, including trisomies 13 and 18. The incidence of chromosomal abnormalities is approximately 10%. Agenesis of the corpus callosum, combined with intracranial cysts or eye anomalies, should suggest Aicardi syndrome, an X-linked dominant disorder with male lethality.

**Inheritance Patterns** Most isolated defects are sporadic. Autosomal dominant, recessive, and X-linked syndromes have been described.

**Teratogens** None known.

**Prognosis** Isolated ACC may be asymptomatic unless associated with other brain abnormalities. Typically, complete agenesis will have a worse prognosis than partial ACC. Associated brain, or extracranial, abnormalities suggest a guarded prognosis.

## SONOGRAPHY

### FREQUENT FINDINGS

- Absence of the cavum septum pellucidum
- Colpocephaly (teardrop-shaped lateral ventricle)
- Widened interhemispheric fissure
- Midline interhemispheric cyst
- Absence of the corpus callosum
- Absent pericallosal artery
- Atypical radiating appearance of the median sulci, which converge toward the third ventricle

### LESS FREQUENT

- Medial intracranial lipoma in the third trimester

### KEY FINDINGS/PITFALLS

- If ACC is diagnosed, a detailed anatomic survey is required for complete evaluation.

- The pericallosal artery follows the superior surface of the corpus callosum. Complete and partial absence of the corpus callosum can be inferred by evaluating the course of the pericallosal artery.
- Three-dimensional (3-D) multiplanar imaging can be employed to obtain appropriate sagittal and coronal images of the corpus callosum.
- Fetal magnetic resonance imaging (MRI) should be considered as an integral part of the assessment of ACC, particularly when isolated ACC is diagnosed. Fetal MRI may detect additional cerebral anomalies (i.e., heterotopias and migration anomalies).

### DIFFERENTIAL DIAGNOSIS

- Isolated absence of the cavum septum pellucidum: There is fusion of the frontal horns of the lateral ventricles with inferior pointing. The corpus callosum is present.
- Lobar holoprosencephaly (HPE): There is absence of both the cavum septum pellucidum and the normal interhemispheric fissure.
- Septo-optic dysplasia must be distinguished from isolated absence of the cavum septum pellucidum. MRI or 3-D ultrasound can be employed to look at the optic chiasm and nerves. Atrophy of the optic chiasm would indicate a diagnosis of septo-optic dysplasia rather than isolated absence of the cavum septum pellucidum.
- Arachnoid cyst: Irregular shape and unlikely to be exactly midline. There is usually no ventricular dilation.
- Mild lateral ventriculomegaly: The entire ventricle is dilated. The third ventricle is normal or slightly dilated.
- Enlarged cavum septum pellucidum and vergae: The corpus callosum is present. The cavum septum pellicudum extends directly into the cavum vergae.
- Aicardi syndrome: This is associated with agenesis or dysgenesis of the corpus callosum and occurs almost exclusively in females.

## PREGNANCY MANAGEMENT

**Investigations and Consultations Required** ACC is a difficult diagnosis, and subsequent pregnancy management depends in part on the certainty of the diagnosis. Many cases of ACC are part of a syndrome, and steps to determine whether a case is isolated or syndromic are warranted. Chromosome studies, including microarrays, of the fetus are essential. Evaluation of the parents by a dysmorphologist for signs of autosomal dominant conditions, such as basal cell nevus syndrome and tuberous sclerosis, may be helpful. Fetal echocardiography should be performed to detect congenital heart disease. Maternal serum viral titers should be drawn. Additional consultations will depend on the associated abnormalities found. If uncertainty about the central nervous system (CNS) findings remains, a fetal MRI may be useful to delineate the CNS anatomy.

**Monitoring** No change in standard obstetric practice is indicated for isolated ACC. The aggressiveness of fetal intervention must be based on the underlying cause, if that can be determined. Isolated ACC should not progress, but if associated with a cyst or with ventriculomegaly or if the diagnosis is in question, a third-trimester examination is desirable to make sure the cyst has not enlarged, the ventricles are stable, and other processes have not been missed.

**Pregnancy Course** Obstetric complications are not expected on the basis of ACC alone.

**Pregnancy Termination Issues** Because many conditions have ACC as a component, an intact fetus should be delivered in an institution with expertise in dysmorphology and fetal pathology.

**Delivery** Because of the high association with other non-CNS abnormalities, delivery should occur in a tertiary center with full capabilities for diagnosis and management of infants with multiple malformations.

## NEONATOLOGY

**Resuscitation** There are no specific issues except in those infants with additional CNS defects, in which case the associated defect will be the dominant factor in decisions regarding intervention.

**Transport** Referral to a tertiary center after birth is not indicated with an isolated lesion and asymptomatic course. Referral to pediatric neurology as an outpatient is indicated for further evaluation. With any neurologic symptoms present or associated CNS lesions, the infant should be referred promptly to a tertiary perinatal center with pediatric neurology capabilities for definitive evaluation.

**Testing and Confirmation** Postnatal confirmation of the defect and evaluation for other associated lesions are best achieved with MRI. Screening for inherited metabolic disorders is indicated with isolated lesions of the corpus callosum.

**Nursery Management** Subsequent course and management are dictated by the associated lesion(s).

**Prognosis** In cases of isolated ACC, there is variability in neurodevelopmental outcome, ranging from within normal limits to moderate-to-severe disability. The presence of associated CNS malformations is associated with an increased risk of significant neurodevelopmental deficits.

### SUGGESTED READINGS

1. Achiron R, Achiron A: Development of the human fetal corpus callosum: a high-resolution, cross-sectional sonographic study. Ultrasound Obstet Gynecol 2001; 18:343-347.
2. Bromley B, Krishnamoorthy KS, Benacerraf BR: Aicardi syndrome: prenatal sonographic findings. A report of two cases. Prenat Diagn 2000; 20:344-346.
3. Chadie A, Radi S, Trestard L, et al. Neurodevelopmental outcome in prenatally diagnosed isolated agenesis of the corpus callosum. Acta Paediatr 2008; 97:420.

4. D'Ercole C, Girard N, Cravello I, et al: Prenatal diagnosis of fetal corpus callosum agenesis by ultrasonography and magnetic resonance imaging. Prenat Diagn 1998; 18:247-253.

5. Goodyear PW, Bannister CM, Russell S, et al: Outcome in prenatally diagnosed fetal agenesis of the corpus callosum. Fetal Diagn Ther 2001; 16:134-145.

6. Gupta JK, Lilford RJ. Assessment and management of fetal agenesis of the corpus callosum. Prenat Diagn 1995; 15:301-312.

7. Kroner BL, Preis LR, Ardini MA, Gaillard WD: New incidence, prevalence and survival in Aicardi syndrome from 408 cases. J Child Neurol 2008; 23:531-535.

8. Malinger G, Lev D, Kidron D, et al: Differential diagnosis in fetuses with absent septum pellucidum. Ultrasound Obstet Gynecol 2005; 25:42-49.

9. Mangione R, Fries N, Godard P, et al: Neurodevelopmental outcome following prenatal diagnosis of an isolated anomaly of the corpus callosum. Ultrasound Obstet Gynecol 2011; 37:290-295.

10. Marszal E, Jamroz E, Pilch J, et al: Agenesis of corpus callosum: Clinical description and etiology. J Child Neurol 2000; 15:401-405.

11. Moutard M-L, Kieffer V, Feingold J, et al: Isolated corpus callosum agenesis: a 10-year follow-up after prenatal diagnosis (How are the children without corpus callous at 10 years of age?). Prenat Diagn 2012; 32:277-283.

12. Paladini D, Pastore G, Cavallaro A, et al: Agenesis of the fetal corpus callosum: sonographic signs change with advancing gestational age. Ultrasound Obstet Gynecol 2013; 42:687-690.

13. Palmer EE, Mowat D: Agenesis of the corpus callosum: a clinical approach to diagnosis. Am J Med Genet C Semin Med Genet 2014; 166C: 184-197.

14. Pilu G, Segata M, Chi T, et al: Diagnosis of midline anomalies of the fetal brain with the three-dimensional median view. Ultrasound Obstet Gynecol 2006; 27:522-529.

15. Santo S., D'Antonio F, Homfray T, et al: Counseling in fetal medicine: agenesis of the corpus callosum. Ultrasound Obstet Gynecol 2012; 40:513-521.

16. Sotiriadis A, Makrydimos G: Neurodevelopment after prenatal diagnosis of isolated agenesis of the corpus callosum: an integrative review. Am J Obstet Gynecol 2012; 206:337-338.

17. Volpe P, Paladini D, Resta M, et al: Characteristics, associations and outcome of partial agenesis of the corpus callosum in the fetus. Ultrasound Obstet Gynecol 2006; 27:509-516.

18. Winter TC, Kennedy AM, Byrne J, Woodward PJ: The cavum septi pellucidi: why is it important? J Ultrasound Med 2010; 29:427-444.

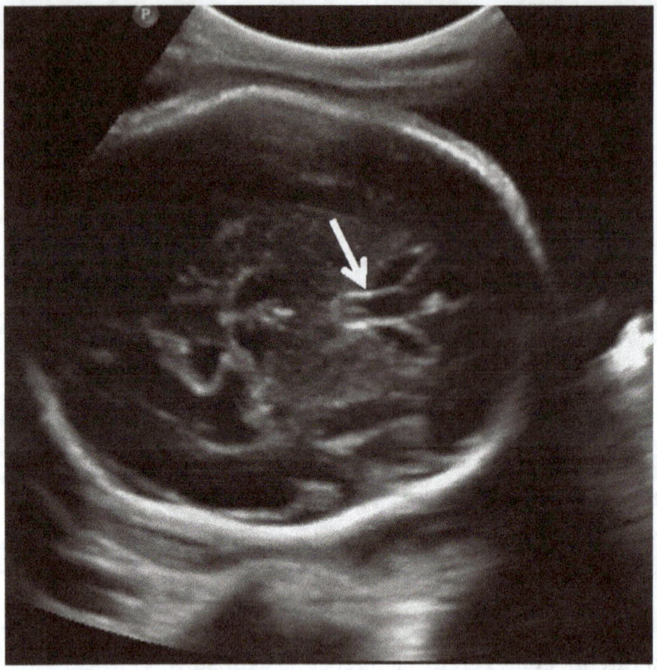

**FIGURE 2.1A** Normal view of cavum septum pellucidum (arrow).

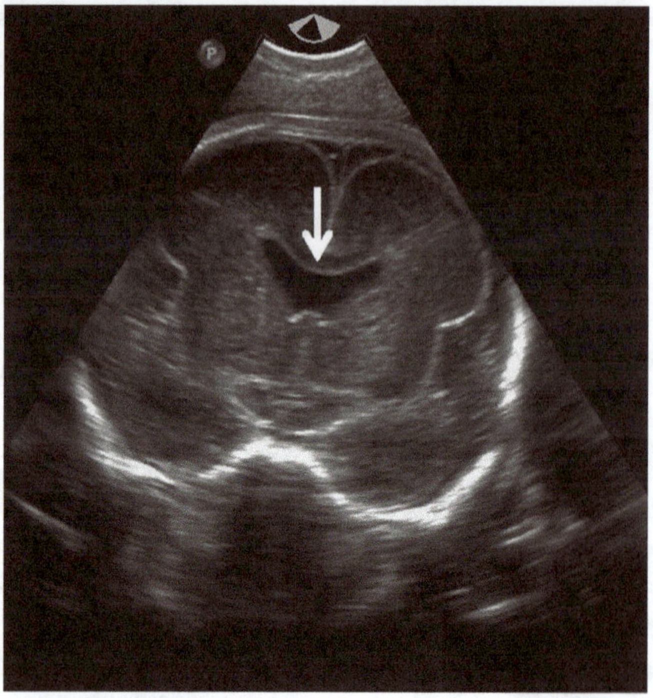

**FIGURE 2.1B** Absent cavum septum pellucidum with corpus callosum (arrow) present.

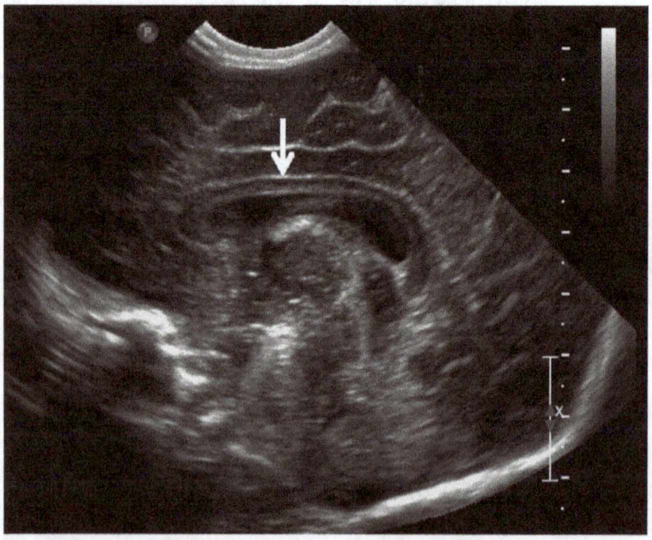

**FIGURE 2.1C** Normal corpus callosum (arrow).

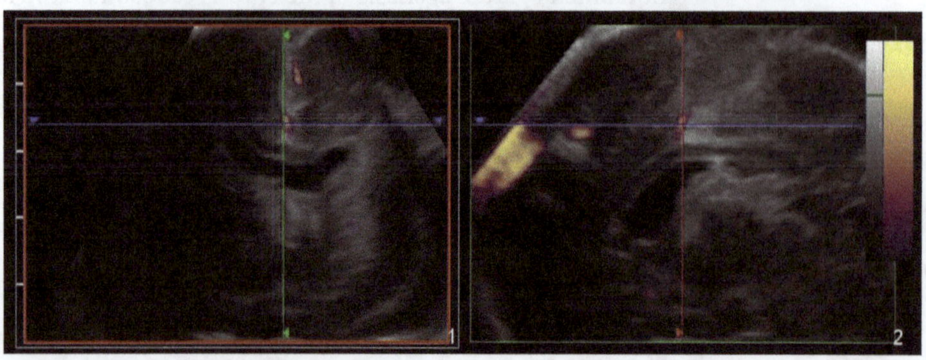

**FIGURE 2.1D** Three-dimensional image of the corpus callosum.

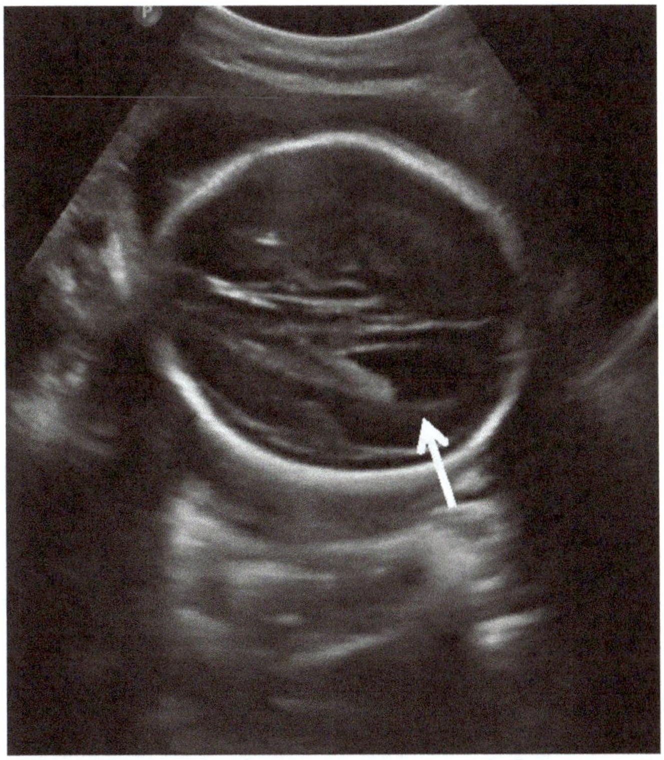

FIGURE 2.1E Agenesis of the corpus callosum with colpocephaly (arrow).

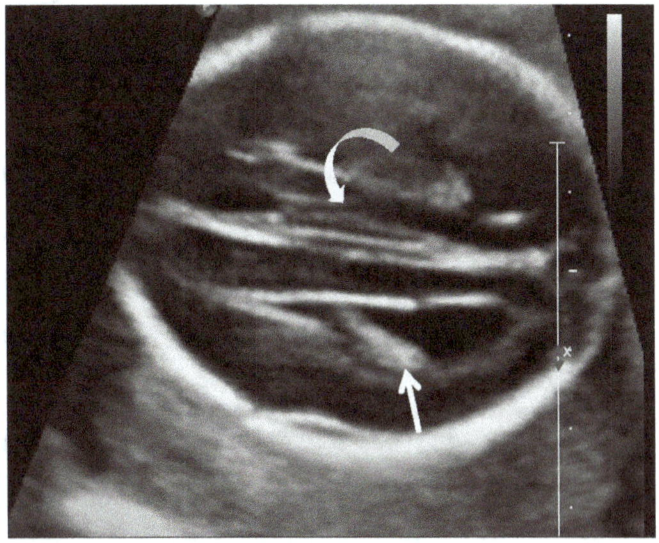

FIGURE 2.1F Agenesis of the corpus callosum illustrating teardrop-shape lateral ventricle (straight arrow) and interhemispheric separation (curved arrow).

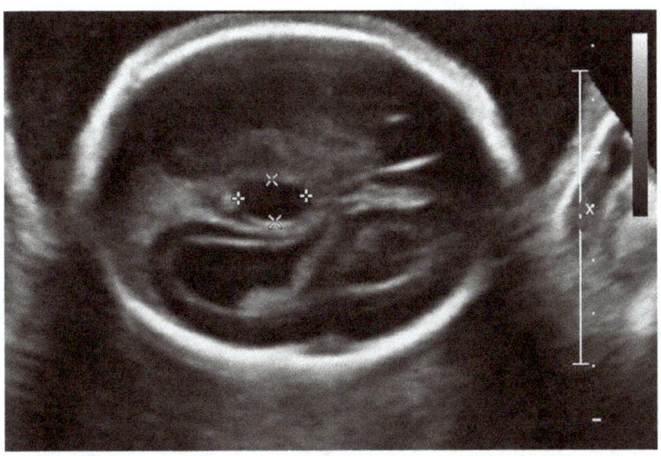

FIGURE 2.1G Agenesis of the corpus callosum with an interhemispheric cyst (markers).

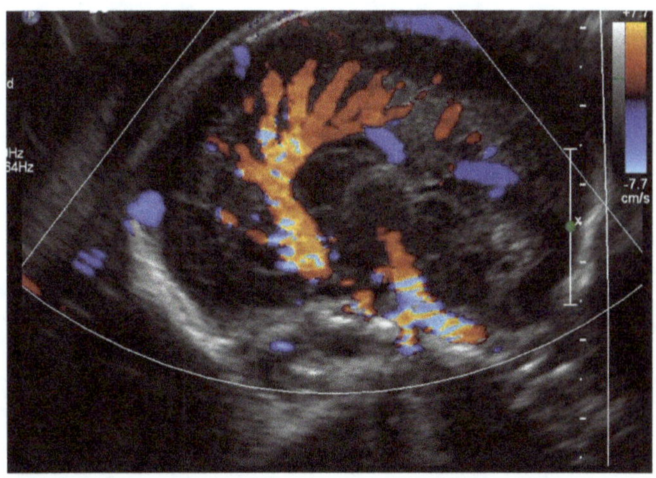

FIGURE 2.1H Normal pericallosal artery at 20 weeks.

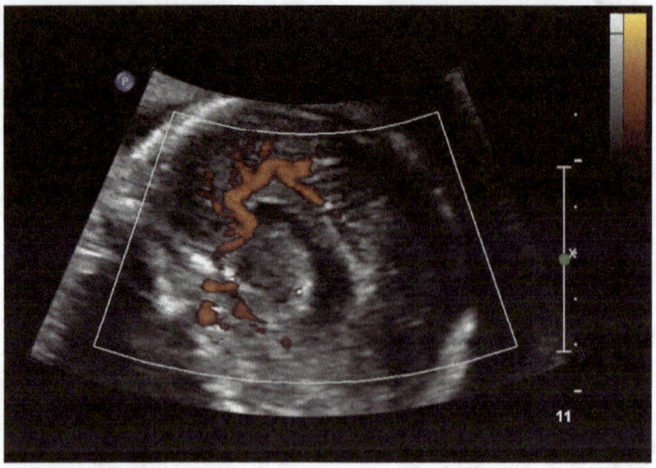

**FIGURE 2.1I** Partial agenesis of the corpus callosum; only genu and rostrum are present. Pericallosal artery follows along the genu and rostrum.

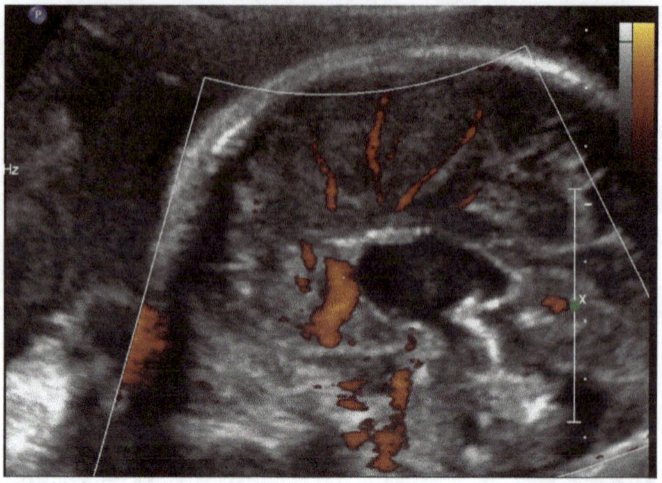

**FIGURE 2.1J** Agenesis of the corpus callosum illustrating the absence of the pericallosal artery.

# 2.2 ANENCEPHALY

## EPIDEMIOLOGY/GENETICS

**Definition** Anencephaly is a defect in closure of the anterior neural tube characterized by complete or partial absence of the forebrain, overlying meninges, skull, and skin.

**Epidemiology** The incidence is geographically and population dependent and ranges from about 1 in 1000 births in the United States to 1 in 100 in parts of the British Isles (M1:F3). Preconceptual supplementation with folic acid has been shown to decrease the incidence of open neural tube defects.

**Embryology** Neural tube closure occurs between 20 and 28 days of pregnancy, with abnormalities of cephalic closure, which occurs late, resulting in anencephaly. Anencephaly is characterized by the absence of the cranial vault with exposed neural tissue and is associated with spina bifida, facial and nasal clefts, and omphalocele. Amniotic band disruptions are also an unusual cause of anencephaly. A small number of cases are associated with chromosomal abnormalities, such as trisomy 18.

**Inheritance Patterns** Multifactorial inheritance with both genetic and environmental factors is implicated. Recurrence risk after one affected pregnancy is 2% to 3% for any open neural tube defect. Rare families have been reported with X-linked inheritance. Periconceptional folic acid supplementation of 0.4 mg/d will decrease the incidence of spina bifida and anencephaly, but a subset of neural tube defects is not prevented by current therapeutic strategies. With folic acid supplementation and food fortification with folic acid, only approximately 50% of cases will be prevented.

**Teratogens** Valproic acid; folic acid antagonists, such as methotrexate and aminopterin; maternal diabetes; hyperthermia; and folic acid deficiency are associated with an increased risk for neural tube defects.

**Screening** Maternal serum α-fetoprotein screening or fetal ultrasonographic screening will detect most cases of anencephaly.

**Prognosis** Anencephaly is invariably lethal, with about 50% of cases being stillborn and the remainder dying in the newborn period.

## SONOGRAPHY

### FINDINGS

- Skull development is usually completed by 10 weeks' gestation in a normal fetus.
- While early first-trimester crown-rump length may be within the normal range, the mean crown-rump length is lower than expected.
- In the first trimester, the brain may appear normal or have varying distorted shapes ("Mickey Mouse" sign of anencephaly at 11-14 weeks' gestation).

- There is gradual degeneration of exposed cerebral tissue, giving rise to the acrania/exencephaly/anencephaly sequence.
  - The sequence begins with a normal-appearing brain (acrania) that progressively degenerates to amorphous cerebral tissue (exencephaly), and finally to absence of cerebral tissue (anencephaly).
- Degenerated cortical tissue is replaced by a vascular mass (area cerebrovasculosa).
- On a coronal second-trimester image, the fetus has a "frog-like" appearance.
- Anencephaly can be divided into "isolated" anencephaly and anencephaly with "multiple anomalies." The chromosomal abnormality rate is higher in the multiple-anomaly group.
- Late second- and third-trimester polyhydramnios is common, but not invariable.

### DIFFERENTIAL DIAGNOSIS

- Acrania: This results from abnormal development of the neurocranium, which ossifies to form the cranial vault.
  - Cortical tissue is still present.
  - Acrania is part of the anencephaly spectrum.
- Large encephalocele: The skull will be visible on close inspection.
- Microcephaly: A small skull will be present.
- Iniencephaly: This is often present with anencephaly.

## PREGNANCY MANAGEMENT

**Investigations and Consultations Required** No specific antenatal evaluations or consultations are necessary.

**Monitoring** In pregnancies that are continued, clinical assessment for the presence of polyhydramnios is indicated. Symptomatic polyhydramnios is an indication for delivery. Tocolysis is never indicated. The most important component of the prenatal care is emotional support for the family.

**Pregnancy Course** Anencephaly is always lethal at or shortly after birth.

**Pregnancy Termination Issues** Suction dilatation and evacuation techniques are appropriate. Karyotyping abortus material is worthwhile to detect the unusual case caused by a chromosome anomaly, such as trisomy 18.

**Delivery** There are no special conditions regarding delivery. The majority of anencephalic infants will deliver in the breech presentation.

## NEONATOLOGY

**Resuscitation** Given the lethal prognosis, neonatal resuscitation is never indicated. Prenatal diagnosis and counseling should focus on preparing the family for nonintervention.

**Transport** Transport is not an issue.

**Testing and Confirmation** The abnormality is obvious at birth. Evidence of amniotic band disruptions should be sought. Cord blood should be obtained for genetic testing.

**Nursery Management** Palliative care with provision of comfort measures and facilitation of parental grief are the principal elements of care. Parents and the health care staff should be counseled that some infants may survive for several days with intermittent periods of stable cardiorespiratory function.

**Organ Donation** Organ donation from anencephalic infants should not be undertaken due to the serious difficulties surrounding the establishment of brain death in these infants and the lack of evidence to date supporting successful organ transplantation. There can be no modification in the medical criteria of brain death and legal standards of pronouncement of death to include infants with anencephaly. Families who request the opportunity to donate organs from their infant with anencephaly should have information and educational material provided that explains why this practice is not supported. The option of tissue donation from an anencephalic infant, including heart valves, cornea, and liver cells, should be discussed as these tissues may be harvested up to several hours after the death of the infant and can be frozen until a recipient is identified.

## SUGGESTED READINGS


1. Becker R, Mende B, Stiemer B, Entezami M: Sonographic markers of exencephaly at 9 + 3 weeks of gestation. Ultrasound Obstet Gynecol 2000; 16:582-584.
2. Canadian Paediatric Society. Use of anencephalic newborns as organ donors. Paediatr Child Health 2005; 10:335-337.
3. Chatzipapas IK, Whitlow BJ, Economides DL: The "MickeyMouse" sign and the diagnosis of anencephaly in early pregnancy. Ultrasound Obstet Gynecol 1999; 13:196-199.
4. Copp AJ, Greene NDE: Neural tube defects—disorders of neurulation and related embryonic processes. Wiley Interdiscip Rev Dev Biol 2013; 2:213-227.
5. Goldstein RB, Filly RA: Prenatal diagnosis of anencephaly: spectrum of sonographic appearances and distinction from the amniotic band syndrome. Am J Roentgenol 1988; 151:547-550.
6. Johnson SP, Sebire NJ, Snijders RJM, Tunkel S, Nicolaides KH: Ultrasound screening for anencephaly at 10-14 weeks of gestation. Ultrasound Obstet Gynecol 1997; 9:14-16.
7. Obeidi N, Russell N, Higgins JR, O'Donoghue K: The natural history of anencephaly. Prenat Diagn 2010; 30:357-360.
8. Salamanca A, Gonzalez-Gomez F, Padilla MC, et al: Prenatal ultrasound semiography of anencephaly: sonographic-pathological correlations. Ultrasound Obstet Gynecol 1992; 2:95-100.
9. Sepulveda W, Corral E, Ayala C, Be C, Gutierraz J, Vasquez P: Chromosomal abnormalities in fetuses with open neural tube defects: prenatal identification with ultrasound. Ultrasound Obstet Gynecol 2004; 23:352-356.

10. Van Allen MI, Kalousek DK, Chernoff GF, et al: Evidence for multi-site closure of the neural tube in humans. Am J Med Genet 1993; 47:723-743.
11. Wilkins-Haug L, Freedman W: Progression of exencephaly to anencephaly in the human fetus: an ultrasound perspective. Prenat Diagn 1991; 11:227-233.
12. Yang YC, Wu CH, Chang FM, et al: Early prenatal diagnosis of acrania by transvaginal ultrasonography. J Clin Ultrasound 1992; 20:343-345.

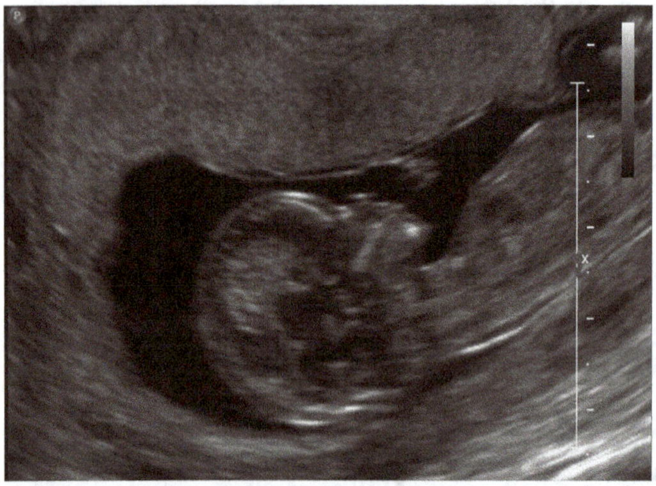

**FIGURE 2.2A** Normal calvarium and brain architecture at 12 weeks' gestation.

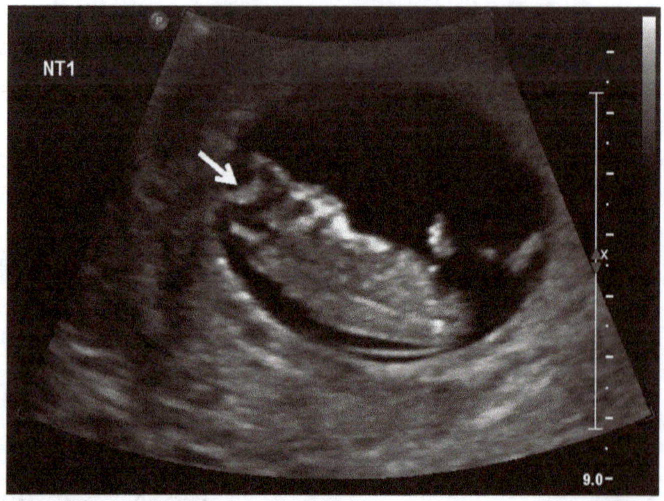


**FIGURE 2.2B** Acrania (arrow).

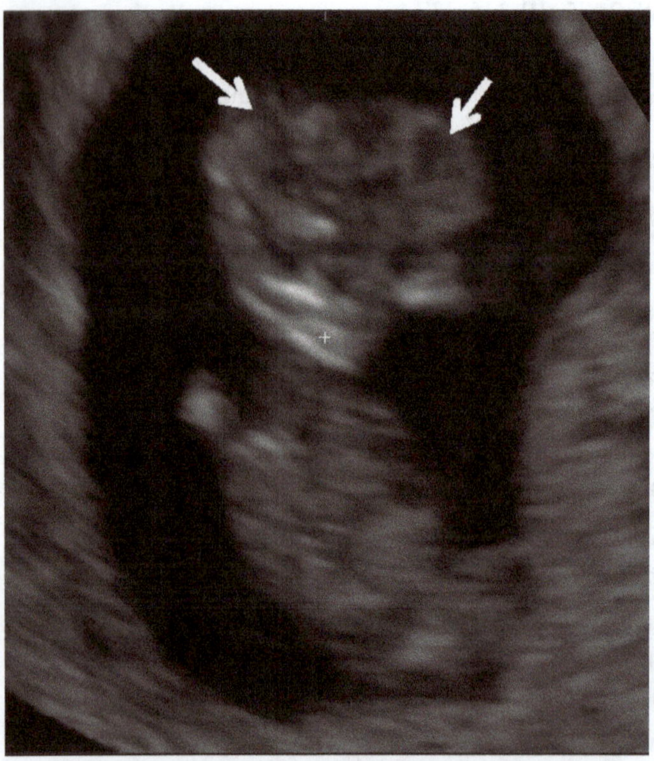

**FIGURE 2.2C** Anencephaly: bilobed brain, "Mickey Mouse" appearance (arrows).

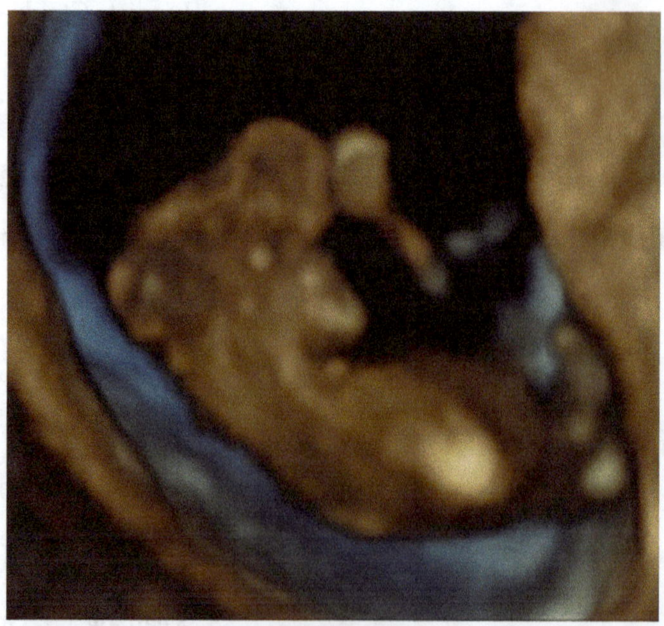

**FIGURE 2.2D** Three-dimensional image of a first-trimester anencephalic fetus.

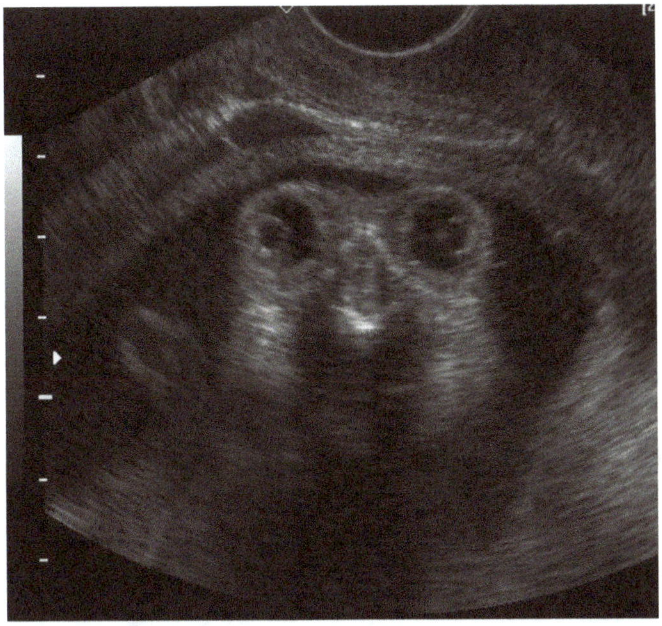

**FIGURE 2.2E** Anencephaly: "frog-like" appearance.

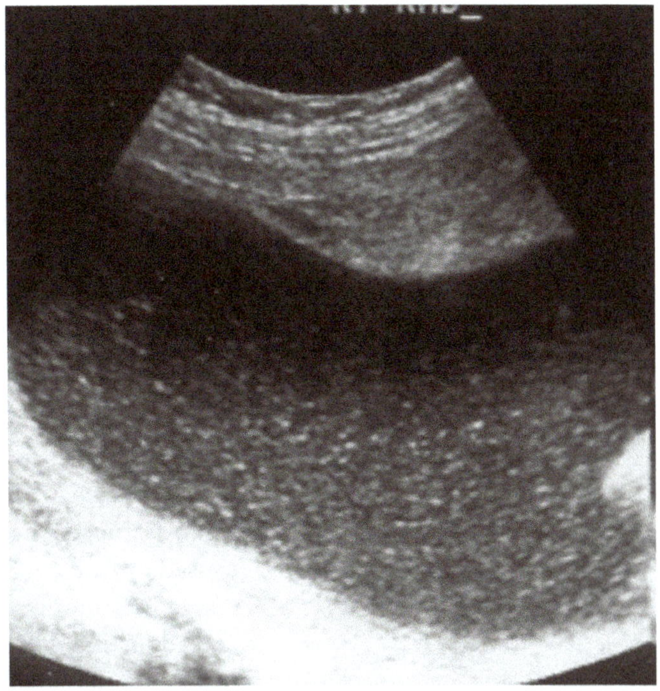

**FIGURE 2.2F** Anencephaly: debris in amniotic fluid from degeneration of cortical tissue.

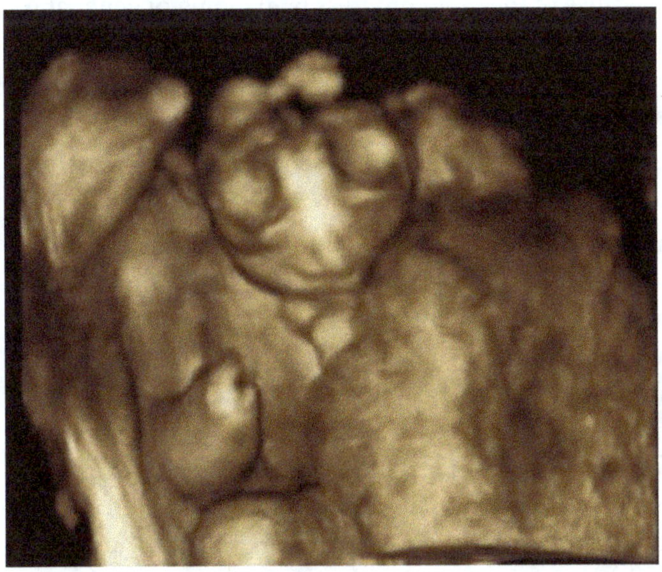

**FIGURE 2.2G** Three-dimensional image of second-trimester fetus with anencephaly.

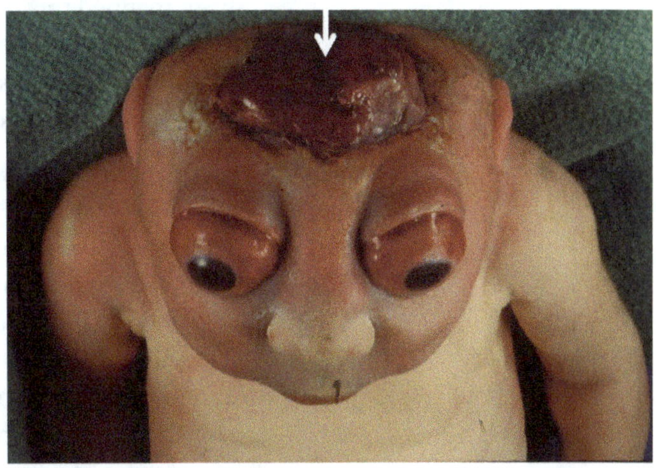

**FIGURE 2.2H** Fetus with anencephaly, illustrating the cerebrovasculosa (arrow).

# 2.3 AQUEDUCTAL STENOSIS

## EPIDEMIOLOGY/GENETICS

**Definition** Aqueductal stenosis is an obstruction or maldevelopment of the aqueduct of Sylvius, resulting in congenital hydrocephalus.

**Epidemiology** One in 2000 (M1.8: F1). Ninety percent of cases of congenital hydrocephalus are the result of Arnold-Chiari malformations, whereas 3% to 5% have aqueductal stenosis.

**Embryology** The aqueduct of Sylvius is the connection between the third and fourth ventricles in the brain and develops at about 6 weeks' gestation. Histologic evidence of gliosis is found in approximately 50% of cases of aqueductal stenosis, suggesting inflammatory or infectious causes. Some cases may be caused by true congenital atresia. The etiology is heterogeneous and includes congenital tumors, hemorrhage, infections, and genetic syndromes. Flexion and adduction deformities of the thumbs are present in 20% of boys with X-linked aqueductal stenosis.

**Inheritance Patterns** Most cases are sporadic. Estimates suggest that 2% to 5% of cases of hydrocephalus not associated with neural tube defects have X-linked recessive inheritance. The gene for X-linked aqueductal stenosis has been mapped to Xq28. Because of the rapid progress in mapping of genes and subsequent development of genetic testing, consultation with a medical geneticist or genetic counselor to determine the availability of clinical genetic testing for this disorder is advised.

**Teratogens** Teratogens are congenital infections, including cytomegalovirus, rubella, and toxoplasmosis.

**Prognosis** The neonatal detection of aqueductal stenosis is associated with normal development in 24%-86% of cases. However, prenatal diagnosis has a worse prognosis, and "normal" development occurs in only 10% of neonates. There is a 10% to 30% neonatal mortality rate, partly dependent on associated abnormalities. Up to half of fetuses with apparently isolated aqueductal stenosis will have other abnormalities found postnatally or at autopsy. The difference in outcome between a fetal and a neonatal diagnosis of aqueductal stenosis is due to the presence of undetected additional anomalies/chromosomal abnormalities in the fetal group. Approximately 50% of survivors will have an IQ greater than 70. The X-linked recessive form is associated with profound mental retardation and a poor prognosis.

## SONOGRAPHY

### FREQUENT FINDINGS

- Ventriculomegaly
- Symmetrical ventricular enlargement
- Dangling choroid

- Dilated third ventricle (>2 mm)
- Normal posterior fossa

### LESS FREQUENT

- Macrocephaly (head circumference > 2 SD above the mean)
- Symmetric parenchymal thinning
- Absence of aqueduct distal to the third ventricle

### KEY FINDINGS/PITFALLS

Ventriculomegaly is a descriptive term indicating a lateral ventricle measurement greater than 10 mm at the level of the cavum septum pellucidum. The calipers are positioned on the internal borders of the medial and lateral ventricles at the globus of the choroid plexus.

- An atrial width between 10 and 15 mm is considered mild and width greater than 15 mm severe ventriculomegaly.
- Ventriculomegaly is associated with different disease processes. Hence, prognosis varies.
- Cerebral spinal fluid flows from the lateral ventricles through the foramen of Monro to the third ventricle and then to the fourth ventricle via the aqueduct of Sylvius. The more distal the obstruction is, the greater the involvement of the ventricle system.
- The aqueduct of Sylvius is the narrowest passageway in the ventricular system.
- While aqueductal stenosis can result in severe ventriculomegaly, brain anatomy may be otherwise preserved.
- The sizes of the lateral and third ventricle are not useful predictors of long-term outcome.

### DIFFERENTIAL DIAGNOSIS

- Isolated aqueductal stenosis is, by necessity, a diagnosis of exclusion and accounts for only 1%-2% of patients with diagnosed ventriculomegaly.
- A 3-D multiplanar view can reconstruct the midsagittal view to evaluate both the corpus callosum and the posterior fossa. The presence of a normal cavum septum pellucidum on a transaxial view is presumptive evidence for an intact corpus callosum.

## PREGNANCY MANAGEMENT

**Investigations and Consultations** A family history should be taken and gender determined to evaluate for possible X-linked aqueductal stenosis. In the absence of a previous affected child, the evaluation should exclude other causes of hydrocephalus. Chromosome evaluation and viral studies (both maternal serum and amniotic fluid) should be performed. If ultrasound features are consistent with aqueductal stenosis, gene testing for this disorder should be done. Pediatric neurologic or neurosurgical consultation should be obtained to plan management. Fetal MRI may be helpful to confirm the diagnosis if expertise with this modality is available locally.

**Fetal Intervention** Theoretically, aqueductal stenosis should be the perfect situation for in utero shunt placement. However, the experience to date has been disappointing. There are many reasons for the relatively poor outcomes that have been seen. Misdiagnosis has been a common finding in all series, as has been failure to detect associated abnormalities. Morbidity has been high, reflecting the difficulties of exact shunt placement in the fetus. For these reasons, and the lack of data to support a clear benefit of fetal surgical intervention, in utero ventriculo-amniotic shunts are not indicated in the management of fetal ventriculomegaly from presumed aqueductal stenosis at the present time.

**Monitoring** Ventriculomegaly caused by aqueductal stenosis may abruptly increase in severity over a few weeks, so ultrasonographic monitoring is desirable. In addition, follow-up ultrasound may be used to exclude other comorbidities, such as growth delay, and to monitor head size. Otherwise, few pregnancy complications are expected, and pregnancy management should be unchanged.

**Pregnancy Termination Issues** The method of termination should be a nondestructive one as confirmation of etiology is necessary. Termination should be undertaken at a site with special expertise in neuropathology.

**Delivery** Although, in theory, early delivery followed by shunt placement could improve outcome, neonatal data do not support the benefit of this approach. Further study is needed before clear recommendations can be made. Mode of delivery can be vaginal if the head is of relatively normal size and the fetus is in a vertex presentation. Macrocephaly or breech presentation are common and often require cesarean section. Delivery should occur in a center where appropriate neonatal and neurologic services are available.

## NEONATOLOGY

**Resuscitation** The decision regarding management following the onset of respiration should be discussed with the family prior to delivery. Except in circumstances of extreme enlargement of the head or presence of other severe CNS abnormalities, initial resuscitation is indicated.

**Transport** Immediate referral to a tertiary perinatal center with pediatric neurology and neurosurgery capabilities is indicated. Precautions during transport are dictated by the maturity of the infant, presence of respiratory distress, and other associated abnormalities.

**Testing and Confirmation** At the time of delivery, cord blood should be sent for genetic testing if antenatal testing was not performed. Head ultrasound and MRI are useful to establish a definite anatomic diagnosis. Further imaging studies to be considered are echocardiography and abdominal sonography if physical examination findings suggest other abnormalities and studies were not obtained prenatally.

**Nursery Management** Infants require admission to the neonatal intensive care unit for stabilization and evaluation. Pediatric neurology and pediatric neurosurgery consultation should be obtained to determine management plans.

## SURGERY

**Preoperative Assessment** Issues of importance with respect to the surgical management of aqueductal stenosis are as follows:

1. The presence of other anomalies (i.e., cardiac, renal, spinal, or limb deformities), which may be associated with a poor overall prognosis.
2. The presence of a posterior fossa mass or compressive lesion, such as congenital tumor or tectal mass.
3. Rate of ventricular enlargement and head growth.

**Operative Indications** Evidence of progressive ventricular enlargement or accelerated head growth is indication for surgical intervention.

**Types of Procedures** Standard surgical therapy for aqueductal stenosis is ventricular shunting with either a ventriculoperitoneal (VP) or a ventriculoatrial shunt using a pressure-regulated valve system. An alternative therapy is endoscopic third ventriculostomy (ETV), a procedure that opens an alternative pathway for cerebrospinal fluid (CSF) to exit the third ventricle by a fenestration in the tuber cinereum of the floor of the third ventricle.

**Surgical Results/Prognosis** In the absence of associated CNS or non-CNS abnormalities, children with aqueductal stenosis have a good overall prognosis.

## SUGGESTED READINGS

1. Cardoza JD, Filly RA, Podrasky AE: The dangling choroid plexus: a sonographic observation of value in excluding ventriculomegaly. Am J Roentgenol 1988; 151:767-770.
2. Emery S, Hogge A, Hill L: Accuracy of prenatal diagnosis of isolated aqueductal stenosis. Prenat Diagn 2015; 35:319-324.
3. Gupta JK, Boyce FC, Lilford RJ: Management of apparently isolated fetal ventriculomegaly. Obstet Gynecol Surv 1994; 49:716-721.
4. Hata T, Yanagihara T, Matsumoto M, et al: Three-dimensional sonographic features of fetal central nervous system anomaly. Arch Obstet Gynecol Scand 2000; 79:635-639.
5. Hertzberg BS, Kliewer MA, Freed KS, et al: Third ventricle: size and appearance in normal fetuses through gestation. Radiology 1997; 203:641-644.
6. Levitsky DB, Mack LA, Nyberg DA, et al: Fetal aqueductal stenosis diagnosed sonographically: how grave the prognosis? Am J Roentgenol 1995; 164:725-730.
7. Pilu G, Falco P, Gabrielli S, et al: The clinical significance of fetal isolated cerebral borderline ventriculomegaly: report of 31 cases and review of the literature. Ultrasound Obstet Gynecol 1999; 14:320-326.
8. Rosenthal A, Jonet M, Kenwrick S: Aberrant splicing of neural cell adhesion molecule L1 mRNA in a family with X-linked hydrocephalus. Nat Genet 1992; 2:107-112.

9. Senat MV, Bernard JP, Schwarzler P, et al: Prenatal diagnosis and follow-up of 14 cases of unilateral ventriculomegaly. Ultrasound Obstet Gynecol 1999; 14:327-332.

10. Tomlinson MW, Treadwell MC, Bottoms SF: Isolated mild ventriculomegaly: associated karyotypic abnormalities and in utero observations. J Matern Fetal Med 1997; 6:241-244.

11. Vergani P, Locatelli A, Strobelt N, et al: Clinical outcome of mild fetal ventriculomegaly. Am J Obstet Gynecol 1998; 178:218-222.

12. Vinchon M, Rekate H, Kulkarni AV: Pediatric hydrocephalus: a review. Fluids Barriers CNS 2012; 2:9-18.

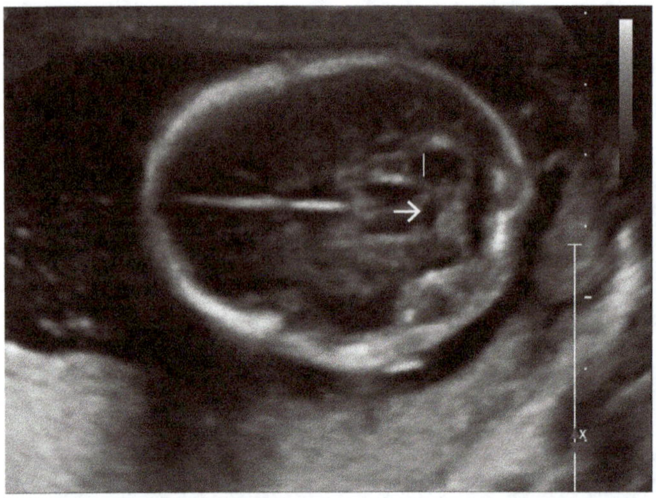

**FIGURE 2.3A** Normal fourth ventricle at 19 weeks' gestation (arrow).

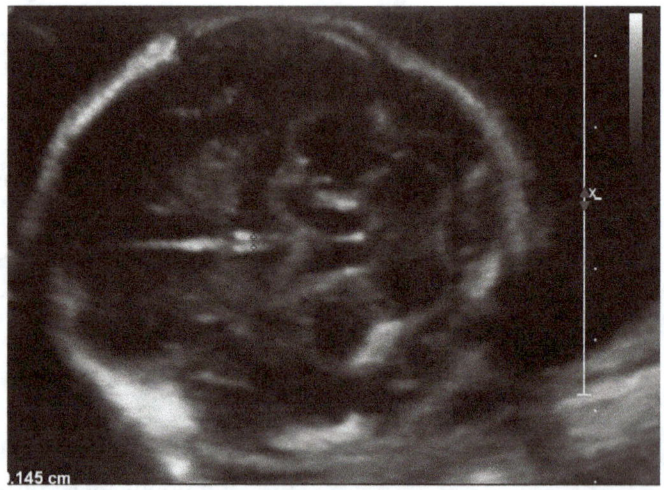


**FIGURE 2.3B** Normal third ventricle (TV) (1.5 mm).

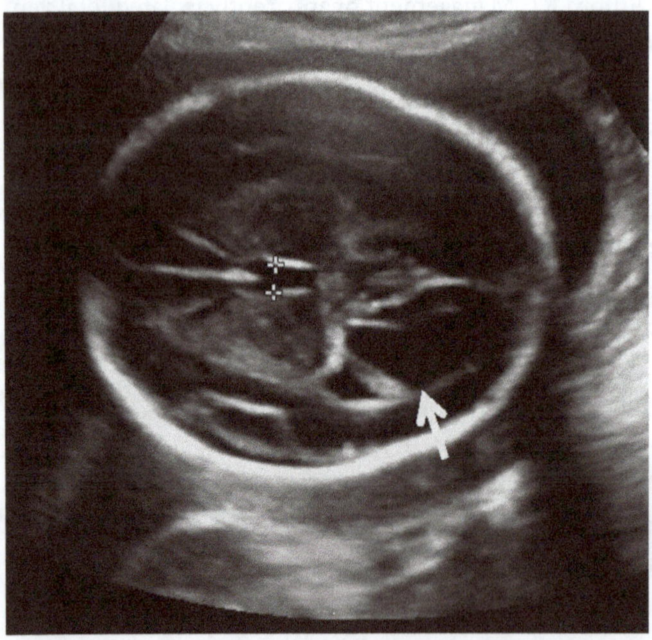

**FIGURE 2.3C** Dilated third ventricle (+ … +) (5.2 mm) with ventriculomegaly (arrow).

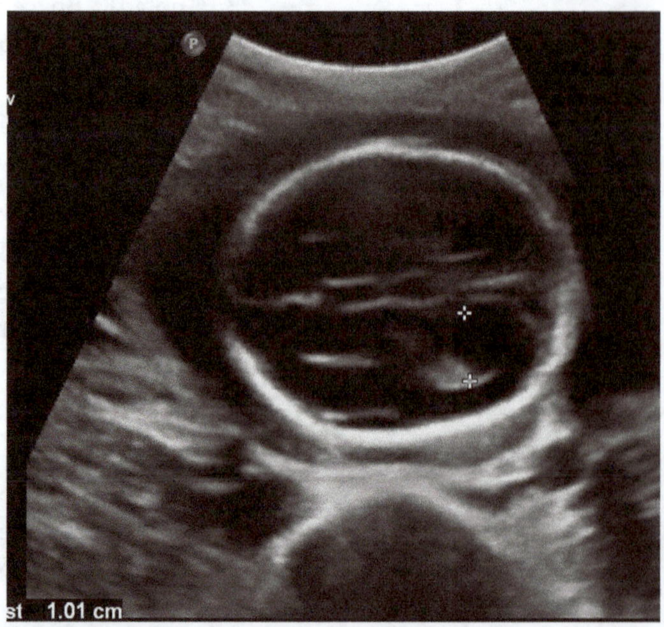


**FIGURE 2.3D** Borderline ventriculomegaly in aqueductal stenosis (+ … +).

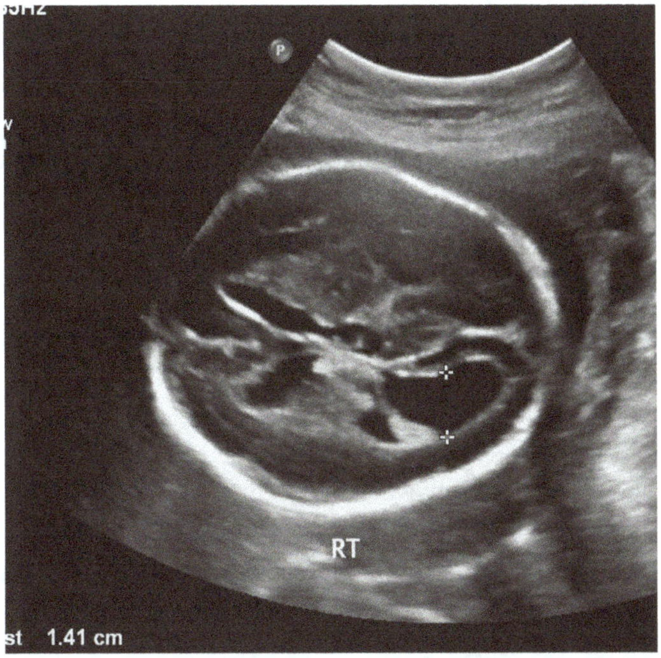


**FIGURE 2.3E** Case of aqueductal stenosis with moderate ventriculomegaly (+ … +).

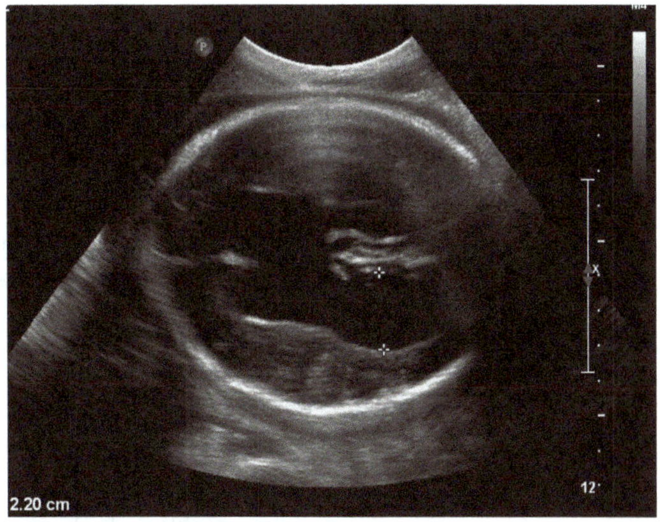


**FIGURE 2.3F** Severe ventriculomegaly in aqueductal stenosis (+ … +).

# 2.4 ARACHNOID CYST

## EPIDEMIOLOGY/GENETICS

**Definition** Arachnoid cysts are membrane-lined, fluid-filled cavities that may occur anywhere within the brain or spinal cord in association with the arachnoid or ventricular lining.

**Epidemiology** These are relatively rare neonatally because most are asymptomatic, but with prenatal ultrasound screening, more are being detected. They account for 1% of intracranial masses found prenatally and are more common in males than females.

**Embryology** Arachnoid cysts can occur anywhere in the lining of the brain or spinal cord. They may arise postnatally and are usually associated with trauma or infection, and they may communicate with the subarachnoid space. The cause of congenital cysts is unclear. They most likely represent maldevelopment of the leptomeninges.

**Inheritance Patterns** Rare autosomal recessive families with isolated arachnoid cysts have been described.

**Teratogens** Congenital infections.

**Prognosis** Because these cysts generally compress normal brain structures, the outcome is usually favorable unless associated with other congenital anomalies or there are significant complications related to treatment. The association of intracranial cysts with ACC should suggest the Aicardi syndrome, an X-linked dominant disorder with male lethality.

## SONOGRAPHY

### FREQUENT

- Interhemispheric cyst
  - Unilocular or containing thin septa

### LESS FREQUENT

- Macrocephaly
- Ventriculomegaly

### KEY FINDINGS/PITFALLS

- Fifty percent occur in the midcranial fossa.
  - They may also occur in the supracellar cisterna, posterior fossa, or surface of the brain at the level of the fissures.
- Most arachnoid cysts are diagnosed between 20 and 30 weeks' gestation.
  - When arachnoid cysts are diagnosed after 30 weeks, there is frequently a normal second-trimester examination, indicating that arachnoid cysts may develop quickly.
  - Occasional diagnoses in the first trimester have been reported.

- Interhemispheric fissure cysts may be associated with partial ACC.
- With large intrahemispheric cysts, it is difficult to distinguish between compression and ACC.
- Associated anomalies increase the likelihood of a karyotypic abnormality.
- Arachnoid cysts may spontaneously resolve.
  - While regression is rare in the fetus, it is common in the neonate.
  - The cyst regression may result from spontaneous rupture into the subdural or subarachnoid spaces or ventricles.
- Of antenatally diagnosed arachnoid cysts, 20% increase in size; approximately 4% regress.
- Three-dimensional scanning can show an arachnoid cyst in 3 orthogonal views and confirm its location.
- MRI can determine the exact location of arachnoid cysts and their relationship to adjacent brain.

### DIFFERENTIAL DIAGNOSIS

- Vein of Galen aneurysm: Utilize color Doppler to distinguish from an arachnoid cyst.
- Porencephalic cyst: The cystic area will border on the ventricle.
- Intracranial bleed: There will be internal echoes in the apparent cyst if the gain is increased.
- Schizencephaly: A disorganized cystic area extends across the midline and involves both hemispheres.

## PREGNANCY MANAGEMENT

**Investigations and Consultations Required** Despite the low reported incidence of chromosome abnormalities, cytogenetic studies should be performed. No other diagnostic evaluations are indicated unless the diagnosis is in question. Fetal MRI is a useful tool to confirm the diagnosis if the diagnosis is in doubt. Consultation with a pediatric neurosurgeon should be arranged.

**Fetal Intervention** Fetal intervention is not indicated because of the relatively benign course of this malformation.

**Monitoring** Serial ultrasound examinations should be performed to detect or follow ventriculomegaly, to follow the cyst size, and to detect evolving macrocephaly, which could affect delivery mode. If the cyst enlarges, the diagnosis may need to be reevaluated.

**Pregnancy Course** Obstetric complications are not expected.

**Pregnancy Termination Issues** The method of termination should be nondestructive as confirmation of etiology is necessary. Termination should be undertaken at a site with special expertise in neuropathology.

**Delivery** The site of delivery should be at a location with expertise in the management of neonates with CNS malformations.

## NEONATOLOGY

**Resuscitation** In the majority of cases, arachnoid cysts do not cause symptoms in the immediate newborn period, and resuscitation is not necessary.

**Transport** Referral to a tertiary center with pediatric neurology and neurosurgery capabilities is indicated.

**Testing and Confirmation** Although the majority of infants are asymptomatic at birth, infants may present with macrocephaly or a bulging fontanelle with widened sutures. The cysts cause their symptoms through pressure and mass effect. Small-to-moderate cysts are frequently asymptomatic. Postnatal MRI will accurately define these abnormalities.

**Nursery Management** Infants with asymptomatic arachnoid cysts require no treatment in the immediate newborn period. Consultation with pediatric neurology is recommended with periodic outpatient follow-up. When treatment is necessary, the specific intervention depends on the size of the cyst and the specific location of the cyst within the skull.

## SURGERY

**Preoperative Assessment** Location of the arachnoid cyst with respect to the ventricular system, the basal cisterns, and the structures of the posterior fossa is important for surgical planning. MRI scanning is useful to define the surgical anatomy.

**Operative Indications** Small arachnoid cysts without mass effect on surrounding neural structures warrant observation only with periodic head ultrasound or MRI. If stable over time, then no surgical intervention is indicated. Larger cysts that present with hydrocephalus, the presence of a neurologic deficit, increase in cyst size, or poorly controlled seizures require surgical intervention.

### TYPES OF PROCEDURES

1. Shunting of the cyst to the peritoneal cavity or the right atrium.
2. Marsupialization of the cyst into the basal cisterns or surrounding subarachnoid space. This technique is useful only for arachnoid cysts that present at the skull base adjacent to the basal cisterns.
3. Fenestration of the cyst into an adjacent ventricle, which may be accomplished endoscopically.

**Surgical Results/Prognosis** Arachnoid cysts in general have an excellent outcome and are not typically associated with neurologic or cognitive impairment.

## SUGGESTED READINGS

1. Bannister CM, Russell SA, Rimmer S, Mowle DH: Fetal arachnoid cysts: their site, progress and differential diagnosis. Eur J Pediatr Surg 1999; 1:27-28.
2. Blaicher W, Prager D, Kuhle S, et al: Combined prenatal ultrasound and magnetic resonance imaging in two fetuses with suspected arachnoid cysts. Ultrasound Obstet Gynecol 2001; 18:166-168.

3. Bretelle F, Senat M-V, Bernard J-P, et al: First-trimester diagnosis of fetal arachnoid cyst: prenatal implication. Ultrasound Obstet Gynecol 2002; 20:400-402.

4. Bromley B, Krishnamoorthy K, Benacerraf BR: Aicardi syndrome: prenatal sonographic findings. A report of two cases. Prenat Diagn 2000; 20:344-346.

5. Chen CY, Chen FH, Lee CC, et al: Sonographic characteristics of the cavum velum interpositum. Am J Neuroradiol 1998; 19:1631-1635.

6. DiRocco C: Arachnoid cysts. In: Youmans JR, ed. Neurological Survey. Vol 2, 4th ed. Philadelphia: Saunders; 1996: 967-994.

7. Elbers SEL, Furness ME: Resolution of presumed arachnoid cysts in utero. Ultrasound Obstet Gynecol 1999; 14:353-355.

8. Gedikbosi A, Palabiyi KF, Oztarhan A, et al: Prenatal diagnosis of a suprasellar arachnoid cyst with 2- and 3-dimensional sonography and fetal magnetic resonance imaging. J Ultrasound Med 2010; 29:1487-1493.

9. Hogge WA, Schnatterly P, Ferguson JE II: Early prenatal diagnosis of an infratentorial arachnoid cyst: association with an unbalanced translocation. Prenat Diagn 1995; 15:186-188.

10. Pierre-Kahn A, Sonigo P: Malformative intracranial cysts: diagnosis and outcome. Child's Nerv Syst 2003; 19:477-483.

11. Pilu G, Falco P, Perolo A, et al: Differential diagnosis and outcome of fetal intracranial hypochoic lesions: report of 21 cases. Ultrasound Obstet Gynecol 1997; 9:229-236.

12. Weber R, Volt T, Lumenta C, Lenard H-G: Spontaneous regression of a temporal arachnoid cyst. Child's Nerv Sys 1991; 7:414-415.

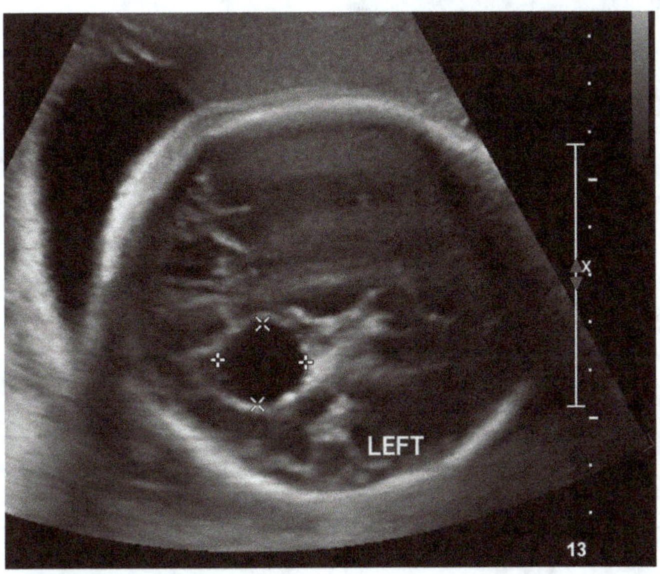


**FIGURE 2.4A** A 9 × 7 mm left arachnoid cyst.

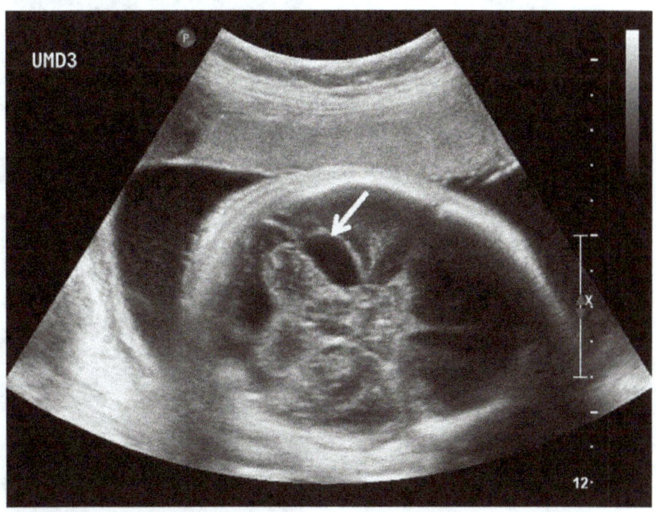


**FIGURE 2.4B** Supratentorial arachnoid cyst (arrow).

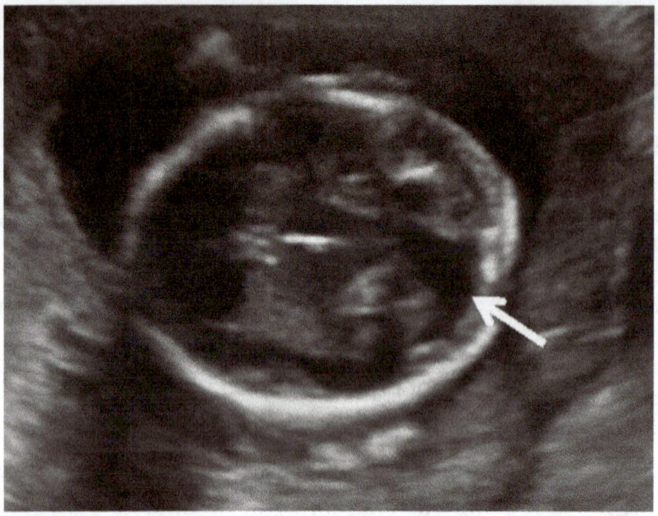

**FIGURE 2.4C** Posterior fossa arachnoid cyst (arrow).

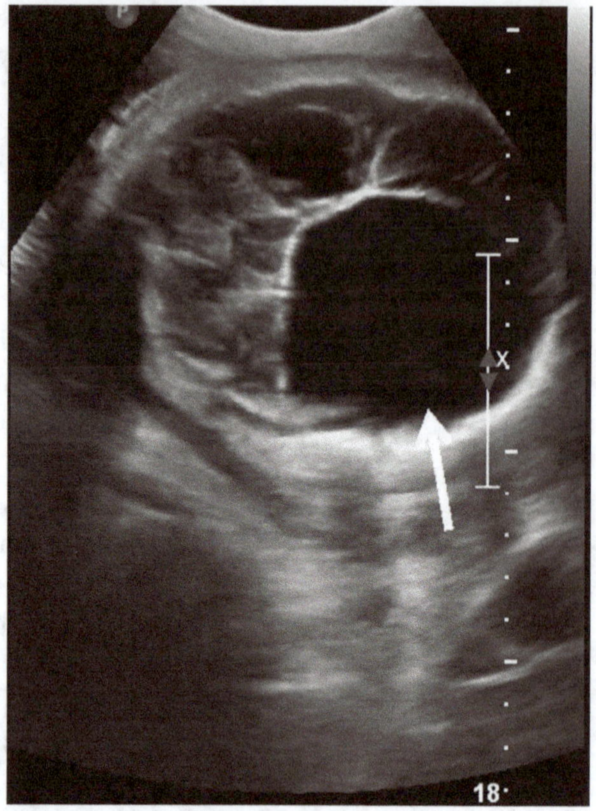


**FIGURE 2.4D** Arachnoid cyst (arrow) on ultrasound.

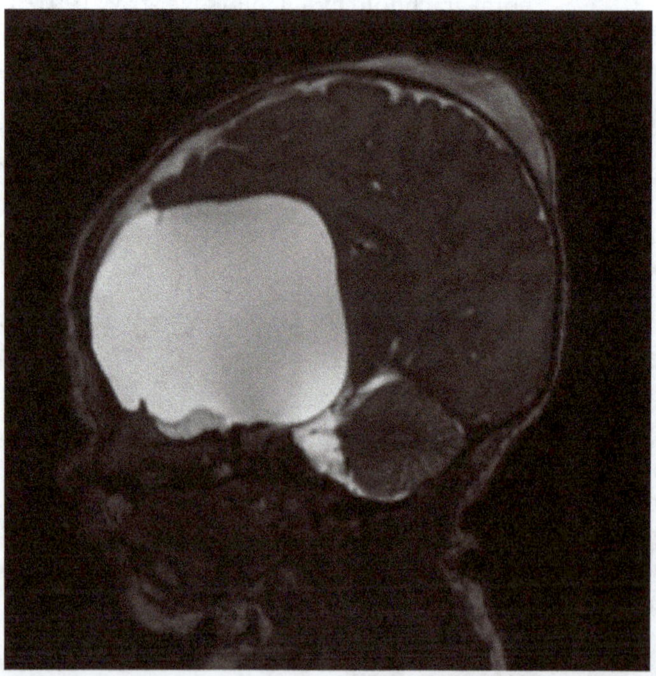

**FIGURE 2.4E** Arachnoid cyst seen in Figure 2.4D visualized on MRI.

# 2.5 CAUDAL APLASIA/DYSPLASIA (REGRESSION) SEQUENCE

## EPIDEMIOLOGY/GENETICS

**Definition** Caudal aplasia/dysplasia sequence (caudal regression) is the total or partial agenesis of the distal neural tube resulting in sacral agenesis/dysgenesis with associated abnormalities of the lower extremities and gastrointestinal or genitourinary tracts. It is a continuum from partial agenesis of the sacrococcygeal spine to complete absence of the sacrum, lumbar, and lower thoracic vertebrae.

**Epidemiology** The sequence occurs in about 1 to 5 of 100,000 births (M1:F1).

**Embryology** Differentiation of the lower spine is usually complete before the seventh week of pregnancy. The term *caudal regression* is probably inaccurate, as the caudal defects in this condition are primary malformations rather than the result of regression of structures. Sirenomelia may represent one end of the spectrum of this condition or may be etiologically separate. Heart defects are common associated malformations. This condition may overlap with the VACTERL (vertebral defects, anal atresia, cardiac defects, tracheoesophageal fistula, renal anomalies, limb abnormalities) association, making evaluation for other VACTERL association findings important.

**Inheritance Patterns** Most often, inheritance is sporadic. Rare families showing autosomal and X-linked dominant inheritance have been reported. It is often seen in association with maternal diabetes.

**Teratogens** Approximately 16% of cases are seen in infants of diabetic mothers. Individuals with poorly controlled diabetes have an incidence of caudal regression that is 200-fold higher than the general population.

**Prognosis** Prognosis is dependent on the severity of the defect and presence of associated abnormalities. Bowel and urinary complications are common and may not be compatible with life. If not part of a genetic or chromosomal syndrome, cognitive function is usually normal.

## SONOGRAPHY

### FREQUENT FINDINGS

- Conical termination of the spine with absent sacral and lower lumbar vertebrae
- Disproportion between the upper and lower portions of the body
- Shortened lower extremities
- Femurs fixed in a V pattern
- Decreased/absent movement of the lower extremities
- Distal leg atrophy
- Clubbed feet

- Sacral agenesis
  - Absence of the sacrum results in approximation of the iliac blades, giving a "shield-like" appearance.

### LESS FREQUENT

- Distended bladder
- Imperforate anus
- Bladder exstrophy
- Renal dysplasia
- Holoprosencephaly
- Myelomeningocele
- Single umbilical artery
- Renal agenesis
- Kyphoscoliosis
- Congenital heart disease
- Absent fibula

### KEY FINDINGS/PITFALLS/DIFFERENTIAL DIAGNOSIS

- Incomplete ossification of the sacrum in the first trimester makes the diagnosis difficult, but not impossible.
- A 3-D ultrasound can accurately determine the level at which the spine is suddenly interrupted.
- Sirenomelia is a related condition in which both legs are fused. In sirenomelia, there is oligohydramnios or absent fluid, and the kidneys may appear to be absent, obstructed, or dysplastic. There may be a single lower extremity, or both legs may be fused and lie alongside each other.

## PREGNANCY MANAGEMENT

**Investigations and Consultations Required** Evaluation of the mother for diabetes should be performed. Fetal echocardiography should be performed to evaluate for associated cardiac defects. Pediatric surgical consultations should be obtained to plan neonatal management with the family.

**Monitoring** No specific alterations in obstetric care are necessary unless diabetes is diagnosed. The diagnosis is difficult to make, so repeat ultrasound examinations may be worthwhile. In addition, following fetal growth and amniotic fluid volume may be helpful in ongoing cases.

**Pregnancy Termination Issues** In the patient with known diabetes, no special autopsy requirements are necessary. In the absence of maternal diabetes, full autopsy of an intact fetus should be performed to establish the diagnosis.

**Delivery** Breech presentation is common and may warrant cesarean section, particularly as marked body/head discrepancy may be present. The complex neonatal issues that will be encountered require delivery at a tertiary center.

## NEONATOLOGY

**Resuscitation** Except for the issues related to prematurity and to infants of diabetic mothers, there are no special concerns in planning for resuscitation. In a small number of cases, there may be other serious anomalies (CNS or cardiac) that could govern approach. If other life-threatening and potentially uncorrectable defects are known to be present, prenatal discussion with the parents regarding nonintervention is appropriate. If caudal regression is associated with bilateral renal agenesis, the defect is lethal.

**Transport** Referral to a tertiary center with multiple pediatric subspecialty capabilities is indicated.

**Testing and Confirmation** The physical findings are apparent at birth. Imaging studies, including echocardiography, to exclude concomitant cardiac anomalies, skeletal survey, abdominal ultrasound, head ultrasound, or cranial MRI should be obtained prior to invasive interventions.

**Nursery Management** Approach and management are governed by the suspected cause (i.e., maternal diabetes), associated anomalies, and the location of the defect. Caudal regression syndromes with lumbosacral agenesis may range from absent coccyx, as an isolated finding without neurologic sequelae, to sacral or lumbosacral agenesis. There are five types of caudal regression sequence. Types I and II are considered mild forms with coccyx absence, but without deficits in functionality. Type I involves total or partial unilateral sacral agenesis. Type II involves total sacral agenesis with variable lumbar agenesis. Types III and IV are the most severe, with total absence of the sacrum and systemic and neurological complications. Type III involves variable lumbar and total sacral agenesis, with the caudal end plate of the lowest vertebra often resting above fused ilia. Type IV involves fusion of soft tissues of both the lower limbs. Type V, also known as "sirenomelia" or "mermaid syndrome," is associated with a single femur and tibia and may not have the same etiology as the other types. Depending on the type of sacral agenesis, bowel or urinary bladder deficiencies may be present. Associated orthopedic anomalies may include deformities of the feet, flexion contractures of the lower extremities, dislocation of the hips, kyphoscoliosis, and absence of ribs.

Management requires a multidisciplinary approach by neurosurgeons, urologists, nephrologists, physical therapists, and psychologists. Surgical interventions, such as transureteroureterostomy and cutaneous vesicostomy, may be necessary if clean intermittent catheterization or anticholinergic drug administration is not adequate to treat urological disorders. Colostomy is performed to treat an imperforate anus. Depending on the severity of the syndrome, orthopedic interventions may also be required. Treatment is supportive only when the primary pathology is irreversible.

Prognosis is poor in many cases. Early neonatal death in the severe forms occurs from cardiac, renal, and respiratory complications. Surviving infants usually have normal cognitive function.

## SUGGESTED READINGS


1. Bashiri A, Sheizaf B, Burstein E, et al: Three dimensional ultrasound diagnosis of caudal regression syndrome at 14 gestational weeks. Arch Gynecol Obstet 2009; 280:505-507.
2. Baxi L, Warren W, Collins MH, Timor-Tritsch IE: Early detection of caudal regression syndrome with transvaginal scanning. Obstet Gynecol 1990; 75:486-489.
3. Fukada Y, Yasumizu T, Tsurugi Y, et al: Caudal regression syndrome detected in a fetus with increased nuchal translucency. Acta Obstet Gynaecol Scand 1999; 78:655-656.
4. Gonzalez-Quintero VH, Lama T, Dibe M, et al: Case report—sonographic diagnosis of caudal regression in the first trimester of pregnancy. J Ultrasound Med 2002; 21:1175-1178.
5. Pang D: Sacral agenesis and caudal spinal malformations. Neurosurgery 1993; 32:755-779.
6. Passarge E, Lenz W: Syndrome of caudal regression in infants of diabetic mothers: observation of further cases. Pediatrics 1966; 37:672-675.
7. Renshaw TS. Sacral agenesis. In: Weinstein SL, ed. The Pediatric Spine—Principles and Practice. New York: Raven Press; 1994: 1:2214.
8. Torre M, Buffa P, Jasonni V, Cama A: Long-term urologic outcome in patients with caudal regression syndrome, compared with meningomyelocele and spinal cord lipoma. J Pediatr Surg 2008; 43:530-533


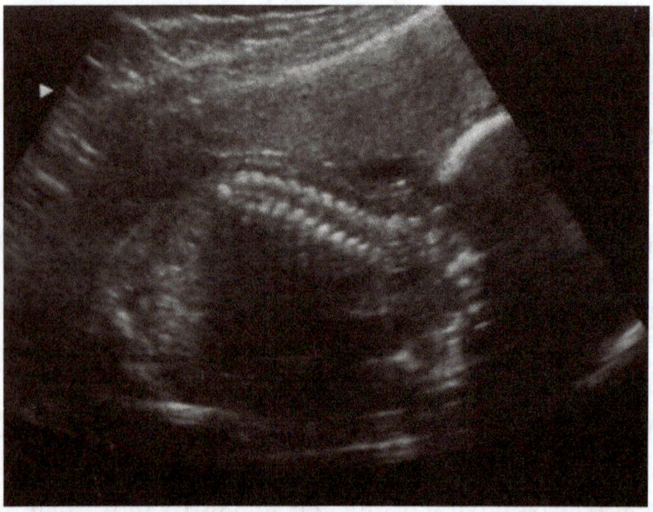

**FIGURE 2.5A** Caudal regression illustrating abrupt end to spine and absent sacrum.

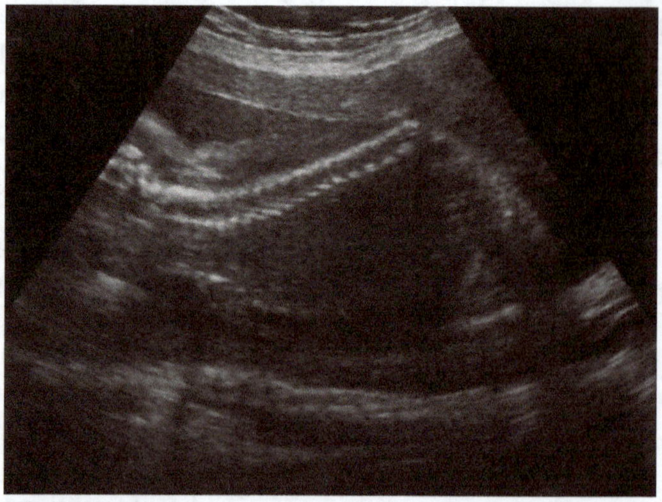

**FIGURE 2.5B** Caudal regression with absence of the lower spine.

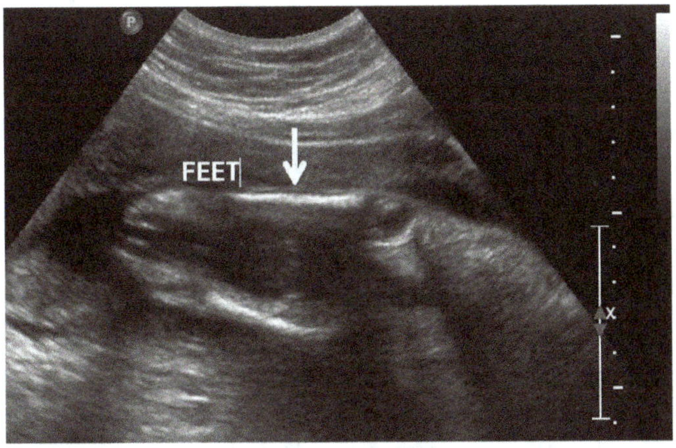


**FIGURE 2.5C** Bilateral clubfeet; muscular atrophy (arrow) in caudal regression.

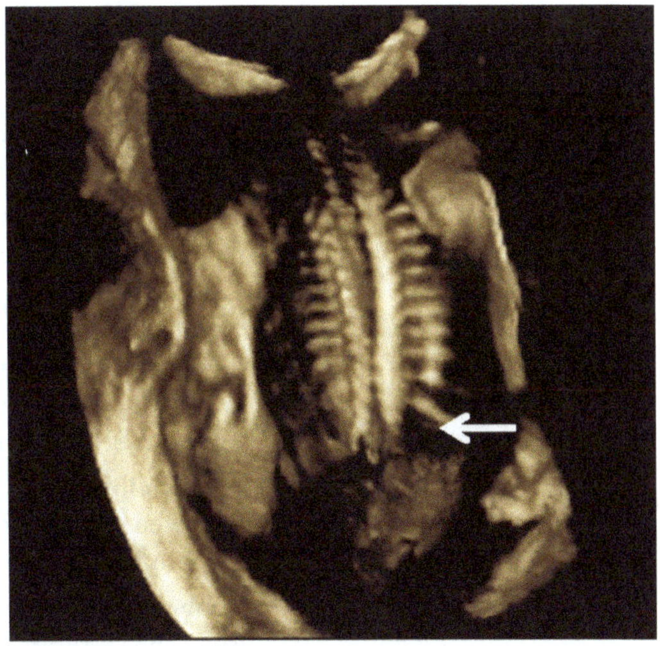

**FIGURE 2.5D** Three-dimensional image showing complete absence of sacrum and lower lumbar vertebrae (arrow).

# 2.6 INTRACRANIAL TUMORS

## EPIDEMIOLOGY/GENETICS

**Definition** There are over 100 types of intracranial tumors, but the majority of antenatally detected cranial tumors are teratomas derived from totipotent cells, including embryonic ectodermal, endodermal, and mesodermal tissue derivatives. Other more common fetal brain tumors are astrocytoma, ependymoma, choroid plexus papilloma, medulloblastoma, craniopharyngioma, and meningioma. It is difficult, however, to reliably separate these tumors from other intracranial neoplasms and benign cystic lesions.

**Epidemiology** Intracranial tumors are rare, with 50% of antenatally detected tumors being teratomas that show a very high male-to-female preponderance.

**Embryology** Teratomas occur most often in a midline location and have mixed solid and cystic areas. Only 3% of all teratomas occur intracranially. Other brain tumors form from specific areas of the developing nervous system. Most are located supratentorially.

**Inheritance Patterns** Sporadic.

**Teratogens** None.

**Differential Diagnosis** Benign intracranial lesions such as arachnoid cysts and lipomas. Teratomas and other intracranial neoplasms generally show progression and distortion of normal structures.

**Prognosis** Prognosis depends on the size and location of the tumor. The majority of antenatally detected tumors have been lethal.

## SONOGRAPHY

### FREQUENT FINDINGS

- Distortion of brain anatomy
  - Cystic or solid appearance
- Macrocephaly
  - Tumor occupies a variable volume of the intracranial cavity
  - Size may result in dystocia at time of delivery
- Midline shift

### LESS FREQUENT

- Polyhydramnios
- Hydrops from high output failure
- Hemorrhage into the cerebral mass

### KEY FINDINGS/PITFALLS/DIFFERENTIAL DIAGNOSIS

- Sonographic detection usually occurs in the third trimester. However, detection in the second trimester has been reported.

- Teratoma
  - Heterogeneous appearance
    - Rapid growth results in necrotic components that appear cystic.
- Astrocystoma
  - This is the second most common brain tumor.
  - Glioblastoma is a type of astrocytoma and develops rapidly.
- Ependymoma
  - Arises from the fourth ventricle
  - Has a poor prognosis
- Choroid plexus papilloma
  - Rapid onset of ventriculomegaly and macrocephaly
  - Extends into the lateral ventricle
  - Secretes a large amount of CSF
  - Less commonly arises in third and fourth ventricles
- Medulloblastoma
  - Originates from vermis
  - Tumor inception: 14-23 weeks' gestation
- Craniopharyngioma
  - Arises from Rathke's pouch—an extodermal extension from the roof of the mouth
  - Centrally located
  - When large, sonographically similar to a teratoma
- Prenatal ultrasound cannot accurately diagnosis tumor histology.
  - Ultrasound can distinguish the few potentially curable lesions (i.e., a localized choroid plexus papilloma) from a rapidly expanding fatal tumor.
  - A neonatal brain biopsy is required to obtain a definitive diagnosis.
- Color Doppler can evaluate an intracranial mass for vascularity and displacement of normal vessels.
  - Choroid plexus papillomas and astrocytomas demonstrate internal vascular flow.
  - Gangliomas generally present as an avascular mass.
- To determine the extent of an intracranial tumor, MRI should be considered.

## PREGNANCY MANAGEMENT

**Investigations and Consultations Required** Because of the inability to make a precise diagnosis in some cases, other causes must be considered for the sonographic features, particularly intracranial hemorrhage. Consultation with a neurosurgeon or neurologist and with a neonatologist is essential to provide the family full information regarding the grave prognosis for the neonate and to develop a plan of management.

**Fetal Intervention** None is indicated.

**Monitoring** These tumors tend to grow quickly, and there may be massive macrocephaly. In addition to being a part of the differential diagnosis, intracranial hemorrhage may occur within a tumor, contributing to both uncertainty in interpreting the ultrasonographic findings and rapid head growth.

Fetal hydrops and polyhydramnios are common complications of intracranial tumors. Serial ultrasound examinations are useful to monitor for the development of these complications, as well as to assess fetal head size.

**Pregnancy Course** The pregnancy may be complicated by polyhydramnios and resulting preterm labor. Symptomatic polyhydramnios is an indication for delivery, and tocolysis is not indicated.

**Pregnancy Termination Issues** The excessive growth of the head may complicate both forms of pregnancy termination. An intact fetus is not necessary for confirmation of the diagnosis.

**Delivery** The significant head size reported in these infants may require elective cesarean section for maternal indications, despite the grave prognosis. Attempts at cranial decompression are not likely to be successful. The decision to use a vertical or horizontal incision on the uterus will depend on the fetal lie and the status of the lower uterine segment. Spontaneous rupture of the fetal head has been reported.

## NEONATOLOGY

**Resuscitation** Because progressive cranial enlargement is the primary fetal manifestation of an intracranial tumor, operative delivery prior to full gestation may be indicated. Assistance with the onset of respiration will be determined by both the gestational age at delivery and the difficulties encountered intrapartum. The most common intracranial mass presenting in fetal life is a teratoma, which has an almost uniform perinatal mortality. Therefore, if prenatal diagnosis suggests that the mass is a teratoma, it is appropriate for the option of nonintervention to be presented to the parents.

**Transport** Transfer to a tertiary center with neonatology, pediatric neurosurgery, pediatric neurology, and pediatric oncology subspecialty capabilities is essential.

**Testing and Confirmation** MRI is used to determine tumor location, morphology, relationship to surrounding structures, and presence of ventricular enlargement. On occasion, Doppler flow studies are useful to define the impact on cerebral vasculature. Biochemical markers obtained from CSF may aid in making a diagnosis. The definitive diagnosis requires tissue histopathologic examination from either tumor resection or biopsy.

**Nursery Management** The management of a neonate with an intracranial tumor in general involves three issues beyond those that are relative to preterm delivery, if such has been required. These are as follows:

- hydrocephalus—if and when to place a shunt
- tumor removal—timing, approach, and feasibility of complete resection
- adjuvant therapy—chemotherapy, radiotherapy, or both

The most common clinical presentation in the newborn is increased cranial size with or without hydrocephalus. Certain tumors, especially astrocytomas, may be complicated by intraventricular hemorrhage. In addition, in the immediate newborn period, infants may present with apneic episodes, increased irritability, neurological deficits, and in some cases seizures. The approach chosen for a given infant depends directly on the specific tumor cell type, the size and location of the mass, and the general condition of the infant.

## SURGERY

**Preoperative Assessment** Congenital tumors usually occur in the midline and may reach a very large size. Tumors diagnosed antenatally are usually aggressive and have a poor prognosis. Therefore, a careful assessment to determine the extent of disease and a search for metastatic lesions in the spine or outside the CNS are necessary preoperatively.

**Operative Indications and Procedures** The decision to proceed with surgery depends on the preoperative assessment and the predicted histology. Neonates with large tumors that involve vital structures or that have replaced the majority of the developing brain are usually not surgical candidates because of their poor prognosis. Teratomas are associated with a poor outcome. Mortality rates in these infants generally exceed 90%, principally because the lesions are usually extensive at the time of presentation. Medulloblastoma at birth also has a poor prognosis. Astrocytomas and ependymomas are associated with variable outcomes, depending primarily on the degree of differentiation of the tumor and its location. Markedly anaplastic lesions and deep diencephalic and brainstem locations are rarely curable. After complete surgical resection, choroid plexus papillomas have a highly favorable prognosis. Some tumors, such as lipomas or hamartomas of the brain, may not require surgical intervention unless symptomatic. Tumors that are highly vascular, or of malignant histology, may be treated with chemotherapy prior to attempted definitive resection.

The goal of surgical intervention is to decrease the tumor load by either complete or partial resection. Surgery may be endoscopic or open. The surgical approach and extent of resection are determined by the size, position, histology, relationship of the tumor to other structures in the brain, and the level of risk acceptable to the parent and surgeon on behalf of the infant. Before embarking on surgical treatment, parents must be informed of the prognosis and the morbidity and mortality associated with the particular type of tumor. They should be offered the option of nonintervention and provision of palliative care, if deemed appropriate by the multidisciplinary team.

**Surgical Results/Prognosis** The prognosis of infants with antenatally diagnosed brain tumors is poor. The majority of infants expire within 5 years of diagnosis. Survivors are likely to experience long-term morbidities, including endocrine or neurologic deficits. The size and histologic type of the tumor and the neurologic status of the child at birth will ultimately determine prognosis.

### SUGGESTED READINGS

1. Armstrong GT, Liu Q, Yasui Y, et al: Long-term outcomes among adult survivors of childhood central nervous system malignancies in the Childhood Cancer Survivor Study. J Natl Cancer Inst 2009; 101:946-958.

2. Buetow P, Smirniotopoulos JG, Done S: Congenital brain tumors: a review of 45 cases. AJR Am J Roentgenol 1990; 155:587-93.
3. Cassart M, Bosson N, Garel C, et al: Fetal intracranial tumors: a review of 27 cases. Eur Radiol 2008; 18:2060-2066.
4. Fort DW, Rushing EJ: Congenital central nervous system tumors. J Child Neurol 1997; 12:157-164.
5. Hirakawa K, Suzuki K, Ueda S, Handa J: Fetal origin of the medulloblastoma: evidence from growth analysis of two cases. Acta Neuropathol 1986; 70:227-234.
6. Isaacs H Jr: II Perinatal brain tumors: a review of 250 cases. Pediatr Neurol 2002; 27:333-342.
7. Isaacs H Jr: Fetal brain tumors: a review of 154 cases. Am J Perinatol 2009; 26:453-466.
8. Magdum SA: Neonatal brain tumors: a review. Early Hum Dev 2010; 86:627-631.
9. Mapstone TB, Warf BC: Intracranial tumor in infants: characteristics, management, and outcome of a contemporary series. Neurosurgery 1991; 28:343.
10. Sherer DM, Abramowicz JS, Eggers PC, et al: Prenatal ultrasonographic diagnosis of intracranial teratoma and massive craniomegaly with associated high-output cardiac failure. Am J Obstet Gynecol 1993; 168:97-99.
11. Sosa-Olavarria A, Diaz-Guerrero L, Reigoza A, et al: Fetal craniopharyngioma. Early prenatal diagnosis. J Ultrasound Med 2001; 20:803-806.

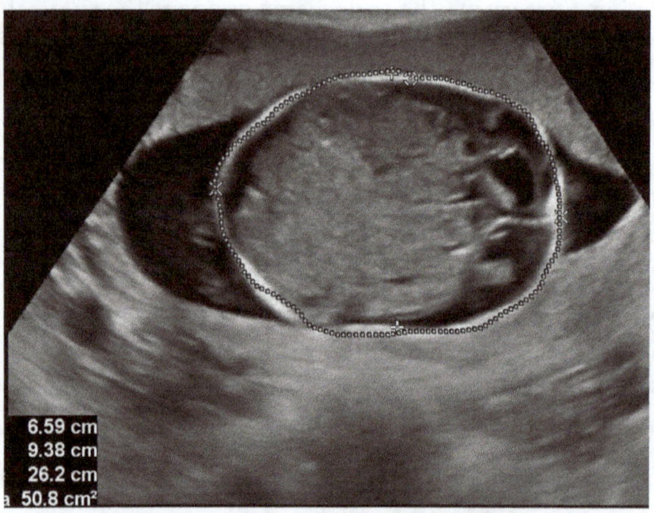


**FIGURE 2.6A** Intracranial teratoma at 21 weeks with a head circumference consistent with 28 weeks.

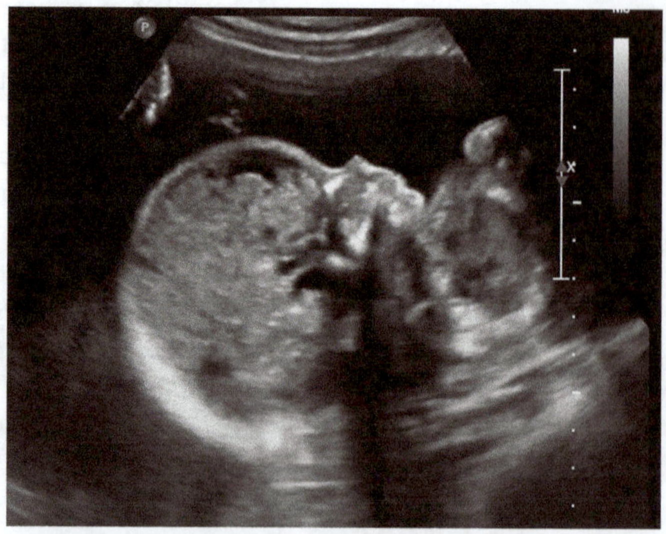

**FIGURE 2.6B** Intracranial teratoma with macrocephaly.

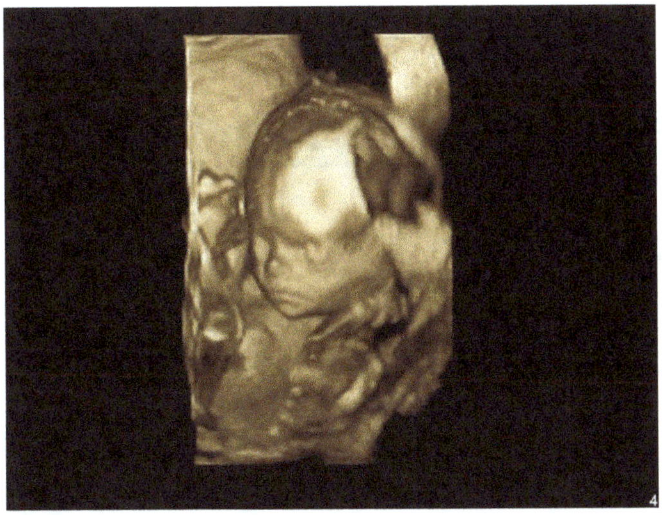

**FIGURE 2.6C** Three-dimensional image illustrating macrocephaly at 21 weeks.

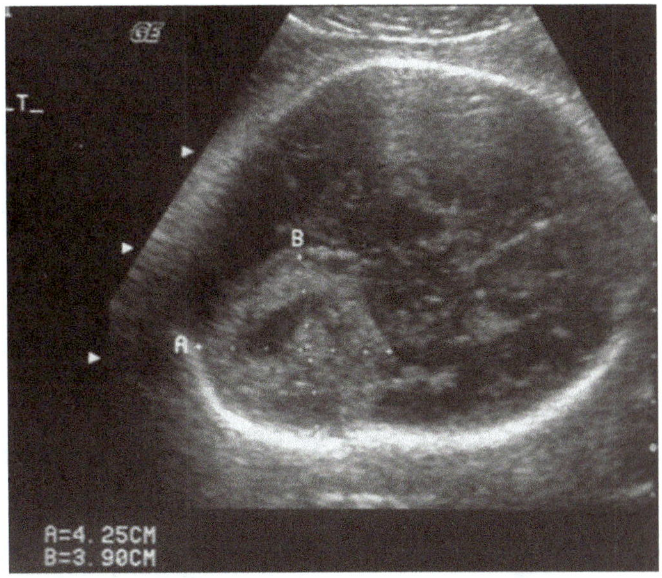


**FIGURE 2.6D** Astrocytoma.

# 2.7 CRANIOSYNOSTOSIS

## EPIDEMIOLOGY/GENETICS

**Definition** Craniosynostosis is abnormal development or premature closure of one or more of the cranial sutures, resulting in an abnormal head shape. More than 150 syndromes with craniosynostosis have been described.

**Epidemiology** Isolated craniosynostosis is relatively common (3.4 in 1000 live births, M2:F1), but most craniosynostosis syndromes are rare (<1 in 50,000–100,000).

**Embryology** The abnormal head shape ranges from plagiocephaly caused by a single fused suture to a trilobar skull deformity referred to as a cloverleaf skull (kleeblattschädel) caused by multiple suture synostosis.

- Head shape is dependent on which suture or sutures are closed and the timing of closure.
  - Scaphocephaly
    - Most common nonsyndromic single-suture fusion
    - Premature closure of the sagittal suture
      - Short biparietal diameter
      - Long occipital frontal diameter
      - Frontal bossing
  - Brachycephaly
    - Premature closure of the coronal sutures
    - Short occipital frontal diameter
    - Large biparietal diameter
  - Trigonocephaly
    - Premature closure of metopic suture
    - Triangular-shaped head
    - Hypertelorism
  - Acrocephaly
    - Premature closure of the coronal suture
    - "Cone" shape
    - High cranial vault
    - Reduced midfacial bone growth
    - Concave, flat face
  - Oxycephaly
    - Fusion of coronal and lambdoidal sutures
  - Plagiocephaly
    - Unilateral fusion of coronal suture
    - Restricts growth of one side of the face, resulting in facial asymmetry
    - Eye socket on the affected side pulled back with compensatory overgrowth of the unaffected side

There is often associated syndactyly of the hands and feet or other abnormalities. Currently, six syndromes are associated with abnormalities of fibroblast growth factor receptors (FGFRs) for which molecular testing is available: Crouzon, Jackson-Weiss, Apert, and Pfeiffer syndromes (FGFR2); Crouzon with acanthosis nigricans (FGFR3); and Pfeiffer II (FGFR1). Those with thanatophoric dysplasia type II (FGFR3) can have a cloverleaf skull but this is distinguished by severe short-limbed dwarfism.

**Inheritance Patterns** Most isolated cases of craniosynostosis have multifactorial or sporadic inheritance, although some families show autosomal dominant or autosomal recessive inheritance. Craniosynostosis as part of a syndrome is often autosomal dominant. The inheritance pattern depends on the specific syndrome diagnosis.

**Teratogens** Aminopterin, methotrexate, hydantoin, retinoic acid, valproic acid, and intrauterine mechanical restraint (abnormal pressure on the skull approximates the bone, resulting in a bony bridge across the suture and subsequent fusion) are teratogenic.

**Prognosis** Prognosis for isolated craniosynostosis is usually very good with reconstructive surgery. Prognosis for individuals with a genetic syndrome featuring craniosynostosis varies from very good (Crouzon, Jackson-Weiss syndromes) to developmental delay and mental retardation (Apert and Pfeiffer syndromes) or lethality (thanatophoric dysplasia type II).

## SONOGRAPHY

### FREQUENT FINDINGS

- Dolichocephaly
- Brachycephaly
- Abnormal skull configuration
- Hyperechoic bony ridge when a suture is fused
- Asymmetric skull shape depending on which suture closes prematurely

### LESS FREQUENT

- Ventriculomegaly
- Proptosis
- Hypertelorism
- Hypotelorism

### SPECIFIC FINDINGS IN COMMON SYNDROMES

- Crouzon
  - Sutures fuse simultaneously.
  - Skull proportions are normal.
  - There is midface hypoplasia and proptosis.
- Apert
  - Coronal sutures fuse first.
  - Metopic sutures are widely separated.
  - The brain expands away from the midline.
  - There is a bulging forehead.
- Pfeiffer
  - The time of craniosynostosis is variable.
  - Cloverleaf skull formation is due to early fusion of multiple sutures.

- Carpenter
    - There is asymmetric premature closure of all sutures.
    - Characteristic findings in addition to acrocephaly include
        - Preaxial polydactyly of the hands and feet
        - Syndactyly of the toes
        - Omphalocele
        - Congenital heart defects
        - Proptosis
        - Ventriculomegaly
        - Hypertelorism
        - Flat nasal bridge
- Saethre-Chotzen syndrome
    - The gene mutation is TWIST 1.
    - Both coronal sutures are fused.
        - High forehead
        - Brachycephaly
        - Polysyndactyly

### KEY FINDINGS/PITFALLS

- To distinguish etiologies of craniosynostosis, evaluate the face, skeleton, hands, and feet.
- A routine 20-week ultrasound examination will not reliably detect craniosynostosis except in severe cases.
- A 3-D ultrasound is able to demonstrate the echogenic lines of fusion rather than characteristic sutures.
- A 3-D ultrasound may demonstrate facial features associated with craniosynostosis.

## PREGNANCY MANAGEMENT

**Investigations and Consultations Required** Craniosynostosis may be associated with several different genetic syndromes, and imaging to distinguish these may be aided by molecular testing. Depending on the shape of the head, chromosome studies also may be indicated. Many of the craniosynostosis syndromes are caused by mutations in either FGFR2 or FGFR3. For some, such as those with Apert syndrome, the limited number of responsible mutations may allow a precise molecular diagnosis. Collaboration between the sonologist and a pediatric dysmorphologist may be helpful in determining which molecular studies may be useful for a more definitive diagnosis.

**Fetal Intervention** None is indicated.

**Monitoring** Because of the association of ventriculomegaly with many of the disorders, serial ultrasound examinations should be performed to monitor ventricular size.

**Pregnancy Course** Polyhydramnios has been reported in a number of syndromes with craniosynostosis and may result in preterm labor.

**Pregnancy Termination Issues** Unless a precise diagnosis has been established prenatally, an intact fetus should be delivered for complete pathologic evaluation.

**Delivery** Abnormal head shape or significant enlargement of the head due to ventriculomegaly may prevent vaginal delivery.

## NEONATOLOGY

**Resuscitation** In general, respiratory depression at birth is not expected with isolated craniosynostosis; therefore, there is no contraindication to full resuscitation following delivery. If the premature suture closure is one manifestation of a rare syndrome or systemic disorder, the need for resuscitation is predicated on the specific disorder and its implications for long-term prognosis.

**Transport** In the absence of systemic disease, prematurity, or other need for neonatal intensive care, transfer to a tertiary center is not indicated in the immediate neonatal period. Early referral to a center with pediatric neurosurgery and preferably with a multidisciplinary craniofacial reconstructive program is recommended.

**Testing and Confirmation** Identification of a closed suture or sutures can be suspected from the physical findings of a nonmobile suture, a closed fontanel, or an abnormal cranial shape. While plain radiographs may further characterize the structural abnormality, computed tomographic (CT) scanning is the recommended imaging technique for more accurately assessing the extent of fusion and its effect on adjacent bones. A careful physical examination will reveal concomitant abnormalities, suggesting a syndrome or metabolic cause, the incidence of which is related to the specific suture involved. Additional diagnostic testing and imaging will be dictated by the concomitant abnormalities.

**Nursery Management** Beyond careful assessment to exclude multiple congenital anomaly syndromes, no special care requirements are indicated in the immediate newborn period. The decision for surgical correction and the appropriate timing for correction are influenced by the anatomic involvement, the apparent pathophysiology, associated anomalies, and the presence of increased intracranial pressure (ICP).

Optimal care of patients with craniofacial anomalies requires a multidisciplinary approach. This approach has been supported by a consensus conference of the American Cleft Palate–Craniofacial Association. The team consists of specialists from anesthesiology, audiology, cardiology, dermatology, radiology, genetic counseling, medical genetics, neurology, neurosurgery, nursing, ophthalmology, oral and maxillofacial surgery, nutrition, orthodontics, orthopedics, otolaryngology, pediatrics, pediatric dentistry, physical anthropology, plastic surgery, prosthodontics, psychiatry, psychology, social work, and speech and language pathology.

## SURGERY

**Preoperative Assessment** Some mild forms of single-suture craniosynostosis may not be readily appreciated at birth but become more apparent as the cranium grows and a more unusual cranial configuration becomes evident. Ridging along the involved suture often will accompany this process. Early obliteration of the anterior and posterior fontanelles can also occur with this process and signal possible increased ICP. In cases of multiple-suture craniosynostosis and syndromic forms of craniosynostosis, the physical and neurologic problems are often evident. Many of these will involve the coronal sutures and the cranial base. Frontal bone bossing may also be seen in conjunction with an abnormal cranial configuration.

**Operative Indications/Types of Procedures** Surgical repair of craniosynostosis is performed to prevent intracranial hypertension and improve socialization by normalizing the appearance of the face and head. The preferred time for surgical intervention is 8 to 12 months of age. At that age, there is adequate intracranial volume and the calvarium is thicker, which allows for more stable fixation. Signs of intracranial hypertension, such as papilledema, a beaten copper appearance on skull radiograph (called "fingerprinting" or "thumbprints" of the skull), or increased ICP measured transcutaneously, require urgent neurosurgical intervention and decompression. The different types of craniosynostosis require specific surgical approaches.

**Surgical Results/Prognosis** Surgical results are good and usually restore normal craniofacial aesthetics and reduce any possibility of neurologic sequelae.

Children with nonsyndromic craniosynostosis demonstrate an increased incidence of speech/language, cognitive, behavioral, and neurodevelopmental abnormalities. The exact relationship between structural and developmental abnormalities, as well as the relationship between surgical correction of craniosynostosis and changes in neurodevelopment, remains equally unclear.

### SUGGESTED READINGS

1. Becker DB, Petersen JD, Kane AA, et al. Speech, cognitive, and behavioral outcomes in nonsyndromic craniosynostosis. Plast Reconstr Surg 2005; 116:400-407.
2. Benacerraf BR, Spiro R, Mitchell AG: Using three-dimensional ultrasound to detect craniosynostosis in a fetus with Pfeiffer syndrome. Ultrasound Obstet Gynecol 2000; 16:391-394.
3. Buchanan EP, Hollier LJ. Overview of Craniosynosotsis. UpToDate. http://www.uptodate.com/contents/overview-of-craniosynostosis?source=search_result&search=craniosynostosis&selectedTitle=1~42.
4. Chaoui R, LeVaillent JM, Benoit B, et al: Three-dimensional sonographic description of abnormal metopic suture in second- and third-trimester fetuses. Ultrasound Obstet Gynecol 2005; 26:761-764.
5. Chieffo D, Tamburrini G, Massimi L, et al. Long-term neuropsychological development in single-suture craniosynostosis treated early. J Neurosurg Pediatr 2010; 5:232-237.

6. Cohen SR, Cho DC, Nichols SL, et al: American Society of Maxillofacial Surgeons outcome study: preoperative and postoperative neurodevelopmental findings in single-suture craniosynostosis. Plast Reconstr Surg 2004; 114:841-847.
7. De Jong T, Bannink N, Bredero-Boelhouwer HH, et al: Long-term functional outcome in 167 patients with syndromic craniosynostosis; defining a syndrome-specific risk profile. J Plast Reconstr Aesthet Surg 2010; 63:1635-1641.
8. Delahaye S, Bernard JP, Renier D, Ville Y: Prenatal ultrasound diagnosis of fetal craniosynostosis. Ultrasound Obstet Gynecol 2003; 21:347-353.
9. Faro C, Chaoui R, Wegrzyn P, et al: Metropic sutures in fetuses with Apert syndrome at 22-27 weeks of gestation. Ultrasound Obstet Gynecol 2006; 27:28-33.
10. Huang MHS, Mouradian WE, Cohen SR, Gruss JS: The differential diagnosis of abnormal head shapes: separating craniosynostosis from positional deformities and normal variants. Cleft Palate Craniofac J 1998; 35:204-211.
11. Johnson D, Wilkie AOM: Craniosynostosis. Eur J Hum Genet 2011; 19:369-376.
12. Lam H, Lo T-K, Lau E, et al: The use of 2- and 3-dimensional sonographic scans in the evaluation of cranial sutures. Prenatal diagnosis of Apert syndrome. J Ultrasound Med 2006; 25:1481-1484.
13. Miller C, Losken HW, Towbin R, et al: Ultrasound diagnosis of craniosynostosis. Cleft Palate Craniofac J 2002; 39:73-80.
14. Starr JR, Collett BR, Gaither R, et al. Multicenter study of neurodevelopment in 3-year-old children with and without single-suture craniosynostosis. Arch Pediatr Adolesc Med 2012; 166:536-542.
15. Tonni G, Panteghini M, Rossi A, et al: Cranosynostosis: prenatal diagnosis by means of ultrasound and SSSE-MRI. Family series with report of neurodevelopmental outcome and review of the literature. Arch Gynecol Obstet 2011; 283:909-916.

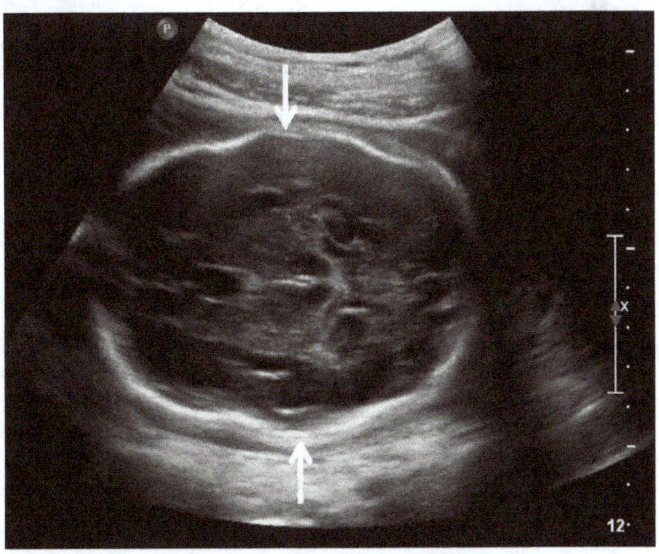

**FIGURE 2.7A** Scaphocephaly: fused sagittal suture; circumscribed calverial bulging on both sides of cranium (arrows).

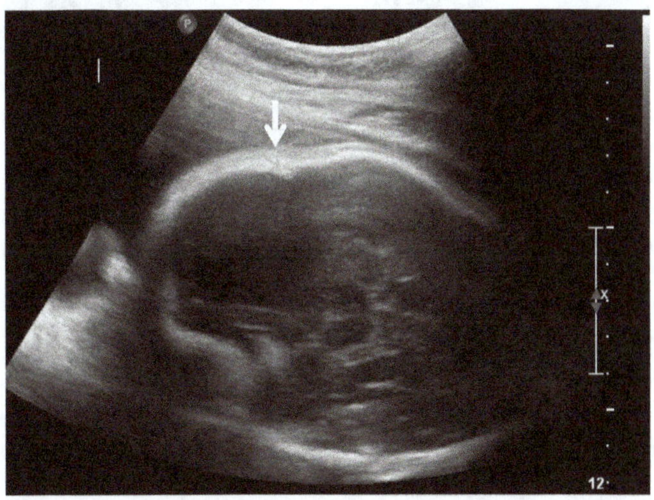

**FIGURE 2.7B** Fused coronal suture (arrow).

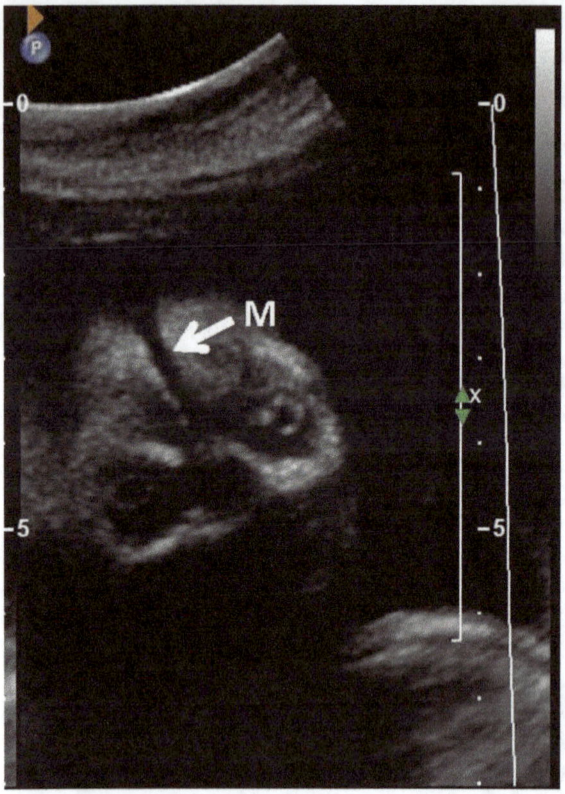


FIGURE 2.7C Normal metopic suture (M); normally spaced orbits.

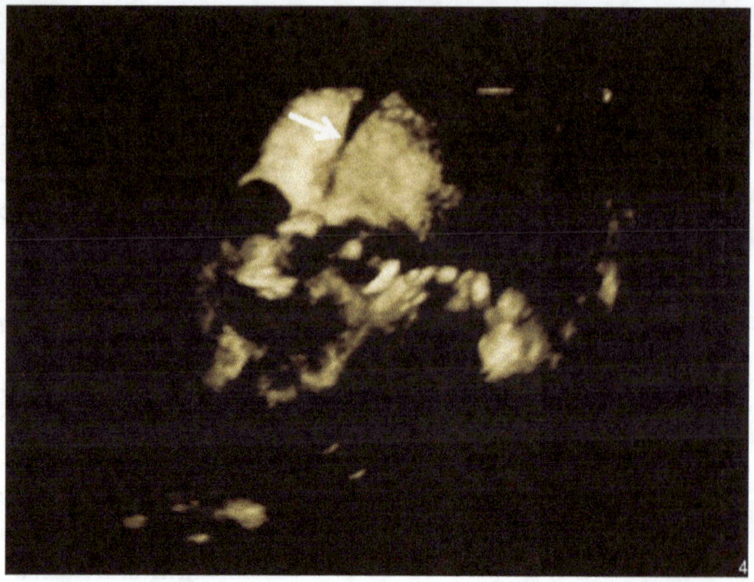

FIGURE 2.7D Three-dimensional image of a normal metopic suture (arrow).

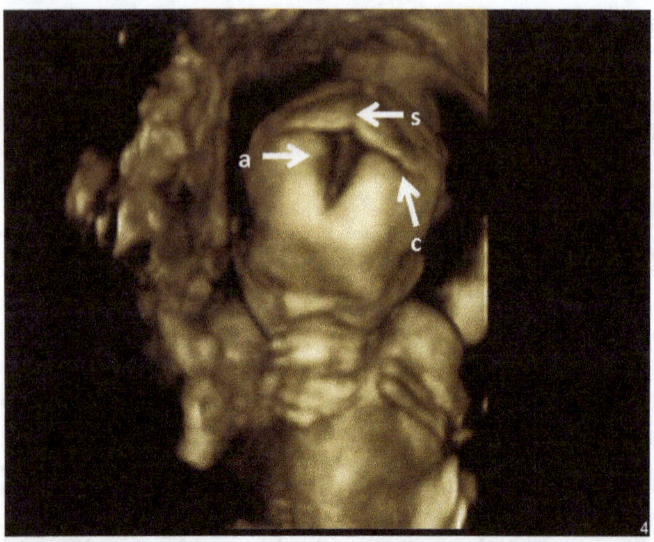


FIGURE 2.7E Three-dimensional image illustrating the normal anterior fontanelle (a) and sagittal (s) and coronal (c) sutures.

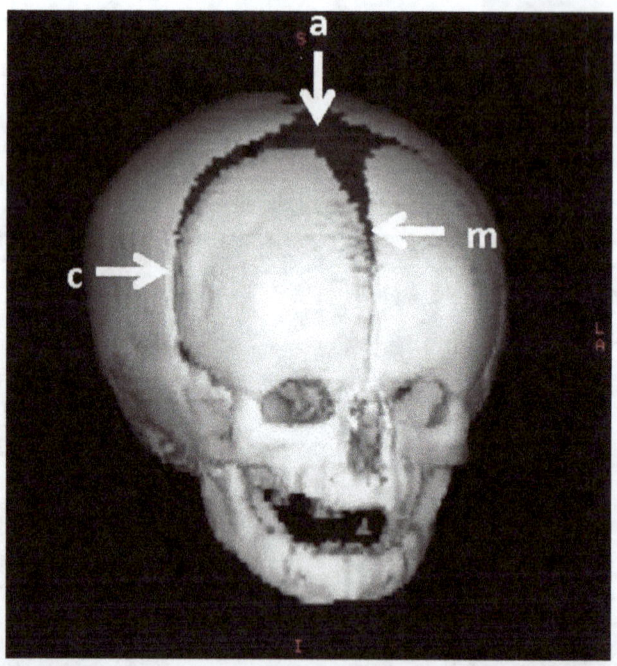


FIGURE 2.7F Skeletal cranial sutures on CT: coronal (c) and metopic (m) sutures; anterior fontanel (a).

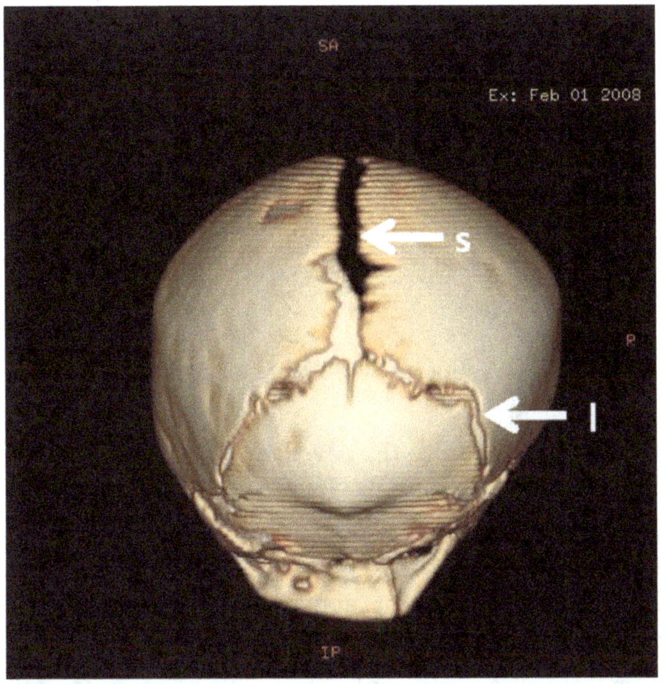


FIGURE 2.7G Sagittal (s) and lambdoid (l) sutures.

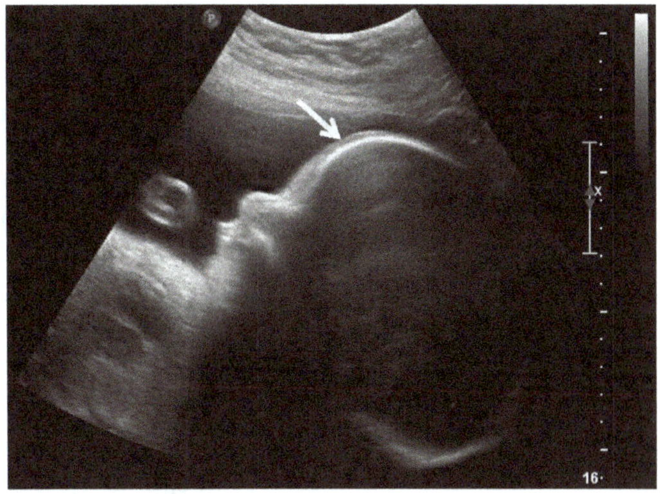


FIGURE 2.7H Image illustrating frontal bossing (arrow).

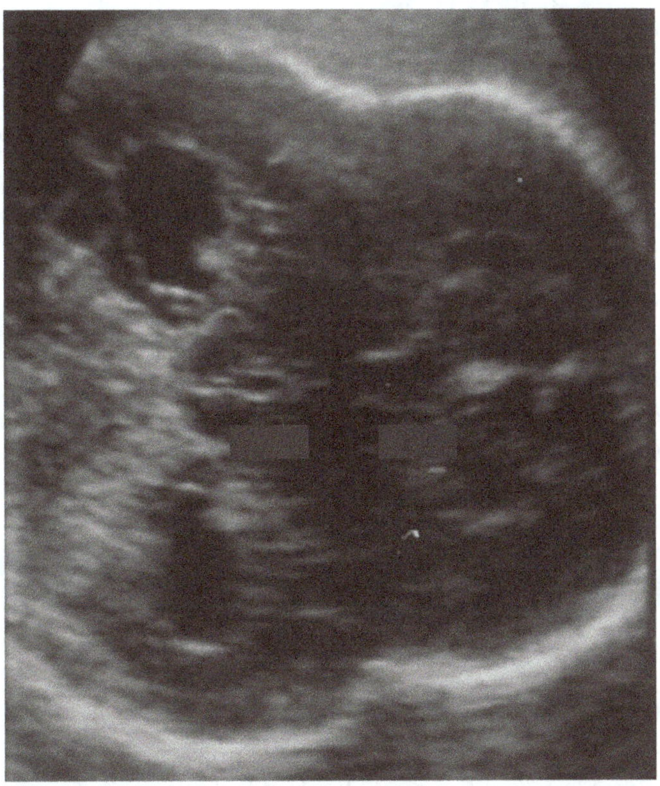

FIGURE 2.7I Cloverleaf skull.

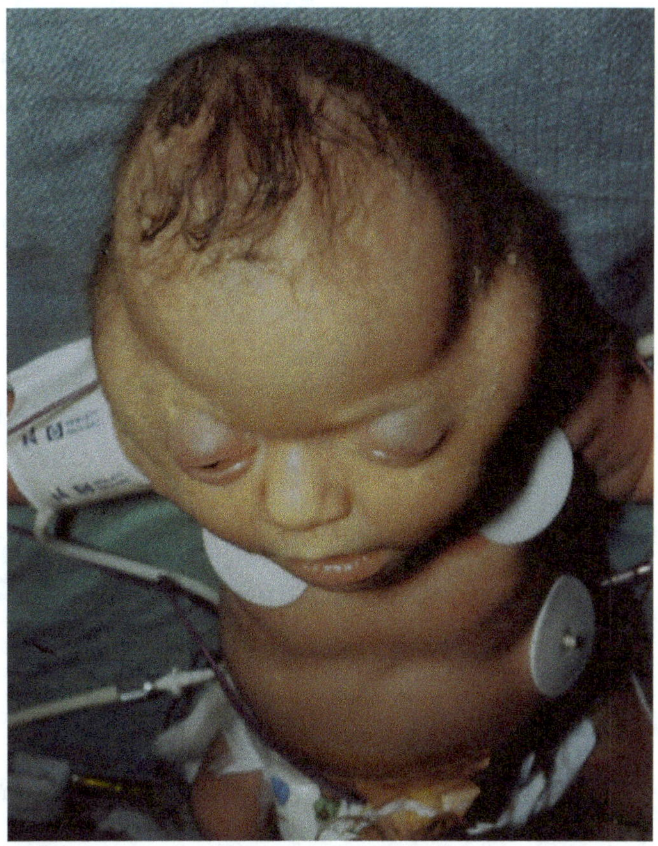

FIGURE 2.7J Infant with a cloverleaf skull.

# 2.8 DANDY-WALKER MALFORMATION

## EPIDEMIOLOGY/GENETICS

**Definition** Dandy-Walker malformations (DWMs) are characterized by (1) a posterior fossa cyst, (2) a defect in the cerebellar vermis that provides a communication between the cyst and the fourth ventricle, and (3) variable hydrocephalus.

**Epidemiology** DWMs occur in 1 in 25,000 to 30,000 live births and in approximately 4% of cases of hydrocephalus.

**Embryology** The DWM is an abnormality in the development of the CNS that probably occurs before the sixth to seventh week of gestation. Associated intracranial abnormalities occur in about 50% of cases and associated extracranial abnormalities in 35% of cases. Common associated defects are ACC, ventricular septal defects, and facial clefts. Chromosomal abnormalities are seen in approximately 30% of cases, including trisomies 13, 18, and 21.

**Inheritance Patterns** Rare familial recurrence of isolated DWM has been seen with possible autosomal or X-linked recessive inheritance. The DWM can be a feature of Mendelian genetic syndromes, including the Meckel-Gruber syndrome (autosomal recessive), Walker-Warburg syndrome (autosomal recessive), and the Aicardi syndrome (X-linked dominant with male lethality). Because of the rapid progress in mapping of genes and the subsequent development of genetic testing, consultation with a medical geneticist or genetic counselor to determine the availability of clinical genetic testing for this disorder or disorders is advised.

**Teratogens** Congenital infections are teratogenic.

**Prognosis** Postnatal mortality is approximately 35% and is dependent on the associated abnormalities. Of survivors with isolated abnormalities, 20% to 30% have IQs above 80. Shunting is usually required for associated hydrocephalus. However, outcome data may be biased, as only fetuses with the most favorable prognosis survive. The degree of vermian hypoplasia has been correlated with the severity of developmental delay.

## SONOGRAPHY

### FREQUENT FINDINGS

- Triad of CNS abnormalities:
  - There is complete or partial agenesis of the cerebellar vermis.
    - A trapezoid-shaped gap between the cerebellar hemispheres is diagnostic.
    - When present, the vermis is rotated counterclockwise.
  - Enlarged posterior fossa with elevated tentorium
  - Cystic dilatation of the fourth ventricle
- Cerebellar hemispheres may be hypoplastic with a "bat-wing" appearance.

- Ventriculomegaly (80%)
  - A complication of, rather than a part of, DWM
- Associated anomalies (85%)

### LESS FREQUENT

- Holoprosencephaly (25%)
- Occipital encephalocele (7%)
- Pontine hypoplasia associated with severity of cerebellar hypoplasia
- Spina bifida

### KEY FINDINGS/PITFALLS

- On the axial plane, a normal posterior fossa is 10 mm or less.
  - An increased fluid space in the posterior fossa may be due to the upward rotation of a normal cerebellar vermis.
- Abnormalities of the vermis include
  - Agenesis
    - Complete
    - Partial
      - The remaining vermis has a normal volume.
  - Hypoplasia
    - Small, but intact, vermis
    - Based on a reduced transverse cerebellar diameter
  - Atrophy
    - Secondary reduction in cerebellar volume
    - Distinct from hypoplasia (i.e., congenital reduction in cerebellar size)
- When an axial view of the CNS indicates a potential posterior fossa abnormality, a 3-D ultrasound examination, using multiplanar imaging, is required to more accurately evaluate anatomic relationships and narrow the differential diagnosis. Vermian size can be assessed and compared to established normal ranges.
  - The position of the tentorium can be evaluated to help in the differential diagnosis.
- A "keyhole" in contrast to a trapezoid gap between the cerebellar hemispheres is not diagnostic of DWM and is likely a false positive.
  - The poor correlation between prenatal sonographic diagnosis of DWM and autopsy findings is, in part, due to the utilization of the keyhole sign as a marker of DWM.
- MRI can be added to the diagnostic armamentarium in specific, difficult cases.

### DIFFERENTIAL DIAGNOSIS

Dandy-Walker variant (DWV)

- Partial vermis hypoplasia
- Fourth ventricle not enlarged

- Connection between fourth ventricle and cisterna magna has appearance of a cleft
  - The space between cerebellar hemispheres may not close until 18 weeks' gestation.
    - Occasionally, fetuses may have further delay in normal vermian development.
      - Vermian hypoplasia may not be diagnosed until 24 weeks' gestation.
    - The diagnosis of a DWV (i.e., agenesis of the inferior cerebellar vermis) is especially difficult prenatally.
      - Scanning in an exaggerated semicoronal plane may result in an incorrect diagnosis of DWV.
    - There is a similar constellation of congenital anomalies and chromosomal abnormalities as with DWM.
    - DWV may represent cerebellar hypoplasia rather than a mild form of DWM.
      - Some authors therefore recommend abandoning DWV in favor of vermian agenesis and vermian hypoplasia.

Megacisterna magna

- Enlarged posterior fossa
- Normal cerebellar vermis
- Normal fourth ventricle
- Absence of ventriculomegaly
- Associated with trisomy 18

Arachnoid cyst

- Developmental in origin
- Displaces cerebellum with fourth ventricle anteriorly
- Demonstrates a mass effect
  - Compression of the cerebellum results in a false impression of DWM.

Blake's pouch cyst

- A transient posterior fossa structure normally perforates, forming the foramen of Magendie.
- Failure of perforation results in a caudal protrusion of the fourth ventricle and displacement of a normal cerebellar vermis.

## PREGNANCY MANAGEMENT

**Investigations and Consultations Required** Many of these malformations are part of a syndrome or have associated anomalies. Therefore, chromosome studies with microarray analysis should be performed and a fetal echocardiogram obtained to detect any associated cardiac lesions. Specific molecular testing may be indicated if ultrasound features or family history suggest a specific genetic syndrome. A pediatric neurosurgeon should be consulted to discuss prenatal and neonatal management.

**Monitoring** Serial ultrasonographic examinations should be performed every 3 to 4 weeks to assess for the presence and degree of ventriculomegaly and for the development of macrocephaly, particularly near to term.

**Pregnancy Course** Many of the syndromes of which the DWM is a component may be associated with intrauterine growth restriction, and decisions regarding management of this complication will be highly dependent on the prognosis of the underlying condition.

**Pregnancy Termination Issues** As with other CNS malformations, special expertise in neuropathology is essential for a precise diagnosis and the resultant counseling that will be necessary following this diagnosis.

**Delivery** Because of the high association with other non-CNS abnormalities, delivery should occur in a tertiary center with full capabilities for diagnosis and management of infants with multiple malformations.

## NEONATOLOGY

**Resuscitation** The major issues relate to fetal distress secondary to dystocia from macrocephaly, or prematurity, if early delivery is chosen because of rapidly advancing hydrocephalus. Given the guarded neurodevelopmental prognosis, if there are associated CNS or other organ system anomalies, a prenatal discussion with the family regarding intervention to initiate respiration is appropriate.

**Transport** Referral to a tertiary center with pediatric neurology, neurosurgery, and neonatology capabilities is indicated.

**Testing and Confirmation** The priority issue is the identification of associated CNS abnormalities by cranial MRI or CT scan. In the majority of infants, hydrocephalus develops by 2 months of age, if not present prenatally. If karyotyping was not performed on the fetus, it should be obtained after birth before invasive interventions are undertaken, especially if there are other dysmorphic features.

**Nursery Management** Hemorrhage into the cyst can occur at any point and should be suspected with an abrupt clinical deterioration.

### SUGGESTED READINGS

1. Ecker JC, Shipp TD, Bromley B, Benacerraf B: The sonographic diagnosis of Dandy-Walker and Dandy-Walker variant: associated findings and outcomes. Prenat Diagn 2000; 20:328-332.
2. Guibaud L, des Portres V: Plea for an anatomical approach to abnormalities of the posterior fossa in prenatal diagnosis (opinion). Ultrasound Obstet Gynecol 2006; 27:477-481.
3. Has R, Ermis H, Yüksel A, et al: Dandy-Walker malformation: a review of 78 cases diagnosed by prenatal sonography. Fetal Diagn Ther 2004; 19:342-347.
4. Kalidasan V, Carroll T, Allcutt D, Fitzgerald RJ: The Dandy-Walker syndrome—a 10-year experience of its management and outcome. Eur J Pediatr Surg 1995; 5:Suppl 1:16-18.

5. Kölbe N, Wisser J, Kuranavicius J, et al: Dandy-Walker malformation: prenatal diagnosis and outcome. Prenat Diagn 2000; 20:318-327.
6. Leibovitz Z, Haratz KK, Malinger G, et al: Fetal posterior fossa dimensions: normal and anomalous development assessed in mid-sagittal cranial plane by three-dimensional midplanar sonography. Ultrasound Obstet Gynecol 2014:43:147-153.
7. Malinger G, Lev D, Lerman-Sagie T: The fetal cerebellum. Pitfalls in diagnosis and management. Prenat Diagn 2009; 29:372-380.
8. Paladina D, Volpe P: Posterior fossa and vermian morphometry in the characterization of fetal cerebellar abnormalities: a prospective three-dimensional ultrasound study. Ultrasound Obstet Gynecol 2006; 27:482-489.
9. Phillips J, Mahony BS, Siebert JR, et al: Dandy-Walker malformation complex. Correlation between ultrasonographic diagnosis and postmortem neuropathology. Obstet Gynecol 2006; 107:685-693.
10. Salihu H, Kornosky JL, Druschel CM: Dandy-Walker syndrome, associated anomalies and survival through infancy: a population-based study. Fetal Diagn Ther 2008; 24:155-160.
11. Sasaki-Adams D, Elbabaa SK, Jewells V, et al: The Dandy-Walker variant: a case series of 24 pediatric patients and evaluation of associated anomalies, incidence of hydrocephalus, and developmental outcomes. J Neurosurg Pediatrics 2008; 2:194-199.
12. Zalel Y, Gilboa Y, Gabis L, et al: Rotation of the vermis as a cause of enlarged cisterna magna on prenatal imaging. Ultrasound Obstet Gynecol 2006; 27:490-493.

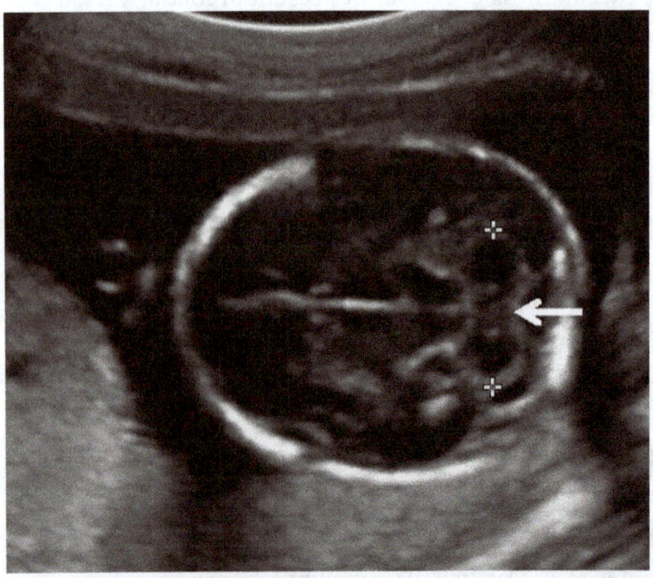

FIGURE 2.8A Normal transverse cerebellar diameter (+ … +); intact vermis (arrow).

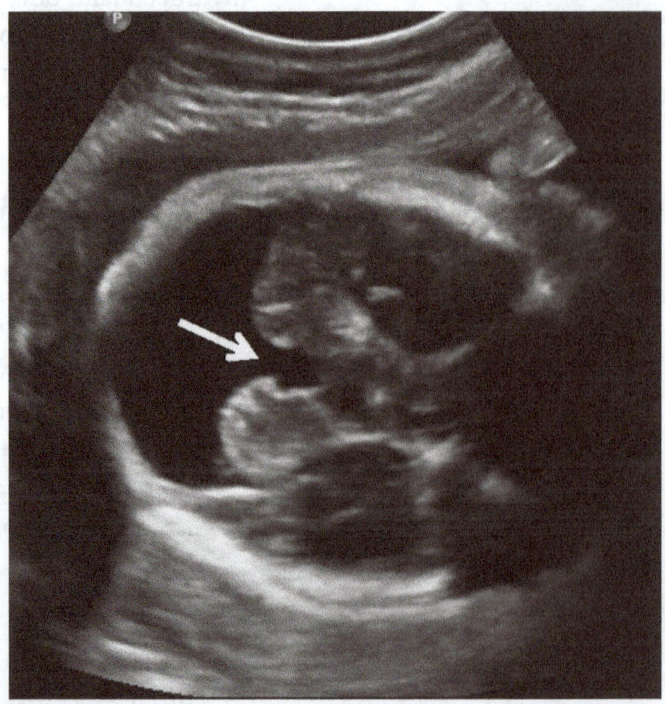

FIGURE 2.8B Dandy-Walker malformation (arrow).

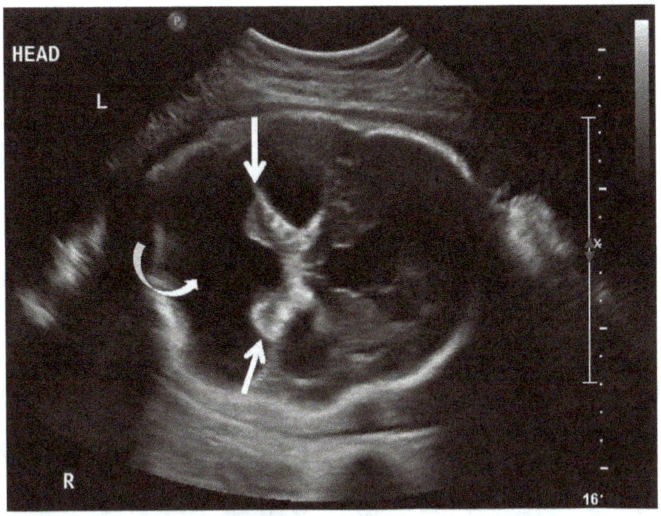


**FIGURE 2.8C** Dandy-Walker malformation (curved arrow). Hypoplastic cerebellar hemispheres with "bat-wing" appearance (straight arrows).

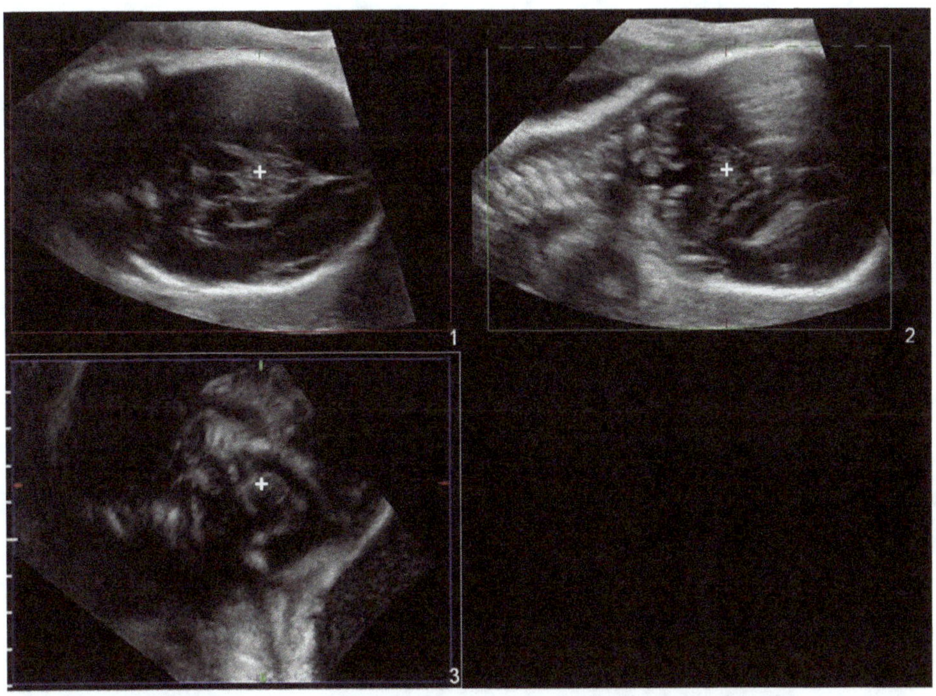

**FIGURE 2.8D** Multiplanar image of a normal vermis (+).

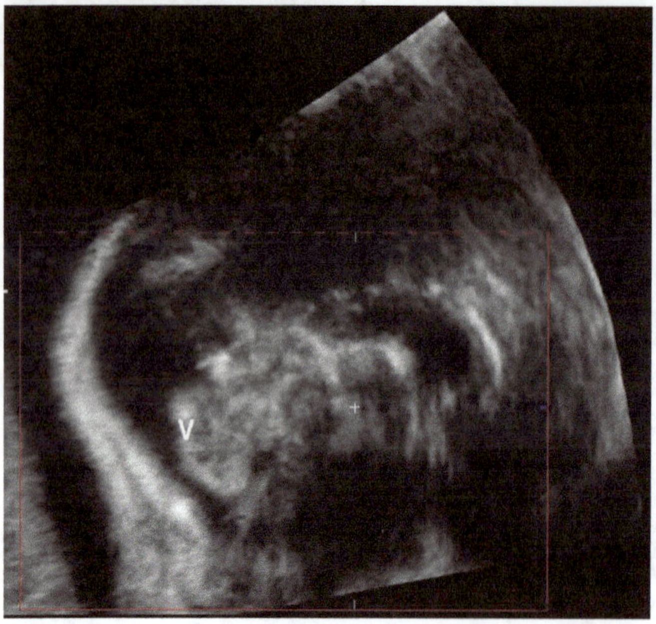


**FIGURE 2.8E** Three-dimensional multiplanar midsagittal image of a normal vermis (V).

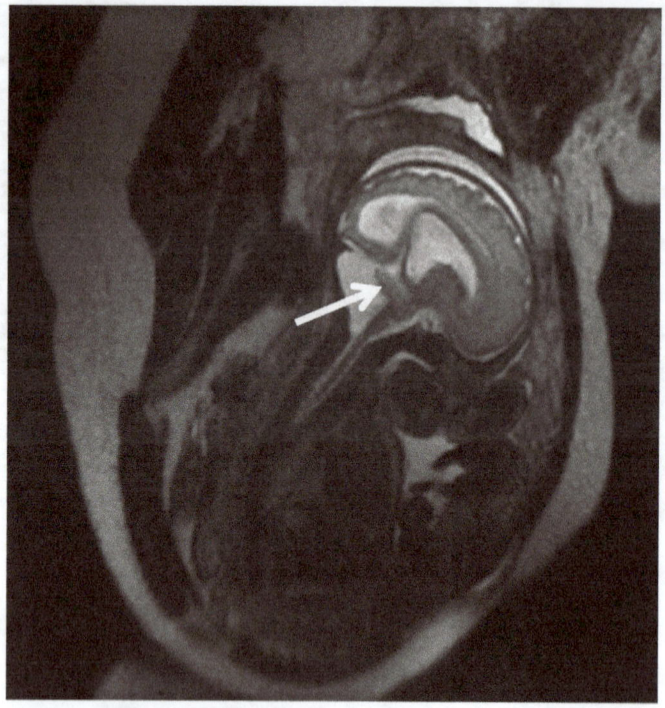

**FIGURE 2.8F** Dandy-Walker variant with agenesis of the inferior portion of the vermis at 31 weeks (arrow).

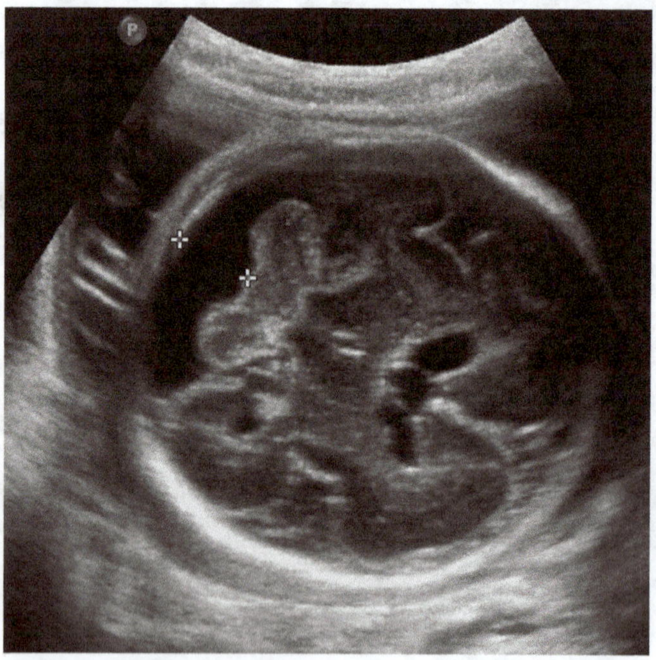

**FIGURE 2.8G** Megacisterna magna: 12 mm (+ … +).

# 2.9 ENCEPHALOCELE

## EPIDEMIOLOGY/GENETICS

**Definition** Encephaloceles are skin-covered neural tube defects affecting the cranium that result in a midline mass overlying a skull defect.

**Epidemiology** Occurrence is 1 in 2000 live births (M1:F1), varying with ethnic group and geographic region.

**Embryology** Encephaloceles are the result of failure of neural tube closure in the cranial region during the first month of fetal development. They are frequently associated with other brain malformations, such as hydrocephalus, iniencephaly; facial clefts; cardiac abnormalities; and genital malformations. More than 30 genetic, sporadic, and chromosomal syndromes have been described with encephaloceles, including trisomy 13; amniotic band disruption syndrome; Meckel-Gruber syndrome (autosomal recessive disorder with encephalocele, polycystic kidneys, and polydactyly); and Walker-Warburg syndrome (autosomal recessive). Because of the rapid progress in mapping of genes and subsequent development of genetic testing, consultation with a medical geneticist or genetic counselor to determine the availability of clinical genetic testing for this disorder or disorders is advised.

**Inheritance Patterns** Most commonly, inheritance is multifactorial with recurrence risk of 2%–3%. In cases of known syndromes, the recurrence risk is that of the specific syndrome diagnosis.

**Teratogens** Maternal diabetes and maternal hyperthermia are teratogenic.

**Prognosis** Prognosis depends on the associated brain malformations and syndrome diagnosis, as well as the anatomic site, volume of brain content within the herniated sac, and coexisting congenital anomalies. Microcephaly with the presence of neural elements in the encephalocele is associated with a poor prognosis.

## SONOGRAPHY

### FREQUENT FINDINGS

- Cranial defect
- Herniation of meninges or meninges with a variable amount of brain tissue

### LESS FREQUENT

- Ventriculomegaly
- Microcephaly
- Open neural tube defect
- Agenesis of the corpus callosum
- Dandy-Walker malformation

### KEY FINDINGS/PITFALLS/ DIFFERENTIAL DIAGNOSIS

- Encephalocele locations: frontal, parietal, and occipital.
- In Asia, frontal encephaloceles predominate. In the Western Hemisphere, occipital encephaloceles are more common.
- An encephalocele in an atypical location may be due to an amniotic band.
- With meningoceles, the underlying brain is usually normal. Hence, the prognosis is generally better than with encephaloceles.
- Approximately 60% of fetuses with an encephalocele have other malformations.
- A 3-D ultrasound improves visualization of encephaloceles and assists in the evaluation of the fetus for other anomalies that may improve the diagnostic accuracy of specific syndromes.
- A 3-D ultrasound can be used to distinguish an occipital meningocele from a fetal scalp cyst.

## PREGNANCY MANAGEMENT

**Investigations and Consultations Required** Many cases of encephalocele are part of a syndrome, and steps to determine whether it is isolated, or not, are warranted. In addition to the sonographic search for associated abnormalities, chromosome studies, including microarrays, should be performed. Specific gene mutation testing should be considered if features are suggestive of a specific syndrome. Fetal echocardiography should be done to exclude cardiac malformations, which are a common feature of many of the syndromes with an encephalocele. The family should also be referred to a pediatric neurosurgeon for discussion regarding prognosis and neonatal management.

**Fetal Intervention** No in utero therapy is indicated. Decompression of the encephalocele under ultrasonographic control prior to delivery may be required, although this is unusual.

**Monitoring** The prognosis depends on the size of the encephalocele, its content, and the degree of disruption of the remaining CNS, as well as the presence of any associated anomalies. As the CNS features (e.g., microcephaly) may change over time, serial ultrasonographic examinations should be done monthly.

**Pregnancy Course** Many of the syndromes of which encephalocele is a feature may also have prenatal growth deficiency as a component. Management should be based on the prognosis for the underlying condition, not the presence of intrauterine growth restriction.

**Pregnancy Termination Issues** Because of the large number of syndromes that may have encephalocele as a component, and the wide range of inheritance patterns seen in these conditions, termination should be done in an institution with special expertise in fetal pathology.

**Delivery** Nonaggressive management is recommended when severe microcephaly is present, the CNS is severely disrupted, or in cases in which the encephalocele is part of a syndrome known to be lethal.

## NEONATOLOGY

**Resuscitation** Most cases do not require assistance with the onset of respiration unless the mass is very large and contains mostly brain tissue. Intubation may be difficult, with large posterior masses impeding proper positioning for visualization of the cords. Bag and mask–assisted ventilation with the infant in a side-lying position is often sufficient.

When prenatal diagnostic evaluations confirm associated intracranial malformations, microcephaly with the bulk of the brain tissue in the mass, or other severe organ abnormalities, a predelivery discussion should be undertaken with the family about nonintervention in the event that spontaneous onset of respiration does not occur.

Special care to avoid trauma to the mass is important when the attachment is pedunculated or there is only a membranous tissue covering the surface.

**Transport** Referral to a tertiary center with pediatric neurology and neurosurgery capabilities is always indicated.

**Testing and Confirmation** Diagnostic imaging, CT scan and MRI, to define the defect and to delineate any associated CNS abnormalities is important. Chromosomal analysis, echocardiography, and abdominal sonography are indicated, contingent on physical findings and clinical course, if not obtained prenatally.

**Nursery Management** Postoperatively, seizures and hydrocephalus are the most common neurologic complications requiring intervention.

## SURGERY

**Preoperative Assessment** The size and location of the encephalocele, its contents, and its relationship to major vascular structures are important for surgical planning. The volume of the remaining intracranial contents, hydrocephalus, and the head circumference are also important information for surgical planning.

Magnetic resonance imaging is useful to define the encephalocele contents and its relationship to vital structures. The relationship of the encephalocele to the structures of the posterior fossa and venous sinuses is important from the surgical standpoint and can be determined by MRI and magnetic resonance angiography.

**Operative Indications** Surgical treatment is appropriate in most cases unless the encephalocele is massive. Small, entirely skin-covered lesions can be repaired electively. Large lesions or those that are leaking CSF need to be repaired urgently to reduce the risk of infection.

**Types of Procedures** Surgical treatment involves resection of the encephalocele contents and closure of the dura, scalp, and skull. Large encephaloceles such as those in which the majority of the brain is in the encephalocele sac, or in which vital structures such as the brain stem are extracranial, cannot be treated surgically and are associated with a very poor outcome.

If hydrocephalus is present, then a ventricular shunt is placed at the time of the initial procedure.

**Surgical Results/Prognosis** Outcome is dependent on the size, location, and contents of the encephalocele, as well as the presence of other brain anomalies. Infants with occipital encephaloceles are at risk for developmental and physical impairment. Large lesions in which the majority of the brain is extracranial or in which essential structures are included in the encephalocele sac have a poor functional outcome and are treated expectantly. Despite this, a good overall prognosis is possible, regardless of the size of the encephalocele, when the encephalocele sac is devoid of vital neural or vascular structures. Seizure disorders are noted in approximately 20% of infants with congenital encephalocele.

## SUGGESTED READINGS


1. Borowski D, Wegrzyn P, Bartkowiak R, et al: First trimester diagnosis of encephaloceles—report of two cases and review of the literature. Ginekol Pol 2011; 82:700-704.
2. Cohen MM, Lemire RJ: Syndromes with cephaloceles. Teratology 1982; 25:161-172.
3. Copp AJ, Stanier P, Greene NDE: Neural tube defects—recent advances, unsolved questions and controversies. Lancet Neurol 2013 A; 12: 799–810.
4. Ickowicz V, Eurin D, Meugay-Laulom B, et al: Meckel-Grüber syndrome: sonography and pathology. Ultrasound Obstet Gynecol 2006; 27:296-300.
5. Kiymaz N, Yilmaz N, Demir I, Keskin S: Prognostic factors in patients with occipital encephalocele. Pediatr Neurosurg 2010; 46:6-11.
6. Liao S-L, Tsai P-Y, Cheng Y-C, et al: Prenatal diagnosis of fetal encephaloceles using three-dimensional ultrasound. J Med Ultrasound 2012; 20:150-154.
7. Lo BW, Kulkarini AV, Rutka JT, et al: Clinical predictors of developmental outcome in patients with encephaloceles. J Neurosurg Pediatr 2008; 2:254-257.
8. Parelkar SV, Kapadnis SP, Sanghvi BV, et al: Meckel-Gruber syndrome: a rare and lethal anomaly with review of literature. J Pediatr Neurosci 2013; 8:154-157.
9. Thompson DNP: Postnatal management and outcome for neural tube defects including spina bifida and encephaloceles. Prenatal Diagn 2009; 29:412-419.
10. Timor-Tritsch IE, Monteagudo A, Santos R: Fine-tuning the diagnosis of fetal scalp cysts. The value of high-frequency sonography. J Ultrasound Med 2008; 27:1363-1368.
11. Tsai PY, Chang CH, Chang FM: Prenatal diagnosis of the fetal frontal encephalocele by three-dimensional ultrasound. Prenat Diagn 2006; 26:378-380.

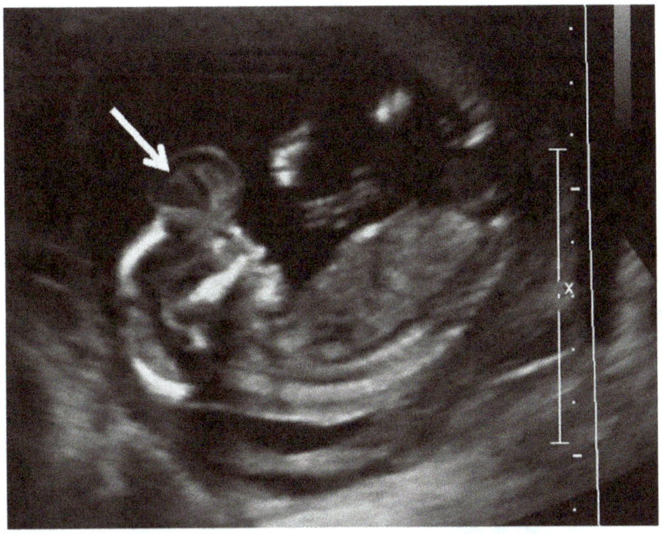

FIGURE 2.9A Anterior encephalocele (arrow).

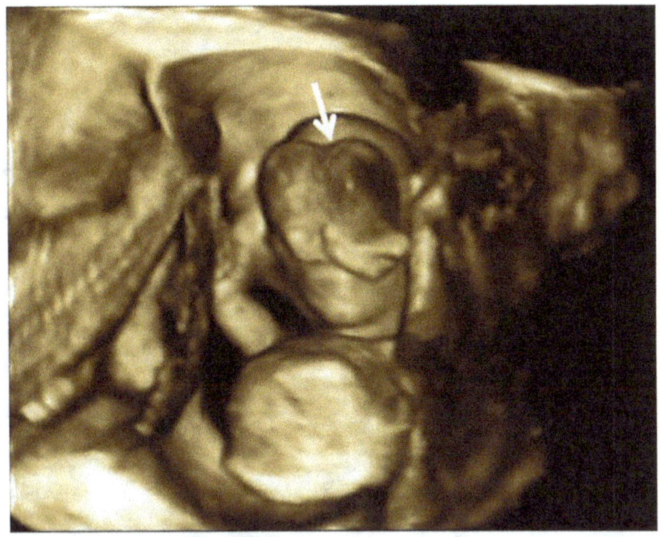

FIGURE 2.9B Three-dimensional image of an anterior encephalocele (arrow).

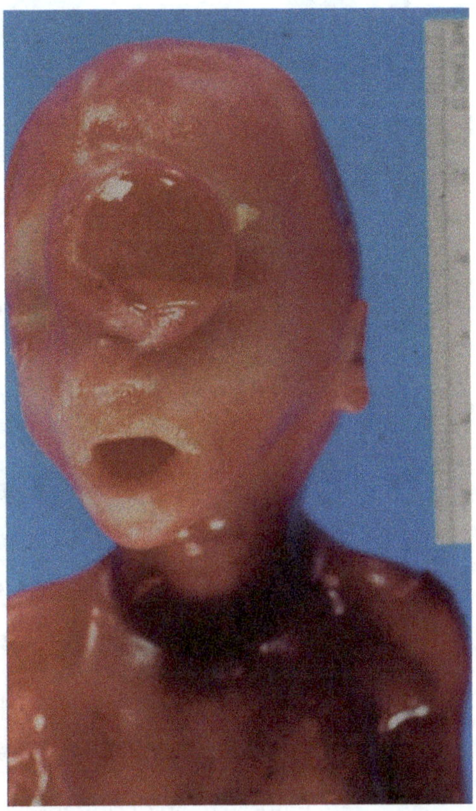

FIGURE 2.9C Fetus with an anterior encephalocele.

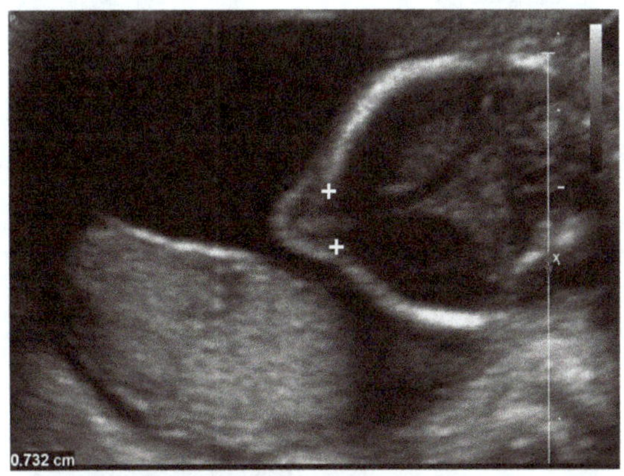


FIGURE 2.9D Occipital meningocele (+ … +).

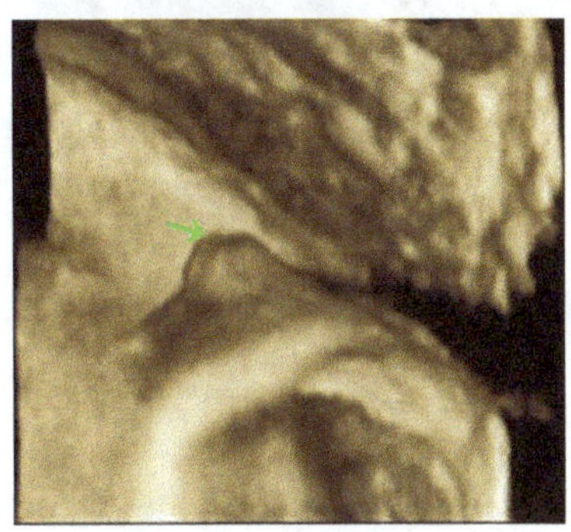

FIGURE 2.9E Occipital meningocele 3-D image (arrow).

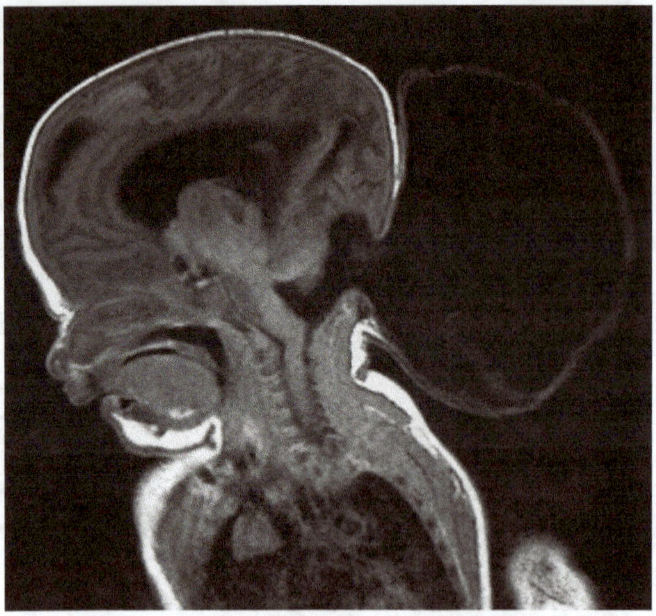

FIGURE 2.9F Large occipital meningocele.

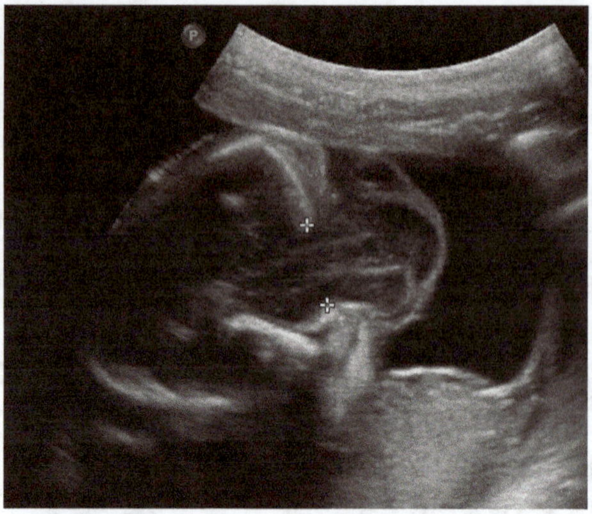

FIGURE 2.9G Occipital encephalocele (+ … +).

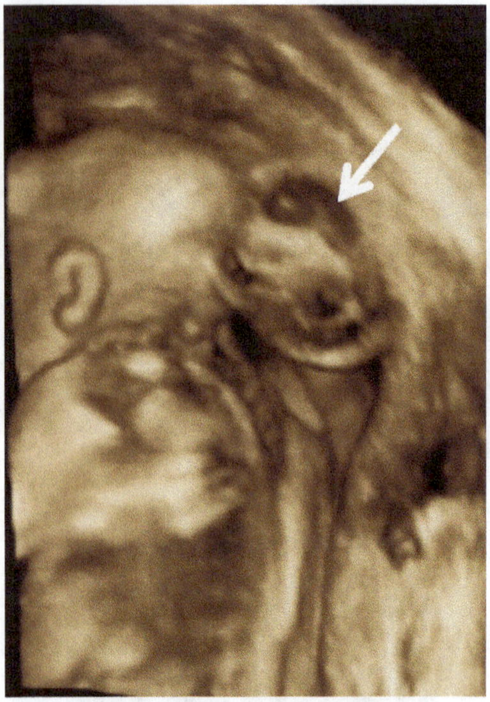

FIGURE 2.9H Three-dimensional image of an occipital encephalocele (arrow).

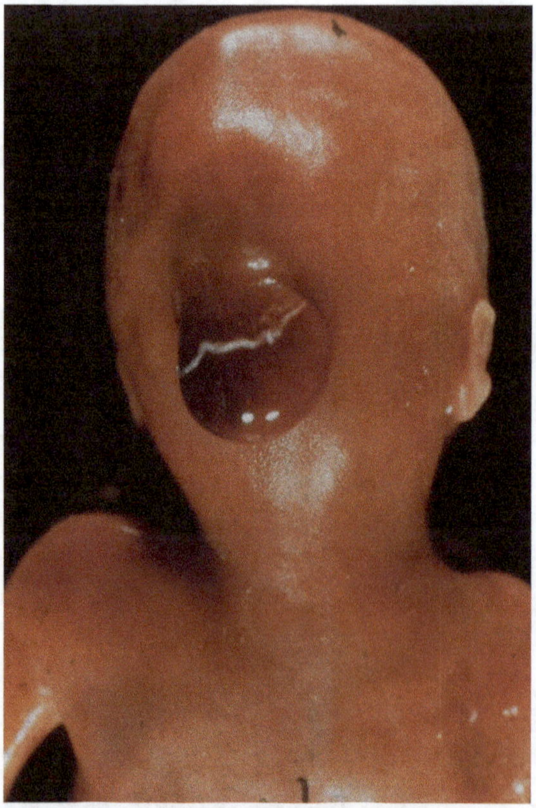

FIGURE 2.9I Fetus with an occipital encephalocele.

# 2.10 HOLOPROSENCEPHALY

## EPIDEMIOLOGY/GENETICS

**Definition** Holoprosencephaly (HPE) is the term used for the spectrum of severe, early abnormalities in forebrain cleavage. These cleavage abnormalities can occur both sagittally, resulting in fusion of the cerebral hemispheres, and horizontally, resulting in abnormalities of the optic and olfactory bulbs.

**Epidemiology** Epidemiologically, HPE affects 1 to 2 per 10,000 liveborns and 1 in 250 conceptuses (M1:F3 for alobar HPE, M1:F1 for lobar form).

**Embryology** Holoprosencephaly is an early arrest in prosencephalon cleavage. The third or fourth week of inception is the critical time for induction of HPE in humans. A defect in development of the rostral neuropore results in an incomplete separation of the cerebral hemispheres. Chromosomal, genetic, and teratogenic causes have been described, but up to 15% have no etiology determined. Chromosomal abnormalities occur in 30%-50% of cases, with trisomy 13, trisomy 18, triploidy, 13q, and 18p the most common. Mutations in at least 12 genetic loci have been mapped for HPE, but only 5%-10% of cases have detectable mutations.

**Inheritance Patterns** The empirical recurrence risk for sporadic cases is approximately 6%. Multiple malformation syndromes, including Smith-Lemli-Opitz syndrome (autosomal recessive), Meckel-Gruber syndrome (autosomal recessive), Aicardi syndrome (X-linked dominant), Fryns syndrome (autosomal recessive), and hydrolethalus syndrome (autosomal recessive), have been described with HPE. The current status of genetic testing should be discussed with a clinical geneticist to determine what gene panel is currently recommended for diagnostic evaluation.

**Teratogens** Alcohol, phenytoin, retinoic acid, statins, and maternal insulin-dependent diabetes are teratogenic.

**Prognosis** Most severely affected patients die at birth or in the first 6 months of life. Survival, with variable mental retardation, occurs in milder cases.

## SONOGRAPHY

### FREQUENT FINDINGS

- Facial anomalies: 80%
  - Midface hypoplasia
  - Hypotelorism
  - Proboscis
  - Single nostril
  - Median cleft
  - Cyclopia
  - Microcephaly

- Associated structural anomalies: 70%
  - Ventriculomegaly
  - Cardiovascular
    - Single umbilical artery
    - Ventricular septal defect
    - Atrial septal defect
    - Hypoplastic left heart
  - Hydrops
  - Omphalocele
  - Diaphragmatic hernia
- HPE is a heterogeneous disease entity.
  - Categories:
    - Alobar
      - One single ventricle
      - Fused thalami
      - Agenesis of the corpus callosum
    - Semilobar
      - Single ventricle
      - Rudimentary cerebral lobes
      - Interhemispheric fissure posteriorly
      - Agenesis of the corpus callosum
    - Lobar
      - Some midline continuity
      - Agenesis of the corpus callosum
    - Midline cleavage of the thalami is incomplete.
      - Middle interhemispheric variant
        - Incomplete separation of the thalami and caudate nucleus
        - Agenesis of the corpus callosum
- Sonographic detection of HPE is based on severity.

| Type | Earliest Gestational Age At Diagnosis (Weeks) |
|---|---|
| Alobar | 9 |
| Semilobar | 13 |
| Lobar | 21 |

- Better visualization of the facial features associated with HPE is achieved with 3-D multiplanar and volumetric scanning.
- Color Doppler in a parasagittal image can view the abnormally positioned anterior cerebral artery that courses under frontal bone.

## PREGNANCY MANAGEMENT

**Investigations and Consultations Required** The high incidence of cytogenetic abnormalities makes chromosome evaluation of the fetus mandatory, even late in pregnancy. Maternal evaluation for diabetes should be done.

Fetal echocardiography is useful only to document additional malformations but is not essential. Consultations with the neonatology staff should be arranged to discuss nonaggressive management at birth.

**Fetal Intervention** In utero therapeutic procedures are contraindicated.

**Monitoring** No pregnancy interventions such as early delivery or cesarean section are appropriate. All forms of HPE have a poor prognosis, so monitoring, except at the parents' request, is unwarranted. The head size needs to be assessed before delivery to make sure vaginal delivery is possible.

**Pregnancy Course** Polyhydramnios may be associated with HPE, resulting in preterm labor.

**Pregnancy Termination Issues** The heterogeneous causes for HPE require that a complete external and internal examination of the fetus be performed by individuals with training in fetal pathology and dysmorphology.

**Delivery** Vaginal delivery should be accomplished in all cases.

## NEONATOLOGY

**Resuscitation** With an established diagnosis of HPE, the decision to initiate resuscitative measures should be discussed with the family prior to delivery. If the diagnosis is uncertain or associated anomalies are not delineated, it is appropriate to support respiration to allow time for the diagnostic evaluation and parental adaptation to occur.

**Transport** If the diagnostic evaluation has not been completed prior to delivery, transfer to a tertiary center with neonatology and pediatric neurology capabilities is appropriate to confirm the diagnosis and provide counseling and support to the family.

**Testing and Confirmation** The clinical presentation of HPE includes a spectrum of facial abnormalities, including cyclopia, hypotelorism, and facial clefts. Newborns may have hydrocephalus and signs of neurologic dysfunction. Postnatal CT or MRI clearly defines these abnormalities.

**Nursery Management** The priority is to obtain a definitive diagnosis as promptly as possible. If chromosomal analysis was not performed prenatally, blood should be collected prior to any major invasive procedure or blood transfusion. Respiratory support is indicated pending confirmation of diagnosis. Consultation with pediatric neurology and palliative care should be obtained once the diagnosis is confirmed to give the family time to make a decision about life support and long-term care.

### SUGGESTED READINGS

1. Barchovich AJ, Quint DJ: Middle interhemispheric fusion: an unusual variant of holoprosencephaly. Am J Neuroradiol 1993; 14:431-447.
2. Bernard JP, Drummon CL, Zaarour P, et al: A new clue to the prenatal diagnosis of lobar holoprosencephaly: the abnormal pathway of the anterior cerebral artery crawling under the skull. Ultrasound Obstet Gynecol 2002; 19:605-607.

3. Blaas H-GK, Eik-Nes SH, Vainio T, Isaksen CV: Alobar holoprosencephaly at 9 weeks gestational age visualized by two- and three-dimensional ultrasound. Ultrasound Obstet Gynecol 2000; 15:62-65.

4. Blaas H-GK, Eriksson AG, Salvesen KÅ, et al: Brains and faces in holoprosencephaly: pre- and postnatal description of 30 cases. Ultrasound Obstet Gynecol 2002; 19:24-38.

5. Cohen M Jr, Shiota K: Teratogenesis of holoprosencephaly. Am J Med Genet 2002;109:1-15.

6. Kauvar EF, Muenke M: Holoprosencephaly: recommendations for diagnosis and management. Curr Opin Pediatr 2010; 22:687-695.

7. Ming JF, Muenke M: Multiple hits during early embryonic development: digenic disease and holoprosencephaly. Am J Hum Genet 2002; 71:1017-1032.

8. Pilu G, Sandra F, Perolo A, et al: Prenatal diagnosis of lobar holoprosencephaly. Ultrasound Obstet Gynecol 1992; 2:88-94.

9. Pineda-Alvarez DE, Dubourg C, David V, et al: Current recommendations for the molecular evaluation of newly diagnosed holoprosencephaly patients. Am J Med Genet C Semin Med Genet 2010; 154C:93-101.

10. Solomon BD, Pineda-Alvarez DE, Mercier S, et al: Holoprosencephaly flashcards: a summary for the clinician. Am J Med Genet C Semin Med Genet 2010; 154C:3-7.

11. Wong HS, Lam YH, Tang MHY, et al: First-trimester ultrasound diagnosis of holoprosencephaly: three case reports. Ultrasound Obstet Gynecol 1999; 13:356-359.

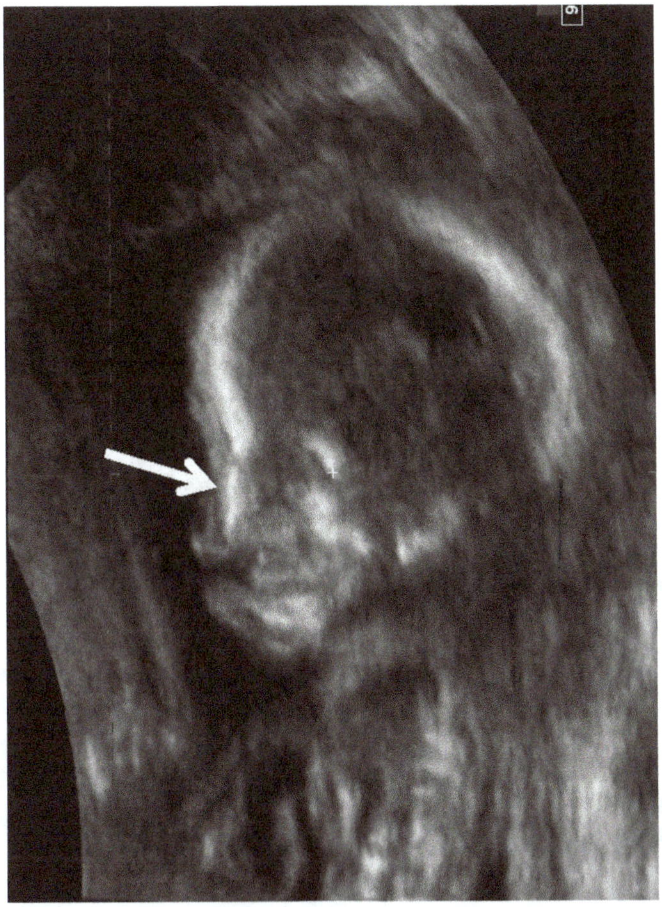

FIGURE 2.10A Midface hypoplasia (arrow).

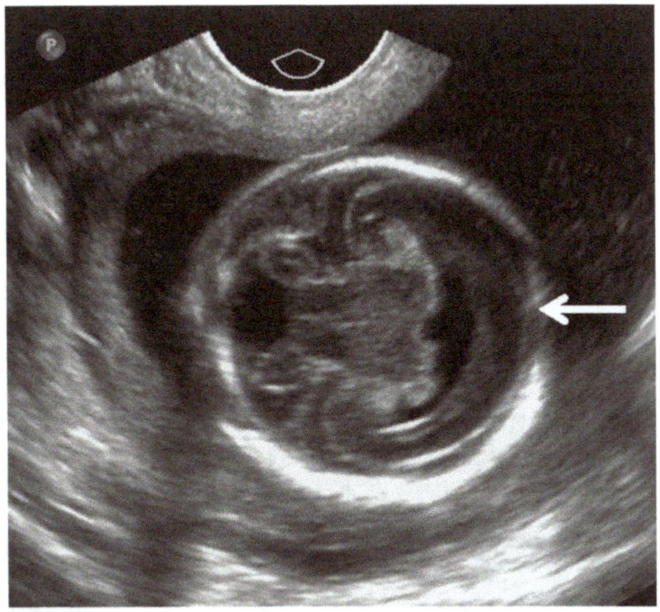

FIGURE 2.10B Alobar holoprosencephaly showing a single ventricle (arrow).

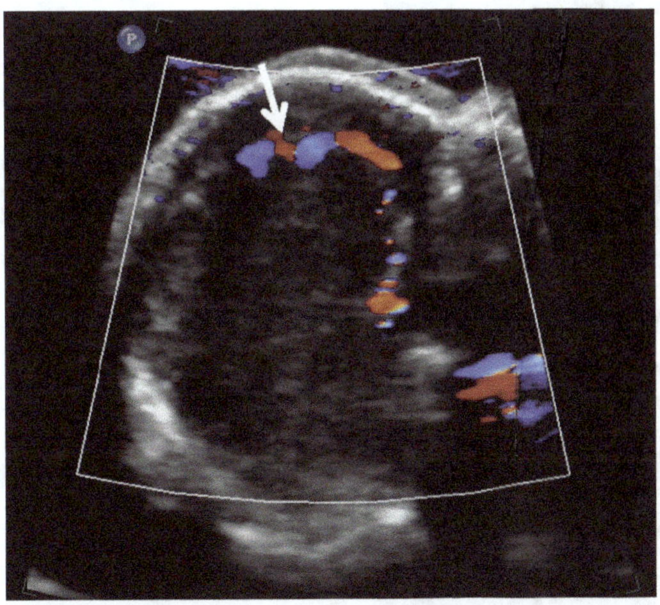

FIGURE 2.10C Holoprosencephaly illustrating the abnormal course along the frontal bone of the anterior cerebral artery (arrow).

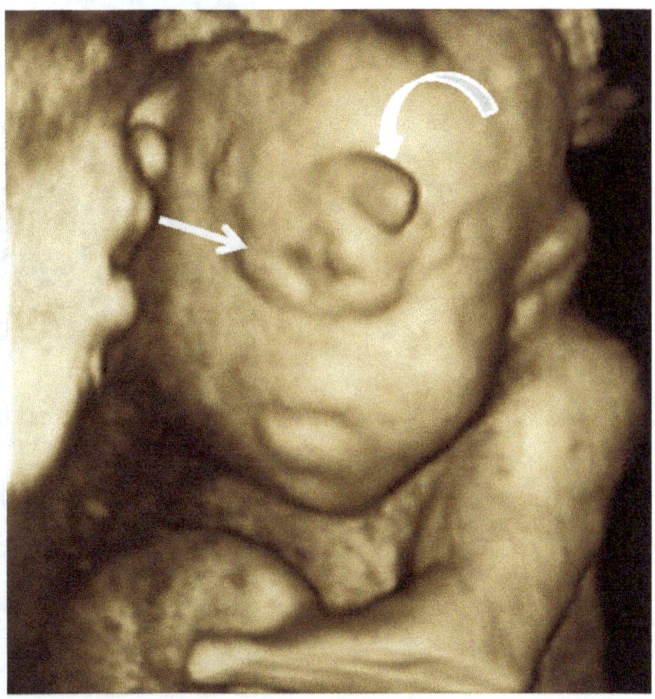

FIGURE 2.10D Three-dimensional image of cyclops with two eye anlagen (straight arrow); proboscis (curved arrow).

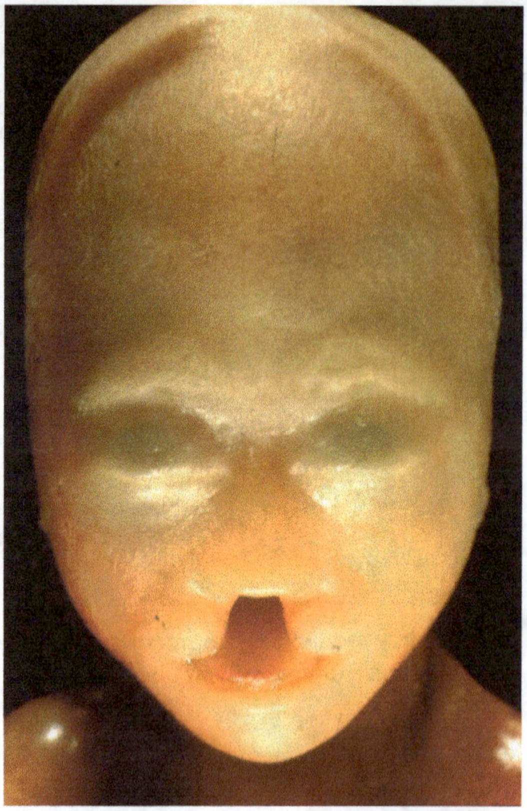

**FIGURE 2.10E** Median cleft lip/palate and hypotelorism in fetus with holoprosencephaly.

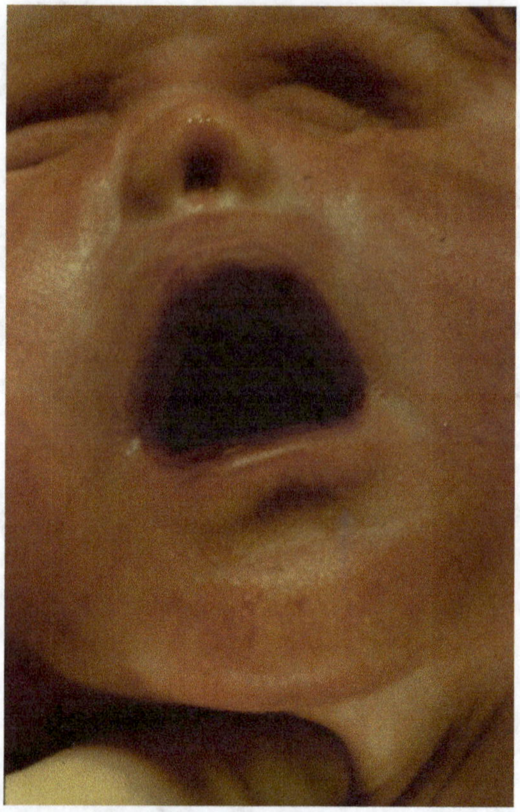

**FIGURE 2.10F** Fetus with cebocephaly: single nostril and ocular hypotelorism.

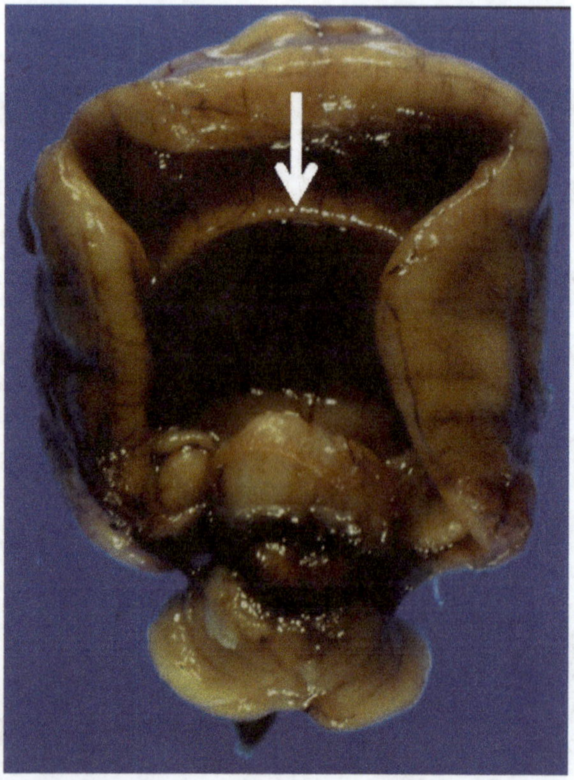

**FIGURE 2.10G** Pathologic brain specimen showing alobar holoprosencephaly. Note the single ventricle (arrow).

# 2.11 HYDRANENCEPHALY

## EPIDEMIOLOGY/GENETICS

**Definition** Hydranencephaly is a severe brain abnormality in which most or all of the cerebral hemispheres are absent and the cranium is filled with fluid.

**Epidemiology** Prevalence is 1 to 2.5 per 10,000 births (M1:F1).

**Embryology** Classic hydranencephaly is due to bilateral internal carotid obstruction, resulting in hemispheric necrosis. The internal carotid occlusion likely occurs between 8 and 11 weeks' gestation. However, there may be many variations of "hydranencephaly" and a heterogeneous group of etiologies that result in destruction of brain parenchyma secondary to ischemia. The ischemia may be due to hypotension, vascular agenesis/dysgenesis, or arterial occlusion. The etiologies reported include abdominal trauma, chromosomal abnormalities, congenital infection, genetic disorders, hypercoagulable states, and monochorionic twins with a fetal demise. Extreme hydrocephalus differs from hydranencephaly in having a lining of cortex at the outside of its sac.

**Inheritance Patterns** Rare familial recurrence has been reported. About 20 multiple malformation syndromes have been reported with hydranencephaly or porencephaly.

**Teratogens** Congenital infections (herpes, cytomegalovirus, rubella, toxoplasmosis), cocaine, and warfarin are teratogenic.

**Prognosis** Hydranencephaly is usually lethal, with neonatal survivors having profound mental retardation.

## SONOGRAPHY

### FREQUENT FINDINGS

- Cerebral hemispheres are replaced with CSF.
- There is preservation of the thalami and cerebellum.
  - The cerebellum is usually hypoplastic.
- There is debris within the cerebral membranous sacs.
- A midline falx is present but may be disrupted.
- Generally, there is a normal head circumference for gestational age.
- Color Doppler demonstrates an absence of the middle cerebral arteries.

### LESS FREQUENT

- Scattered preserved regions of cerebral cortical tissue occur due to collateral circulation.
  - The ophthalmic artery preserves portions of the frontal lobe.
  - Posterior communicating arteries preserve portions of the occipital lobe.

### KEY FINDINGS/PITFALLS

- Earliest sonographic detection is at 12 weeks' gestation.

- The basilar artery preserves the cerebellum, brainstem, basal ganglia, and thalamus.
- The choroid plexus continues to produce CSF, which is not adequately absorbed. As a result, the head is characteristically normocephalic, but can rarely be macrocephalic. The finding of macrocephaly makes the diagnosis of hydranencephaly much less likely.

### DIFFERENTIAL DIAGNOSIS

- Intracranial neoplasm: Disorganized necrotic tissue may initially have an architectural pattern consistent with clot. Serial ultrasound examinations will differentiate the evolution of an intracranial hemorrhage from an intracerebral neoplasm.
- Alobar HPE: A cortical mantle excludes a diagnosis of hydranencephaly. Additional sonographic findings associated with alobar HPE include a proboscis, hypotelorism, microopthalmia, and fused thalami.
- Porencephaly: The remaining cortical tissue excludes a diagnosis of hydranencephaly.
- Severe hydrocephalus: The presence of any frontal cerebral cortex excludes hydranencephaly. Depending on the level of obstruction, the third or fourth ventricle may be dilated in hydrocephalus. MRI may help to distinguish hydranencephaly from severe hydrocephalus.

## PREGNANCY MANAGEMENT

**Investigations and Consultations Required** Although rare, disseminated fetal viral infections can cause extensive cerebral destruction. Therefore, viral titers should be done. Chromosome studies should also be performed because of the potential for a misclassification of severe hydrocephalus as hydranencephaly.

**Monitoring** Serial ultrasound examinations should be performed to monitor head size. Because hydranencephaly should not be an "increased-pressure" form of ventriculomegaly, an enlarging head, relative to other fetal parameters, should prompt a reassessment of the diagnosis.

**Pregnancy Course** Hydranencephaly should not be associated with specific obstetric complications.

**Pregnancy Termination Issues** Termination of pregnancy is an appropriate option, and it should be done by a nondestructive procedure at an institution with expertise in fetal neuropathology.

**Delivery** Vaginal delivery is appropriate in all cases. In the presence of a relatively large head, cephalocentesis may be indicated to accomplish vaginal delivery of the infant.

## NEONATOLOGY

**Resuscitation** The decision to initiate resuscitative efforts should be discussed with the family prior to delivery. With a definitive diagnosis of hydranencephaly of known cause, nonintervention is appropriate if spontaneous onset of respiration does not occur. If the diagnosis is uncertain, support is indicated to allow time for confirmation.

**Transport** Transfer to a tertiary center with pediatric neurology and neurosurgery capabilities is indicated for confirmation of the diagnosis.

**Testing and Confirmation** Postnatally, the diagnosis is confirmed by MRI or CT scan. Serologic and microbiologic testing for congenital infections is indicated if not obtained prenatally.

**Nursery Management** The major priorities are confirmation of the diagnosis and etiology and facilitation of parental adaptation to the severe prognosis. Decisions regarding long-term custodial care may be required, as some infants may survive the neonatal period.

## SUGGESTED READINGS


1. Belfar HL, Kuller JA, Hill LM, Kislak S: Evolving fetal hydranencephaly mimicking intracranial neoplasm. J Ultrasound Med 1991; 10:231-233.
2. Byers BD, Barth WH, Stewart TL, Pierce BT: Ultrasound and MRI appearance and evolution of hydranencephaly in utero. A case report. J Reprod Med 2005; 50:53-56.
3. Cecchetto G, Milanase L, Giordano R, et al: Looking at the missing brain: hydranencephaly case series and literature review. Pediatr Neurol 2013; 48:152-158.
4. Dixon A: Hydranencephaly. Radiography 1988; 54:12-13.
5. Hahn JS, Lewis AJ, Barnes P: Hydranencephaly owing to twin-twin transfusion: serial ultrasonography and magnetic resonance imaging findings. J Child Neurol 2003; 18:367-370.
6. Kurtz AB, Johnson PT: Case 7: Hydranencephaly. Radiology 1999; 210:419-422.
7. Lam YH, Tang MH: Serial sonographic features of a fetus with hydranencephaly from 11 weeks to term. Ultrasound Obstet Gynecol 2000; 16:77-79.
8. Lin YS, Chang FM, Liu CH. Antenatal detection of hydranencephaly at 12 weeks menstrual age. J Clin Ultrasound 1992; 20:62-65.
9. Sepulveda W, Cortes-Yepes H, Wong AE, et al: Prenatal sonography of hydranencephaly. Findings during the early stages of disease. J Ultrasound Med 2012; 31:789-804.
10. Witters I, Moerman P, Devriendt K, et al: Two siblings with early onset fetal akinesia deformation sequence and hydranencepahly: further evidence for autosomal recessive inheritance of hydranencephaly, fowler type. Am J Med Genet 2002; 108:41-44.

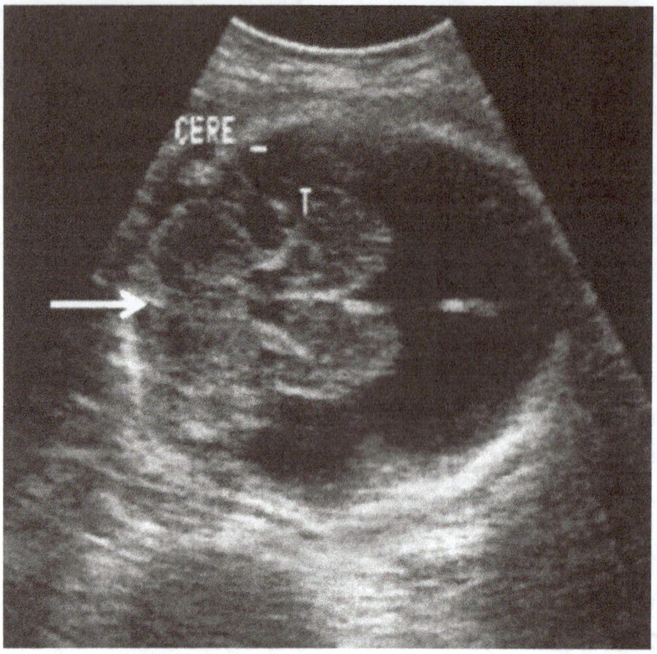


**FIGURE 2.11A** Hydranencephaly showing preservation of cerebellum (arrow) (CERE) and thalami (T).

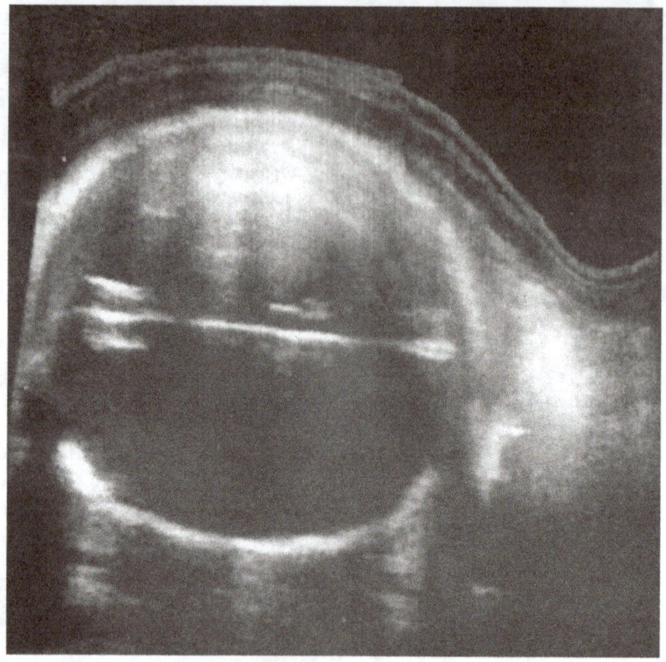

**FIGURE 2.11B** Hydranencephaly illustrating macrocephaly and an intact falx.

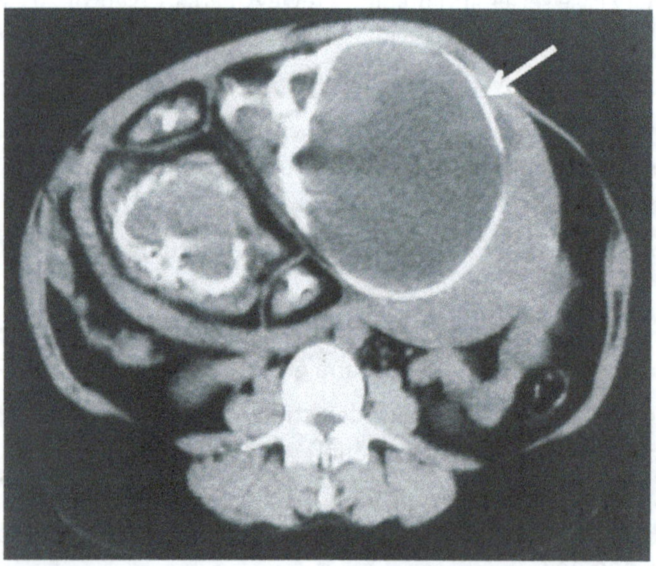

**FIGURE 2.11C** Magnetic resonance image of fetal hydranencephaly (arrow).

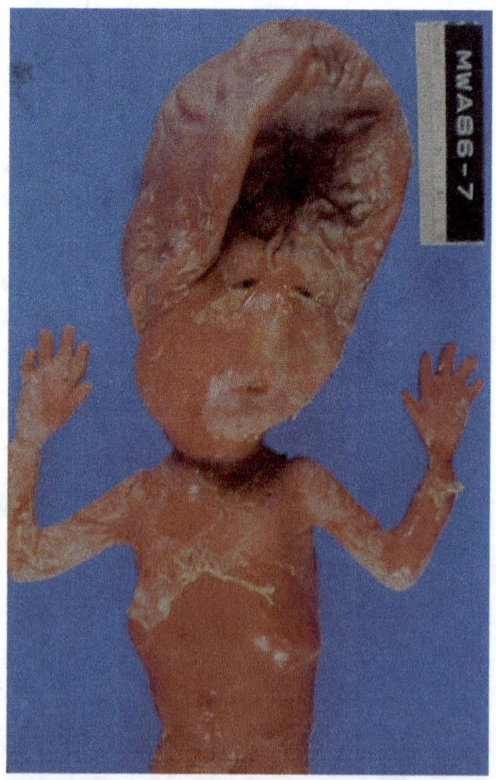


**FIGURE 2.11D** Fetus with hydranencephaly and macrocephaly.

# 2.12 INIENCEPHALY

## EPIDEMIOLOGY/GENETICS

**Definition** Iniencephaly is an abnormality in cervical vertebrae associated with an excessive lordosis of the cervicothoracic spine and neural tube closure defects.

**Epidemiology** Rare (M1:F10). Preconceptual supplementation with folic acid may be of use in decreasing the incidence, or recurrence, of iniencephaly.

**Embryology** The pathogenesis is unknown. It is possible that iniencephaly is a primary defect in fetal cervical development, and the resulting lordosis causes a failure of neural tube closure. Alternatively, it may be a primary defect in neural tube closure. Anencephaly, encephalocele, microcephaly, and other anomalies have been associated with iniencephaly. Currently, it is thought that iniencephaly is likely a neural tube defect, with the time of onset being a few days later than anencephaly and secondary to an arrest or imperfect development of the base of the skull. It has been associated with trisomy 18 and partial monosomy 6p.

**Inheritance Patterns** Inheritance is sporadic, with no known syndrome associations.

**Teratogens** Folic acid antagonists (methotrexate and aminopterin), vitamin A, thalidomide, maternal diabetes, hyperthermia, and folate deficiency are associated with an increased risk for neural tube abnormalities.

**Screening** Alpha-fetoprotein elevation may be present, but only if there is an open defect present.

**Prognosis** Iniencephaly, when diagnosed in utero, is almost always lethal.

## SONOGRAPHY

### FREQUENT FINDINGS

- Short cervical spine
- Fixed retroflexion of the head
  - Face looks upward ("stargazing")
- Uninterrupted skin covering the retroflexed head
- Short/absent neck
  - Mandibular skin continuous with the chest
- Shortened spinal length
- Polyhydramnios common in the late second and third trimesters

### LESS FREQUENT

- Diaphragmatic hernia
- Omphalocele
- Myelomeningocele

- Holoprosencephaly
- Single umbilical artery
- Clubfoot

### KEY FINDINGS/PITFALLS

- In the first trimester, the crown-rump length may be smaller than expected due to the position of the head.
- A 3-D ultrasound image provides a better evaluation of any external cranial defect, as well as the cervical and upper thoracic regions.

### DIFFERENTIAL DIAGNOSIS

- Anencephaly with spinal retroflexion. The affected spinal region is not covered with skin.

## PREGNANCY MANAGEMENT

**Investigations and Consultations Required** The distinctive ultrasonographic features should preclude the need for any additional evaluation.

**Monitoring** There are no special considerations for prenatal care. This is almost always a lethal anomaly, so ultrasonographic monitoring is not necessary except to ensure that massive hydrocephalus preventing vaginal delivery does not occur and to document fetal lie and the presenting part.

**Pregnancy Course** Polyhydramnios and preterm labor are common, as is antenatal stillbirth. The incidence of complicated labor and delivery is high with iniencephaly because of the high likelihood of fetal malpresentation.

**Pregnancy Termination Issues** There are no indications for special pathologic examination. Nondestructive methods of termination may be complicated by obstructed labor secondary to malpresentation of these fetuses.

**Delivery** If obstructed labor occurs, cesarean section may be necessary for maternal indications.

## NEONATOLOGY

**Resuscitation** This is not indicated, as the lesion is uncorrectable.

**Transport** Transport is not indicated, as the lesion is uncorrectable.

**Testing and Confirmation** The abnormality is obvious at birth.

**Nursery Management** Provision of comfort care and support of family are the only appropriate care measures.

### SUGGESTED READINGS

1. Bianchi DW, Crombleholme TM, D'Alton ME: Iniencephaly. In: Bianchi DW, Crombleholme TM, D'Alton ME, eds. Fetology: Diagnosis and Management of the Fetal Patient. New York: McGraw-Hill; 2000: 141-146.

2. Chen CP: Prenatal diagnosis of iniencephaly. Taiwan J Obstet Gynecol 2007; 46:199-208.
3. Copp AJ, Stanier P, Greene NDE: Neural tube defects—recent advances, unsolved questions and controversies. Lancet Neurol 2013 A; 12: 799–810.
4. Cullier F, Loenig P, Lagarde L, Cartaulty JF: Transvaginal sonographic diagnosis of iniencephaly apertus and cranioraschischisis at 9 weeks' gestation (Letters). Ultrasound Obstet Gynecol 2003; 22:656-658.
5. Dogan MM, Ekici E, Yapar EG, et al: Iniencephaly: sonographic-pathologic correlation of 19 cases. J Perinat Med 1990; 24:501-511.
6. Joo JG, Bake A, Papp C, et al: Major diagnostic and pathological features of iniencephahy based on twenty-four cases. Fetal Diagn Ther 2008; 24:1-6.
7. Lemire RJ, Beckwith JB, Shepard TH: Iniencephaly and anencephaly with spinal retroflexion. A comparative study of eight human specimens. Teratology 1972; 6:27-36.
8. Sahid S, Sepulveda W, Dezereya V, et al: Iniencephaly: prenatal diagnosis and management. Prenat Diagn 2000; 20:202-205.

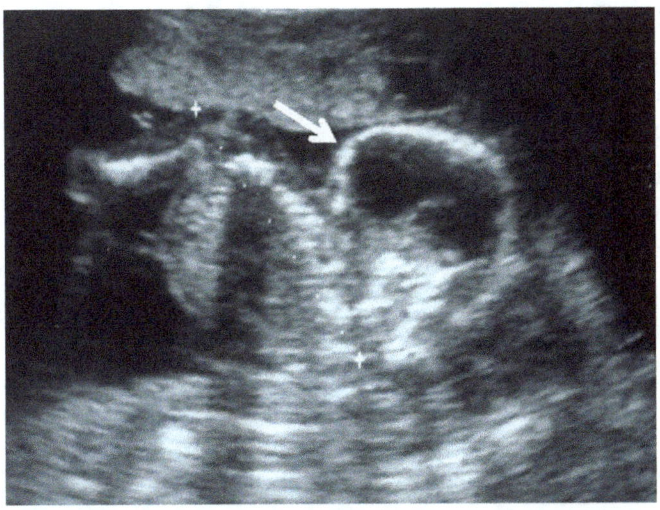

**FIGURE 2.12A** Shortened spine length (+ ... +); marked retroflexion of the head (arrow).

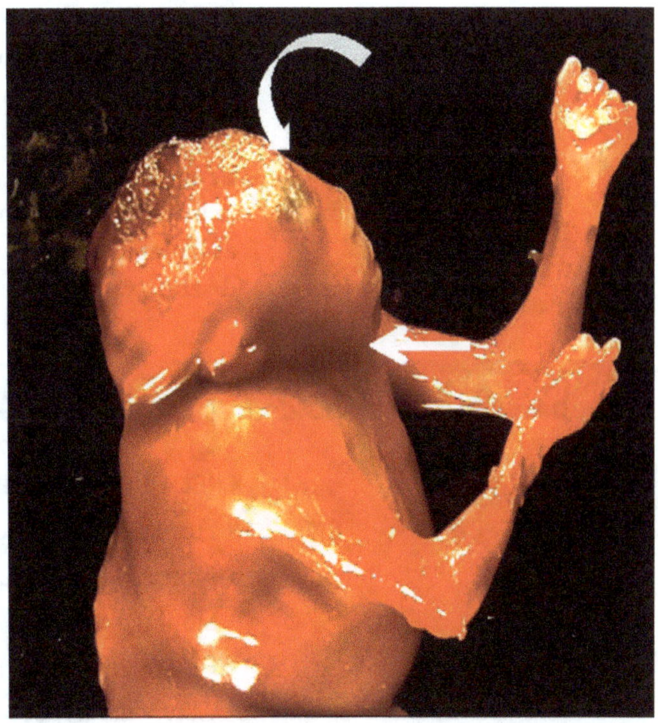

**FIGURE 2.12B** Fetus with iniencephaly: stargazing (curved arrow). Mandibular skin is continuous with chest (straight arrow).

# 2.13 MICROCEPHALY

## EPIDEMIOLOGY/GENETICS

**Definition** Microcephaly is defined as a head circumference three standard deviations below the mean.

**Epidemiology** Occurrence is 1 in 10,000 births (M1:F1) for isolated microcephaly; it is much more commonly seen as an associated abnormality.

**Embryology** Microcephaly most often occurs secondary to a small brain. It can have antenatal or postnatal onset and is associated with various brain malformations, disruptions, and more than 300 sporadic, genetic, and chromosomal syndromes.

**Inheritance Pattern** Both autosomal recessive and autosomal dominant families have been reported with isolated microcephaly. A number of different loci have been identified. Because of the rapid progress in mapping of genes and subsequent development of genetic testing, consultation with a medical geneticist or genetic counselor to determine the availability of clinical genetic testing for this disorder or disorders is advised.

**Teratogens** Most human teratogens, including intrauterine infection (cytomegalovirus, rubella, and toxoplasmosis), radiation, drugs, hypoxia, and alcohol, can cause microcephaly.

**Prognosis** Prognosis is dependent on the cause of the microcephaly and any associated brain malformations. Most microcephaly syndromes, as well as isolated microcephaly, result in moderate-to-severe intellectual disability.

## SONOGRAPHY

### FREQUENT FINDINGS

- Head circumference less than 3 standard deviations below the mean
- Normal facial features
- Sloping forehead
- Frontal lobe less than 2 standard deviations below the mean
- Cerebellar hypoplasia

### LESS FREQUENT

- Encephalocele
- Enlarged subarachnoid space overlying the frontal horns

### KEY FINDINGS/PITFALLS

- Because of the rarity of microcephaly, 3 standard deviations below the mean, rather than 2 standard deviations, should be utilized to define microcephaly.

- The use of multiple diagnostic parameters improves diagnostic accuracy:

| Sonographic Parameter | Definition |
|---|---|
| Head circumference | –3 SD |
| Head circumference/abdominal circumference ratio | –3 SD |
| Femur length/head circumference | +3SD |

- Microcephaly cannot be excluded by normal second-trimester biometry.
- Isolated microcephaly is more difficult to diagnosis and may have a better prognosis than microcephaly with associated congenital anomalies.
- In most cases, there is no adverse neuropsychological outcome when the fetal head circumference is between minus 2 SD and minus 3 SD.
- In microcephaly, power Doppler evaluation demonstrates a discrepancy in the diameter of the vessels derived from the posterior cerebral artery, compared to the anterior/middle cerebral complex.
    - The smaller anterior brain mass requires a smaller blood supply.

## PREGNANCY MANAGEMENT

**Investigations and Consultations Required** Microcephaly may be a difficult diagnosis to make, particularly in mild cases, as there is significant overlap with normal. Subsequent pregnancy management and the extent of the evaluation depend in part on the certainty of the diagnosis. Many cases of microcephaly are part of a syndrome, and steps to determine whether a given case is isolated or syndromic are warranted. A careful history should be taken, including family history, maternal drug or environmental exposures, maternal illnesses and medications, radiation exposure, and other risk factors aimed at possible underlying etiologies. Chromosome evaluation, including microarrays, and viral studies (both maternal serum and amniotic fluid) should be performed. Congenital heart defects are commonly associated with conditions having microcephaly as a feature; therefore, fetal echocardiography should be a part of the initial evaluation. Prenatal consultations with a multidisciplinary team, including neurology and neonatology, may be helpful, depending on the etiology determined with the antenatal evaluation.

**Monitoring** There are no specific needs beyond usual obstetrical care. Because the diagnosis is difficult to make, repeat ultrasonographic studies are helpful to confirm diminished cranial growth, to look at overall fetal growth patterns, and to assess for additional anomalies.

**Pregnancy Course** No specific obstetric complications would be expected.

**Pregnancy Termination Issues** If a diagnosis has not been established, a nondestructive procedure should be performed, and a careful external examination of the fetus by a dysmorphologist should be a part of the autopsy protocol.

**Delivery** Delivery at a tertiary center is appropriate if a precise diagnosis has not been made prenatally. Special care and evaluation may be necessary following birth.

## NEONATOLOGY

**Resuscitation** No specific measures are required with isolated microcephaly. However, when microcephaly is associated with the confirmed antenatal diagnosis of a lethal chromosomal anomaly, such as trisomy 13, or a severe neuroanatomical abnormality, such as a large encephalocele with the bulk of the brain tissue in the mass, a predelivery discussion should be undertaken with the family about nonintervention in the event that spontaneous onset of respiration does not occur.

**Transport** Although isolated microcephaly may not require transfer to a tertiary center at the time of birth, an outpatient evaluation in the immediate newborn period is indicated. In the presence of a suspected congenital infection, syndromic features, or abnormal neurologic exam, the infant should be referred promptly to a perinatal tertiary center with neonatology, pediatric neurology, pediatric genetics, and pediatric infectious disease capabilities for definitive evaluation.

**Testing and Confirmation** Microcephaly is confirmed when a single head circumference (occipital frontal circumference, OFC) measurement is more than 2-3 standard deviations below the mean at birth. Evaluation in the newborn period includes a thorough history and physical exam of the infant, evaluation of parental OFC to assess for autosomal dominant microcephaly, history of antenatal insult, and assessment for syndromic features. Serial measurements of OFC and neuroimaging studies (head ultrasound, CT scan, or MRI) to evaluate brain morphology are indicated. Additional screening should be done for genetic, infectious, and metabolic etiologies, including chromosome analysis and microarray, TORCH titers (toxoplasmosis, rubella, cytomegalovirus, herpes), urine or saliva for cytomegalovirus, and urine and serum testing for metabolic disorders. Ophthalmologic evaluation in the newborn may reveal abnormalities associated with either congenital infection or genetic abnormalities. Hearing screening is indicated to assess for possible deficits.

**Nursery Management:** As noted, microcephaly is often associated with other malformations or diseases that will dictate the neonatal management.

**Prognosis:** Prognosis depends on underlying etiology and the severity of the microcephaly. Infants with microcephaly are at risk for cerebral palsy and neurodevelopmental disability.

### SUGGESTED READINGS


1. Abuelo D: Microcephaly syndromes. Semin Pediatr Neurol 2007; 14:118-127.
2. Ashwal S, Michelson D, Plawner L, et al: Practice parameter; evaluation of the child with microcephaly (an evidence-based review); report of the Quality Standards Subcommittee of the American Academy of Neurology and the Practice Committee of the Child Neurology Society. Neurology 2009; 73:887-897.
3. Barbelanne M, Tsang WY: Molecular and cellular basis of autosomal recessive primary microcephly. Biomed Res Int 2014; 2014: 547986. Published online 2014 December 8. doi:10.1155/2014/547986.
4. Den Hollander NS, Wessels MW, Los FJ, et al: Congenital microcephaly detected by prenatal ultrasound: genetic aspects and clinical significance. Ultrasound Obstet Gynecol 2000; 15:282-287.
5. Leroy JG, Frias JL: Nonsyndromic microcephaly: an overview. Adv Pediatr 2005; 52:261-293.

6. Pilu G, Falco P, Milano V, et al: Prenatal diagnosis of microcephaly assisted by vaginal sonography and power Doppler. Ultrasound Obstet Gynecol 1998; 11:357-360.
7. Rees AEJ, Bates A, Clarke H: Cerebellar hypoplasia in the second trimester associated with microcephaly at birth. Ultrasound Obstet Gynecol 1995; 5:206-208.
8. Stoler-Poria S, Lev D, Schweiger A, et al: Development outcome of isolated fetal microcephaly. Ultrasound Obstet Gynecol 2010; 36:154-158.
9. Woods CG, Bond J, Enard W: Autosomal recessive primary microcephaly (MCPH): a review of clinical, molecular, and evolutionary findings. Am J Hum Genet 2005; 76:717-728.

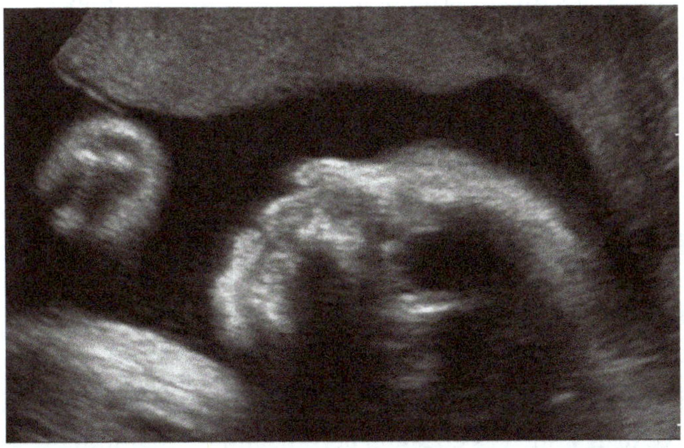

**FIGURE 2.13A** Microcephaly illustrating sloping forehead.

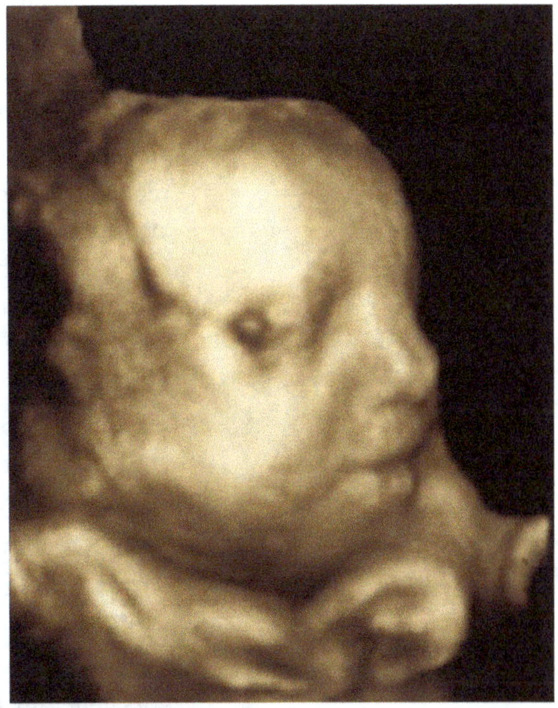

**FIGURE 2.13B** Image illustrating microcephaly and sloping forehead.

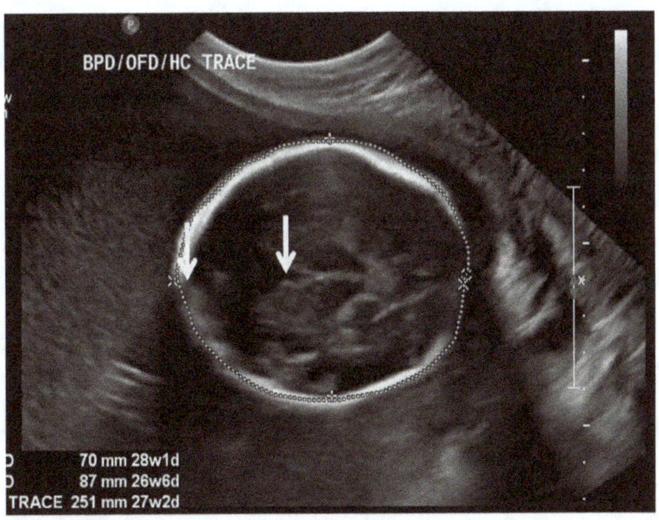


**FIGURE 2.13C** Microcephaly with a 27-week frontal lobe (arrows) at 34 weeks.

# 2.14 PORENCEPHALY

## EPIDEMIOLOGY/GENETICS

**Definition** Porencephaly is generally thought to be a destructive process resulting in cystic cavities within the brain that may communicate with the lateral ventricles or the subarachnoid space.

**Epidemiology** Uncommon.

**Embryology** Most people differentiate extensive porencephaly from hydranencephaly by the latter's symmetry and lack of cavities, although they most likely represent varying severities of similar pathologic processes. The etiology of porencephaly is heterogeneous, but most cases are thought to be due to generalized or localized brain ischemia caused by hypotension, vascular agenesis, twin-to-twin emboli, or overwhelming antenatal infection.

**Inheritance Patterns** Generally, inheritance is sporadic with presumed low recurrence. However, there are families with collagen IV mutations that have an autosomal dominant inheritance, and some genetic disorders, such as Fabry disease, are inherited in an X-linked fashion. Other disorders, such as inherited thrombophilias and alloimmune thrombocytopenia, should be considered when counseling patients regarding recurrence.

**Teratogens** Congenital infections, including cytomegalovirus and toxoplasmosis, and vasoconstrictive drugs, such as cocaine, heroin, and methamphetamines, are teratogenic.

**Differential Diagnosis** Possibilities for differential diagnosis include lissencephaly/pachygyria syndromes, such as Walker-Warburg syndrome and Miller-Dieker (microdeletion 17p) syndrome, arachnoid cysts, and other intracranial cystic abnormalities.

**Prognosis** The prognosis is dependent on the severity of CNS damage. Survivors generally have moderate-to-severe intellectual disability with seizures and other focal signs of neurologic damage.

## SONOGRAPHY

### FREQUENT FINDINGS

- Unilateral round cysts with jagged internal walls
- Cyst may communicate with the lateral ventricle

### LESS FREQUENT

- Asymmetric ventriculomegaly
- Midline shift
- Absence/destruction of the cavum septum pellucidum

### KEY FINDINGS/PITFALLS

- The areas of brain destroyed are replaced with cerebral spinal fluid.

- One or more of the intracranial cysts may communicate with the ventricular system or the subarachnoid space.
- Porencephalic cysts are characteristically detected sonographically in the third trimester.
- Usually, there is no association with other congenital anomalies.
- Asymmetric ventriculomegaly with a midline shift suggests porencephaly.
- An MRI can be used to determine if a cyst is lined with white matter (porencephaly) or gray matter (schizencephaly).
  - In porencephaly, parenchymal destruction occurs after neuronal migration. Hence, the defect is lined by white matter.
- Three-dimensional imaging can be utilized more accurately to delineate the location of brain cysts and their relationship to the lateral ventricles.

## PREGNANCY MANAGEMENT

**Investigations and Consultations Required** Existence of a porencephalic cyst may be a diagnosis of exclusion in some cases. Further evaluation depends on the size and location of the cyst and the timing of its diagnosis. If thought to be related to a fetal intracranial hemorrhage, consideration should be given to alloimmune thrombocytopenia, and appropriate maternal antibody studies should be drawn. If there is diagnostic uncertainty, a fetal MRI may be useful. Amniocentesis should be performed for chromosome analysis, microarray, and viral studies.

**Fetal Intervention** None is indicated.

**Monitoring** Normal obstetric management is appropriate. Serial ultrasound examinations are useful to exclude progression.

**Pregnancy Course** The course should be uncomplicated.

**Pregnancy Termination Issues** An intact fetus should be delivered to confirm the diagnosis.

**Delivery** Because of the possibility of neurologic deficits, delivery in a tertiary center may be prudent.

## NEONATOLOGY

**Resuscitation** Generalization regarding the appropriateness of intervention following birth for a nonbreathing infant in whom an antenatal diagnosis of a cortical destructive lesion has been made is difficult at best. The timing in gestation of the insult, the location and extent of the injury, and the intervening pregnancy history all have an effect on the potential for serious adverse neurologic outcomes. Discussion with the parents prior to delivery of the treatment options in the event of initial respiratory depression is important. Such a discussion should be based on the specific clinical situation, taking into account all of the previously cited factors.

**Transport** Transfer of an infant to a tertiary center with pediatric neurology and neuroradiology diagnostic capabilities is appropriate to confirm the diagnosis and delineate the extent of cortical injury.

**Testing and Confirmation** Computed tomography and MRI, in some circumstances with vascular contrast, are the imaging techniques of choice to describe the pathologic anatomy.

**Nursery Management** Beyond a thorough diagnostic evaluation and routine supportive care for a newborn, the other elements of care are dictated by the specific neurologic deficits manifested by a given infant. These may, but do not always, include respiratory control, feeding difficulties, neonatal seizures, and focal motor deficits.

**Prognosis** The prognosis depends on the size and location of the cyst and the presence of other abnormalities. Long-term sequelae may include delayed growth and development, spastic hemiplegia, hypotonia, seizures, and cognitive impairment.

## SUGGESTED READINGS

1. Blumkin L, Watemberg N, Lev D, et al: Nonprogressive familial leukoencephalopathy with porencephalic cyst and focal seizures. J Child Neurol 2006; 21:145-148.
2. Debus O, Koch HG, Kurlemann G, et al: Factor V Leiden and genetic defects of thrombophilia in childhood porencephaly. Arch Dis Child Fetal Neonatal Ed 1998: 78:F121-F124.
3. Eller KM, Kuller JA: Fetal porencephaly: a review of etiology, diagnosis, and prognosis. Obstet Gynecol Surv 1995; 50:684-687.
4. Kalache KD, Eder K, Essar T, et al: Three-dimensional ultrasonographic reslicing of the fetal brain to assist prenatal diagnosis of central nervous system anomalies. J Ultrasound Med 2006; 25:509-514.
5. Monteagudo A, Timor-Tritsch I: Prenatal diagnosis of CNS anomalies other than neural tube defects and ventriculomegaly. UpToDate. 2016. http://www.uptodate.com/contents/prenatal-diagnosis-of-cns-anomalies-other-than-neural-tube-defects-and-ventriculomegaly.
6. Pilu G, Falco P, Perolo A, et al: Differential diagnosis and outcome of fetal intracranial hypoechoic lesions: report of 21 cases. Ultrasound Obstet Gynecol 1997; 9:229-236.
7. Scher MS, Belfar H, Martin J, Painter MJ: Destructive brain lesions of presumed fetal onset: antepartum causes of cerebral palsy. Pediatrics 1991; 88:898-906.
8. Verbeek E, Meuwissen MEC, Verheijen FW, et al: COL4A2 mutation associated with familial porencephaly and small-vessel disease. Eur J Hum Genet 2012; 20:844-851.

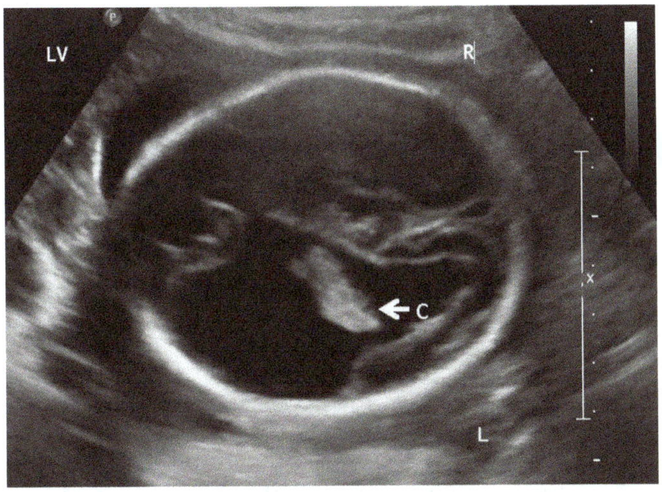


**FIGURE 2.14A** Left porencephalic cyst extending to the ventricle. Choroid plexus (c).

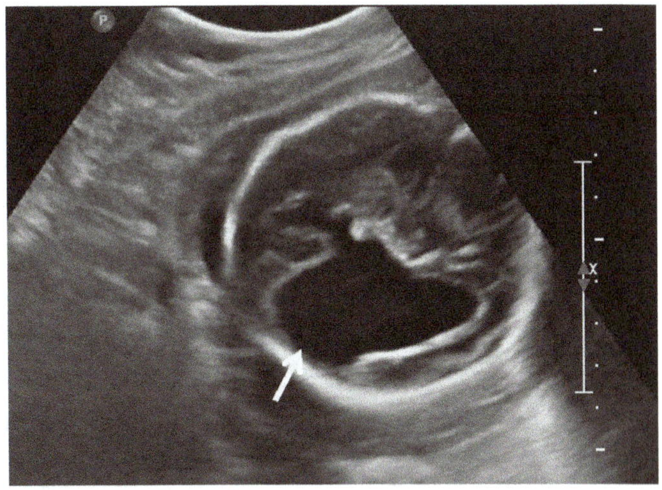

**FIGURE 2.14B** Porencephalic cyst (arrow).

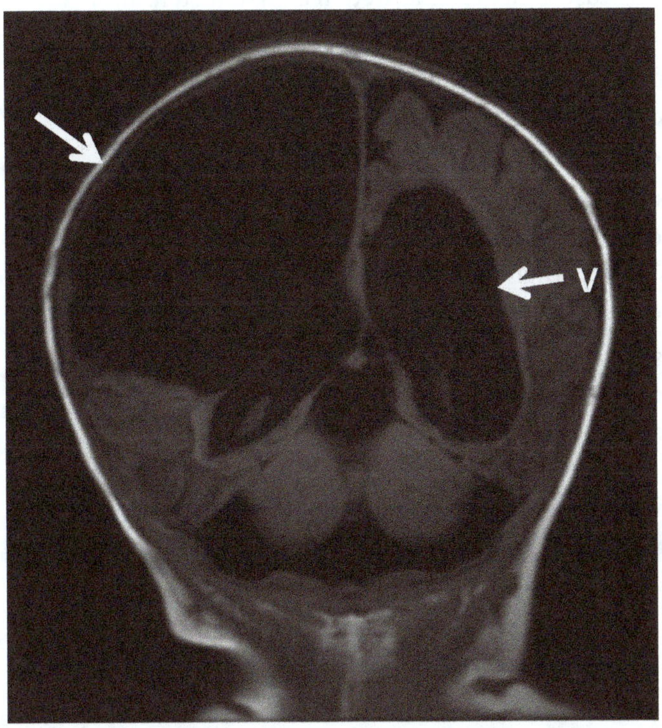


**FIGURE 2.14C(1)** Magnetic resonance image of porencephalic cyst (arrow) with ventriculomegaly (v).

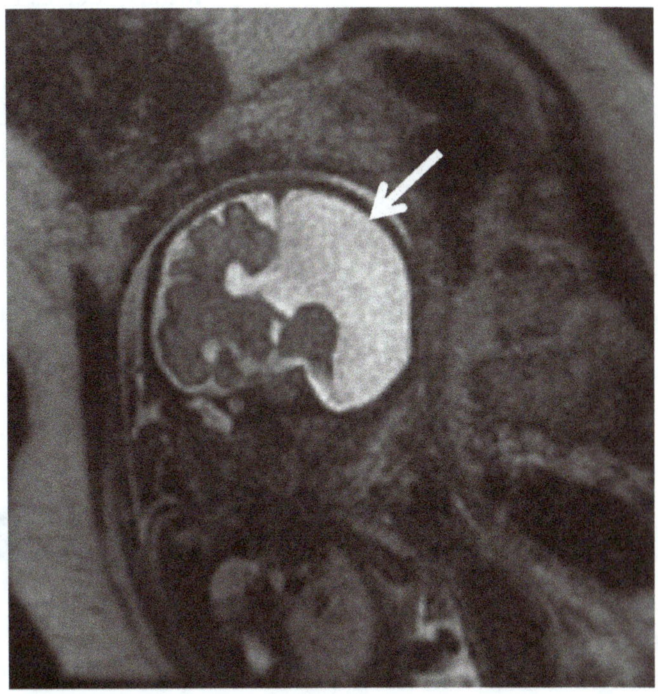

**FIGURE 2.14C(2)** Fetal MRI illustrating a porencephalic cyst (arrow).

# 2.15 SCHIZENCEPHALY

## EPIDEMIOLOGY/GENETICS

**Definition** Schizencephaly (split brain) is a brain abnormality in which cortical gray matter extends from the lateral ventricle to the surface of the brain. There may be either an open communication (open lip) or the abnormal gray matter extending through the brain parenchyma (closed lip).

**Epidemiology** Uncommon.

**Embryology** The brain shows cleft-like lesions, in contrast to the cyst-like structures in porencephaly. The etiology is heterogeneous, and similar to porencephaly, with most cases due to generalized or localized brain ischemia. Some cases of schizencephaly likely represent primary cerebral dysgenesis.

**Inheritance Patterns** Generally, inheritance is sporadic with presumed low recurrence. However, because in porencephaly there are families with collagen IV mutations that have an autosomal dominant inheritance and some genetic disorders, such as Fabry disease, that are inherited in an X-linked fashion, the workup for schizencephaly should be the same as that for porencephaly.

**Teratogens** Congenital infections, including cytomegalovirus and toxoplasmosis, and vasoconstrictive drugs, such as cocaine, heroin, and methamphetamines, may be causative.

**Differential Diagnosis** Lissencephaly/pachygyria syndromes, such as the Walker-Warburg syndrome and Miller-Dieker (microdeletion 17p) syndrome, as well as arachnoid cysts, and other intracranial cystic abnormalities should be considered in the differential diagnosis.

**Prognosis** The prognosis for this group of conditions is dependent on the severity of CNS damage. Survivors generally have moderate-to-severe intellectual disability with seizures and other focal signs of neurologic damage.

## SONOGRAPHY

### FREQUENT FINDINGS

- Cleft between the lateral ventricle and brain surface
  - Often bilateral and symmetrical

### LESS FREQUENT

- Ventriculomegaly
- Absent cavum septum pellucidum

### KEY FINDINGS/PITFALLS

- In schizencephaly, one or more clefts extend from the lateral ventricle to the surface of the brain.
- The sides of the cleft may be in contact with one another (closed lips; type I) or widely separated (open lips; type II).

- Most cases are detected sonographically in the early third trimester; no cases have been detected prior to 20 weeks' gestation.
- The majority of antenatally detected cases of schizencephaly are open (type II).
- The clefts in schizencephaly are associated with the course of the middle cerebral arteries.
- Three-dimensional imaging can be utilized to more accurately evaluate cases of suspected schizencephaly.
- A fetal MRI can determine if a brain cyst is lined with white matter (porencephaly) or gray matter (schizencephaly).
  - In porencephaly, parenchymal destruction occurs after neuronal migration. Hence, the defect is lined by white matter.

## PREGNANCY MANAGEMENT

**Investigations and Consultations Required** Because of the limited number of cases of schizencephaly that have been diagnosed prenatally and the potential for misdiagnosis, a complete evaluation is required to exclude other causes of enlarged ventricles. Amniocentesis should be performed for chromosome analysis, including microarray testing, and for viral studies.

**Fetal Intervention** None is indicated.

**Monitoring** Normal obstetric management is appropriate. Serial ultrasound examinations are useful to document progression, which has been reported.

**Pregnancy Course** The course should be uncomplicated.

**Pregnancy Termination Issues** Because of the rarity of making this diagnosis in the second trimester, an intact fetus should be delivered to confirm the diagnosis.

**Delivery** Because of the significant likelihood of neurologic deficits, delivery in a tertiary center may be prudent.

## NEONATOLOGY

**Resuscitation** Generalization regarding appropriateness of intervention following birth for a nonbreathing infant in whom an antenatal diagnosis of a cortical destructive lesion has been made is difficult at best. The timing in gestation of the insult, the location and extent of the injury, and the intervening pregnancy history all have an effect on the potential for serious adverse neurologic outcomes. Discussion with the parents prior to delivery of the treatment options in the event of initial respiratory depression is important. Such a discussion should be based on the specific clinical situation, taking into account all of the previously cited factors.

**Transport** Transfer of an infant to a tertiary center with pediatric neurology and neuroradiology diagnostic capabilities is appropriate to confirm the diagnosis and delineate the extent of cortical injury.

**Testing and Confirmation** Computed tomography and MRI, in some circumstances with vascular contrast, are the imaging techniques of choice to describe the pathologic anatomy.

**Nursery Management** Beyond a thorough diagnostic evaluation and routine supportive care for a newborn, the other elements of care are dictated by the specific neurologic deficits manifested by a given infant. These may, but do not always, include respiratory control, feeding difficulties, neonatal seizures, and focal motor deficits.

**Prognosis** In infants with schizencephaly, the degree of impairment depends on the location of the cleft, whether it is unilateral or bilateral, and the presence of other anatomic anomalies. Long-term sequelae may include delayed growth and development, spastic hemiplegia, hypotonia, seizures, and cognitive impairment.

## SUGGESTED READINGS

1. Eller KM, Kuller JA: Fetal porencephaly: a review of etiology, diagnosis, and prognosis. Obstet Gynecol Surv 1995; 50:684-687.
2. Kalache KD, Eder K, Essar T, et al: Three-dimensional ultrasonographic reslicing of the fetal brain to assist prenatal diagnosis of central nervous system anomalies. J Ultrasound Med 2006; 25:509-514.
3. Monteagudo A, Timor-Tritsch I Prenatal diagnosis of CNS anomalies other than neural tube defects and ventriculomegaly. UpToDate. 2016. http://www.uptodate.com/contents/prenatal-diagnosis-of-cns-anomalies-other-than-neural-tube-defects-and-ventriculomegaly.
4. Pilu G, Falco P, Perolo A, et al: Differential diagnosis and outcome of fetal intracranial hypoechoic lesions: report of 21 cases. Ultrasound Obstet Gynecol 1997; 9:229-236.
5. Scher MS, Belfar H, Martin J, Painter MJ: Destructive brain lesions of presumed fetal onset: antepartum causes of cerebral palsy. Pediatrics 1991; 88:898-906.

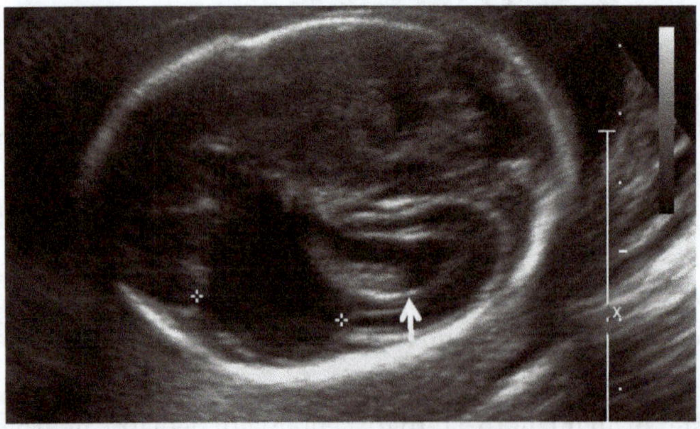

FIGURE 2.15A Schizencephaly (+ … +); ventriculomegaly (arrow).

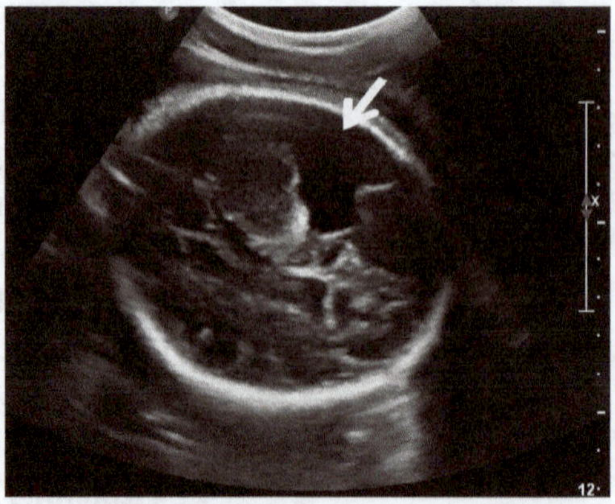

FIGURE 2.15B Ultrasound of open lip schizencephaly at 31 weeks (arrow).

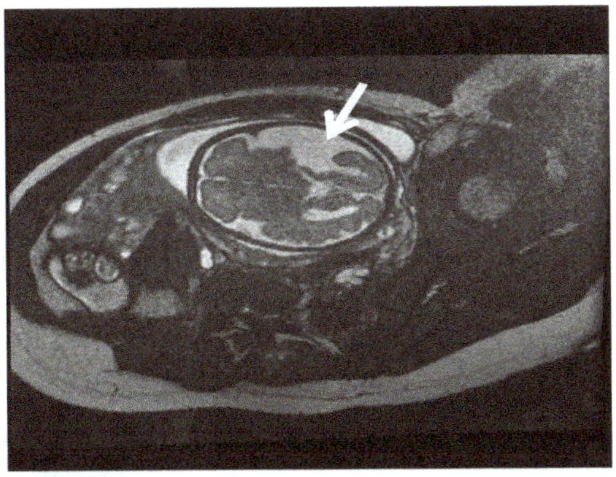

**FIGURE 2.15C** Magnetic resonance image of open lip schizencephaly at 31 weeks (arrow).

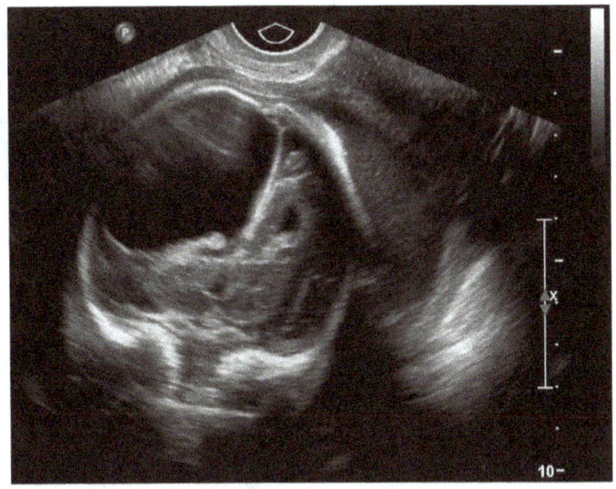

**FIGURE 2.15D** Ultrasound of open lip schizencephaly at 27 weeks.

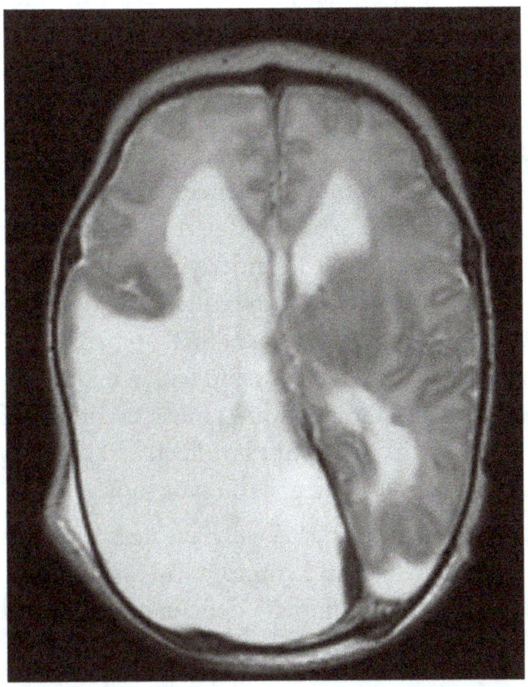

**FIGURE 2.15E** Magnetic resonance image of open lip schizencephaly at 27 weeks.

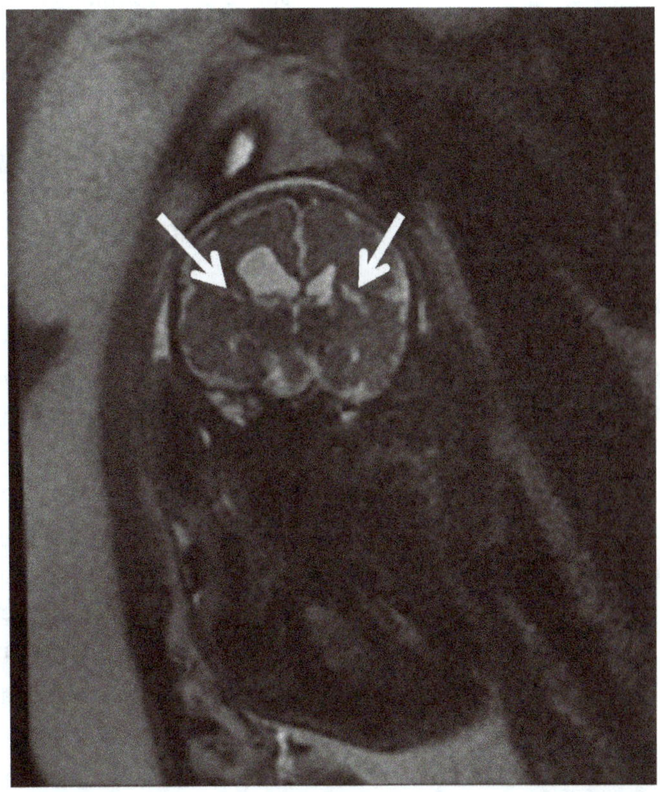

**FIGURE 2.15F** Magnetic resonance image of closed lip schizencephaly (arrows) at 34 weeks.

# 2.16 SPINA BIFIDA (MYELOMENINGOCELE)

## EPIDEMIOLOGY/GENETICS

**Definition** Myelomeningocele, the most common type of neural tube defect, is defined by (1) protrusion of neural elements or meninges through open vertebral arches and (2) associated neurologic deficits.

**Epidemiology** The incidence is very geography and population dependent and ranges from about 1 in 500 to 1 in 2000 births in the United States (M1:F>1).

**Embryology** Meningomyeloceles result from the failure of the vertebral arches to close prior to the sixth week of pregnancy. The location of the defect is most commonly lumbar (75%), followed by sacral (15%), thoracic (9%), and cervical (1%). Hydrocephalus due to an Arnold-Chiari malformation occurs postnatally in 90% of patients. The incidence is lower prenatally, but increases following closure of the lesion. Genitourinary tract and cardiac abnormalities are the most frequently associated malformations. Although most myelomeningoceles are isolated abnormalities, more than 25 genetic, sporadic, and chromosomal multiple malformation syndromes have been described, including trisomy 18.

**Inheritance Patterns** Isolated defects are due to multifactorial inheritance, with a combination of genetic and environmental influences. The risk of recurrence after one affected pregnancy is about 2% to 3%. If part of an underlying genetic syndrome, the recurrence risk is that of the underlying syndrome. Folic acid supplementation (400 μg/d) prior to conception reduces the risk of isolated spina bifida by 60%-70% but has no effect on cases that are part of a genetic syndrome. For women who have had a prior child with a neural tube defect, the folic acid recommendation is 4.0 mg/d for 1 month before and for the first 3 months of pregnancy. Folic acid would not be effective if the previous affected pregnancy was because of an underlying genetic syndrome.

**Teratogens** Of fetuses exposed to valproic acid, 1% will have neural tube defects. Folic acid antagonists (methotrexate and aminopterin), vitamin A, thalidomide, maternal diabetes, hyperthermia, and folate deficiency also have been associated with an increased risk for neural tube defects.

**Screening** Maternal serum α-fetoprotein screening will detect approximately 80% of meningomyeloceles.

**Prognosis** Prognosis depends on the size and location of the defect and the presence of associated abnormalities. In simple isolated defects, there is a 10% risk for developmental delay. Modern surgical and medical treatment has resulted in better long-term function, but urinary tract and orthopedic disability are common long-term problems.

## SONOGRAPHY

### FREQUENT FINDINGS

- Cerebellar compression
  - Banana sign: cerebellum curves with the contour of the calvarium

- Small/absent cisterna magna
- Scalloping of the frontal bones (lemon sign)
- Ventriculomegaly
  - Atrial width 10 mm or more
- Splayed ossification centers

### LESS FREQUENT

- Kyphoscoliosis
- Absent leg movement
  - Limb atrophy
- Clubfoot
- First trimester: midsagittal plane: absent fourth ventricle
- Diastematomyelia (split-cord malformation)

### KEY FINDINGS/PITFALLS

- The scalloping of the frontal bone is first detected at 12 weeks' gestation.
- The "cerebellar" sign of an absent posterior fossa and "banana" cerebellum are first detected around 13 weeks, 4 days.
- The spinal canal may be exposed or covered by a thin membranous sac.
- The second-trimester sonographic detection rate with a thorough evaluation of the calvarium, cerebellum, and spine is greater than 95%.
- Diastematomyelia refers to a division of the spinal cord into two columns by a fibrous, cartilaginous, or bony mass anterior to the vertebral body. The posterior ossification centers of the vertebral column are widened at this level. Of the spinal cord clefts, 80% occur at the lower thoracic or upper lumbar regions.
- Three-dimensional ultrasound can be utilized to optimize imaging of a spinal defect.
- The pathologic level of a spinal defect can accurately be determined by antenatal sonography.

## PREGNANCY MANAGEMENT

**Investigations and Consultations Required** A careful history should be taken that includes a family history; maternal drug exposures; maternal illnesses (diabetes mellitus, seizure disorder, etc.); and medications. An amniocentesis will confirm the ultrasound diagnosis by elevated amniotic fluid α-fetoprotein and positive acetylcholinesterase. Although this is no longer considered a requirement to make the diagnosis if the ultrasound is definitive, this will also allow chromosome analysis. Karyotyping, and microarray analysis, should be performed, particularly if fetal intervention is considered. Congenital heart defects are commonly associated with underlying conditions, such as maternal diabetes; therefore, fetal echocardiography should be a part of the initial evaluation. Consultation with a neurosurgeon and a developmental pediatrician will prepare the family for the multidisciplinary approach necessary for the most favorable outcome in their child.

**Fetal Intervention** Several large centers and a large multidisciplinary study have reported success with in utero fetal repair in cases of isolated meningomyelocele. Outcomes for neonates, including need for early shunt placement and mental and motor development in early childhood, are improved with in utero repair. Longer term outcomes are not yet available, and maternal morbidity is substantial. Fetal risks associated with prematurity are more common with invasive in utero surgery. There are careful selection criteria for intervention, and as such, this is not an option in many cases. Nonetheless, evaluation of patients for this potential treatment should be undertaken, and patients apprised of this option. Parents should have extensive counseling regarding risks and benefits before referral to a center with expertise in fetal surgery.

**Monitoring** If in utero surgery is performed, special monitoring may be suggested by the surgery group. In cases managed expectantly, ventriculomegaly may increase in severity, and ultrasonographic monitoring is recommended. In addition, follow-up ultrasound may be used to exclude other comorbidities, such as growth delay, and to monitor head size. At the time of these examinations, lower leg movements and the presence or absence of clubfeet can be examined. Otherwise, few pregnancy complications are expected, and pregnancy management should be unchanged.

**Pregnancy Termination Issues** If chromosome studies can be completed on abortus material and no associated anomalies are seen by ultrasonography, suction dilation and evacuation procedures are appropriate.

**Delivery** Mode of delivery can be vaginal if the head is of relatively normal size and the fetus is in a vertex presentation. Macrocephaly and breech presentation are common and often require cesarean section. Delivery should occur in a center where appropriate neonatal and neurologic services are available.

## NEONATOLOGY

**Resuscitation** Nonselective management describes the practice of providing full surgical and medical intervention for all patients and is the standard of care in the United States for infants with myelomeningocele. At the time of delivery, the lesion should be briefly assessed to note its location and size. Sterile nonlatex gloves should be used to minimize the risk of latex sensitization. The defect is then covered with a sterile saline-soaked dressing to prevent heat loss and prevent infection. Larger lesions may require coverage with a plastic wrap. The infant should be placed in the prone or lateral position to avoid placing pressure on the lesion.

**Transport** Referral to a tertiary center for management with a multidisciplinary team, including neonatology, pediatric neurology, neurosurgery, urology, and orthopedics, is always indicated. Protection of the lesion, as described previously, during transport is essential.

**Testing and Confirmation** The first priority is the complete assessment of the infant to identify all abnormalities and determine severity of dysfunction. This should include thorough neurologic examination, cranial imaging to detect the likely hydrocephalus due to the associated Chiari type II malformation, and evaluation for other organ system anomalies. Common associated anomalies include cardiac defects, renal anomalies, gastrointestinal tract anomalies, clubfeet, kyphosis, and congenital hip dysplasia.

**Nursery Management** Surgical closure of the defect should occur preferably within 72 hours after birth. Broad-spectrum antibiotic therapy is instituted until surgical closure to reduce the risk of CNS infection. Following closure of the defect, the three primary management issues, depending on the location and extent of the spinal defect, are

- concomitant hydrocephalus in about 90% of infants, requiring placement of a VP shunt;
- urinary tract structural and functional abnormalities; and
- orthopedic deformities and dysfunction.

All require management by the appropriate subspecialties. Referral to a spina bifida clinic at a tertiary center is recommended. Most individuals with myelomeningocele will have intelligence within the normal range, but almost all experience significant learning disabilities.

## SUGGESTED READINGS

1. Adzick NS: Fetal surgery for spina bifida: past, present, future. Semin Pediatr Surg 2013; 22:10-17.
2. Adzick NS, Thom EA, Spong CY, et al: A randomized trial of prenatal versus postnatal repair of myelomeningocele. N Engl J Med 2011; 364:993-1004.
3. Blaas H-G, Eik-Nes SH, Isaksen CV: The detection of spina bifida before 10 gestational weeks using two- and three-dimensional ultrasound. Ultrasound Obstet Gynecol 2000; 16:25-29.
4. Chaoui R, Benoit G, Mitkowska-Wozniak H, et al: Assessment of intracranial translucencey (IT) in the detection of spina bifida at the 11-13 week scan. Ultrasound Obstet Gynecol 2009; 34:249-252.
5. Cohen AR, Couto J, Cummings JJ, et al: Position statement on fetal myelomeningocele repair. Am J Obstet Gynecol 2014; 210:107-111.
6. Copp AJ, Brook FA, Estibeiro JP, et al: The embryonic development of mammalian neural tube defects. Prog Neurobiol 1990; 35:363-403.
7. Kullias SS, Goldstein RB, Cogen PH, Filly RA: Prenatally detected myelomeningoceles: sonographic accuracy in estimation of the spinal level. Radiology 1992; 185:109-112.
8. Lindquist B, Persson EK, Uvebrant P, Carlsson G: Learning, memory, and executive functions in children with hydrocephalus. Acta Paediatr 2008; 97:596-601.
9. Lumley J, Watson M, Bower C: Periconceptional supplementation with folate and/or multivitamins for preventing neural tube defects. Cochrane Database Syst Rev 2001; (3):CD001056.
10. McLone DG: Care of the neonate with a myelomeningocele. Neurosurg Clin N Am 1998; 9:111-120.
11. Nicolaides KH, Gebbe SG, Campbell S, Guidetti R: Ultrasound screening for spina bifida: cranial and cerebellum signs. Lancet 1986; 2:72-74.

12. Sonigo-Cohen P, Schmit P, Zerah M, Chat L, et al: Prenatal diagnosis of diastematomyelia. Childs Nerv Syst 2003; 19:555-560.

13. Van den Hof MC, Nicolaides KH, Campbell J, Campbell S: Evaluation of the lemon and banana signs in one hundred thirty fetuses with an open spina bifida. Am J Obstet Gynecol 1990; 162:332-337.

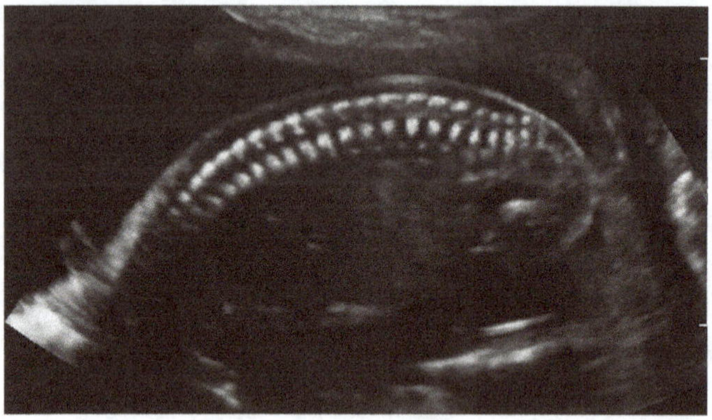

**FIGURE 2.16A** Normal fetal spine.

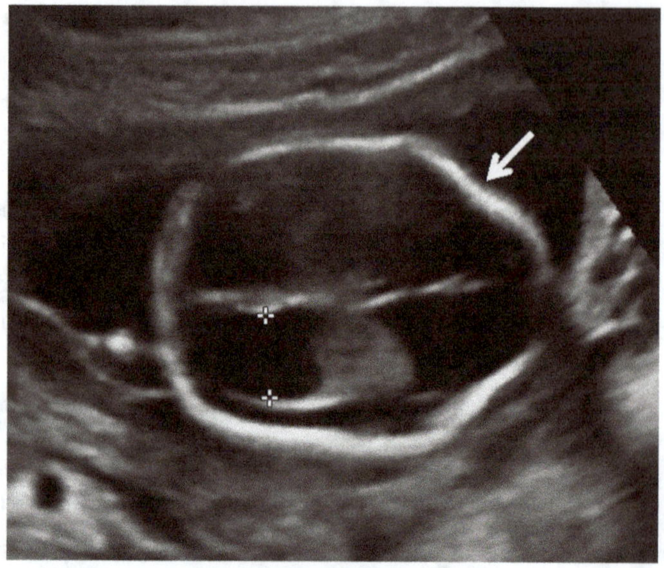

**FIGURE 2.16B** "Lemon sign": scalloping anterior calvarium (arrow) and ventriculomegaly (+ … +).

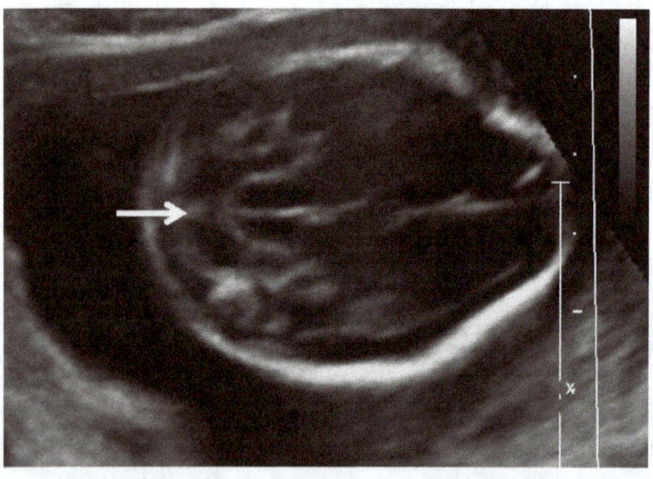

**FIGURE 2.16C** Absent cisterna magna; "banana" cerebellum (arrow).

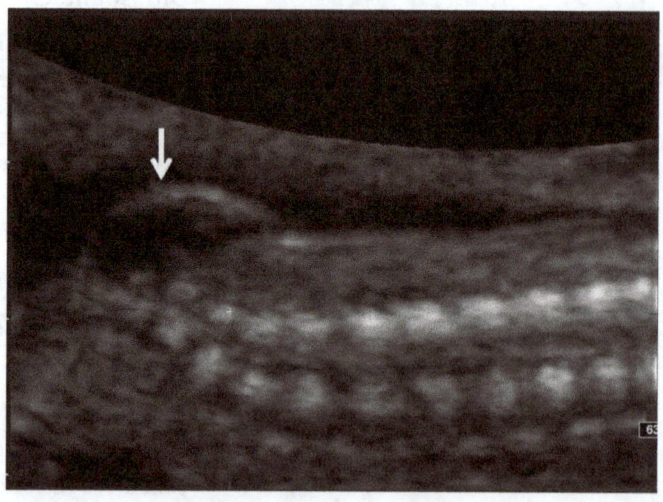

**FIGURE 2.16D** Sacral meningocele (arrow).

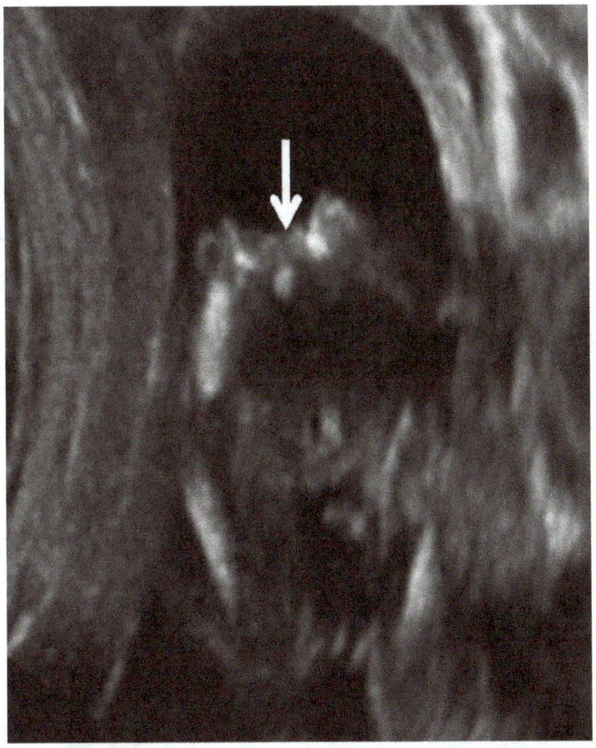

**FIGURE 2.16E** Open spina bifida illustrating splaying of the posterior facets (arrow).

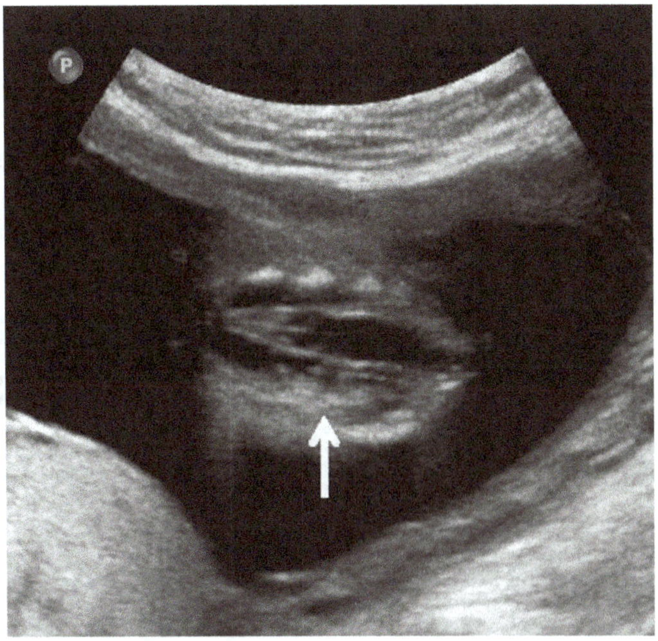


**FIGURE 2.16F** Coronal view of a spinal defect (arrow).

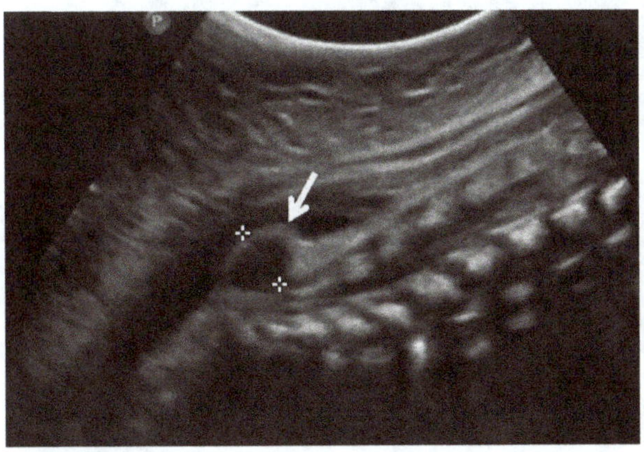


**FIGURE 2.16G** Closed spina bifida (+ … +). Note the skin covering (arrow) of the defect.

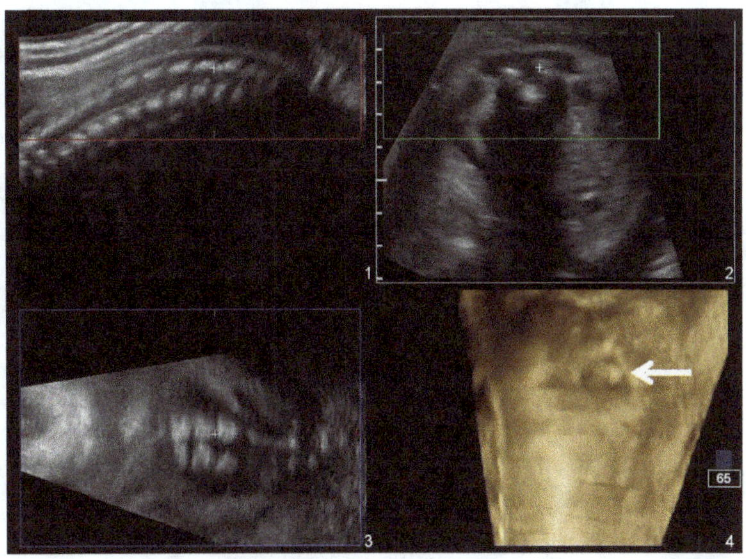


**FIGURE 2.16H** Three-dimensional image taken after in utero spinal repair (arrow).

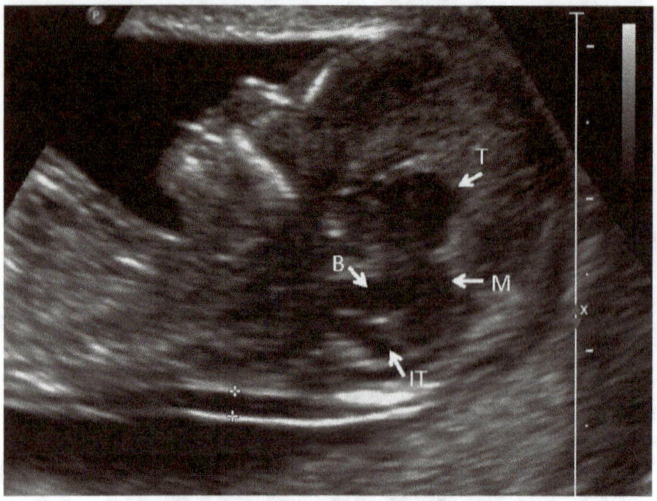


**FIGURE 2.16I** Normal first-trimester intracranial anatomy: midsagittal (I) thalamus (T); midbrain (M); brainstem (B); fourth ventricle (IT).

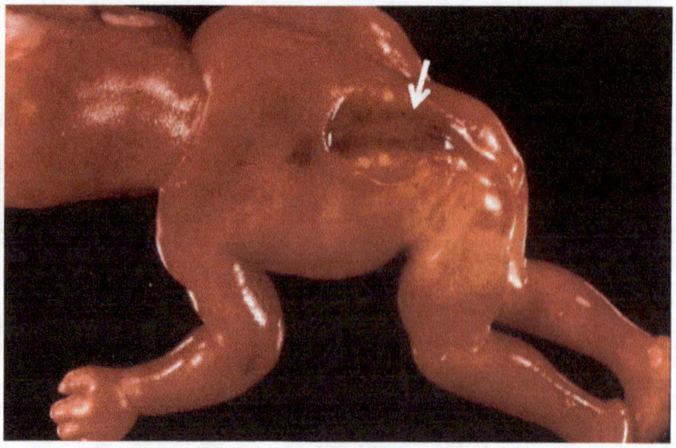

**FIGURE 2.16J** Fetus with open spina bifida (arrow) and spinal kyphoscoliosis.

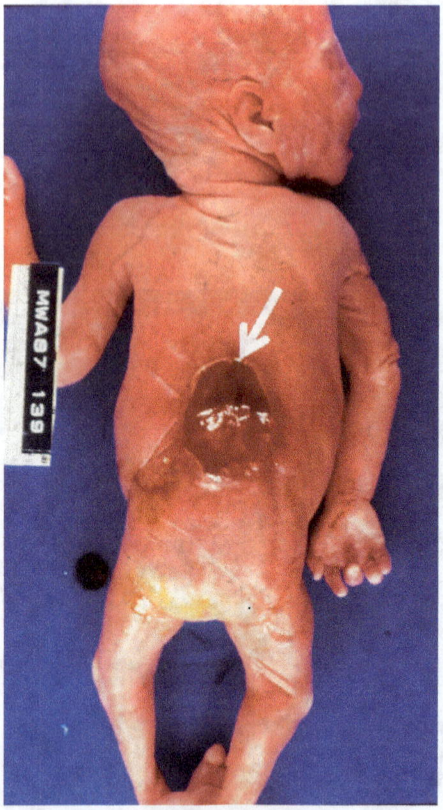

**FIGURE 2.16K** Fetus with a lumbar myelomeningocele (arrow).

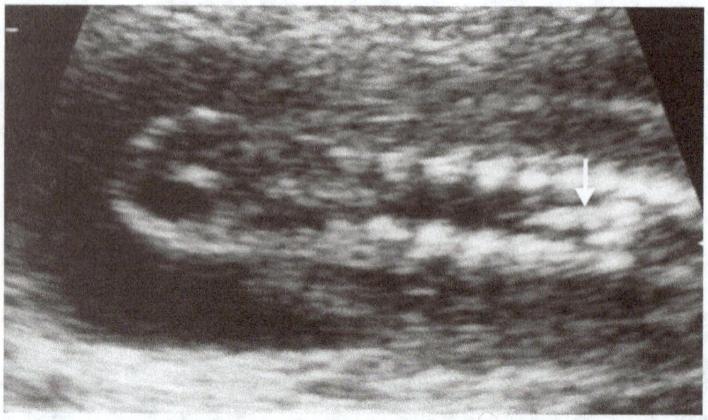

**FIGURE 2.16L** Diastematomyelia: central bony spicule (arrow).

# 2.17 VENTRICULOMEGALY

## EPIDEMIOLOGY/GENETICS

**Definition** Ventriculomegaly is not a specific diagnosis but a term describing a lateral ventricle greater than 10 mm at any gestational age in the second or third trimester. Hydrocephalus refers to a dilated ventricular system due to increased CSF pressure. Because CSF pressure is not measured in utero, ventriculomegaly is the preferred antenatal term.

**Epidemiology** Incidence of ventriculomegaly at 18-24 weeks' gestation is 7.8/10,000 live births.

**Embryology** The increase in ventricular size can be due to obstruction, loss of cerebral tissue, or underdevelopment of the cerebral hemispheres. Therefore, the etiology is heterogeneous and includes chromosomal abnormalities, genetic syndromes, hemorrhage, and infections. One of the most common causes is the presence of a myelomeningocele. A lateral ventricular measurement between 10 and 12 mm is associated with a 3.7% rate of an abnormal karyotype, with trisomy 21 the most common karyotypic abnormality. Additional structural anomalies are associated with ventriculomegaly in 40%-80% of cases, with CNS and cardiac the most common.

**Inheritance Patterns** Inheritance patterns are dependent on the underlying etiology.

**Teratogens** Congenital infections are teratogenic.

**Prognosis** Prognosis depends on the underlying cause of the ventriculomegaly and associated abnormalities. When the karyotype is normal and the ventriculomegaly apparently isolated, there is an approximately 10%-15% incidence of developmental delay. The size of the ventricles does not correlate with the likelihood of developmental delay.

## SONOGRAPHY

### FREQUENT FINDINGS

- Lateral ventricle greater than 10 mm at the level of the atria
- "Dangling" choroid plexus
- Intact interhemispheric fissure

### KEY FINDINGS/PITFALLS

- Errors in measurement of the lateral ventricle:
  - Measuring at the wrong portion of the lateral ventricle.
  - Measuring obliquely rather than perpendicular to the long axis of the lateral ventricle.
  - Measuring the lateral ventricle outer-to-outer border rather than from the internal borders of the lateral ventricle.
  - The false-positive rate for ventriculomegaly (incorrect measurement) is 15%.

- The 10-mm upper limit of normal for a lateral ventricular measurement is clinically, rather than statistically, based.
- A lateral ventricle measurement of 10 mm is between the third and fourth standard deviation above the mean.

| Ventriculomegaly Lateral Ventricle (mm) |
|---|
| Mild 10-12 |
| Moderate 13-15 |
| Severe >15 |

- Of cases with mild second-trimester ventriculomegaly, 60% resolve by term.
- Prenatal MRI has been shown to detect additional brain abnormalities in 5%-17% of cases of "isolated" ventriculomegaly based on antenatal sonography.
- Three-dimensional ultrasound can be used to reconstruct the brain in three planes: sagittal, coronal, and axial. This technique can help to assess both lateral ventricles.
- A major pitfall is pseudoventriculomegaly. In the second trimester, the brain parenchyma is hypoechoic and may be confused with ventriculomegaly. In the absence of ventriculomegaly, the choroid plexus remains parallel to the lateral border of the lateral ventricle; that is, there is an absence of a dangling choroid.

## PREGNANCY MANAGEMENT

**Investigations and Consultations Required** Ventriculomegaly initially may present in mild or severe forms and has a wide spectrum of outcomes, but the initial evaluation and testing are similar in all cases. Many cases of ventriculomegaly are part of a syndrome, and steps to determine whether a given case is isolated or syndromic are warranted. A careful history should be taken, including family history, maternal drug or environmental exposures, maternal illnesses and medications, radiation exposure, and other risk factors for possible underlying etiologies. Chromosome evaluation with microarray testing and viral studies (both maternal serum and amniotic fluid) should be performed. Fetal echocardiography should be a part of the initial evaluation. If local expertise with fetal MRI is available, a fetal MRI may be useful to delineate the CNS anatomy and to look for associated CNS pathology. Prenatal consultations with a multidisciplinary team, including neurology and neonatology, may be helpful, depending on the etiology determined with the antenatal evaluation.

**Monitoring** There are no specific needs beyond usual obstetrical care. Repeat sonographic studies every 4 weeks are helpful to monitor the ventriculomegaly, as both progression and resolution are common.

**Pregnancy Course** There are no specific obstetric complications expected. However, because of the multiple potential etiologies of ventriculomegaly, a specific etiology may result in an obstetric complication. For example, the onset of polyhydramnios may result in preterm labor. Similarly, the development of severe ventriculomegaly with macrocephaly could affect delivery options.

**Pregnancy Termination Issues** If a diagnosis has not been established, a nondestructive procedure should be performed, and a careful external examination of the fetus should be performed by a pathologist, with special expertise in fetal dysmorphology.

**Delivery** Delivery at a tertiary center is appropriate if a precise diagnosis has not been made prenatally. Special care and evaluation may be necessary following birth.

## NEONATOLOGY

**Resuscitation** No specific measures are required with isolated mild-to-moderate ventriculomegaly. However, when ventriculomegaly is associated with the confirmed antenatal diagnosis of a lethal chromosomal anomaly or a severe neuroanatomical abnormality, a predelivery discussion should be undertaken with the family about nonintervention in the event that spontaneous onset of respiration does not occur.

**Transport** Transport to a tertiary center with neonatology, pediatric neurology, and pediatric neurosurgery is indicated for further evaluation and treatment.

**Testing and Confirmation** The first priority is the complete assessment of the infant to identify any other associated abnormalities. This should include a thorough neurologic examination, cranial imaging to distinguish noncommunicating from communicating hydrocephalus, and evaluation for other organ system anomalies. The diagnosis can be confirmed by head ultrasound, MRI, or CT scan. While the hydrocephalus may be isolated, common associated anomalies include cardiac anomalies, neural tube defects, chromosomal abnormalities, genetic syndromes, intraventricular hemorrhage, and congenital infection.

**Surgery Management** In the majority of cases, the hydrocephalus will progress if the hydrocephalus is not effectively treated by placement of a ventriculoperitoneal (VP) shunt or endoscopic third ventriculostomy (ETV). An ETV is typically employed in the treatment of pure noncommunicating hydrocephalus. Ventriculoperitoneal shunting is used for patients with communicating hydrocephalus or for those in whom ETV is not successful. In cases of hydrocephalus with both communicating and noncommunicating components, the outcome of ETV is inconsistent. Long-term neurodevelopment follow-up is indicated due to the increased incidence of developmental delay.

### SUGGESTED READINGS

1. Almog B, Gamzu R, Achiron R, et al: Fetal lateral ventricular width: what should be its upper limit? A prospective cohort study and reanalysis of the current and previous data. J Ultrasound Med 2003; 22:39-43.
2. Cardoza JD, Goldstein RB, Filly RA: Exclusion of fetal ventriculomegaly with a single measurement: the width of lateral ventricular atrium. Radiology 1988; 169:711-714.
3. Correa FF, Lara C, Bellver J, et al: Examination of the fetal brain by transabdominal three-dimensional ultrasound: potential for routine neurosonographic studies. Ultrasound Obstet Gynecol 2006; 27:503-508.

4. Griffiths PD, Reeves MJ, Morris JE, et al: A prospective study of fetuses with isolated ventriculomegaly investigated by antenatal sonography and in utero MR imaging. Am J Neuroradiol 2010; 31:106-111.
5. Heiserman J, Filly RA, Goldstein RB: The effect of measurement errors on the sonographic evaluation of ventriculomegaly. J Ultrasound Med 1991; 10:121-124.
6. Melchiorre K, Bhide A, Gika AD, et al: Counseling in isolated fetal ventriculomegaly. Ultrasound Obstet Gynecol 2009; 34:212-224.
7. Nicolaides KH, Berry S, Snijders RJM, et al: Fetal lateral cerebral ventriculomegaly: associated malformations and chromosomal defects. Fetal Diagn Ther 1990; 5:5-14.
8. Nyberg DA, Mack LA, Hirsch J, et al: Fetal hydrocephalus: sonographic detection and clinical significance of associated anomalies. Radiology 1987; 163:187-191.
9. Salamon LJ, Ouahbe J, Delezoide AL, et al: Third-trimester fetal MRI in isolated 10-to-12 mm ventriculomegaly: is it worth it? Br J Obstet Gynaecol 2006; 113:942-947.
10. Sethna F, Tennant PWG, Rankin J, Robson SC: Prevalence, natural history, and clinical outcome of mild to moderate ventriculomegaly. Obstet Gynecol 2011; 117:867-876.
11. Signorelli M, Tiberti A, Valsariati D, et al: Width of the fetal lateral ventricular atrium between 10 and 12 mm: a simple variation of the norm? Ultrasound Obstet Gynecol 2004; 23:14-18.

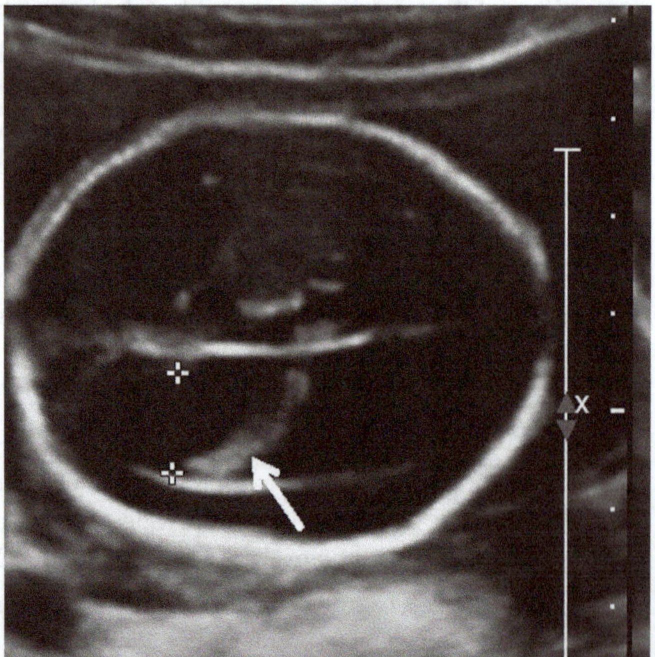

FIGURE 2.17A Moderate ventriculomegaly (+ … +); dangling choroid (arrow).

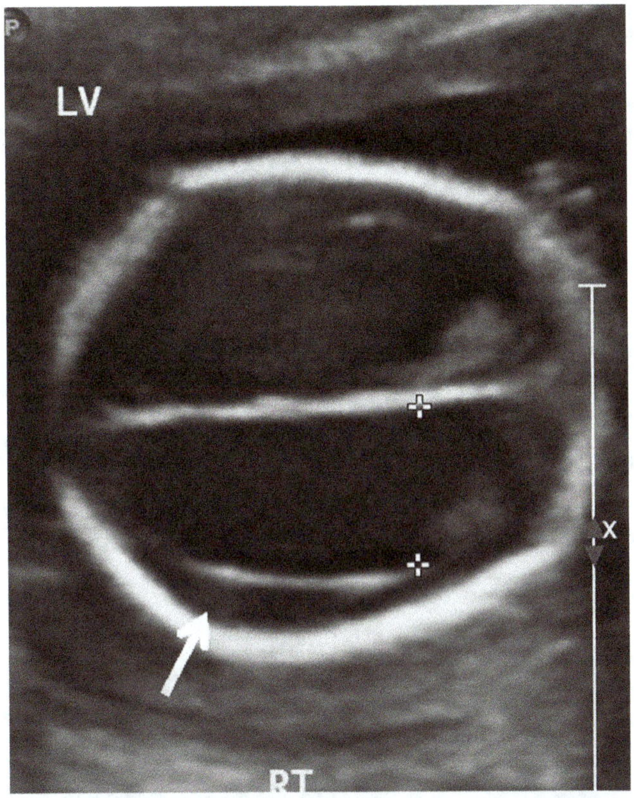


**FIGURE 2.17B** Ventriculomegaly (+ … +) illustrating residual cerebral mantle (arrow).

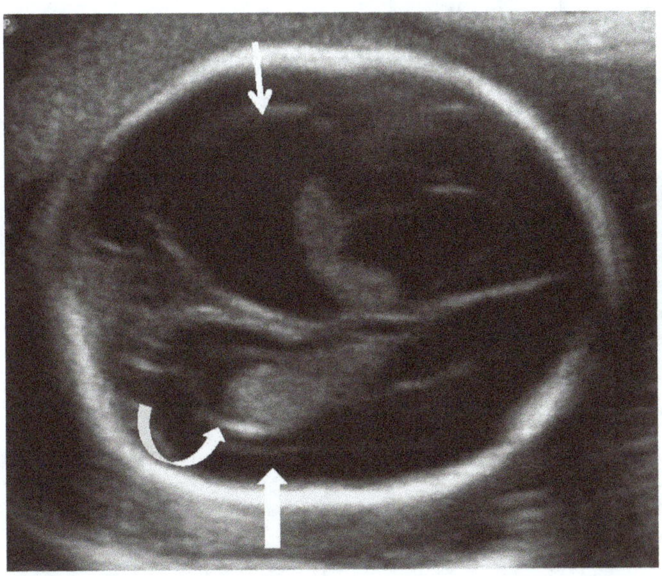

**FIGURE 2.17C** Unilateral ventriculomegaly (straight arrow); normal ventricle (curved arrow); hypoechoic brain (broad arrow).

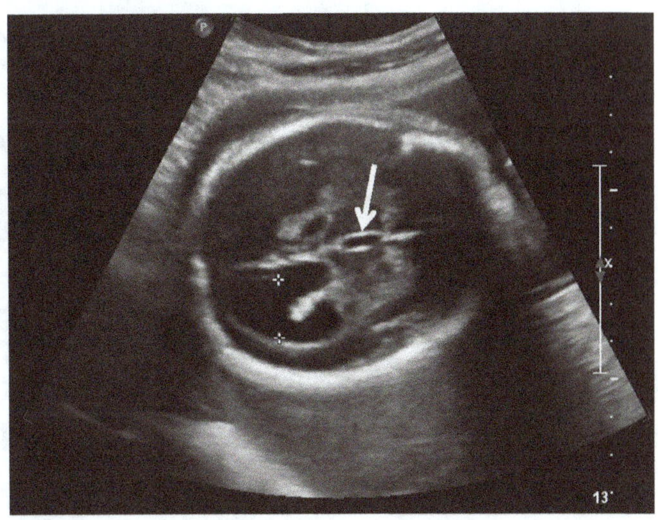


**FIGURE 2.17D** Ventriculomegaly (+ … +) with a dilated third ventricle (arrow).

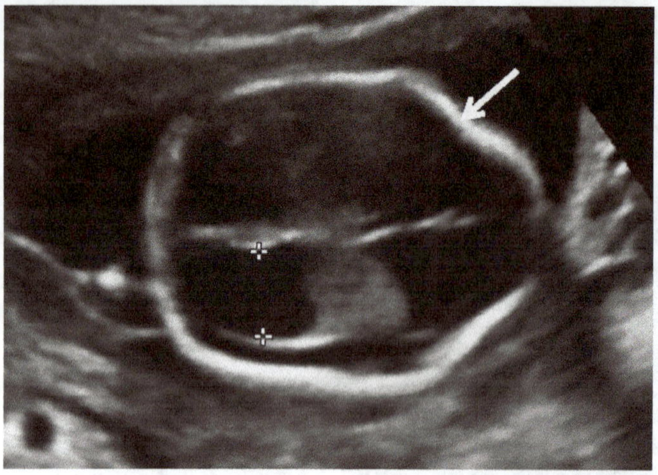

**FIGURE 2.17E** Mild ventriculomegaly due to spina bifida. Note the lemon-shape calvarium (arrow).

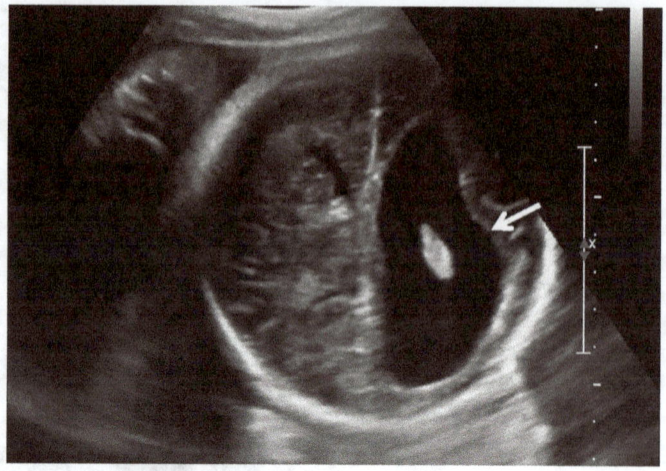

**FIGURE 2.17F** Unilaterally enlarged ventricle (arrow) due to compression by arachnoid cyst.

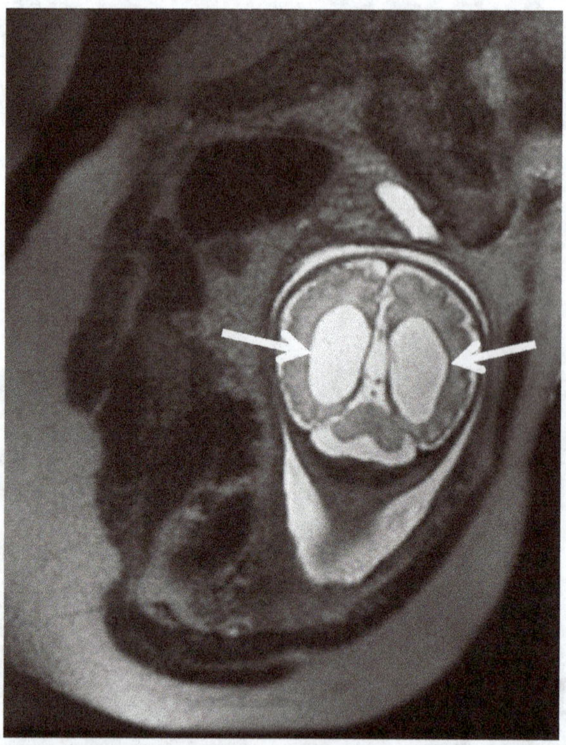

**FIGURE 2.17G** Fetal MRI showing ventriculomegaly (arrows).

# CHAPTER 3

# CARDIAC ENTITIES

# 3.1 AORTIC COARCTATION

## EPIDEMIOLOGY/GENETICS

**Definition** Aortic coarctation (AC) is a narrowing of the aorta; greater than 90% occur between the left subclavian artery and the ductus arteriosus (aortic isthmus). The most severe form of AC is complete interruption of the aortic arch, with most interruptions occurring between the left carotid artery and the left subclavian artery.

**Epidemiology** The prevalence is 0.6 per 1000 live births and has a M2:F1 ratio. AC accounts for 7% of all congenital cardiac disease. Of AC, 32% are isolated, while the remaining 68% have additional anomalies, including cardiovascular (24%), genitourinary (20%), central nervous system (12%), and skeletal (6%) anomalies.

**Embryology** There are two theories to explain the different types of AC. A preductal AC is theorized to result from decreased blood flow through the left ventricle and aorta leading to impaired growth of the isthmus. A ductal, or postductal, AC is suspected to result from ductal tissue present around the posterior aspect of the proximal descending aorta. This tissue constricts along with the ductus, causing aortic constriction.

**Inheritance Pattern** The inheritance pattern is thought to be polygenic. There is a strong association with monosomy X (Turner syndrome). At least 5% of girls with coarctation may be found to have monosomy X; thus, the prevalence may be higher prenatally. The recurrence risk for isolated coarctation is 2% when one sibling is affected and 6% when two siblings are affected. The recurrence risk for congenital heart defects in offspring given one affected parent is 4% when the mother is affected and 2% when the father is affected. Coarctation also occurs in mosaic trisomy 16, DiGeorge syndrome (deletion 22q), Noonan syndrome, and many other syndromes.

**Teratogens** Maternal diabetes mellitus.

**Prognosis** With isolated coarctation of the aorta, surgical management generally results in a good long-term outcome. When coarctation occurs along with other, more complex intracardiac disease, it is often the associated disease that more strongly influences the prognosis. If the AC goes undetected in the newborn, severe heart failure and acidosis can occur.

## SONOGRAPHY

### FINDINGS

- Ultrasound identification of a discrete narrowing of the aortic arch is limited due to compensation from the ductus arteriosus.
- Indirect signs of AC can lead to a very strong suspicion in the mid-second and early third trimester. These include the following:
  - Discrepant ventricular size with the right larger than the left. This finding is more useful in the second compared to the third trimester.

  - The ratio of the diameter of the ascending aorta to the diameter of the main pulmonary artery is a helpful clue to AC, with a normal ratio being 1.25. One study found that AC was associated with a ratio greater than 2.
  - At 14 to 16 weeks, a significant discrepancy between a large ductus arteriosus and a smaller aorta may be seen.
  - Left-to-right flow across the atrial septum occurs in AC when the left heart is significantly hypoplastic and may be a marker for a ductal-dependent lesion.
- Ventricular septal defects (VSDs) are present in approximately 50% of patients.
  - When there is a posterior misalignment type of defect, there is often critical arch obstruction or even an interrupted aortic arch.
  - In a posterior misalignment type of defect, the conal septum is deviated posteriorly under the aortic valve, resulting in a VSD with subaortic stenosis.
- Other morphologic abnormalities of the left heart are common in coarctation.
  - The aortic valve is abnormal in approximately 60% of infants, with a bicuspid valve the most common. Color and pulse Doppler interrogation of the aortic valve may show accelerated flow if there is significant stenosis.
  - On detailed fetal echocardiography, closely spaced papillary muscles or a single left ventricular papillary muscle (a "parachute" mitral valve) may be detected. This is recognized in short-axis scans of the left ventricle.
- A left superior vena cava is present in approximately 18% of patients with AC.
- An increased nuchal translucency is frequently identified at 11 to 14 weeks.
- Fetal echocardiography can diagnose AC when it is severe, but the test has weak sensitivity, particularly with mild AC.

### KEY FINDINGS/PITFALLS

- One needs to realize the inadequacy of prenatal echocardiography in reliably predicting all cases of AC.
- The severity of left heart hypoplasia can progress during the second and third trimester. If there is a family history of left-sided disease, such as hypoplastic left heart syndrome (HLHS), valvular aortic stenosis, or AC, it is wise to reexamine the fetus at 28 weeks, even if the initial study results are normal.

### DIFFERENTIAL DIAGNOSIS

- AC needs to be distinguished from interrupted aortic arch. Most commonly, interruptions occur between the left carotid and left subclavian arteries.

## PREGNANCY MANAGEMENT

**Investigations and Consultations Required** Karyotype analysis (with microarray for the chromosome 22q deletion) should be considered when AC or interrupted aortic arch is suspected because of the association with Turner syndrome and DiGeorge syndrome. With interrupted aortic arch, chromosome 22q deletion may be present in more than 50% of patients. In this situation, the interruption is most often between the left common carotid artery and left subclavian artery. A complete fetal survey is indicated. The family should meet with a pediatric cardiologist to discuss the cardiac findings and to coordinate a prenatal and postnatal management plan.

**Pregnancy Course** Generally, the pregnancy course is routine.

**Fetal Intervention** No fetal intervention is available.

**Pregnancy Termination Issues** If termination is chosen, an intact fetus is necessary to confirm the cardiac findings and to assess for other noncardiac abnormalities.

**Monitoring** No special fetal monitoring is usually required. Follow-up fetal echocardiography should be performed in the third trimester to confirm the diagnosis and discuss delivery plans.

**Delivery** Delivery should occur at a tertiary care center where prostaglandin $E_1$ therapy can be administered if the lesion is ductus dependent.

## NEONATOLOGY

**Resuscitation** Assistance with respiration is usually not required. However, if there is delay in the spontaneous onset of breathing, oxygen supplementation should be limited to 40% to 60% maximum, and only for the time needed to establish adequate color, to avoid closing the ductus. If a severe coarctation is diagnosed prenatally, therapy with prostaglandin $E_1$ infusion should be started as soon as possible. Coarctation clinically presents after the first few days of life, when the ductus closes. Therefore, infants who are suspected to have AC by antenatal echocardiogram should be closely monitored in the neonatal intensive care unit. If the femoral pulses diminish or there are significant blood pressure changes, then prostaglandin $E_1$ can be started, even before echo confirmation.

**Transport** Immediate transport to a tertiary center with neonatology and pediatric cardiac diagnostic and surgical capabilities is essential for infants with AC with congestive heart failure (CHF), low cardiac output, or evidence of ductus-dependent systemic perfusion. Consultation with a pediatric cardiologist prior to transport to determine appropriate supportive measures is indicated. Management during transport should be by personnel experienced in neonatal transport with capability for mechanical ventilation and delivery of cardiotonic infusions.

**Testing and Confirmation** AC should be considered when lower-extremity pulses are decreased or when there is a gradient of more than 10 mm Hg between upper and lower extremity systolic blood pressures. Oxygen saturation of 94% or less in the lower extremity is suggestive of right-to-left shunting at the ductal level, which can occur in severe arch obstruction. Echocardiography should be definitive in making the diagnosis of coarctation.

**Nursery Management** Babies with a suspicion of AC prenatally should not go home until the echo shows the ductus arteriosus has closed and the arch is normal. In infants with AC, the goal of initial neonatal management is to achieve and sustain a balance between pulmonary and systemic blood flow by maintaining patency of the ductus and a pulmonary-to-systemic shunt across the ductus that can provide adequate perfusion to the lower body, particularly the liver and kidneys. Hyperventilation and supplemental oxygen decrease pulmonary resistance and thereby alter the direction and magnitude of ductal, or intracardiac, shunting through associated lesions. Both should be avoided. Acidosis should be treated aggressively with buffer. Dopamine infusion may be needed to improve cardiac output and renal perfusion. Limiting organ damage from inadequate perfusion prior to surgery enhances recovery from surgical repair.

Developmental follow-up is recommended in infants with critical neonatal coarctation requiring surgery in the first few weeks of life, as they are at risk for developmental delay.

## SURGERY

**Preoperative Assessment** Echocardiography is sufficient for preoperative diagnosis in most cases of AC.

**Operative Indications** Surgery is indicated during the newborn period when the lesion is ductal dependent or when the AC is severe. In less-severe cases of AC, surgery is usually performed after 2 months of age.

**Types of Procedures** One of two procedures can be performed. The AC can be resected and an end-to-end anastomosis performed. An alternative approach is the left subclavian flap plasty procedure in which the proximal left subclavian artery is used to augment the area of coarctation.

**Surgical Results and Prognosis** Operative mortality for AC is less than 5%. Recurrent AC can develop in approximately 10% of patients and is usually successfully treated with balloon angioplasty.

### SUGGESTED READINGS


1. Bronshtein M, Zimmer EZ: Sonographic diagnosis of fetal coarctation of the aorta at 14-16 weeks of gestation. Ultrasound Obstet Gynecol 1998; 11:254-257.
2. Gomez-Montes E, Herraiz I, Mendoza A, et al: Prediction of coarctation of the aorta in the second half of pregnancy. Ultrasound Obstet Gynecol 2013; 41:298-305.
3. Gurwitz A, Rosner J, Narine B, Anderson V: External aortic diameter ratios: a reliable method to diagnose preductal aortic coarctation. Fetal Pediatr Pathol 2011; 30:286-295.
4. Jowett V, Aparicio P, Santhakumaran S, et al: Sonographic predictors of surgery in fetal coarctation of the aorta. Ultrasound Obstet Gynecol 2012; 40:47-54.
5. Kenny D, Hijazi ZM: Coarctation of the aorta: from fetal life to adulthood. Cardiol J 2011; 18:487-495.
6. Matsui H, Mellander M, Roughton M, et al: Morphological and physiological predictors of fetal aortic coarctation. Circulation 2008; 118:1793-1801.
7. Punukollu M, Harnden A, Tulloh R: Coarctation of the aorta in the newborn. BMJ 2011; 343:d6838.

8. Quarello E, Trabbia A: High-definition flow combined with spatiotemporal image correlation in the diagnosis of fetal coarctation of the aorta. Obstet Gynecol 2009; 33:365-367.
9. Sharland GK, Chan KY, Allan LD: Coarctation of the aorta: difficulties in prenatal diagnosis. Br Heart J 1994; 71:70-75.
10. Wiechec M, Knafel A, Nocun A: Prenatal detection of congenital heart defects at the 11- to 13-week scan using a simple color Doppler protocol including the 4-chamber and 3-vessel and trachea views. J Ultrasound Med 2015; 34:585-594.
11. Wong SC, Burgess T, Cheung M, Zacharin M: The prevalence of Turner syndrome in girls presenting with coarctation of the aorta. J Pediatr 2014; 164:259-263.
12. Zhou J, Zhou Q, Zhang M, et al: Echocardiographic follow-up and pregnancy outcome of fetuses with cardiac asymmetry at 18-22 weeks of gestation. Prenat Diagn 2014; 34:900-907.


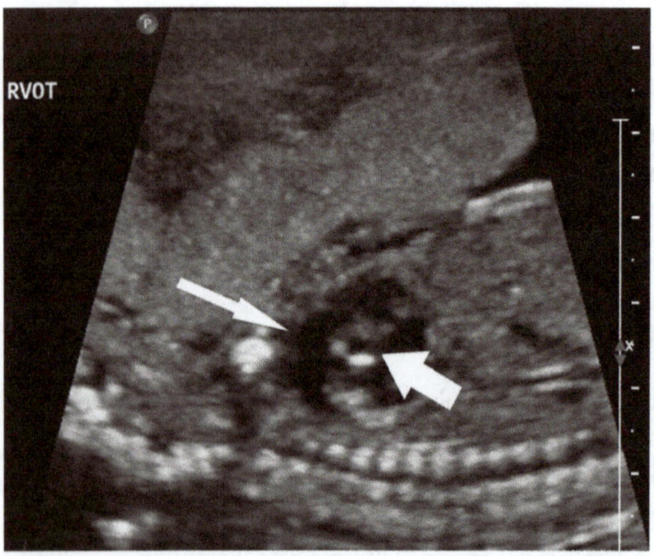


**FIGURE 3.1A** Short-axis view of the great vessels. The aorta (thick arrow) is smaller than the pulmonary artery (thin arrow), suspicious for coarctation.

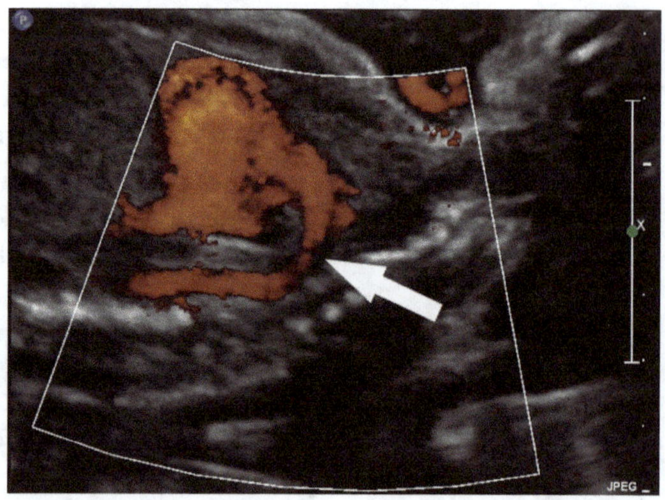


**FIGURE 3.1B** Power Doppler view of the aortic arch demonstrating a narrowing of the isthmus portion (arrow) of the arch consistent with a coarctation.

# 3.2 ATRIOVENTRICULAR SEPTAL DEFECT (ATRIOVENTRICULAR CANAL DEFECTS OR ENDOCARDIAL CUSHION DEFECT)

## EPIDEMIOLOGY/GENETICS

**Definition** Atrioventricular septal defects (AVSDs) include a spectrum of lesions ranging from a complete common atrioventricular (AV) canal to an isolated primum type of atrial septal defect. A **complete** canal defect consists of good-size ventricular and atrial defects associated with a common AV valve. **Intermediate** AVSDs differ from **complete** defects in that there are distinct and separate left AV ("mitral") and right AV ("tricuspid") valves, and any combination of (1) VSD; (2) cleft anterior mitral defect; and (3) cleft septal tricuspid leaflet. An **intermediate** AVSD has anterior and posterior septal bridging leaflets between the two AV valves that are fused over the ventricular septum, giving rise to separate mitral and tricuspid valves. Of the two types of AVSDs described, the **intermediate** type is the most infrequent. AVSDs that are mostly contiguous with one ventricle result in the majority of the blood flow into the ventricle with minimal flow into the opposite ventricle, causing this ventricle to become hypoplastic. This results in an **unbalanced** defect. When there is a **balanced** AVSD, an equal amount of blood enters both ventricular cavities.

**Epidemiology** The prevalence is 0.19 per 1000 live births and accounts for approximately 5% of patients followed with congenital heart disease postnatally. AVSDs are slightly more common in female fetuses (1.3:1), and 60%-70% of these fetuses have a chromosomal abnormality. When complete AVSDs occur as isolated lesions, trisomy 21 is present in 56% to 72% of fetuses. AVSDs also occur, but less commonly, in trisomies 13 and 18, Turner syndrome, and other chromosome abnormalities.

**Embryology** Abnormalities of the AV canal result from malformation in the development of the endocardial cushions. The endocardial cushions are involved in the closure of both the atrial and the ventricular septa and in the development of both AV valves.

**Inheritance Pattern** When isolated, the pattern of inheritance generally appears to be multifactorial; however, a single gene pattern has been suggested in some families. The recurrence risk for congenital heart disease is 3% when one sibling is affected with an endocardial cushion defect and 10% when two siblings are affected. When a parent is affected, the recurrence risk is 14% when the mother is affected and only 1% when the father is affected.

**Teratogens** Maternal diabetes mellitus.

**Prognosis** AVSDs occurring in isolation generally have a good prognosis in terms of the cardiac disease, but surgery is required. When occurrence is associated with chromosomal abnormalities or as a part of a heterotaxy syndrome, the prognosis is frequently poor.

## SONOGRAPHY

### FINDINGS

- An evaluation of the heart can distinguish
  - A complete from an incomplete AVSD
  - The severity of regurgitation of AV valve/valves
  - A balanced from an unbalanced AVSD
- Valve abnormalities are nearly always present with endocardial cushion defects.
  - A common AV valve is well demonstrated in short-axis imaging of the ventricles.
  - In an isolated primum atrial septal defect, the AV valves are separate, but aligned at the same level. Normally, the tricuspid valve is offset slightly toward the apex of the ventricle.
  - Although a cleft mitral valve can be a feature of an intermediate AVSD, it is rarely identified in the fetal period.

### KEY FINDINGS/PITFALLS

- Color Doppler interrogation for AV valve regurgitation is important because the outcome is worse when there is a severely regurgitant AV valve (or valves).
- A comparison of the ventricles provides an initial assessment of the balance of the AVSD.
  - If one ventricle appears hypoplastic, the AVSD is most likely unbalanced.
  - The orientation of the defect over the interventricular septum and color Doppler mapping of blood flow can confirm the diagnosis.
- Increased nuchal translucency is often present at 11 to 14 weeks.
- Transabdominal imaging reveals AVSDs at 16 to 18 weeks, and transvaginal imaging can demonstrate a defect as early as 10 to 14 weeks.
- False dropout can mimic atrial septal defects and VSDs.
  - Imaging in a scan plane perpendicular to the suspected defect and identification of the abnormalities of the AV valve (which are nearly always present in true AVSDs) are important.
  - Cine clips can be used to assess AV valve motion and establish that there is a single large valve.
- Because both are located near the level of the AV valve, a dilated coronary sinus may be easily confused for a primum type of atrial septal defect.
  - The dilated coronary sinus is more posterior (along the posterior AV valve groove) than the primum atrial septal defect, which is located just posterior to the aortic root.
  - Atrioventricular valve abnormalities are also nearly always present in primum defects and are not present with isolated coronary sinus dilation.
  - The most common reason for a dilated coronary sinus is a left superior vena cava.
- An AVSD can occur in the heterotaxy syndrome. Conotruncal abnormalities, such as double-outlet right ventricle (DORV), are frequent in heterotaxy. Therefore, abnormalities of the outflow tracts and venous return should be excluded.

## PREGNANCY MANAGEMENT

**Investigations and Consultations Required** An extended fetal anatomy survey should be completed to assess for additional associated anomalies. A fetal echocardiogram and pediatric cardiology consultation should be obtained to provide prenatal counseling and to help exclude the association of more complex congenital heart disease. Consultation with a geneticist should be obtained. A fetal karyotype and microarray should be performed on amniocytes.

**Pregnancy Course** Unless there are associated anomalies or other congenital heart defects, fetuses with isolated balanced AVSDs do well, and pregnancy complications are not expected. Delivery should be anticipated at term, with cesarean section reserved for the usual obstetrical indications.

**Fetal Intervention** Fetal intervention is not indicated.

**Pregnancy Termination Issues** If termination is chosen, an intact fetus should be delivered for confirming the diagnosis and performing a chromosome analysis with microarray.

**Monitoring** With significant AV valve regurgitation, hydrops may develop. These fetuses are at increased risk for heart block, so monitoring with interval ultrasound examinations is warranted. A follow-up fetal echocardiogram to assess AV valve function in the third trimester is recommended.

**Delivery** A defect that is isolated, balanced, and without regurgitation could be considered for delivery in the patient's community. However, in any fetus with an unbalanced or regurgitant AVSD, delivery should be performed at a center where immediate neonatology and pediatric cardiac consultation is available.

## NEONATOLOGY

**Resuscitation** Assistance with the onset of respiration is usually not required for infants with an isolated defect. In the presence of other defects, particularly those involving the central nervous system or the respiratory tract, spontaneous breathing may be affected and assistance required.

**Transport** Infants with isolated AVSDs do not require referral in the immediate neonatal period.

**Testing and Confirmation** Postnatal diagnosis is confirmed with echocardiography.

**Nursery Management** Mild oxygen desaturation is typical while the pulmonary vascular resistance remains elevated. As the pulmonary resistance falls, the oxygen saturation will gradually increase, there is increased blood flow to the right ventricle, and symptoms of CHF may develop. However, with complete AVSD, resistance takes longer to fall than normal, and CHF does not occur in the immediate newborn period, but later. A significant percentage of these newborns will not drop their resistance. Hence, CHF will not develop. AV valve regurgitation will make failure occur sooner. While failure with a partial AVSD is rare, it may occur if there is significant left AV valve regurgitation.

## SURGERY

**Preoperative Assessment** Echocardiography is usually definitive in assessing AVSDs.

**Operative Indications** Nearly all AVSDs require surgery. Infants with complete AVSDs should undergo elective repair by 4 months of age, earlier if CHF limits growth. Primum atrial septal defects should be closed between 6 and 18 months of age. When there is pulmonary artery hypertension, surgery should take place earlier.

**Types of Procedures** Canal defects are generally approached through a right atriotomy, and septal defects are closed with either a single- or a double-patch technique. The common AV valve is divided at the time of the repair. A pulmonary artery band is sometimes used as a palliative procedure, instead of performing a complete repair to control pulmonary blood flow, when the repair cannot be performed at acceptable risk (i.e., with other more complex lesions or if the patient is too small).

**Surgical Results and Prognosis** Repair of isolated complete AVSD carries a good prognosis, with operative survival in excess of 97%. A minority of patients will have significant AV canal regurgitation postoperatively, and some may require mitral valve replacement or reoperation. There is a less than 5% incidence of postoperative complete heart block, which would require a pacemaker.

### SUGGESTED READINGS


1. Bader RS, Punn R, Silverman NH: Evaluation of risk factors for prediction of outcome in fetal spectrum of atrioventricular septal defects. Congenit Heart Dis 2014; 9:286-293.
2. Beaton AZ, Pike JI, Stallings C, Donofrio MT: Predictors of repair and outcome in prenatally diagnosed atrioventricular septal defects. J Am Soc Echocardiogr 2013; 26:208-216.
3. Calcagni G, Digilio MC, Sarkozy A, et al: Familial recurrence of congenital heart disease: an overview and review of the literature. Eur J Pediatr. 2007; 166:111-116.
4. Craig B: Atrioventricular septal defect: from fetus to adult. Heart 2006; 92:1879-1885.
5. Fesslova V, Villa L, Nava S, et al: Spectrum and outcome of atrioventricular septal defect in fetal life. Cardiol Young 2002; 12:18-26.
6. Friedberg MK, Kim N, Silverman NH: Atrioventricular septal defect recently diagnosed by fetal echocardiography: echocardiographic features, associated anomalies, and outcomes. Congenit Heart Dis 2007; 2:110-114.
7. Hartman RJ, Rasmussen SA, Botto LD, et al: The contribution of chromosomal abnormalities to congenital heart defects: a population-based study. Pediatr Cardiol 2011; 32:1147-1157.
8. Huggon IC, Cook AC, Smeeton NC, et al: Atrioventricular septal defects diagnosed in fetal life: associated cardiac and extra-cardiac abnormalities and outcome. J Am Coll Cardiol 2000; 36:593-601.

9. Langford K, Sharland G, Simpson J: Relative risk of abnormal karyotype in fetuses found to have an atrioventricular septal defect (AVSD) on fetal echocardiography. Prenat Diagn 2005; 25:137-139.
10. Mogra R, Zidere V, Allan LD: Prenatally detectable congenital heart defects in fetuses with Down syndrome. Ultrasound Obstet Gynecol 2011; 38:320-324.
11. Mone F, Walsh C, Mulcahy C, et al: Prenatal detection of structural cardiac defects and presence of associated anomalies: a retrospective observational study of 1262 fetal echocardiograms. Prenat Diagn 2015; 35:577-582.
12. Rasiah SV, Ewer AK, Miller P, et al: Outcome following prenatal diagnosis of complete atrioventricular septal defect. Prenat Diagn 2008; 28:95-101.
13. Yildirim G, Gungorduk K, Yazicioglu F, et al: Prenatal diagnosis of complete atrioventricular septal defect: perinatal and neonatal outcomes. Obstet Gynecol Int 2009; 2009:958496.

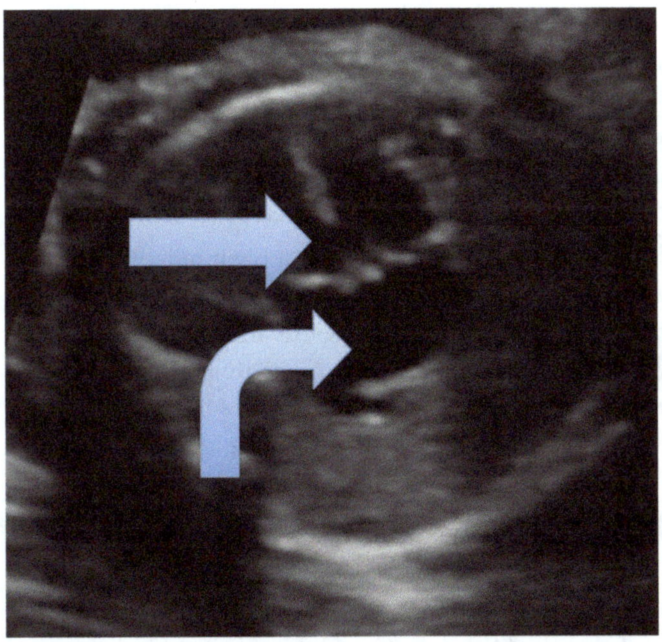

**FIGURE 3.2A** Partial atrioventricular canal defect (curved arrow); ventricular septal defect (straight arrow).

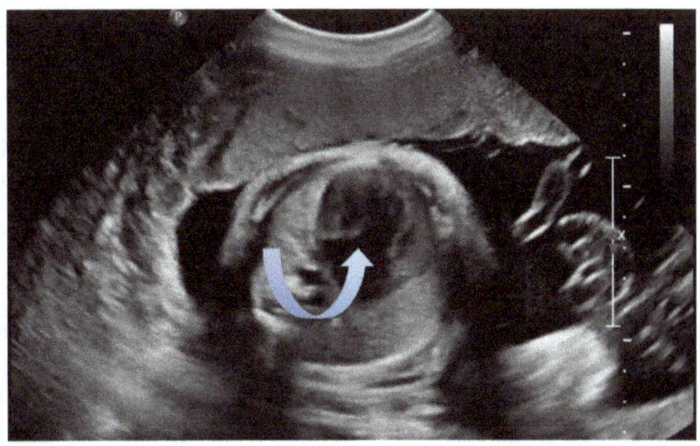

**FIGURE 3.2B** Complete atrioventricular canal defect. Single AV valve (curved arrow).

# 3.3 DOUBLE-OUTLET RIGHT VENTRICLE

## EPIDEMIOLOGY/GENETICS

**Definition** Double-outlet right ventricle (DORV) is commonly defined as a defect in which greater than 50% of both the aorta and the pulmonary arteries are contiguous with a single ventricle that has a right morphological appearance. A VSD is almost always present. DORV is most commonly divided into four types: (1) VSD type, DORV with a subaortic VSD; (2) Fallot type, DORV with subaortic or double committed VSD and pulmonic stenosis; (3) Transposition of the great arteries type (Taussig-Bing), DORV with a subpulmonic VSD; and (4) noncommitted VSD type, DORV with a remote VSD. A double committed VSD consists of two VSDs, one below the aorta and one below the pulmonary artery. A noncommitted VSD is a VSD that is not located near the aorta or pulmonary artery.

**Epidemiology** The prevalence is 0.033 to 0.09 per 1000 live births. It accounts for 1%-3% of children with congenital heart defects.

**Embryology** The primitive right ventricle starts out as a DORV with a conotruncus. In the absence of normal migration of the aortic side of the conotruncus toward the mitral valve, the primitive DORV anatomy persists. It is assumed that DORV is a spectrum of complex defects that are the consequence of failure of a normal, expected sequence of developmental events.

**Inheritance Pattern** The sibling recurrence rate has not been reliably reported but is probably low. Karyotype abnormalities are present in up to 41% of fetuses with DORV. It has been reported in trisomies 13 and 18 and in duplication 3p. Chromosome 22q11 deletion occurs in approximately 5% of patients with DORV. In addition, a variety of genetic syndromes have been reported, including Adams-Oliver, Ellis–van Creveld, Melnick-Needles, Noonan, Opitz, and Robinow syndromes.

**Teratogens** Maternal diabetes mellitus, alcohol, isotretinoin, thalidomide, and trimethadione.

**Prognosis** DORV requires surgical treatment. The prognosis varies considerably depending on the complexity of the defect and the presence, or absence, of associated congenital and karyotypic abnormalities. Overall, DORV has a poor prognosis.

## SONOGRAPHY

### FREQUENT FINDINGS

- The principle feature is demonstration of the connection of the aorta and the pulmonary artery to the right ventricle.
- The apical four-chamber view frequently appears normal. The long-axis views of the left and right outflow tracts tend to be the most helpful in determining DORV.

- The most common orientation of the great arteries is side to side (64%).
- The VSD in DORV tends to be a malalignment defect that is most commonly subaortic (68%).
- A common feature is subvalvular or valvular obstruction of either outflow tract.
  - With aortic stenosis, there is frequently hypoplasia of the ascending aorta and the association of aortic coarctation (AC) or interrupted aortic arch.
  - With pulmonary stenosis, there may be hypoplasia of the branch pulmonary arteries.
  - The three-vessel view can be helpful to compare the relative sizes of the aorta and pulmonary artery.
  - The presence, or absence, of antegrade flow should be evaluated.

## LESS FREQUENT

- Significant valvular stenosis has been associated with nonimmune hydrops.
- Polyhydramnios may develop with the onset of hydrops.

## KEY FINDINGS/PITFALLS

- The manner by which both vessels connect with the right ventricle is variable and important for definitive counseling regarding prognosis.
  - The VSD can be subaortic, subpulmonary, doubly committed, or uncommitted, and more than one VSD may be present.
  - Although the location of the VSD is important for directing surgical consultation, the exact location of the VSD can be difficult to accurately determine on fetal ultrasound.
  - Color and power Doppler can help identify the VSD; however, equal pressures in the ventricles limit identification of small defects.
- DORV sometimes occurs with abnormalities of the AV valves, including atresia, straddling (in which the AV valve attaches into the contralateral ventricles), or overriding (in which the annulus overrides both ventricles but does not necessarily attach to both ventricles).
- DORV can occur with complete common AV canal defects, particularly in heterotaxy syndrome.
- Heterotaxy syndrome should be considered when DORV is suspected. Clear determination of abdominal and atrial situs, as well as pulmonary and systemic venous return, should be performed.
- Chromosomal abnormalities (21%), additional structural abnormalities (40%), and heterotaxy (35%) are associated with DORV.
- DORV is detectable at 16 to 18 weeks by transabdominal imaging and potentially at 14 weeks with transvaginal imaging.

## DIFFERENTIAL DIAGNOSIS

- DORV should be distinguished from transposition, as they are mutually exclusive.
  - In transposition, the aorta arises from the right ventricle, and the pulmonary artery arises from the left ventricle. It is inaccurate to say that transposition of the great arteries and DORV are present in the same heart.
  - If more than one and a half great vessels connect with the right ventricle, the convention is to label the heart as double outlet.

- Tetralogy of Fallot (TOF) with considerable aortic overriding may appear similar to DORV with a subaortic VSD.
  - In tetralogy, the aorta arises predominantly from the left ventricle (i.e., is more than 50% above the left ventricle), and the aortic valve is typically in direct continuity with the anterior leaflet of the mitral valve.
  - In DORV with subaortic VSD, more than one and a half great vessels arise from the right ventricle, and usually there is discontinuity between the aortic and mitral valves due to subaortic conal muscle.

## PREGNANCY MANAGEMENT

**Investigations and Consultations Required** An extended fetal anatomy survey should be completed to assess for additional associated anomalies. A fetal echocardiogram and pediatric cardiology consultation should be obtained to provide prenatal counseling and to exclude the association of more complex congenital heart disease. Consultation with a geneticist should be obtained. Amniocentesis for karyotyping and microarray should be done, especially looking for the 22q11 deletion.

**Pregnancy Course** Pregnancies complicated by isolated DORV tend to do well and have no associated pregnancy complications. However, many cases of DORV are associated with other congenital and karyotypic abnormalities, which may lead to pregnancy complications. Delivery should be anticipated at term, with cesarean section reserved for the usual obstetrical indications. Serial ultrasound assessment is recommended in those subjects with valvular stenosis, given the increased risk for nonimmune hydrops.

**Fetal Intervention** No fetal intervention is available.

**Pregnancy Termination Issues** If termination is chosen, an intact fetus should be delivered for confirmation of diagnosis and karyotyping with microarray.

**Monitoring** With significant valvular regurgitation, hydrops may develop; therefore, serial monitoring with interval ultrasound examinations is warranted. A follow-up fetal echocardiogram to assess valve function in the third trimester may also be helpful.

**Delivery** There is a significant association of DORV with other anomalies and neonatal cyanosis requiring prostaglandin $E_1$ therapy. Delivery should be performed at a center where immediate neonatology and pediatric cardiac consultation and treatment are available.

## NEONATOLOGY

**Resuscitation** Initial resuscitation is generally not required. When there is significant pulmonary outflow tract obstruction, persistent cyanosis may be present from birth, which may be confusing in the immediate transition following delivery. If significant outflow tract obstruction is suspected, venous access should be established to allow administration of prostaglandin $E_1$ as required. Placement of umbilical catheters may be helpful.

**Transport** Transport to a tertiary center with full pediatric cardiac diagnostic and surgical capability is essential. If the infant presents with cyanosis, consultation with a pediatric cardiologist prior to transport is recommended to determine the need for prostaglandin $E_1$ infusion during the transport.

**Testing and Confirmation** Echocardiography provides definitive diagnosis, and preoperative catheterization is generally not required.

**Nursery Management** Management depends on establishing an appropriate balance of systemic and pulmonary blood flow. If there is severe obstruction to pulmonary blood flow, prostaglandin $E_1$ therapy may be indicated to maintain ductal patency and ensure adequate pulmonary blood flow. When there is severe obstruction to systemic blood flow, prostaglandin E1 therapy is necessary to maintain adequate systemic perfusion. When there is no significant obstruction to either outflow tract, CHF may develop with the normal fall in pulmonary vascular resistance. In these cases, anticongestive medications are used to control CHF.

Developmental follow-up is recommended in infants with cyanotic heart disease requiring surgery in the first few weeks of life as they are at risk for developmental delay.

## SURGERY

**Preoperative Assessment** Echocardiography provides definitive diagnosis, and preoperative catheterization is generally not required.

**Operative Indications** All forms of DORV require surgical treatment. The purpose of all operations is to establish unobstructed blood flow of saturated blood to the aorta (preferably from the left ventricle), closure of the VSD, and establishment of unobstructed effective pulmonary blood flow (preferably from the right ventricle). In some cases, a homograft is required to connect the right ventricle with the branch pulmonary arteries

**Types of Procedures** Because of the spectrum of DORV, the methods of surgical correction vary considerably. When the VSD is subaortic, the surgical treatment resembles that used for treatment of TOF. When the VSD is subpulmonary and there is no pulmonary stenosis, the treatment is similar to that used in transposition of the great arteries with VSD. In cases with an uncommitted VSD, it may be impossible to connect the left ventricle with either great vessel. In these unusual cases, single-ventricle management may be necessary. Baffling the left ventricle to the aorta is relatively straightforward in DORV with a subaortic VSD. DORV with a subpulmonary VSD may still allow treatment with a relatively low rate of operative mortality, but the surgery often involves an arterial switch operation as with transposition of the great arteries.

**Surgical Results and Prognosis** The operative mortality rate varies, depending on the complexity of the form of DORV and the presence of associated lesions. In general, the operative mortality rate ranges between 3% and 10%.

### SUGGESTED READINGS

1. Corrigan N, Brazil DP, McAuliffe F: Fetal cardiac effects of maternal hyperglycemia during pregnancy. Birth Defects Res A Clin Mol Teratol 2009; 85:523-530.

2. Gedikbasi A, Oztarhan K, Gul A, et al: Diagnosis and prognosis in double-outlet right ventricle. Am J Perinatol 2008; 25:427-434.
3. Gelehrter S, Owens ST, Russell MW, et al: Accuracy of the fetal echocardiogram in double-outlet right ventricle. Congenit Heart Dis 2007; 2:32-37.
4. Hartge DR, Niemeyer L, Axt-Fliedner R, et al: Prenatal detection and postnatal management of double outlet right ventricle (DORV) in 21 singleton pregnancies. J Matern Fetal Neonatal Med 2012; 25:58-63.
5. Hartman RJ, Rasmussen SA, Botto LD, et al: The contribution of chromosomal abnormalities to congenital heart defects: a population-based study. Pediatr Cardiol 2011; 32:1147-1157.
6. Kim N, Friedberg MK, Silverman NH: Diagnosis and prognosis of fetuses with double outlet right ventricle. Prenat Diagn 2006; 26:740-745.
7. Lee MY, Won HS, Baek JW, et al: Variety of prenatally diagnosed congenital heart disease in 22q11.2 deletion syndrome. Obstet Gynecol Sci 2014; 57:11-16.
8. Obler D, Juraszek AL, Smoot LB, Natowicz MR: Double outlet right ventricle: aetiologies and associations. J Med Genet 2008; 45:481-497.
9. Patel CR, Steele MA, Stewart JW: Double-outlet right ventricle with partial anomalous pulmonary venous connection: prenatal diagnosis. J Ultrasound Med 2005; 24:861-864.
10. Tongsong T, Chanprapaph P, Sittiwangkul R, Khunamornpong S: Antenatal diagnosis of double outlet of right ventricle without extracardiac anomaly: a report of 4 cases. J Clin Ultrasound 2007; 35:221-225.
11. Wu H, Cai A, Zhang Y, et al: Prenatal diagnosis of a fetal double-outlet right ventricle with tricuspid valve atresia, a straddling mitral valve, and a hypoplastic left ventricle. J Ultrasound Med 2012; 31:654-656.
12. Zidere V, Pushparajah K, Allan LD, Simpson JM: Three-dimensional fetal echocardiography for prediction of postnatal surgical approach in double outlet right ventricle: a pilot study. Ultrasound Obstet Gynecol 2013; 42:421-425.


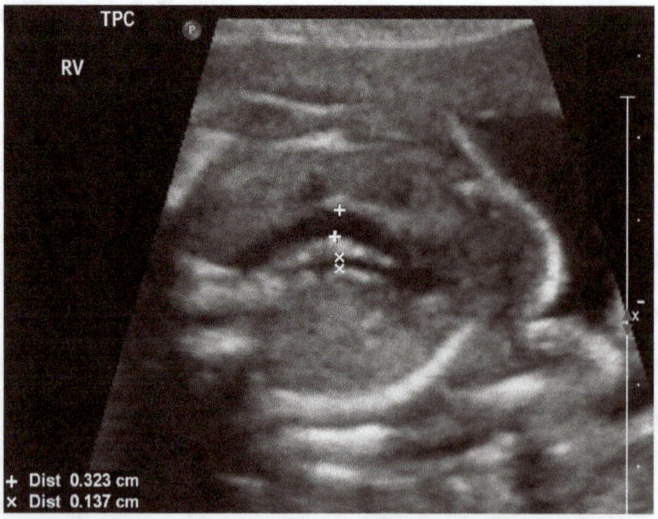


**FIGURE 3.3** Double-outlet right ventricle. Aorta (+ ... +) and stenotic pulmonary artery (x ... x) exit the right ventricle.

# 3.4 DYSRHYTHMIAS

## EPIDEMIOLOGY/GENETICS

**Definition/Epidemiology**

- Fetal dysrhythmias occur in 2% of pregnancies: 90% are ectopic beats, 8% are tachyarrhythmias, and 2% are bradyarrhythmias (BAs).
  - Atrial ectopic beats (extrasystoles)
    - These most frequently occur in the third trimester.
    - On M-mode, the space between an ectopic beat and the prior normal beat is shortened.
    - Two percent become a bradycardia or tachycardia.
- The majority of tachyarrhythmias are either supraventricular tachycardia (80%) or atrial flutter (17%).
- Congenital heart block (CHB) is the most common fetal BA (80%).
  - Five percent of fetuses exposed to maternal lupus develop CHB, usually between 18 and 38 weeks' gestation; approximately 50% are identified prior to 24 weeks' gestation.
  - In CHB secondary to maternal lupus, anti-SSA-Ro or anti-SSB-La antibodies are causative.
    - The same antibodies are present in Sjogren syndrome, which can result in CHB.
  - CHB in the first trimester is due to a structural cardiac defect.

| TACHYARRHYTHMIAS | | |
|---|---|---|
| **Type** | **Rate (beats per minute)** | **Comments** |
| Sinus tachycardia | 170-220 | • Due to a change in autonomic tone<br>• 1-to-1 AV conduction<br>◦ 2 electrical pathways between the atria and ventricles |
| Supraventricular tachycardia | 220-280 | • Reentrant tachycardia is the predominant pathway<br>◦ 2 electrical pathways between the atria and ventricles with 1-to-1 conduction |
| Atrial flutter | Atria: 240-400<br>Ventricle: 150 | • Single reentry circuit around tricuspid valve<br>• 2-to-1 block characteristic<br>◦ Variable degrees of AV block may occur |
| Atrial fibrillation | Atria: 300-600<br>Ventricle: 100-200 | • Multiple atrial impulses through AV node<br>• Rate: irregularly irregular<br>◦ Variable block at AV node |
| Ventricle tachycardia | 150-250 | • Due to reentry mechanism<br>• Rare in the fetus |

| BRADYARRHYTHMIAS | | |
|---|---|---|
| **Type** | **Rate(beats per minute)** | **Comments** |
| Sinus bradycardia | Ventricular: 70-100 | • Underlying conduction abnormality<br>◦ Associated with maternal Ro antibodies |
| Complete Heart Block (third-degree block) | Ventricular: <100 | • Dysfunction at AV node or bundle of His<br>• May be due to a structural cardiac anomaly<br>• Associated with maternal autoimmune disease<br>◦ High association with hydrops |
| Second-degree block (Mobitz, type I) | Ventricular: usually normal depending on P-to-QRS ratio | • Time to travel through AV node gradually increases until it does not penetrate the AV node<br>• Atrial rate regular; ventricular rate regularly irregular<br>◦ Does not progress to CHB |
| Second-degree block (Mobitz, type II) | Atria: 60-100<br>Ventricular: slower than atria based on number of impulses conducted. | • AV conduction time constant<br>• Distal conduction system in ventricle affected<br>• May progress to CHB |

**Inheritance Pattern** Most cases of dysrhythmia are sporadic. There is a small subgroup of patients with familial preexcitation syndromes for which an accessory pathway is found in 1.06% of first-degree relatives, compared to 0.15% in the general population. CHB is unlikely to recur in future pregnancies unless associated with maternal lupus, in which the recurrence risk is 14%-18%.

**Teratogens** None are known.

**Prognosis**

- Survival and prognosis are most highly correlated with the development of hydrops.
- Sustained supraventricular tachycardia (>12 h) and early gestational age at presentation correlate with hydrops.
- One-third of fetuses with CHB do not survive.
- Risk factors for mortality include a ventricular rate less than 55 beats per minute (bpm), a rapid decrease in ventricular rate, the severity of any associated structural cardiac defect, and the development of hydrops.

## SONOGRAPHY

### FREQUENT FINDINGS

- Identify relationship between atrial and ventricular rate to assess type of arrhythmia.
  - M-mode echocardiography of the atrial wall and a ventricular event (free wall motion or semilunar valve motion) are reliable for determining timing.
  - Supraventricular tachycardia and atrial flutter have an abrupt onset and offset.
- Cardiomegaly
- AV valvular regurgitation
- Poor myometrial contractility
- Structural cardiac defects, congenitally corrected transposition (with ventricular inversion)
- Heterotaxy

### LESS FREQUENT

- Hydrops
- Polyhydramnios, if hydrops develops

### KEY FINDINGS/PITFALLS

- Supraventricular tachycardia is frequently intermittent.
  - During the echocardiogram, tachycardia may not be present, even though at other times there are periods of sustained tachycardia.
  - Continuous fetal heart rate monitoring may be useful to confirm, and determine, the frequency and duration of tachycardia episodes.
  - Intermittent tachycardia does not usually lead to hydrops.
- Make sure a bradycardia is not preterminal or related to a central nervous system anomaly.
- Detectible by transabdominal imaging at 16 to 18 weeks. With transvaginal imaging, arrhythmias have been determined during the first trimester.

## PREGNANCY MANAGEMENT

**Investigations and Consultations Required**

- Fetuses with a dysrhythmia are usually best managed in consultation with a perinatalogist, and a pediatric cardiologist skilled in the analysis and treatment of arrhythmias.
- In all cases of CHB, autoantibodies to anti-SSA/Ro and/or anti-SSB/La should be measured in the mother.
  - In cases of maternal lupus, management should be coordinated with a rheumatologist with experience in lupus and a pediatric cardiologist with experience in the management of arrhythmias.
- Fetal karyotype and microarray are recommended in cases of structural cardiac anomalies.

**Pregnancy Course**

- Once AV node disease has been recognized, the fetus should be examined weekly for progression of the disease or the development of either hydrops or ventricular dysfunction.
  - With atrial bigeminy and no evidence of AV node disease, the fetus should be evaluated weekly for evidence of supraventricular tachycardia or sequelae of this arrhythmia that may be intermittent and missed on the weekly fetal evaluation.
- Sinus bradycardia requires an evaluation of overall fetal well-being.
  - Maternal thyroid status should be screened.
  - Since Romano-Ward syndrome has been recognized prenatally, a family history for long QT syndrome should be sought.
    - Sinus bradycardia is one feature of the long QT syndrome.

**Fetal Intervention**

- Complete heart block
  - In the fetus greater than 32-34 weeks' gestational age with CHB, early delivery and postnatal pacing can be considered.
  - In fetuses of mothers with lupus, maternal treatment with fluorinated steroids could be considered when the fetus is diagnosed with second- or third-degree block. However, treatment with high-dose steroids, as well as intravenous immunoglobulin (IVIG), is controversial. Caution must be emphasized if steroids are to be considered in treatment, given the maternal and fetal consequences and the lack of any strong evidence that treatment makes a clinically significant impact on the outcome of CHB.
- With CHB, β-agonists can increase the fetal heart rate approximately 10%.
  - If hydrops is present, the addition of β-agonists will not improve hydropic status.
- Hydrops is unlikely with a ventricular rate of 55-60 bpm in the absence of a cardiac anomaly.
- Hydroxychloroquine may prevent recurrence of autoantibody-related CHB in families with a previously affected child, but there are no controlled studies. The recurrence risk is 18% with no treatment.
- Fetal tachycardia
  - Check maternal thyroid function.
  - Obtain a middle cerebral artery peak systolic velocity to exclude fetal anemia.
  - First-/second-line therapy: digoxin, flecainide, or sotolol. Third-line therapy: amiodarone.
  - Intermittent tachycardia, without evidence of hydrops, does not require treatment.
    - Ventricular tachycardia greater than 200 bpm is the exception due to the potential for rapid progression to hydrops.
  - If there is hydrops with supraventricular tachycardia that is unresponsive to medical therapy, then intramuscular injection of digoxin into the fetal thigh can be considered.

**Pregnancy Termination Issues** If the etiology is unclear, an intact fetus should be delivered for a complete examination due to the potential presence of associated abnormalities.

**Monitoring** Until effective rate control is achieved, the fetus with sustained tachycardia should be reexamined daily. In most cases, the mother should be hospitalized until effective rate control is achieved. Maternal drug levels should be drawn to ensure adequacy of dosing.

**Delivery** A fetus with CHB or second-degree block should be delivered at a center where pediatric cardiology consultation and ventricular pacing are available. If the fetal size allows epicardial pacing, early delivery should be considered if hydrops develops. Cesarean section is recommended, as the fetal heart rate cannot be monitored in labor to assess fetal well-being.

## NEONATOLOGY

**Resuscitation** Infants generally breathe spontaneously and do not require resuscitation. In cases in which hydrops is present secondary to CHB, isoproterenol at very low doses may be helpful to increase the ventricular rate. Equipment should be available for ventricular pacing.

**Transport** Transfer to a center with a pediatric cardiology service is recommended.

**Testing and Confirmation** The mechanism of the arrhythmia can generally be confirmed with a surface electrocardiogram. Occasionally, transesophageal electrocardiography helps to identify the mechanism of the arrhythmia. Invasive electrophysiologic studies are not indicated during infancy.

**Nursery Management** Indications for ventricular pacing include a ventricular rate less than 55 bpm in neonates, ventricular dysfunction related to low heart rate or ventricular ectopy, or increased QT interval. Hemodynamically unstable infants may require electrical cardioversion. Reentry tachycardia is frequently terminated with adenosine.

## SURGERY

**Preoperative Assessment/Types of Procedures/Prognosis** In the majority of patients, supraventricular tachycardia can be controlled with pharmacologic therapy. In patients requiring long-term antiarrhythmic therapy, radiofrequency ablation is successful in extinguishing the accessory pathway. Temporary transvenous ventricular pacing can achieve an adequate ventricular rate for the short term in newborns with BAs. When long-term pacing is required, epicardial pacing leads are placed, and the results are satisfactory unless the newborn is premature or has a low birth weight.

### SUGGESTED READINGS

1. Abel DE: Fetal dysrhythmias: a primer for the obstetrician/gynecologist. Obstet Gynecol Surv 2013; 68:521-525.

2. Api O, Carvalho JS: Fetal dysrhythmias. Best Pract Res Clin Obstet Gynaecol 2008; 22:31-48.
3. Bravo-Valenzuela NJ: Fetal bradycardia and sinus node dysfunction. Pediatr Cardiol 2013; 34:1250-1253.
4. Cuneo BF, Strasburger JF: Management strategy for fetal tachycardia. Obstet Gynecol 2000; 96:575-581.
5. Di Mauro A, Caroli Casavola V, Favia Guarnieri G, et al: Antenatal and postnatal combined therapy for autoantibody-related congenital atrioventricular block. BMC Pregnancy Childbirth 2013; 13:220.
6. Donofrio MT, Moon-Grady AJ, Hornberger LK, et al: Diagnosis and treatment of fetal cardiac disease: a scientific statement from the American Heart Association. Circulation 2014; 129:2183-2242.
7. Hornberger LK: Echocardiographic assessment of fetal arrhythmias. Heart 2007; 93:1331-1333.
8. Hornberger LK, Sahn DJ: Rhythm abnormalities of the fetus. Heart 2007; 93:1294-1300.
9. Jaeggi ET, Hornberger LK, Smallhorn JF, Fouron JC: Prenatal diagnosis of complete atrioventricular block associated with structural heart disease: combined experience of two tertiary care centers and review of the literature. Ultrasound Obstet Gynecol 2005; 26:16-21.
10. Pike JI, Krishnan A, Kaltman J, Donofrio MT: Fetal and neonatal atrial arrhythmias: an association with maternal diabetes and neonatal macrosomia. Prenat Diagn 2013; 33:1152-1157.
11. Saxena A, Izmirly PM, Mendez B, et al: Prevention and treatment in utero of autoimmune-associated congenital heart block. Cardiol Rev 2014; 22:263-267.
12. Sekarski N, Meijboom EJ, Di Bernardo S, et al: Perinatal arrhythmias. Eur J Pediatr 2014; 173:983-996.
13. Sonesson SE: Diagnosing foetal atrioventricular heart blocks. Scand J Immunol 2010; 72:205-212.
14. Srinivasan S, Strasburger J: Overview of fetal arrhythmias. Curr Opin Pediatr 2008; 20:522-531.
15. Wacker-Gussmann A, Strasburger JF, Cuneo BF, Wakai RT: Diagnosis and treatment of fetal arrhythmia. Am J Perinatol 2014; 31:617-628.

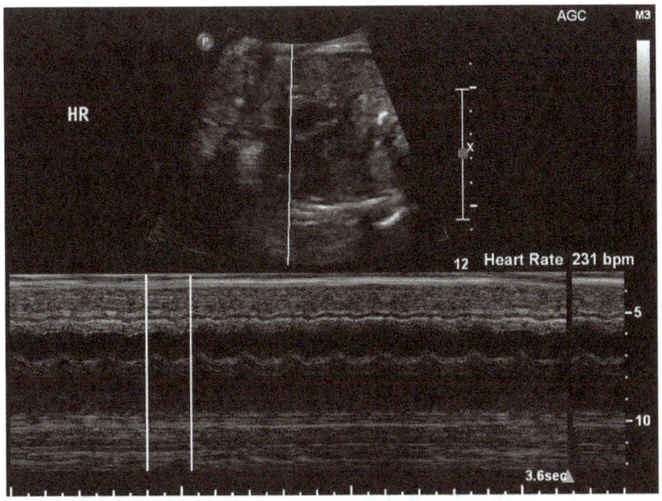


FIGURE 3.4A Atrial flutter with a rate of 231 beats per minute.

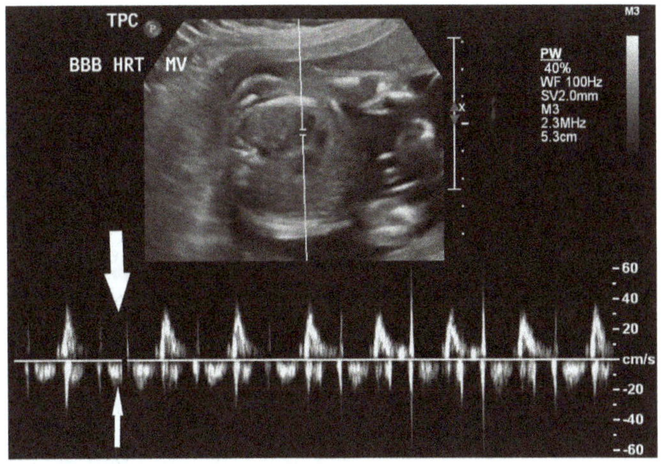


FIGURE 3.4B Atrial premature contractions. Absence of a ventricular contraction (large arrow) after an atrial contraction (small arrow).

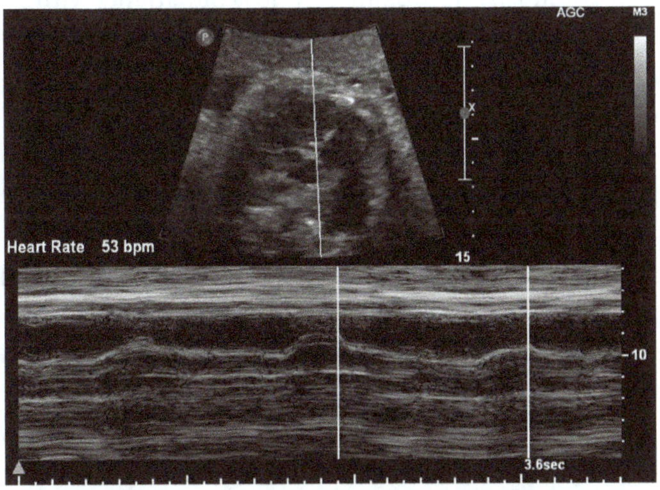


FIGURE 3.4C Complete heart block. Ventricular rate of 53 beats per minute.

# 3.5 EBSTEIN ANOMALY

## EPIDEMIOLOGY/GENETICS

**Definition** Ebstein anomaly refers to an abnormal tricuspid valve with apical displacement of the attachment of the septal leaflet.

**Epidemiology** Prevalence is approximately 1 to 5 per 20,000 live births (M1:F1). It accounts for less than 1% of congenital heart disease.

**Embryology** The tricuspid valve and chordae tendineae most likely develop from the inner layers of the right ventricular inlet in a process called delamination. In Ebstein anomaly, the delamination process is incomplete, resulting in the abnormal apical insertion of the posterior and septal leaflets. This commonly results in tricuspid regurgitation and, much less commonly, tricuspid stenosis. The right heart, mainly the right atrium, is frequently dilated, and there is often an associated atrial septal defect and, rarely, pulmonary stenosis. Approximately 30% of patients with Ebstein anomaly have Wolff-Parkinson-White syndrome.

**Inheritance Pattern** The majority of cases are sporadic. Recurrence risk is 1% when one sibling is affected and 3% when two siblings are affected. Familial cases have been documented, including an autosomal dominant condition with Ebstein anomaly and mild skeletal abnormalities. It also has been reported in association with deletions of 1p36 and 8p23.1.

**Teratogens** Older reports suggested an increased risk for Ebstein anomaly with maternal lithium exposure. More recent data suggest that this risk is much lower, with relative risks of 1.2 to 7.7. Maternal diabetes also been reported to be associated with Ebstein anomaly.

**Prognosis** There is a wide spectrum of severity and in prognosis. Those with less-severe findings are likely to do well and may be asymptomatic. Among fetuses with severe tricuspid regurgitation and marked right atrial dilation, the prognosis is poor. One study reported that, among 20 fetuses with severe tricuspid regurgitation, 48% died in utero and 35% of the live-born infants died, despite vigorous medical and surgical treatment.

## SONOGRAPHY

### FREQUENT FINDINGS

- The displacement of the tricuspid valve (i.e., the septal leaflet and sometimes the posterior leaflet) into the right ventricle is quantified by measuring the distance from the septal leaflet of the tricuspid valve to the anterior leaflet of the mitral valve. This distance has been found to be less than 4 mm at term in normal fetuses.
- In mild cases, the four-chamber view may appear normal. Angling posteriorly accentuates the offset of the AV valves and can be used to improve visualization of the actual insertion site of the septal leaflet.

- Severe levorotation of the fetal heart is common.
- Cardiomegaly is seen due to right atrial and ventricular dilation with coexisting right ventricular dysfunction or dysplasia.
- Most commonly, it is associated with severe tricuspid regurgitation and rarely tricuspid stenosis.
- Some degree of tricuspid valve dysplasia is present with valvular thickening or nodularity.
- Associated findings can include (1) valvular pulmonary stenosis or pulmonary atresia; (2) branch pulmonary artery hypoplasia; (3) atrial septal defect; (4) limitation of left ventricular filling when there is severe right ventricular volume overload with diastolic bowing of the interventricular septum; and (5) reversed ductal flow from aorta to pulmonary artery when there is pulmonary atresia, which can be anatomic or functional.

## LESS FREQUENT

- With severe tricuspid regurgitation or severe right ventricular outflow tract obstruction, polyhydramnios and hydrops may develop.
- Pulmonary hypoplasia can occur when there is severe cardiomegaly, especially when severe cardiomegaly is present by 20 weeks' gestation.
- Supraventricular tachycardia can occur, especially when there is Wolff-Parkinson-White syndrome.
- Associated abnormalities include low-set ears, micrognathia, cleft lip and palate, absent kidney, megacolon, and undescended testes.

## KEY FINDINGS/PITFALLS

- With severe tricuspid regurgitation, the right ventricle may be unable to generate sufficient pressure to open the pulmonary valve, even though the valve is patent. This is termed functional pulmonary atresia, in contrast to anatomic pulmonary atresia, in which the valve leaflets may actually be fused closed. Both functional and anatomic pulmonary valve atresia can occur in Ebstein anomaly. Functional pulmonary atresia can be distinguished from anatomic atresia if even a small amount of pulmonary regurgitation is noted. The pulmonary regurgitation is evidence that the leaflets are patent, even if no antegrade flow is present. Postnatally, when the pulmonary vascular resistance falls, antegrade pulmonary flow may be possible.
- The dilated right heart may be mistakenly interpreted as hypoplastic left heart syndrome (HLHS). This mistake should easily be avoided if measurements of the mitral and tricuspid valve annuli are made and identification of the morphologic and functional abnormality of the tricuspid valve is determined.
- Color Doppler assessment of tricuspid regurgitation can be optimized by first turning the gain down completely and then gradually increasing the gain until background noise begins to appear. Excessively low gain will underestimate regurgitation because of the elimination of low-velocity signals. An excessively high gain will result in "noise" masking the true regurgitant jet. A good estimate of severity is the size of the right atrium. A normal size right atrium suggests that the severity of tricuspid regurgitation is only mild to moderate.

- Ebstein anomaly is detectable by transabdominal imaging at 16 to 18 weeks. Although the fetal heart can be examined by transvaginal echocardiography at 11 to 13 weeks, the diagnosis of Ebstein anomaly has not yet been reported.

### DIFFERENTIAL DIAGNOSIS

- Mild tricuspid regurgitation can occur in 6% to 7% of normal fetuses. In such cases, the tricuspid valve morphology and annulus size are normal and should be easily distinguishable from Ebstein anomaly. There is no right heart dilation.
- Tricuspid regurgitation can also be present with critical right heart obstruction, such as pulmonary stenosis or atresia. This can be distinguished from Ebstein anomaly by recognizing the absence of septal displacement of the tricuspid valve and the presence of obstruction at the pulmonary valve.
- Tricuspid valve dysplasia can result in significant, and even severe, tricuspid regurgitation. Generally, the leaflet tips are thickened. However, the septal displacement of the tricuspid valve found in Ebstein anomaly is not present.
- Giant right atrium as an isolated finding can occur without tricuspid valve disease.

## PREGNANCY MANAGEMENT

**Investigations and Consultations Required** If suspected on an ultrasound examination, a fetal echocardiogram should be obtained to confirm the diagnosis, look for associated cardiac findings, and assess cardiac function. An extended examination to assess possible associated anomalies should be performed. A fetal karyotype and microarray should be done. Pediatric cardiology consultation should be obtained for confirmation of the diagnosis and to coordinate the prenatal and postnatal cardiac plans.

**Pregnancy Course** Unless severe tricuspid regurgitation develops, fetuses are generally delivered at term. In the case of cardiac decompensation, early delivery should be weighed against risks of prematurity, but may be warranted.

**Fetal Intervention** None.

**Pregnancy Termination Issues** If termination is chosen, an intact fetus should be delivered for confirmation of diagnosis.

**Monitoring** With significant tricuspid regurgitation, particularly in the presence of pulmonary stenosis or atresia, hydrops may develop. In addition, the fetus is at risk for supraventricular tachycardia. Monitoring with interval ultrasound examinations should be performed. A follow-up fetal echocardiogram to assess cardiac function and tricuspid valve function in the third trimester should be performed.

**Delivery** Unless the lesion is mild, delivery should be performed at a center where immediate neonatology and pediatric cardiac consultation is available.

## NEONATOLOGY

**Resuscitation** In the absence of fetal hydrops or cardiac dysrhythmia, assistance with the onset of breathing is usually not required. Neonates with Ebstein anomaly who are asymptomatic may exhibit intense cyanosis early after birth. Initial measures are directed toward lowering pulmonary vascular resistance and maintaining cardiac output.

**Transport** If the newborn is asymptomatic at birth except for cardiomegaly, referral for evaluation can be done at nursery discharge. If there is cyanosis, congestive failure, or rhythm disturbance, immediate referral to a tertiary perinatal center with full pediatric cardiac diagnostic capabilities is necessary. Consultation with a pediatric cardiologist prior to transport to determine management requirements during transport is recommended.

**Testing and Confirmation** Echocardiography will confirm anatomic and functional abnormalities. A 12-lead electrocardiogram is necessary to exclude a dysrhythmia. Assessment of oxygenation by arterial $PO_2$ or pulse oximetry is indicated.

**Nursery Management** In most cases, the ductus arteriosus should be allowed to close. With the fall in pulmonary vascular resistance, the systemic oxygen saturation will increase as the right-to-left shunt decreases. If there is markedly diminished pulmonary blood flow due to elevated pulmonary vascular resistance, nitric oxide may be efficacious. When there is critical right heart obstruction, prostaglandin $E_1$ may be required to maintain ductal patency. With cyanosis, prostaglandin $E_1$ may be needed to maintain ductal patency until pulmonary resistance lowers.

Developmental follow-up is recommended in infants with cyanotic heart disease requiring surgery in the first few weeks of life, as they are at risk for developmental delay.

## SURGERY

**Preoperative Assessment** In the majority of cases, echocardiography provides definitive anatomic and physiologic information. In rare cases, however, single-ventricle management may be necessary. In such cases, cardiac catheterization may be needed to assess pulmonary artery anatomy and physiology.

**Operative Indications** In general, one should avoid surgery in a newborn when the oxygen saturation exceeds 75%. The saturation will usually increase as pulmonary resistance falls. However, when the oxygen saturation is less than 75% or when there is anatomic right heart obstruction, surgery is necessary to achieve adequate oxygenation. Beyond infancy, patients are referred for surgery when the tricuspid regurgitation results in significant right ventricular volume load or when there is disadvantageous shunting at the atrial level.

**Types of Procedures** Two-ventricle management is possible in most patients but requires adequate right ventricular and tricuspid valve function. In such cases, tricuspid valve surgery is directed toward decreasing tricuspid regurgitation with annuloplasty or, later in childhood, tricuspid valve replacement. In general, the atrial septal defect is also closed. When there is severe right heart obstruction, the surgical options are more complicated, and the results are less favorable. With anatomic pulmonary valve atresia, a systematic shunt is indicated to establish a reliable source of pulmonary blood flow. The volume load of tricuspid regurgitation may compromise left ventricular filling.

**Surgical Results and Prognosis** In cases of mild-to-moderate Ebstein anomaly without critical right heart obstruction, the results are generally good. Infants requiring neonatal surgery because of severe Ebstein anomaly have a poor prognosis.

## SUGGESTED READINGS


1. Barre E, Durand I, Hazelzet T, David N: Ebstein's anomaly and tricuspid valve dysplasia: prognosis after diagnosis in utero. Pediatr Cardiol 2012; 33:1391-1396.
2. Cohen LS, Friedman JM, Jefferson JW, et al: A reevaluation of risk of in utero exposure to lithium. JAMA 1994; 271:146-150.
3. Connolly HM, Warnes CA: Ebstein's anomaly: outcome of pregnancy. J Am Coll Cardiol 1994; 23:1194-1198.
4. Geerdink LM, Kapusta L: Dealing with Ebstein's anomaly. Cardiol Young 2014; 24:191-200.
5. Lasa JJ, Tian ZY, Guo R, Rychik J: Perinatal course of Ebstein's anomaly and tricuspid valve dysplasia in the fetus. Prenat Diagn 2012; 32:245-251.
6. Osiro S, Tiwari KJ, Mathenge N, et al: When lithium hurts: a look at Ebstein anomaly. Cardiol Rev 2013; 21(5):257-263.
7. Paranon S, Acar P: Ebstein's anomaly of the tricuspid valve: from fetus to adult: congenital heart disease. Heart 2008; 94:237-243.
8. Schreiber C, Cook A, Ho SY, et al: Morphologic spectrum of Ebstein's malformation: revisitation relative to surgical repair. J Thorac Cardiovasc Surg 1999; 117:148-155.
9. Shetty RK, Vivek G, Nayak K, Pai UM: Fetal Ebstein's anomaly. BMJ Case Rep 2012; Aug 24:2012.
10. Song TB, Lee JY, Kim YH, et al: Prenatal diagnosis of severe tricuspid insufficiency in Ebstein's anomaly with pulmonary atresia and intact ventricular septum: a case report. J Obstet Gynaecol Res 2000; 26:223-226.
11. Yu JJ, Yun TJ, Won HS, et al: Outcome of neonates with Ebstein's anomaly in the current era. Pediatr Cardiol 2013; 34:1590-1596.
12. Zhao W, Liu H, Feng R, Lin J: Pregnancy outcomes in women with Ebstein's anomaly. Arch Gynecol Obstet 2012; 286:881-888.
13. Zimmer EZ, Blazer S, Lorber A, et al: Fetal Ebstein's anomaly: early and late appearance. Prenat Diagn 2012; 32:228-233.

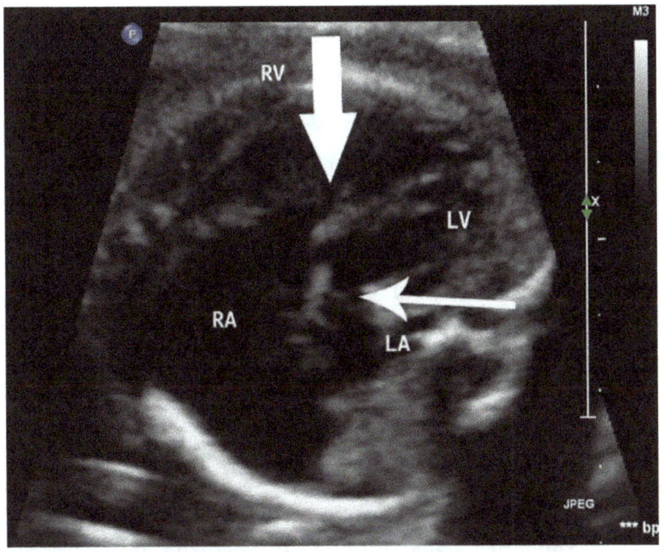


**FIGURE 3.5** Ebstein anomaly. Large right atrium (RA) resulting in levorotation; apically displaced tricuspid valve (thick arrow) and normally positioned mitral valve (thin arrow).

# 3.6 ECTOPIA CORDIS AND PENTALOGY OF CANTRELL

## EPIDEMIOLOGY/GENETICS

**Definition** Ectopia cordis (EC) is the partial or complete displacement of the fetal heart outside the thoracic cavity. There are five types: (1) cervical, for which the heart is in the neck with an intact sternum; (2) thoracocervical, with the heart protruding through a defect in the upper sternum; (3) thoracic, in which the heart herniates through a sternal defect and lies outside the thorax; (4) thoracoabdominal, also known as pentalogy of Cantrell (POC); and (5) abdominal, in which the heart herniates through a diaphragmatic defect into the abdomen. EC can also be part of a limb-body wall complex.

In POC, the most frequent presentation with EC, there is a deficient or absent pericardium, a lower sternal defect, a ventral diaphragmatic defect, a supraumbilical defect (usually an omphalocele), and congenital heart defects.

**Epidemiology** The incidence of EC is 0.55 to 0.79 per 100,000 live births (M1.4:F1).

**Embryology** The specific cause of EC is not known. It is suspected that the cervical type is due to a lack of descent of the heart from its embryologic location. Other forms of EC may be the result of abnormal mesodermal development with failure of fusion of the paired anterior body folds. EC can also be secondary to amniotic bands.

**Inheritance Pattern** Most cases are sporadic, although familial recurrence has been reported. Trisomies 13, 18, and 21, as well as Turner syndrome, have been associated with EC. The Goltz-Gorlin syndrome (X-linked dominant with male lethality) may have EC as a feature.

**Teratogens** None are known.

**Prognosis** EC has a poor prognosis. Postnatal survival is uncommon, given the extent of the abnormality and the numerous viscera involved. Attempts at returning the heart into the small fetal chest are usually unsuccessful due to cardiac compression and kinking of the great arteries. Death usually occurs within days of birth.

## SONOGRAPHY

### FREQUENT FINDINGS

- The classic feature is identification of the beating fetal heart outside the fetal chest.
- Structural intracardiac defects are frequently associated with EC. Tetralogy of Fallot (TOF) can complicate both thoracic and thoracoabdominal types of EC. Atrial septal defects and VSDs have both been commonly associated with EC; however, any type of congenital cardiac defect can coexist with EC.

- Further imaging can identify additional sternal or abdominal wall defects, which can extend down below the fetal umbilicus. An umbilical mass can be seen, consistent with an omphalocele.

### LESS FREQUENT

- Assess for amniotic bands, which can be associated with sternal and abdominal wall defects.
- Other anomalies that can be associated with EC include:
  - gastroschisis;
  - neural tube defects;
  - cleft lip/cleft palate; and
  - skeletal deformities.

### KEY FINDINGS/PITFALLS

- In some types of the limb-body wall complex, the thoracic anatomy may be so distorted that the EC defect may be overlooked. It may be difficult to determine whether a portion of the heart is outside the chest with a large omphalocele.
- In addition to EC, other congenital cardiac defects such as TOF or atrial septal defects and VSDs may be present and can be missed.
- EC is detectible as early as 12–14 weeks' gestation with transvaginal imaging.

### DIFFERENTIAL DIAGNOSIS

- EC and POC are both distinct presentations but can be part of other syndromes, such as limb-body wall or amniotic band.

## PREGNANCY MANAGEMENT

**Investigations and Consultations Required** An extended anatomy survey should be performed to assess the fetus for additional anomalies. A fetal karyotype and microarray should be done. Because of the association with neural tube defects, both amniotic fluid α-fetoprotein and acetylcholinesterase studies should be done. Fetal echocardiography must be performed to determine the extent of cardiac defects. Pediatric surgery and pediatric cardiology consultations should be obtained to assess prognosis and plan neonatal management.

**Pregnancy Course** No specific obstetric complications are to be expected.

**Fetal Intervention** None are currently available.

**Pregnancy Termination Issues** If termination is chosen, an intact fetus should be delivered for confirmation of diagnosis and karyotyping with microarray, if not previously performed.

**Monitoring** The overall dismal prognosis for this disorder should preclude aggressive pregnancy intervention in most cases. If the structural cardiac malformation and the degree of heart displacement are relatively minor, then surgical correction may be successful, and standard obstetric management is appropriate.

**Delivery** A nonaggressive approach without fetal monitoring should be considered. The site for delivery should be a tertiary center, where an immediate evaluation of the neonate can be undertaken to assess whether surgical correction should be attempted. The optimal routine of delivery has not been clearly determined; however, given the poor prognosis, a cesarean section delivery should be avoided.

## NEONATOLOGY

**Resuscitation** Given the almost total lethality of this lesion, the decision to provide support following birth should be discussed with the family prior to delivery. When there is uncertainty regarding the prognosis, it is appropriate to provide at least assisted ventilation, pending full evaluation and determination of the prognosis.

**Transport** Immediate referral to a tertiary center with full pediatric cardiac diagnostic and surgical capabilities is essential, particularly for the infant with a minor, or limited, defect. The exposed viscera should be protected with a warm, moist, sterile dressing against trauma and contamination during transit.

**Testing and Confirmation** Careful physical examination, postnatal echocardiography, and abdominal ultrasonography will confirm the nature and severity of the lesions. If not obtained prenatally, neonatal karyotyping and microarray are important.

**Nursery Management** Provision of respiratory support during the interval between birth and completion of the diagnostic evaluation is appropriate to allow time for parental adaptation and clarification of the feasibility of surgical correction.

## SURGERY

**Preoperative Assessment** The initial goal of assessment is to determine the extent of the sternal defect and the severity of the associated anomalies, particularly cardiac, as the latter determines the survival prognosis. Three postnatal categories of defects have been described based on the approach for surgical management:

- Cleft sternum: either a partial or complete cleft beginning superiorly, and without associated anomalies
- EC with the exposed heart presenting outside the chest wall through a cleft sternum and the anterior chest wall
- POC: an association of defects, including cleft distal sternum, absent anterior crescent of the diaphragm, midline anterior abdominal wall defect above the umbilicus (omphalocele), defect of the apical pericardium with communication into the peritoneum, and a cardiac anomaly, most commonly a VSD or left ventricular diverticulum

Careful physical examination, echocardiography, chest radiography, and, if necessary, cardiac catheterization may be used to define the anatomic and functional defects.

**Operative Indications** Experience has shown that surgical repair of the cleft sternum is best achieved in the newborn period, while elasticity of the chest wall is such that it allows approximation of the separated sternal bands. The presence of an omphalocele mandates immediate surgical intervention to place an appropriate prosthetic covering for prevention of infection and fluid losses. Use of such a prosthetic covering to protect the exposed heart in a true EC has been reported as a temporizing measure to facilitate completion of the evaluation of the associated cardiac lesion. Staging of cardiac repair may be necessary in both the true EC and the POC because of severe and unusual anatomic abnormalities.

**Types of Procedures** For the isolated cleft-sternal defect, usually a direct approximation of the sternal halves is done after appropriate excision or wedging to prevent buckling. If the thoracic volume is inadequate after approximation, sliding chondrotomy of several ribs on either side will provide further volume. Return of the ectopic and exposed heart to the thoracic cavity and sternal closure, although technically possible, has not resulted in improved survival, usually because of the severity of the associated cardiac lesions. If a life-sustaining corrective or palliative procedure for the cardiac defect is possible in the newborn period, chest wall closure, using prosthetic material to increase thoracic volume, is usually required. Both primary and staged repair of the various defects present in the POC have been reported. Small defects are more amenable to primary closure if the cardiac anomaly is limited to either a septal defect or ventricular diverticulum. The latter can be amputated during the primary procedure. For extensive defects, such as large omphaloceles, staged closure with an initial Silastic silo may be necessary.

**Surgical Results and Prognosis** The prognosis is contingent primarily on the presence and severity of an accompanying cardiac defect. For an isolated cleft sternum repair, the prognosis for survival is good, although recurrence of the cleft has been reported. For the true EC and for POC, reported survival after surgical closure is poor, perhaps no more than 5% to 10%, with the underlying cardiac defect being the primary determinant of survival.

## SUGGESTED READINGS

1. Amitabh P, Sharan R, Talapatra A: Ectopia cordis. J Clin Neonatol 2012; 1:166-167.
2. Chandran S, Ari D: Pentalogy of Cantrell: an extremely rare congenital anomaly. J Clin Neonatol 2013; 2:95-97.
3. Falkensammer CB, Ayres NA, Altman CA, et al: Fetal cardiac malposition: incidence and outcome of associated cardiac and extracardiac malformations. Am J Perinatol 2008; 25:277-281.
4. Hannoun A, Usta IM, Sawaya F, Nassar AH: First trimester sonographic diagnosis of ectopia cordis: a case report and review of the literature. J Matern Fetal Neonatal Med 2011; 24:867-869.
5. Humpl T, Huggan P, Hornberger LK, McCrindle BW: Presentation and outcomes of ectopia cordis. Can J Cardiol 1999; 15:1353-1357.

6. Mallula KK, Sosnowski C, Awad S: Spectrum of Cantrell's pentalogy: case series from a single tertiary care center and review of the literature. Pediatr Cardiol 2013; 34:1703-1710.
7. Pepper MA, Fishbein GA, Teitell MA: Thoracoabdominal wall defect with complete ectopia cordis and gastroschisis: a case report and review of the literature. Pediatr Dev Pathol 2013; 16:348-352.
8. Repondek-Liberska M, Janiak K, Wloch A: Fetal echocardiography in ectopia cordis. Pediatr Cardiol 2000; 21:249-252.
9. Restrepo MS, Cerqua A, Turek JW: Pentalogy of Cantrell with ectopia cordis totalis, total anomalous pulmonary venous connection, and tetralogy of Fallot: a case report and review of the literature. Congenit Heart Dis 2014; 9:E129-E134.
10. Sepulveda W, Andreeva E, Machado LE: Sonographic diagnosis of ectopia cordis before 9 weeks of gestation. Prenat Diagn 2014; 34:1231-1232.
11. Tongsong T, Wanapirak C, Sirivatanapa P, Wongtrangan S: Prenatal sonographic diagnosis of ectopia cordis. J Clin Ultrasound 1999; 27:440-445.
12. van Hoorn JH, Moonen RM, Huysentruyt CJ, et al: Pentalogy of Cantrell: two patients and a review to determine prognostic factors for optimal approach. Eur J Pediatr 2008; 167:29-35.


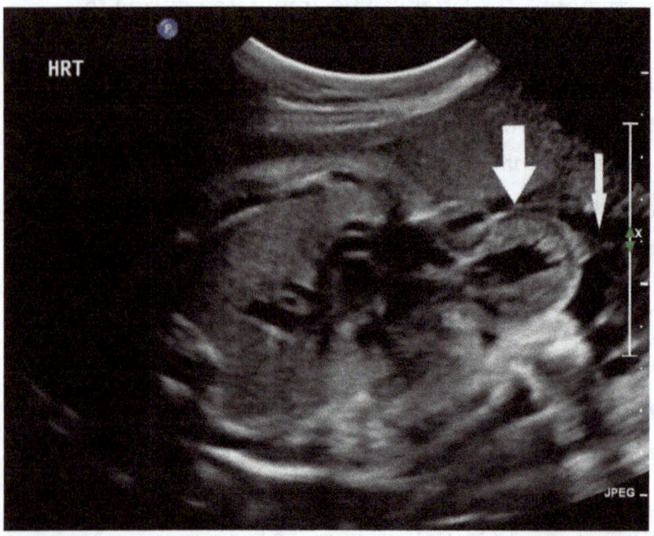


**FIGURE 3.6A** Ectopia cordis (large arrow) secondary to amniotic bands (small arrow).

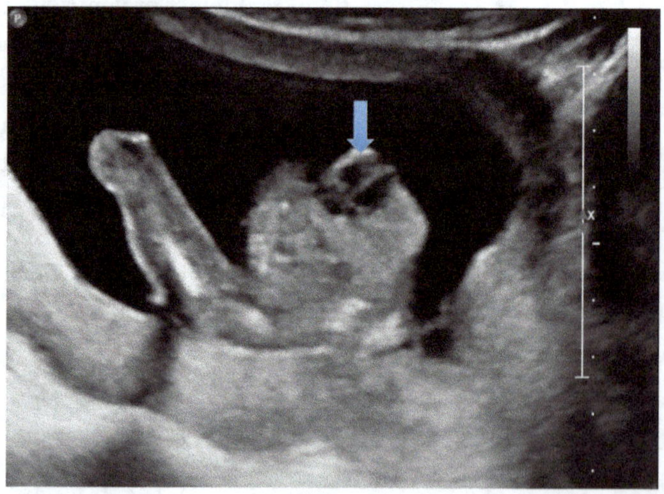

**FIGURE 3.6B** Pentalogy of Cantrell. Ectopia cordis (arrow).

# 3.7 HYPOPLASTIC LEFT HEART SYNDROME

## EPIDEMIOLOGY/GENETICS

**Definition** Hypoplastic left heart syndrome (HLHS) is a spectrum of disorders with underdevelopment of the left ventricle, associated with mitral stenosis or atresia and valvular aortic stenosis or atresia. There is usually hypoplasia of the ascending aorta. The left ventricle is considered critically hypoplastic when it is so small that it is not able to supply an adequate systemic output.

**Epidemiology** Prevalence is 1.5 to 6.7 per 10,000 live births. It accounts for 2% to 3% of children with congenital cardiac disease. Chromosomal abnormalities have been reported in 5%-16% of cases, including trisomies 13 and 18, monosomy X, and a terminal 11q deletion (Jacobsen syndrome, for which 10% of patients have HLHS). One or more extracardiac abnormalities are present in up to 28% of cases. In addition, HLHS has been reported in association with a variety of genetic syndromes, including Adams-Oliver syndrome, Rubinstein-Taybi syndrome, and Holt-Oram syndrome.

**Embryology** The left ventricle forms from the primitive left ventricle, the mitral valve forms from the endocardial cushions, and the aortic valve forms from the truncus arteriosus (TA).

**Inheritance Pattern** The specific inheritance pattern is complex, including multiple loci. In addition, there appears to be a strong association with other left-sided lesions, including aortic coarctation (AC) and bicuspid aortic valve. The recurrence risk for HLHS is reported to be 2% when one sibling is affected and 6% when two siblings are affected. The recurrence risk for any left-sided abnormality may be as high as 10% to 15% among siblings of a proband with HLHS. There are inadequate data to estimate recurrence risk for congenital heart defects in offspring of an affected parent with HLHS.

**Teratogens** None are reported.

**Prognosis** Untreated HLHS is lethal. The syndrome may be associated with other abnormalities, such as chromosomal abnormalities, which would exclude surgery. Palliative surgery generally involves the Norwood operation, with a subsequent Glenn, and finally a Fontan procedure. Among centers with favorable results with this management strategy, the operative survival rate for the Norwood procedure is 76% for all patients and 86% among those at standard risk. The 5-year survival rate including all patients is 70%. Neurobehavioral abnormalities have been noted in infants even prior to surgery, and up to 30% of survivors will have neurologic abnormalities noted at school age.

## SONOGRAPHY

### FREQUENT FINDINGS

- The position of the heart is usually normal, with normal AV and ventriculoarterial connections.

- The tricuspid valve is structurally normal, but the right ventricle is often enlarged, and the pulmonary artery is frequently dilated.
- Critical left ventricle hypoplasia is generally present when the long-axis length of the left ventricle is less than 80% of the long-axis length of the heart.
- The left ventricle endocardium can be hyperechoic because of endocardial fibroelastosis.
- An abnormal mitral valve is always present. With mitral stenosis or atresia, the mitral valve annulus is hypoplastic, and leaflet motion is restricted.
- The ascending aorta is poorly developed. The aortic valve demonstrates either critical aortic stenosis or atresia, with a hypoplastic annulus and restricted leaflet motion.
- Co-existing coarctation of the aorta.
- HLHS is frequently associated with increased nuchal translucency between 11 and 14 weeks.

### LESS FREQUENT

- Conduction disturbances may be present due to abnormalities in the bundle of His.
- Hydrops
- Interrupted aorta
- Extracardiac abnormalities (12%)
  - Duodenal atresia
  - Imperforate anus
  - Vertebral anomalies
  - Single umbilical artery

### KEY FINDINGS/PITFALLS

- Retrograde flow in the transverse aortic arch is a crucial finding and indicates that the left heart is inadequate to supply systemic output and that the lesion will be ductal dependent after delivery.
- Reversed flow across the atrial septum (i.e., from left atrium to right atrium) also suggests that the left heart is inadequate to supply the systemic output postnatally.
- The presence of tricuspid regurgitation increases the chance for the development of hydrops.
- HLHS may be seen by transabdominal imaging as early as 18-20 weeks.
- In cases with a family history of left-sided obstructive disease, the fetus should be reimaged at 28 to 32 weeks because the findings of HLHS-related anatomical defects can be subtle, or absent, in the early second trimester.
- The left ventricle can appear of normal size in the early-to-middle second trimester and become severely hypoplastic later during pregnancy, especially with aortic stenosis. One can avoid being fooled in such cases by carefully measuring the mitral and aortic valves to exclude hypoplasia, by examining for "reversed" flow at the atrial septum and transverse arch, and by demonstrating normal antegrade flow with color Doppler interrogation at the mitral and aortic valves.

- One should assess the adequacy of the foramen ovale. With critical left atrial outflow obstruction, such as with mitral atresia, an inadequate foramen ovale will not allow left atrial decompression. In such cases, the pulmonary veins are dilated, and there is prominent flow reversal with atrial systole. In addition, pulse Doppler interrogation shows restrictive flow from the left to the right atrium. In the neonatal period the foramen ovale usually remains patent. HLHS with an intact septum is lethal.

### DIFFERENTIAL DIAGNOSIS

Mild HLHS can occur with

- Aortic coarctation
- Diaphragmatic hernia
- Omphalocele

## PREGNANCY MANAGEMENT

**Investigations and Consultations Required** At the time of the initial diagnosis, an extended ultrasound examination should be performed to assess for associated anomalies. Chromosome studies, including microarray, should be obtained by amniocentesis. Prenatal consultation with a pediatric cardiologist should occur for a fetal echocardiogram, discussion of options, and coordination of a postnatal management plan, when appropriate. Consultations with genetics and neonatology should be obtained.

**Pregnancy Course** Unless hydrops develops, fetuses will generally go to term and can be delivered vaginally.

**Fetal Intervention** In utero balloon valvuloplasty for the treatment of severe aortic stenosis has had some limited success in allowing left ventricle growth and leading to 2-ventricle circulation at birth, but fetal hemodynamic instability is common during the procedure.

**Pregnancy Termination Issues** If termination is chosen, an intact fetus should be delivered for confirmation of diagnosis.

**Monitoring** Repeat ultrasound examinations are performed every 4 weeks. Fetuses with left heart obstructive disease should have a repeat fetal echocardiogram at 28 and 32 weeks. Close follow-up is needed to monitor for any progression in the severity of left ventricle hypoplasia and obstruction. Hydrops can develop and is more likely to occur when there is severe tricuspid regurgitation or right ventricle dysfunction. Also, the foramen ovale must be assessed to make sure it is open. If it is very restrictive or closed, then the delivery plan will be altered.

**Delivery** Delivery should occur at a center where immediate pediatric cardiology and cardiac surgery consultation are available. This lesion will be ductal dependent, and even more urgent management is necessary if there is a restrictive atrial septal defect. Vaginal delivery is preferred.

## NEONATOLOGY

**Resuscitation** Infants with HLHS will usually breathe spontaneously, without the immediate need for assisted ventilation. Adequate venous and arterial access should be obtained and prostaglandin $E_1$ therapy begun.

**Transport** In most cases, infants should be transported to regional centers skilled in taking care of infants with HLHS. In cases in which an accurate prenatal diagnosis of HLHS is made and in which the family has chosen compassionate care, transport may not be required.

**Testing and Confirmation** The diagnosis of HLHS is definitively made by echocardiography. Neuroimaging should be considered, given recent studies that found that up to 60% of full-term newborns with congenital heart disease have evidence of brain injury.

**Nursery Management** Institution of prostaglandin $E_1$ therapy often stabilizes the infant with HLHS and allows adequate systemic blood flow. As the pulmonary vascular resistance drops, there may be a tendency for excessive pulmonary blood flow and diminished systemic blood flow. In such situations, measures to reduce excessive pulmonary blood flow include avoidance of supplemental oxygen, administration of nitrogen or carbon dioxide to reduce inspired oxygen concentration, and positive-pressure ventilation.

## SURGERY

**Preoperative Assessment** Echocardiography is adequate for preoperative diagnosis whether one pursues the Norwood procedure or heart transplantation. A fetus with a definitive prenatal diagnosis of HLHS can be listed for heart transplantation prenatally and fetal blood samples obtained to allow for typing. If a donor heart becomes available during the late third trimester, induction or cesarean section may be performed to allow heart transplantation.

**Operative Indications** HLHS is fatal without surgical intervention; thus, the diagnosis itself represents an indication for surgery unless the family chooses compassionate care.

**Types of Procedures** Palliative surgery involves three operations. The Norwood procedure is performed soon after birth. The main pulmonary artery is transected proximal to the branch pulmonary arteries and anastomosed to the ascending aorta and transverse arch. The atrial septum is resected to allow unobstructed flow from the left to the right atrium. A modified Blalock-Taussig shunt is placed to supply pulmonary blood flow. A bidirectional Glenn procedure is performed between 3 and 6 months of age. The superior vena cava is anastomosed to the right pulmonary artery and the Blalock-Taussig shunt removed. This allows systemic venous blood from the head and neck vessels to travel directly to the branch pulmonary arteries. A Fontan operation is performed between 1 and 6 years of age. The blood from the inferior vena cava and hepatic veins is baffled directly to the lungs. Therefore, the only blood returning to the atria is pulmonary venous blood, which is routed directly to the aorta. Some centers have chosen to pursue infant heart transplantation. However, securing an adequate number of donor hearts for infant transplantation is problematic.

**Surgical Results and Prognosis** Among centers with favorable results pursuing the Norwood procedure and later Fontan operation, 5-year survival is 70%. Families are now counseled that even with successful three-stage palliation, a transplant will be needed in the future. There is significant attrition in infants waiting for a donor heart. Among infants receiving hearts, the actuarial survival rate after transplantation is 84% at 1 month, 70% at 1 year, and 69% at 2 years.

## SUGGESTED READINGS

1. Allen RH, Benson CB, Haug LW: Pregnancy outcome of fetuses with a diagnosis of hypoplastic left ventricle on prenatal sonography. J Ultrasound Med 2005; 24:1199-1203.
2. Barron DJ, Kilby MD, Davies B, et al: Hypoplastic left heart syndrome. Lancet 2009; 374:551-564.
3. Feinstein JA, Benson DW, Dubin AM, et al: Hypoplastic left heart syndrome: current considerations and expectations. J Am Coll Cardiol 2012; 59:S1-S42.
4. Freud LR, McElhinney DB, Marshall AC, et al: Fetal aortic valvuloplasty for evolving hypoplastic left heart syndrome: postnatal outcomes of the first 100 patients. Circulation 2014; 130:638-645.
5. Galindo A, Nieto O, Villagra S, et al: Hypoplastic left heart syndrome diagnosed in fetal life: associated findings, pregnancy outcome and results of palliative surgery. Ultrasound Obstet Gynecol 2009; 33:560-566.
6. Hinton RB, Andelfinger G, Sekar P, et al. Prenatal head growth and white matter injury in hypoplastic left heart syndrome. Pediatr Res 2008; 64:364-369.
7. Khalil A, Suff N, Thilaganathan B, et al: Brain abnormalities and neurodevelopmental delay in congenital heart disease: systematic review and meta-analysis. Ultrasound Obstet Gynecol 2014; 43:14-24.
8. Rychik J, Szwast A, Natarajan S, et al: Perinatal and early surgical outcome for the fetus with hypoplastic left heart syndrome: a 5-year single institutional experience. Ultrasound Obstet Gynecol 2010; 36:465-470.
9. Simpson JM: Hypoplastic left heart syndrome. Ultrasound Obstet Gynecol 2000; 15:271-278.
10. Tongsong T, Sittiwangkul R, Khunamornpong S, Wanapirak C: Prenatal sonographic features of isolated hypoplastic left heart syndrome. J Clin Ultrasound 2005; 33:367-371.
11. Wilkins-Haug LE, Tworetzky W, Benson CB, et al: Factors affecting technical success of fetal aortic valve dilation. Ultrasound Obstet Gynecol 2006; 28:47-52.

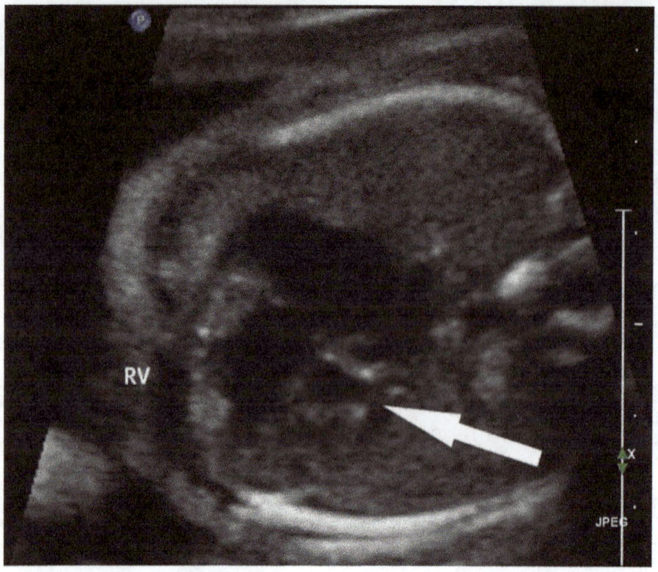


**FIGURE 3.7A** Hypoplastic left heart syndrome. Small left ventricle (arrow).

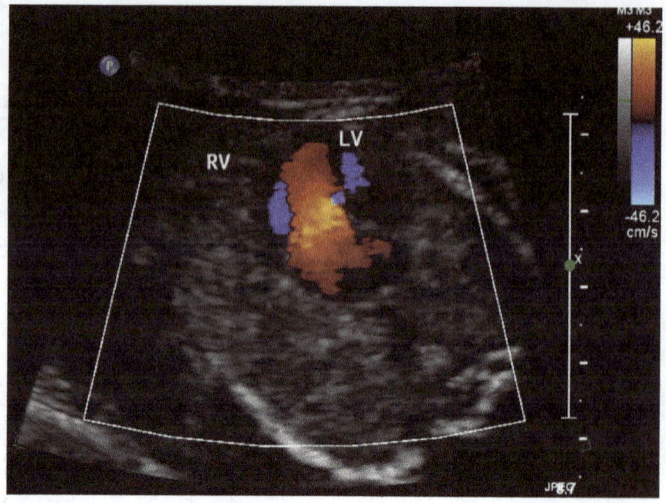


**FIGURE 3.7B** Hypoplastic left heart syndrome. Color Doppler of a small left ventricle (blue) and a large right ventricle (red).

# 3.8 TETRALOGY OF FALLOT

## EPIDEMIOLOGY/GENETICS

**Definition** Tetralogy of Fallot (TOF) is a conoventricular defect with four classic features: (1) ventricular septal defect (VSD), (2) overriding aorta over the VSD, (3) pulmonary stenosis or atresia, and (4) right ventricular hypertrophy (RVH).

**Epidemiology** TOF occurs in 1 in 3600 live births and accounts for 3.5% to 7% of infants with congenital heart disease (CHD). Males are slightly more commonly affected than females (3:2).

**Embryology** TOF develops from a single embryonic anomaly; an unequal division of the conus, or infundibulum, is caused by an anterior displacement of the truncoconal septum. As a result of this anterior displacement, the conus is divided into a smaller anterior right ventricular section and a larger posterior portion. This results in outflow narrowing and hence pulmonary stenosis. The displacement also prevents closure of the interventricular septum, resulting in a VSD. Because the right ventricular outflow is narrowed by the conotruncal malalignment, the aorta is now larger and overrides the septum over the VSD.

**Inheritance Pattern** The recurrence of congenital heart disease in siblings of patients with TOF is 3% if one sibling is affected and 8% if two siblings are affected. The recurrence risk for congenital heart defects in offspring of a parent affected with TOF is 2.5% when the mother is affected and 1.5% when the father is affected. Among patients with TOF, the prevalence of the chromosome 22q11 microdeletion is 25%. When there is a right aortic arch, associated dysplastic pulmonary valve syndrome, or associated pulmonary valve atresia, the risk of chromosome 22q11 microdeletion is greater. TOF can occur in trisomies 21, 18, and 13; Alagille syndrome; and CHARGE (coloboma, heart defect, atresia choanae, retarded growth, genital anomaly, ear abnormality) syndrome, as well as a number of other genetic syndromes.

**Teratogens** Retinoic acid, valproate, amantadine, coumadin, maternal diabetes mellitus, and maternal phenylketonuria.

**Prognosis** Long-term survival is 85%-90%. The prognosis is worse in the subset of infants with pulmonary atresia or with severely hypoplastic branch pulmonary arteries. These patients may require multiple operations and interventional catheterization procedures to recruit an adequate pulmonary bed to allow repair.

## SONOGRAPHY

### FREQUENT FINDINGS

- A VSD is typically seen in the 4-chamber view with an overriding aorta in the long-axis view.
  - The aorta can be dilated, but not always. The left ventricular outflow tract will tend to have a Y appearance in the long-axis view.
  - The first clue to the diagnosis is often the discrepancy between the great vessels, with the aorta larger than the pulmonary artery. This discrepancy can be appreciated on the three vessel view.

- The VSD is perimembraneous and is usually seen on the subcostal view of the heart.
  - Color flow may be necessary to confirm the defect.
- The right ventricular outflow tract will appear small, especially in the short-axis view, compared to the left.
  - The pulmonary valve should be measured and compared to normative data.
  - The smaller the valve is, the greater the obstruction will be and the more severe the RVH.

## LESS FREQUENT

- Hydrops can be found when there is significant pulmonary and tricuspid regurgitation secondary to a dysplastic pulmonary valve.
- Polyhydramnios, usually in association with hydrops, may occur.
- Noncardiac abnormalities (16%) may occur.

## KEY FINDINGS/PITFALLS

- The direction of ductal flow should be assessed. With more severe pulmonary obstruction, ductal flow will reverse and course from aorta to pulmonary artery. Reversed ductal flow suggests that postnatally the fetus will be ductal dependent. A small percentage of infants do not have a ductus arteriosus.
- RVH is rarely seen in the fetus.
- Severe levocardia may be seen in some cases.
- TOF can be associated with various abnormalities of the pulmonary valve, including pulmonary atresia, dysplastic pulmonary valve, and pulmonic stenosis. Pulmonary regurgitation may be seen, especially with the absent pulmonary valve syndrome.
- A left superior vena cava is noted in 15% of patients with TOF. A right aortic arch is seen in 25%.
- TOF is most commonly identified on the anatomy survey performed at 17-22 weeks; however, it is occasionally identified on transvaginal imaging at 13-15 weeks.
- An overriding great vessel above a VSD is a nonspecific finding in TOF and can also be seen in double outlet right ventricle (DORV), transposition of the great arteries with VSD, or truncus arteriosus (TA). One must not assume that the overriding great vessel is the aorta. If more than 50% of the aorta overlies the left ventricle, TOF is present. If more than 50% overlies the right ventricle, DORV is more likely.
- A normal apical or subcostal 4-chamber heart view does not rule out TOF. All four chambers will usually be of equal size.
- TOF can also be confused with TA. In TA, there is a single semilunar root from which both the branch pulmonary arteries and the ascending aorta arise.
- TOF can be confused with transposition of the great arteries with VSD.
- The severity of pulmonary stenosis in TOF can progress in utero, and pulmonary atresia may develop. It may be difficult to identify antegrade flow across the pulmonary valve. Detection of even a small amount of pulmonary regurgitation is a clue that the pulmonary valve is patent.

## PREGNANCY MANAGEMENT

**Investigations and Consultations Required** At the time of the initial diagnosis, an extended ultrasound examination should be performed to assess for associated anomalies. Consultation with a geneticist is important to guide the genetic testing and review the findings. Chromosome studies should include a karyotype with a microarray for 22q11 deletion. Of patients with TOF, 11% to 34% can have this deletion, and up to 27% of prenatally diagnosed cases will have a chromosome abnormality. The family should meet with a pediatric cardiologist to perform a fetal echocardiogram, to discuss the cardiac findings, and to coordinate a prenatal and postnatal management plan.

**Pregnancy Course** There is little, if any, impact on pregnancy course.

**Fetal Intervention** None.

**Pregnancy Termination Issues** If termination is chosen, an intact fetus should be delivered for confirmation of diagnosis and exclusion of noncardiac abnormalities.

**Monitoring** Repeat ultrasound examinations are performed every 4 weeks. A fetal echocardiogram should be repeated at 28 and 34 weeks to assess the growth of the pulmonary valve, main pulmonary artery, and branch pulmonary arteries.

**Delivery** Delivery should be performed at a tertiary care center that has the immediate availability of pediatric cardiology. This lesion can be a ductal-dependent lesion and require initiation of prostaglandin $E_1$ therapy.

## NEONATOLOGY

**Resuscitation** If delivery occurs at term, spontaneous respirations are usually present, and mechanical ventilation is not necessary. Venous access may be needed, depending on the oxygen saturation and the infant's clinical condition. Prostaglandin $E_1$ is not started unless ductal patency is required to achieve adequate pulmonary blood flow. Usually, the need for institution of prostaglandin $E_1$ therapy can be predicted at the 28- to 34-week antenatal echocardiography assessment.

**Transport** Transport to a center with neonatology, pediatric cardiology, and cardiac surgery capability is indicated. If the infant becomes symptomatic in the immediate newborn period, with worsening cyanosis or perfusion, transport should occur immediately. Consultation with a pediatric cardiologist prior to transport is recommended to determine the need for prostaglandin $E_1$ infusion to maintain ductal flow.

**Testing and Confirmation** A definitive diagnosis of TOF and identification of associated findings should be made with echocardiography.

**Nursery Management** If the infant is stable at the time of delivery, the ductus arteriosus is allowed to close, while the baby is observed closely in the neonatal intensive care unit to ensure that there is adequate pulmonary blood flow. If the oxygen saturation exceeds 85% after the ductus is closed, this suggests that there is sufficient antegrade pulmonary blood flow to allow the baby to be safely discharged home.

Developmental follow-up is recommended in infants with cyanotic heart disease requiring surgery in the first few weeks of life, as they are at risk for developmental delay.

## SURGERY

**Preoperative Assessment** In most cases, echocardiography is sufficient for preoperative diagnosis. Cardiac catheterization is rarely needed to exclude coronary artery abnormalities, additional VSDs, or branch pulmonary artery distortion. In TOF with pulmonary atresia, cardiac catheterization is required because associated aorta-to-pulmonary-artery collaterals and distal branch pulmonary artery distortion are not well seen with echocardiography.

**Operative Indications** All patients require surgical repair. Most patients are electively repaired between 2 and 6 months of age, or earlier, if cyanosis worsens, or TOF spells (episodes of bluish skin during crying and feeding) occur. When there is pulmonary atresia with an unreliable source of pulmonary blood flow, surgery will be needed in the newborn period.

**Types of Procedures** Surgical repair involves closure of the VSD, either through a right ventriculotomy or via a transtricuspid valve approach. The subpulmonary obstruction is resected, and frequently an outflow patch is placed to enlarge the subpulmonary area. If the pulmonary annulus is hypoplastic, the patch may need to extend across the annulus and into the main pulmonary artery. Branch pulmonary artery stenoses are addressed at surgery as well.

**Surgical Results and Prognosis** Operative mortality for TOF is less than 5%. Approximately 5% to 10% of patients may require intervention for peripheral pulmonary artery stenosis postoperatively, but these stenoses can often be addressed with interventional catheterization. Balloon dilation or placement of intravascular stents is used to relieve the branch pulmonary artery distortion.

### SUGGESTED READINGS

1. Allan LD, Sharland GK: Prognosis in fetal tetralogy of Fallot. Pediatr Cardiol 1992; 13:1-4.
2. Apitz C, Webb GD, Redington AN: Tetralogy of Fallot. Lancet. 2009; 374:1462-1471.
3. Arya B, Levasseur SM, Woldu K, et al: Fetal echocardiographic measurements and the need for neonatal surgical intervention in tetralogy of Fallot. Pediatr Cardiol 2014; 35:810-816.
4. Bailliard F, Anderson RH: Tetralogy of Fallot. Orphanet J Rare Dis 2009; 4:2.
5. Bhat AH, Kehl DW, Tacy TA, et al: Diagnosis of tetralogy of Fallot and its variants in the late first and early second trimester: details of initial assessment and comparison with later fetal diagnosis. Echocardiography 2013; 30:81-87.

6. Escribano D, Herraiz I, Granados M, et al: Tetralogy of Fallot: prediction of outcome in the mid-second trimester of pregnancy. Prenat Diagn 2011; 31:1126-1133.
7. Friedman K, Balasubramanian S, Tworetzky W: Midgestation fetal pulmonary annulus size is predictive of outcome in tetralogy of fallot. Congenit Heart Dis 2014; 9:187-193.
8. Hartge D, Hoffmann U, Schroer A, Weichert J: Three- and four-dimensional ultrasound in the diagnosis of fetal tetralogy of Fallot with absent pulmonary valve and microdeletion 22q11. Pediatr Cardiol 2010; 31:1100-1103.
9. Marino B, Digilio MC, Toscano A, et al: Anatomic patterns of conotruncal defects associated with deletion 22q11. Genet Med 2001; 3:45-48.
10. Monaco M, Williams I: Tetralogy of Fallot: fetal diagnosis to surgical correction. Minerva Pediatr 2012; 64:461-470.
11. Poon LC, Huggon IC, Zidere V, Allan LD: Tetralogy of Fallot in the fetus in the current era. Ultrasound Obstet Gynecol 2007; 29:625-627.
12. Starr JP: Tetralogy of Fallot: yesterday and today. World J Surg 2010; 34:658-668.
13. Yoo SJ, Lee YH, Kim ES, et al: Three-vessel view of the fetal upper mediastinum: an easy means of detecting abnormalities of the ventricular outflow tracts and great arteries during obstetric screening. Ultrasound Obstet Gynecol 1997; 9:173-182.
14. Yoo SJ, Lee YH, Kim ES, et al: Tetralogy of Fallot in the fetus: findings at targeted sonography. Ultrasound Obstet Gynecol 1999; 14:29-37.
15. Ziolkowska L, Kawalec W, Turska-Kmiec A, et al: Chromosome 22q11.2 microdeletion in children with conotruncal heart defects: frequency, associated cardiovascular anomalies, and outcome following cardiac surgery. Eur J Pediatr 2008; 167:1135-1140.

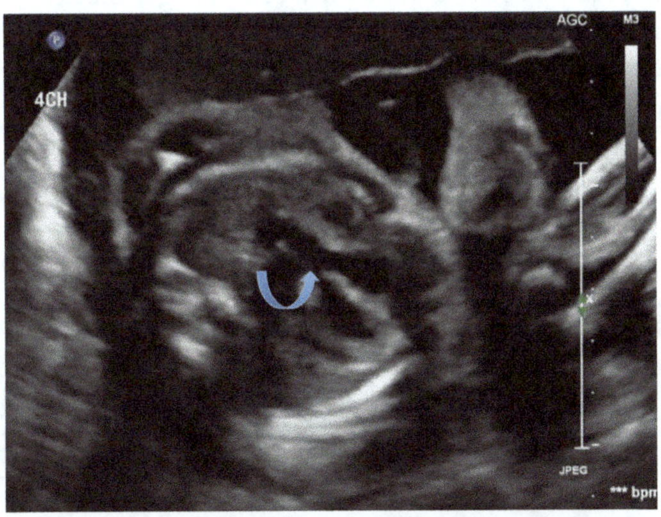


FIGURE 3.8A Tetralogy of Fallot. Ventricular septal defect with an overriding aorta (curved arrow).

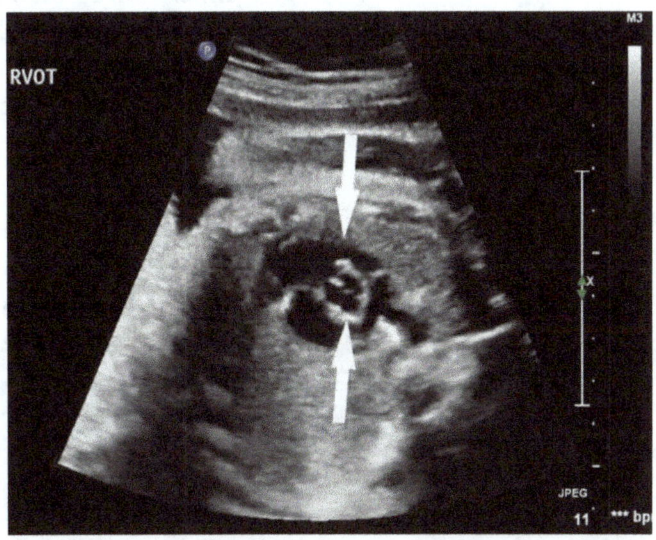


FIGURE 3.8B Tetralogy of Fallot. Enlarged aorta (lower arrow) and narrow main pulmonary artery (upper arrow).

# 3.9 TRANSPOSITION OF THE GREAT ARTERIES (D-TRANSPOSITION OF THE GREAT ARTERIES)

## EPIDEMIOLOGY/GENETICS

**Definition** The aorta connects with the right ventricle, and the main pulmonary artery connects with the left ventricle. The most common form of transposition is complete transposition, also called d-transposition (TGA, transposition of the great arteries). Patients are cyanotic because deoxygenated blood (i.e., systemic venous blood) is pumped by the right ventricle to the body, and oxygenated blood (i.e., pulmonary venous blood) is pumped by the left ventricle to the lungs. The right ventricle is the systemic ventricle, which can lead to hypertrophy and dysfunction. The connections of the atria and ventricles are correct.

Complete transposition should be distinguished from congenitally corrected transposition of the great arteries, sometimes referred to as physiologically corrected or L-TGA. Usually in physiologically corrected transposition, the heart tube loops to the left (L-looping), resulting in ventricular inversion. Anatomically, transposition is present because the right ventricle connects with the aorta and the left ventricle connects with the main pulmonary artery. However, physiologically, the baby is not cyanotic. Systemic venous blood is pumped by the left ventricle to the pulmonary artery, and pulmonary venous blood is pumped by the right ventricle to the aorta.

**Epidemiology** Prevalence is 0.2 to 0.3 per 1000 live births and accounts for 5% to 8% of children with cardiac disease. It has a male predominance.

**Embryology** TGA is due to straight downward growth of the conotruncal ridge instead of the normal spiraling growth at 4 to 5 weeks' gestation. This results in a disruption in the expected relationship of the ventricles to the great vessels.

**Inheritance Pattern** The recurrence risk is 1.5% when one sibling is affected and 5% when two siblings are affected. It is rarely associated with chromosomal abnormalities or other syndromes, except heterotaxy. Approximately 1% of TGA cases are associated with a 22q11 deletion.

**Teratogens** Thalidomide, trifluoperazine, trimethadione, and maternal diabetes mellitus are teratogenic.

**Prognosis** The most common repair is the arterial switch operation, which has an early mortality of 5% or less. Long-term results are limited but suggest a 20-year survival rate approaching 90%.

## SONOGRAPHY

### FREQUENT FINDINGS

- The diagnosis is best made by identifying parallel outflow tracts in a long view of the heart (normal outflow tracts should cross).

- The aortic valve is most commonly to the right of, and anterior to, the pulmonary valve, but the aorta can be side by side with, straight anterior to, or even left of, and anterior to, the pulmonary valve.
- Ventricular septal defects (VSDs) are present in 30% to 50% of patients.

### LESS FREQUENT

- Hypoplastic tricuspid valve or right ventricle
- Pulmonary stenosis
- Subaortic stenosis
- Coarctation or interrupted arch
- Coronary abnormalities

### KEY FINDINGS/PITFALLS

- Once the abnormal ventricular/great vessel connections are identified, each great vessel should be identified. The pulmonary tract will be noted to bifurcate into right and left pulmonary arteries. The aorta can be followed as it develops an arch, and head and neck vessels can be seen extending superiorly off the arch.
- To differentiate d-TGA (dextro-TGA) from l-TGA, the ventricles should be imaged and the moderator band identified to confirm the right ventricle.
- Restrictive patent foramen ovale can be associated with worse postnatal cyanosis.
- Small, or restrictive, ductus arteriosus may also be associated with a worse postnatal outcome.
- The ascending aorta and main pulmonary artery should be measured and compared with normative data. Ascending aortic hypoplasia occurs in association with coarctation, interrupted aortic arch, and subvalvular aortic stenosis. Marked main pulmonary artery hypoplasia is associated with subvalvular and valvular pulmonary stenosis.
- Detectable at 16-18 weeks' gestation.

### DIFFERENTIAL DIAGNOSIS

- Double-outlet right ventricle: One great vessel and the majority of the other arise from the right ventricle. It may be confusing when the aorta arises from the right ventricle and the pulmonary artery straddles the VSD. When the pulmonary artery is more than 50% above the right ventricle, the diagnosis is DORV. When the pulmonary artery is more than 50% above the left ventricle, the diagnosis is transposition with VSD.
- Tetralogy of Fallot (TOF): The aorta overrides a VSD, and the main pulmonary artery arises from the right ventricle. If the great vessels are inaccurately identified (i.e., the main pulmonary artery and the aorta are confused for one another), then TGA with VSD could be confused with TOF.

## PREGNANCY MANAGEMENT

**Investigations and Consultations Required** An extended fetal anatomy survey should be performed to assess for additional anomalies. Chromosomal studies should be done, including microarray for chromosome 22q deletion. Pediatric cardiology consultation should be obtained for a fetal echocardiogram and to coordinate the prenatal and postnatal cardiac plans. Consultations with genetics and neonatology should be obtained.

**Pregnancy Course** No major issues are expected.

**Fetal Intervention** None are available.

**Pregnancy Termination Issues** If chosen, an intact fetus should be delivered for confirmation of diagnosis.

**Monitoring** Repeat echocardiography is indicated at 28 to 30 weeks, primarily to assess the outflow tracts, ductus arteriosus, and foramen ovale. Repeat ultrasound examinations are performed every 4 weeks.

**Delivery** Delivery should be performed at a tertiary center where pediatric cardiology consultation is immediately available and where atrial balloon septostomy can be performed on an emergency basis.

## NEONATOLOGY

**Resuscitation** Spontaneous respirations are generally present, and immediate mechanical ventilation is usually not necessary. Secure venous access is needed, and, depending on the oxygen saturation and clinical condition, placement of arterial and venous umbilical catheters may be indicated as well. Prostaglandin $E_1$ is generally started to improve mixing by maintaining ductal patency. If the diagnosis is TGA and VSD, then prostaglandin is often not required, as the VSD allows mixing of saturated and desaturated blood.

**Transport** The neonate should be transported to a center with expertise in echocardiographic diagnosis, interventional catheterization, pediatric cardiology, and pediatric cardiac surgery.

**Testing and Confirmation** A complete and accurate diagnosis can generally be obtained using echocardiography alone.

**Nursery Management** Oxygen saturations between 70% and 85%, without metabolic acidosis, are desirable. When oxygen saturations are inadequate, supplemental oxygen is administered to increase pulmonary venous saturation. If the oxygen saturation is still inadequate, prostaglandin $E_1$ and atrial balloon septostomy can be helpful. Maintaining systemic blood pressure will often facilitate mixing as well.

Developmental follow-up is recommended in infants with cyanotic heart disease requiring surgery in the first few weeks of life, as they are at risk for developmental delay.

## SURGERY

**Preoperative Assessment** Echocardiographic diagnosis is generally definitive.

**Operative Indications** All patients with transposition require surgery. This generally should be performed after the pulmonary resistance falls, usually within the first week of life. Associated lesions, such as pulmonary stenosis or VSD, may change the timing of surgery.

**Types of Procedures** The arterial switch operation is most commonly used to repair d-TGA. The great vessels are transected and reconnected to the appropriate ventricles. The coronary arteries are removed from the aortic root and translocated to the neoaortic root (i.e., the great vessel arising from the left ventricle). A Rastelli operation is performed when transposition of the great arteries is associated with VSD and subvalvular pulmonary stenosis. In such cases, the pulmonary stenosis does not allow an arterial switch procedure because postoperatively there would be aortic stenosis. In a Rastelli operation, the pulmonary venous blood is baffled from the left ventricle through the VSD to the aorta, and a homograft or conduit is placed from the right ventricle to the pulmonary artery. This allows physiologic correction, and the left ventricle becomes the systemic ventricle (in contrast to the atrial switches). In rare cases, in which there is severe ventricular hypoplasia or straddling of AV valves that does not allow VSD closure, a single-ventricle operation is required.

**Surgical Results/Prognosis** The operative mortality rate for the arterial switch procedure is less than 5%. Subsequent reoperation or interventional catheterization procedures are required in 10% of patients. Late complications of the arterial switch operation include supravalvular pulmonary stenosis, neoaortic root enlargement, aortic regurgitation, left ventricular dysfunction, branch pulmonary artery stenosis, aortic anastomotic stenosis, and coronary artery stenosis or distortion. Long-term survival appears to be excellent. Patients who have undergone the arterial switch have a 10% to 15% probability of significant right ventricular dysfunction or tricuspid regurgitation.

### SUGGESTED READINGS

1. Bartlett JM, Wypij D, Bellinger DC, et al: Effect of prenatal diagnosis on outcomes in D-transposition of the great arteries. Pediatrics 2004; 113:e335-e340.
2. Bertagna F, Rakza T, Vaksmann G, et al: Transposition of the great arteries: factors influencing prenatal diagnosis. Prenat Diagn 2014; 34:534-537.
3. Freire G, Miller M, Huhta J: Foetal echocardiography of transposition of the great arteries and common arterial trunk. Cardiol Young 2012; 22:671-676.
4. Khalil A, Suff N, Thilaganathan B, et al: Brain abnormalities and neurodevelopmental delay in congenital heart disease: systematic review and meta-analysis. Ultrasound Obstet Gynecol 2014; 43:14-24.
5. Li J, Tulloh RM, Cook A, et al: Coronary arterial origins in transposition of the great arteries: factors that affect outcome. A morphological and clinical study. Heart 2000; 83:320-325.

6. Masoller N, Martinez JM, Gomez O, et al: Evidence of second-trimester changes in head biometry and brain perfusion in fetuses with congenital heart disease. Ultrasound Gynecol 2014; 44:182-187.
7. McGahan JP, Moon-Grady AJ, Pahwa A, et al: Potential pitfalls and methods of improving in utero diagnosis of transposition of the great arteries, including the baby bird's beak image. J Ultrasound Med 2007; 26:1499-1510.
8. Rudolph AM: Aortopulmonary transposition in the fetus: speculation on pathophysiology and therapy. Pediatr Res 2007; 61:375-380.
9. Unolt M, Putotto C, Silvestri LM, et al: Transposition of great arteries: new insights into the pathogenesis. Front Pediatr 2013; 1:11.
10. van Velzen CL, Haak MC, Reijnders G, et al: Prenatal detection of transposition of the great arteries reduces mortality and morbidity. Ultrasound Obstet Gynecol 2015; 45:320-325.
11. Williams IA, Fifer WP, Andrews H: Fetal growth and neurodevelopmental outcome in congenital heart disease. Pediatr Cardiol 2015; 36:1135-1144.
12. Zhang Y, Cai A, Sun W: Prenatal diagnosis of fetal transposition of the great arteries. Circulation 2011; 123:1919-1920.


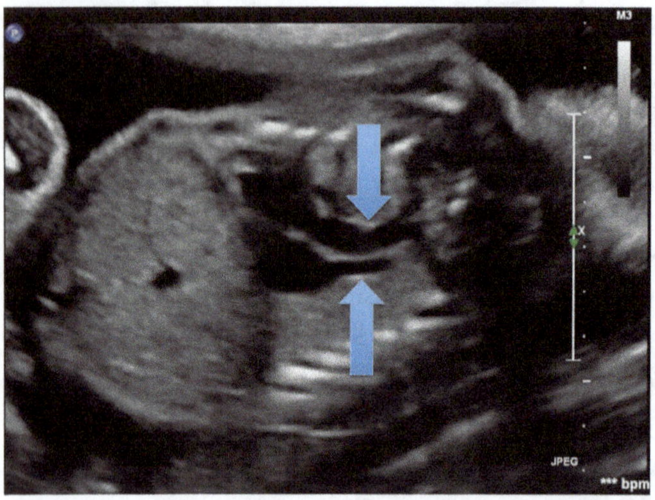


**FIGURE 3.9A** Transposition. Parallel outflow tracts (arrows).

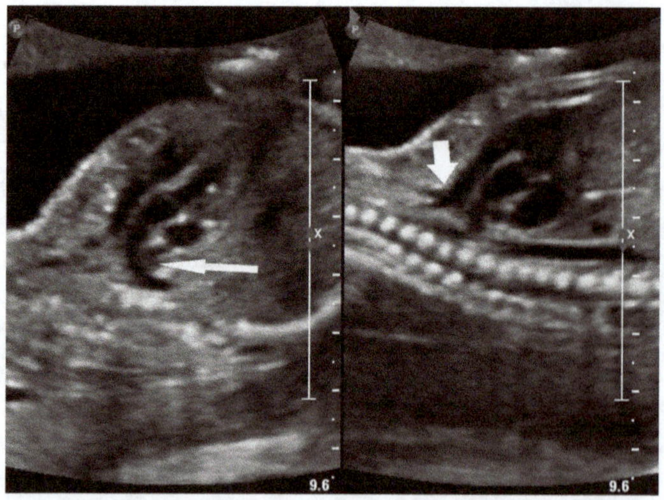


**FIGURE 3.9B** Transposition. Aorta (thin arrow) arising from the right ventricle. The pulmonary artery arises from the left ventricle and bifurcates (thick arrow).

# 3.10 TRUNCUS ARTERIOSUS

## EPIDEMIOLOGY/GENETICS

**Definition** In truncus arteriosus (TA) a single great vessel arises from the heart and supplies the systemic, pulmonary, and coronary blood flow. This single vessel usually arises above a malalignment type of ventricular septal defect (VSD) and straddles the ventricular septum. There is variability in the origins of the branch pulmonary arteries and whether the aortic arch is interrupted. TA with VSD can be classified into four types:

- Type I: A main pulmonary artery arises from the truncal root and bifurcates into the branch pulmonary arteries.
- Type II: The branch pulmonary arteries arise separately from the truncal root.
- Type III: The left pulmonary artery is supplied by collaterals from the aortic arch and does not arise from the truncal root.
- Type IV: The aortic arch is interrupted.

The large, single semilunar valve lies above the VSD in 42% of patients, over the right ventricle in 42%, and over the left ventricle in 16%. The valve to the common vessel is frequently dysplastic, resulting in insufficiency or stenosis.

**Epidemiology** The prevalence is 0.03 to 0.21 per 1000 live births and accounts for 1%-3% of fetal cardiac defects. Males and females are affected equally.

**Embryology** The bulbus cordis differentiates into the right ventricle, conus cordis, and TA. The TA should septate into the aortic and pulmonary valves and the ascending aorta and main pulmonary artery. A persistent TA is the consequence of failure of the truncoconal ridges to fuse. This fusion failure also results in a VSD.

**Inheritance Pattern** The recurrence risk for congenital heart disease in siblings of a patient with nonsyndromic TA is 1.2% when one sibling is affected and 3% when two are affected. The recurrence risk in offspring of parents affected with TA is unknown. Rare familial cases have been reported, showing an autosomal dominant inheritance pattern. Chromosomal abnormalities are common. A microdeletion of chromosome 22q11 occurs in up to 31% of fetuses with TA and up to 41% of affected infants.

**Teratogens** Maternal diabetes mellitus.

**Prognosis** The initial operative mortality rate is between 13% and 50%. Replacement of the conduit, placed during the repair between the right ventricle and pulmonary arteries, is needed in the future. The operative mortality rate for conduit replacement is approximately 1% to 3%. The frequent association of the chromosome 22q11 deletion may have a significant impact on the prognosis. Long-term survival after surgical correction is approximately 30% to 83% by 15 years of age. Left untreated, survival is poor, with a 75% 1-year mortality rate.

# SONOGRAPHY

## FREQUENT FINDINGS

- The primary finding is a single great vessel arising from the ventricles that is associated with a VSD.
  - This vessel supplies both the branch pulmonary arteries and the ascending aorta.
  - The origin of the right and left pulmonary arteries can vary and can even be found off the descending aorta.
  - Identification of their origins is crucial for confirming the diagnosis and identifying the subtype.
- The apical four-chamber view frequently appears normal in fetuses with TA.
  - Imaging of the five-chamber view will provide visualization of the single trunk overriding the associated VSD. There are only two vessels identified in the three vessel view.
- Usually, the truncal root will straddle the muscular septum above a malalignment type of VSD.
- The truncal valve is frequently abnormal and commonly appears dilated.
  - Color and pulse Doppler interrogation should identify truncal stenosis or regurgitation.

## LESS FREQUENT

- Hydrops
- Polyhydramnios, usually in association with hydrops
- Intrauterine growth restriction if there is significant valvular stenosis or regurgitation

## KEY FINDINGS/PITFALLS

- Interrupted aortic arch occurs in 10% to 15% of patients with TA.
  - The ascending aorta supplies the head and neck vessels, but the descending aorta is supplied by the ductus arteriosus and not by continuation of the aortic arch.
  - In TA without interrupted aortic arch, a ductus arteriosus is not present in 50%–75% of cases.
- A right aortic arch is present in 15% to 30% of patients. The probability of the chromosome 22q11 deletion is increased when the arch is right sided.
- TA is detectible by transabdominal imaging at 16 to 18 weeks. Malalignment VSDs have been diagnosed with transvaginal echocardiography at 14 weeks.
- A single great vessel originating over a VSD can be seen in TOF and pulmonary atresia with a VSD. A definitive diagnosis can only be made if more than three leaflets can be identified within the truncal valve. TOF with pulmonary artery atresia would be the most common alternative etiology. In this case, the aorta straddles the septum and the main pulmonary artery is absent. Another cardiac defect that may mimic TA is aortic atresia with VSD, in which the main pulmonary artery straddles the septum and the ascending aorta is tiny. Careful

identification of the branch pulmonary arteries and the origins of the head and neck vessels distinguishes TA from these defects.

- In TA with an interrupted aortic arch, the ductus arteriosus can mimic the transverse arch and might confuse the sonographer into believing that the arch is not interrupted. This mistake is less likely if the origins of the head and neck vessels are identified. They will arise from the transverse arch, not from the ductus arteriosus.

### DIFFERENTIAL DIAGNOSIS

- Tetralogy of Fallot
- Pulmonary atresia or aortic atresia with a VSD

## PREGNANCY MANAGEMENT

**Investigations and Consultations Required** An extended fetal anatomy survey should be completed to assess for additional associated anomalies. A fetal echocardiogram and pediatric cardiology consultation should be obtained to provide prenatal counseling and to exclude the association of more complex congenital heart disease. Consultation with a geneticist should be obtained for fetal karyotyping and microarray, with specific attention to testing for the 22q11 deletion (DiGeorge syndrome).

**Pregnancy Course** Unless associated with other anomalies or complex congenital heart defects, fetuses with isolated TA tend to have no associated pregnancy complications. Delivery should be anticipated at term, with cesarean section reserved for the usual obstetrical indications. In cases with valvular stenosis or regurgitation, there is an increased risk for nonimmune hydrops.

**Fetal Intervention** None are available.

**Pregnancy Termination Issues** If termination is chosen, an intact fetus should be delivered for confirmation of diagnosis obtaining tissue and karyotyping with microarray.

**Monitoring** With significant valvular regurgitation, hydrops may develop. Therefore, serial monitoring with interval ultrasound examinations is recommended. A follow-up fetal echocardiogram to assess valve function in the third trimester may be helpful.

**Delivery** There is a significant association of TA with other anomalies, and congestive heart failure (CHF) can develop within the first days of life in some patients. Delivery should be performed at a center where immediate neonatology and pediatric cardiac consultation and treatment are available.

## NEONATOLOGY

**Resuscitation** Assistance with the onset of respiration is usually not required. Early-onset cyanosis may occur and be confusing in the transition immediately following delivery.

**Transport** Immediate referral to a tertiary center with full pediatric cardiac diagnostic and surgical capability is imperative once a diagnosis of cyanotic congenital heart disease is suspected. Consultation with a pediatric cardiologist prior to transport is recommended to determine the need for initiation of a prostaglandin $E_1$ infusion. Management in transport should be by personnel experienced in neonatal transport and with the capability of mechanical ventilation.

**Testing and Confirmation** Postnatal echocardiography is generally sufficient for preoperative assessment.

**Nursery Management** The critical issues that determine early management are (1) the anatomy of pulmonary blood flow and the potential for early-onset CHF and (2) the anatomy of the aortic arch, including the integrity of systemic flow to the distal body. Infants with the former may require measures to limit pulmonary flow, such as limited fluid intake, decreased inspired oxygen concentration, and diuretics. Infants with an interrupted aortic arch require the administration of prostaglandin $E_1$ to maintain ductal flow and thus blood to the descending aorta.

Developmental follow-up is recommended in infants with cyanotic heart disease requiring surgery in the first few weeks of life, as they are at risk for developmental delay.

## SURGERY

**Preoperative Assessment** Postnatal echocardiography is generally sufficient for preoperative assessment.

**Operative Indications** All infants with TA require surgical treatment.

**Types of Procedures** In most cases, definitive repair is performed within the first 10 days of life. The septal defect is patched such that the truncal root receives blood only from the left ventricle. The branch pulmonary arteries are removed from the truncal root and are connected to the right ventricle, generally using a homograft. The donor pulmonary artery sites are carefully patched so the coronary arteries that are in close proximity are not distorted. When the aortic arch is interrupted, complete repair is still performed within the newborn period. The interrupted segments are directly anastomosed. It is not advisable to palliate infants with TA by banding the branch pulmonary arteries because it may result in long-term problems with branch pulmonary artery distortion or pulmonary vascular disease.

**Surgical Results and Prognosis** With infant reparative surgery, the operative mortality rate is approximately 5%. The mortality rate is higher when the truncal valve is more abnormal. In rare cases, the truncal valve must be replaced, and this considerably elevates the operative mortality rate. Because a homograft is generally used to establish continuity between the right ventricle and the branch pulmonary arteries, the homograft needs to be replaced as the child grows. In general, two replacements are necessary before adulthood. Homograft replacement carries an operative mortality rate of 1% to 3%.

The postoperative outcome is directly related to the presence, or absence, of the DiGeorge syndrome.

## SUGGESTED READINGS


1. Freire G, Miller M, Huhta J: Foetal echocardiography of transposition of the great arteries and common arterial trunk. Cardiol Young 2012; 22:671-676.
2. Galindo A, Mendoza A, Arbues J, et al: Conotruncal anomalies in fetal life: accuracy of diagnosis, associated defects, and outcome. Eur J Obstet Gynecol Repro Biol 2009; 146:55-60.
3. Gomez O, Soveral I, Bennasar M, et al: Accuracy of fetal echocardiography in the differential diagnosis between truncus arteriosus and pulmonary atresia with ventricular septal defect. Fetal Diagn Ther 2016; 39:90-99.
4. Hartman RJ, Rasmussen SA, Botto LD, et al: The contribution of chromosomal abnormalities to congenital heart defects: a population-based study. Pediatr Cardiol 2011; 32:1147-1157.
5. Johnson TR: Conotruncal cardiac defects: a clinical imaging perspective. Pediatr Cardiol 2010; 31:430-437.
6. Momma K: Cardiovascular anomalies associated with chromosome 22q11.2 deletion syndrome. Am J Cardiol 2010; 105:1617-1624.
7. Russell HM, Jacobs ML, Anderson RH, et al: A simplified categorization for common arterial trunk. J Thorac Cardiovasc Surg 2011; 141:645-653.
8. Swanson TM, Selamet Tierney ES, et al: Truncus arteriosus: diagnostic accuracy, outcomes, and impact of prenatal diagnosis. Pediatr Cardiol 2009; 30:256-261.
9. Tometzki AJ, Suda K, Kohl T, et al: Accuracy of prenatal echocardiographic diagnosis and prognosis of fetuses with conotruncal anomalies. J Am Coll Cardiol 1999; 33:1696-1701.
10. Vaidyanathan B, Kumar S, Sudhakar A, et al: Conotruncal anomalies in the fetus: referral patterns and pregnancy outcomes in a dedicated fetal cardiology unit in South India. Ann Pediatr Cardiol 2013; 6:15-20.
11. Volpe P, Paladini D, Marasini M, et al: Common arterial trunk in the fetus: characteristics, associations, and outcome in a multicentre series of 23 cases. Heart 2003; 89:1437-1441.
12. Ziolkowska L, Kawalec W, Turska-Kmiec A, et al: Chromosome 22q11.2 microdeletion in children with conotruncal heart defects: frequency, associated cardiovascular anomalies, and outcome following cardiac surgery. Eur J Pediatr 2008; 167:1135-1140.

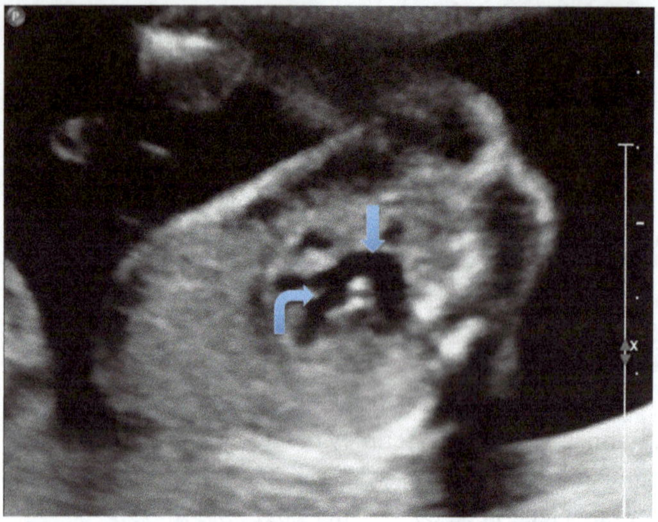

**FIGURE 3.10A** Truncus arteriosus. Single great vessel (straight arrow) with a malaligned ventricular septal defect (curved arrow).

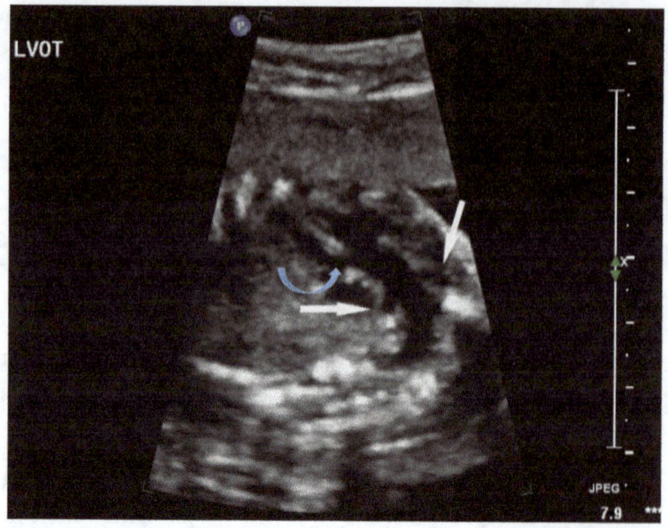


**FIGURE 3.10B** Truncus arteriosus. Single great vessel; malaligned ventricular septal defect (curved arrow); pulmonary branches (straight arrows).

# 3.11 VENTRICULAR SEPTAL DEFECT

## EPIDEMIOLOGY/GENETICS

**Definition** A ventricular septal defect (VSD) is an incomplete septation between the left and right ventricles. VSDs are classified into four major types: conoventricular (also called perimembranous), muscular, inlet (also called AV canal, or posterior), and conal septal or intraconal (also called subpulmonary and, less accurately, supracristal).

**Epidemiology** The prevalence is 0.4 to 2.7 per 1000 live births. VSDs are the most common congenital heart lesion diagnosed during the first year of life and account for up to 50% of congenital heart disease. They are slightly more common in females than males (56% females, 44% males).

**Embryology** The embryology varies depending on the location of the septal defect. Malalignment defects, a subtype of conoventricular defects, represent an abnormality of the conotruncus and are frequently associated with abnormalities of either the pulmonary or the systemic outflow. Muscular defects are thought to be due to excessive excavation during ventricular growth. Inlet defects are thought to be due to a failure of fusion.

**Inheritance Pattern** VSDs may be isolated or may be associated with other cardiac defects. They may also be an inherent part of more complex cardiac anomalies, such as tetralogy of Fallot (TOF). The inheritance pattern is multifactorial. Recurrence risk is 3% when one sibling is affected and 10% when two siblings are affected. The recurrence risk when a parent has a VSD is approximately 6%-10% for affected mothers and 2% for affected fathers. The majority of VSDs are sporadic. However, more than 100 genetic and chromosomal syndromes have been described with a VSD as an component, including trisomy 21, monosomy X, DiGeorge syndrome (22q11 deletion), and Holt-Oram syndrome.

**Teratogens** Alcohol, maternal diabetes, maternal phenylketonuria, rubella, anticonvulsants, retinoic acid, and amphetamines.

**Prognosis** Isolated VSDs usually have an excellent prognosis, with a quality of life for the patient similar to that of the general population. Of isolated VSDs, 74% close spontaneously before birth, and 75% to 90% of those that do not close prenatally will close within the first year of life. Inlet and intraconal defects usually do require surgery. Malalignment defects nearly always require surgery and carry the prognosis of the associated lesion, such as TOF or interrupted aortic arch with VSD. Prognosis is frequently dependent on associated abnormalities or syndrome diagnosis.

## SONOGRAPHY

### KEY FINDINGS

- Although VSDs are the most common congenital heart defect, they are only the fifth most commonly identified on ultrasound.

  - Color and pulsed Doppler can aid in visualization but are not definitive because flow through a fetal VSD may be minimal.
  - The varied locations and small size of many defects also limit identification.
- The four-chamber heart view is the most common view used to detect a VSD. Axial imaging, with the ultrasound beam perpendicular to the septum (subcostal four-chamber view), provides more detail and fewer artifacts than the lateral view (apical four-chamber view).
  - The VSD will present as an anechoic area in the septum and should be demonstrated in more than one plane.
  - The apical four-chamber view can frequently cause a dropout artifact, leading to a false-positive "pseudo"-VSD. A T sign has been described to distinguish an artifact from a real perimembranous VSD. The T sign represents a region of hypoechoic dropout bordering the hyperechogenic blunted edge of the intact interventricular septum at the edge of the defect. Although helpful, it is not 100% sensitive or specific.
- Membranous defects are anatomically located beneath the septal leaflet of the tricuspid valve on the right ventricular septal surface and below the aortic valve along the left ventricular septal surface.
  - These defects are best imaged when the scan plane is perpendicular to this portion of the septum.
  - False dropout can occur in this portion of the septum when viewed from the apical four-chamber view.
- Malalignment defects occur when the conal septum is misaligned in relation to the muscular septum. There are two types of malalignment defects:
  - Anterior malalignment: Malalignment of the conal septum is often best seen when one or both outflows are profiled from a high parasagittal view or an apical view. Short-axis views at the level of great vessels will also demonstrate malalignment of conal septum. An anterior malalignment type of defect in a fetus with normally related great vessels may result in subvalvular pulmonary stenosis and most commonly occurs in TOF. An anterior malalignment type of defect in a fetus with TGA may result in subvalvular aortic stenosis and is frequently associated with arch obstruction.
  - Posterior malalignment: A posterior malalignment defect in a fetus with normally related great vessels may result in subvalvular aortic stenosis and is frequently associated with valvular aortic stenosis and aortic arch obstruction. The posteriorly misaligned conal septum is best profiled from an apical four-chamber view or a high parasagittal view. A posterior malalignment defect in a fetus with transposition of the great arteries may result in subvalvular pulmonary stenosis and is frequently associated with pulmonary valve stenosis and annular hypoplasia.
- Muscular septal defects are further subcategorized based on their location within the muscular septum as anterior, middle, posterior, or apical muscular defects.
  - Muscular defects are difficult to see prenatally when they are small and even occasionally when they are moderate size.
  - Frequently, muscular defects are multiple.
  - Color Doppler echocardiography with appropriate optimization may show biphasic flow across the defects.

- Inlet defects involve the AV canal septum and are immediately adjacent to the AV valves and confluent with the crux of the heart.
  - These defects can be seen in isolation but are more commonly seen in a complete AV canal defect.
- Conal septal defects occur when there is a deficiency of the conal septum and are located immediately below the pulmonary and aortic valves.
  - These defects do not involve malalignment of the conal septum and are rare in North America. They are more common among Asian populations.
- Transabdominal imaging can detect defects between 16 and 18 weeks, and transvaginal imaging has detected malalignment defects as early as 14 weeks.

### PITFALLS

- It may be difficult to distinguish false dropout of the ventricular septum from a true septal defect.
  - This is best avoided by imaging perpendicular to the suspected defect and in multiple views.
  - False dropout is most likely to occur when the beam is parallel to the suspected defect, such as in the apical four-chamber view.
- Color Doppler flow mapping is most reliable when the angle of interrogation is perpendicular to the suspected defect and the machine settings are optimized. Low persistence and achieving a color Doppler frame rate in excess of 20 Hz provide the best imaging.

## PREGNANCY MANAGEMENT

**Investigations and Consultations Required** An extended fetal anatomy survey should be completed to assess for additional associated anomalies. A fetal echocardiogram and pediatric cardiology consultation should be obtained to provide prenatal counseling and to exclude the association of more complex congenital heart disease. If other noncardiac abnormalities are noted or a more complex congenital heart defect is found, consultation with a geneticist should be obtained for fetal karyotyping and microarray, especially looking for the presence of a possible 22q deletion (DiGeorge syndrome).

**Pregnancy Course** Unless associated with other anomalies or more complex congenital heart defects, fetuses with isolated VSDs are not expected to have associated pregnancy complications. Delivery should be anticipated at term, with cesarean section reserved for the usual obstetrical indications.

**Fetal Intervention** Fetal intervention is not indicated.

**Pregnancy Termination Issues** Delivery of an intact fetus is generally necessary to confirm the anatomic findings.

**Monitoring** Conoventricular septal defect should be reimaged between 28 and 30 weeks' gestation to ensure that the outflow tracts are not obstructed. If the VSD is isolated, a follow-up examination is appropriate to assess for any abnormalities that may have been missed on the initial scan. A third-trimester fetal echocardiogram also can assess if the lesion has closed spontaneously.

**Delivery** If the VSD is isolated and not associated with outflow obstruction, it would be acceptable for the fetus to be delivered in a community setting and pediatric cardiology consultation obtained during the first week of life. However, with a conoventricular defect and outflow obstruction, in which there is the potential for a ductus-dependent lesion, delivery at a tertiary care center is recommended for immediate neonatal and cardiology consultations and availability of prostaglandin $E_1$ therapy. Many simple VSDs close spontaneously before delivery.

## NEONATOLOGY

**Resuscitation** Infants will generally breathe spontaneously and not require resuscitation.

**Transport** An infant with a VSD without outflow tract obstruction can be discharged with pediatric cardiology follow-up within the first week of life.

**Testing and Confirmation** The urgency of postnatal testing is determined by the presence of associated cardiac defects and the type of septal defect. If the defect is located in the muscular or membranous septum and is in isolation, pediatric cardiology follow-up can be obtained electively within the first week or two of life. When conotruncal abnormalities are present, an echocardiogram should be performed before discharge.

**Nursery Management** Small muscular VSDs usually remain asymptomatic, whereas moderate-to-large and membranous defects become progressively more symptomatic as pulmonary vascular resistance falls in the first 4 to 6 weeks of life. Sodium and fluid restriction and diuretic therapy are used to control congestive heart failure (CHF).

## SURGERY

**Preoperative Assessment** Noninvasive diagnosis using echocardiography is generally adequate. If it is uncertain whether there is irreversible pulmonary vascular resistance, cardiac catheterization will be required preoperatively. This is rarely needed before age 1 year, as most defects are closed by then either spontaneously or surgically.

**Operative Indications** During infancy, isolated VSDs are closed if CHF results in failure to thrive despite maximum medical management or if there is pulmonary artery hypertension. Long-standing pulmonary artery hypertension can result in the development of pulmonary vascular obstructive disease. A large left ventricular volume overload may represent an indication for surgery during childhood, even if the patient is thriving, and the pulmonary artery pressures are normal.

### SUGGESTED READINGS

1. Allan LD: Atrioventricular septal defect in the fetus. Am J Obstet Gynecol 1999; 181:1250-1253.
2. Craig B: Atrioventricular septal defect: from fetus to adult. Heart 2006; 92:1879-1885.

3. Fesslova V, Villa L, Nava S, et al: Spectrum and outcome of atrioventricular septal defect in fetal life. Cardiol Young 2002; 12:18-26.
4. Gomez O, Martinez JM, Olivella A, et al: Isolated ventricular septal defects in the era of advanced fetal echocardiography: risk of chromosomal anomalies and spontaneous closure rate from diagnosis to age of 1 year. Ultrasound Obstet Gynecol 2014; 43:65-71.
5. Hyett JA, Moscoso G, Nicolaides KH: First-trimester nuchal translucency and cardiac septal defects in fetuses with trisomy 21. Am J Obstet Gynecol 1995; 172:1411-1413.
6. Jin Y, Wang A, Wang Y, et al: Natural history of prenatal ventricular septal defects and their association with foetal echocardiographic features. Cardiol Young 2012; 22:323-326.
7. Minette MS, Sahn DJ: Ventricular septal defects. Circulation. 2006; 114:2190-2197.
8. Mosimann B, Zidere V, Simpson JM, Allan LD: Outcome and requirement for surgical repair following prenatal diagnosis of ventricular septal defect. Ultrasound Obstet Gynecol 2014; 44:76-81.
9. Orie J, Flotta D, Sherman FS: To be or not to be a VSD. Am J Cardiol 1994; 74:1284-1285.
10. Paladini D, Palmieri S, Lamberti A, et al: Characterization and natural history of ventricular septal defects in the fetus. Ultrasound Obstet Gynecol 2000; 16:118-122.
11. Paladini D, Tartaglione A, Agangi A, et al: The association between congenital heart disease and Down syndrome in prenatal life. Ultrasound Obstet Gynecol 2000; 15:104-108.
12. Yagel S, Benachi A, Bonnet D, et al: Rendering in fetal cardiac scanning: the intracardiac septa and the coronal atrioventricular valve planes. Ultrasound Obstet Gynecol 2006; 28:266-274.

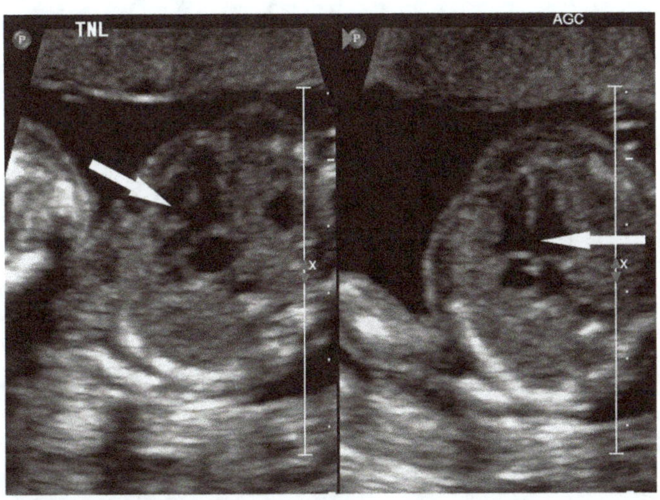


**FIGURE 3.11A** Perimembranous ventricular septal defect (arrows) on the left ventricular outflow tract view (left) and the four-chamber view (right).

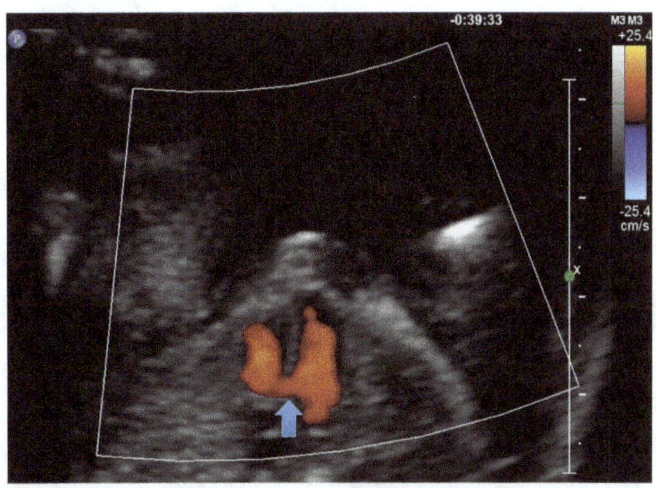


**FIGURE 3.11B** Power Doppler of four-chamber view. Perimembranous ventricular septal defect (arrow).

# CHAPTER 4

# THE GENITOURINARY SYSTEM

# 4.1 AMBIGUOUS GENITALIA

## EPIDEMIOLOGY/GENETICS

**Definition** *Ambiguous genitalia* is a term used to describe the clinical situation when examination of the external genitalia does not allow a clear gender assignment. Those conditions where chromosomal sex and phenotypic sex do not correspond are called disorders of sexual development.

**Epidemiology** The condition occurs in 1 in 5000 live births.

**Embryology** The term *ambiguous genitalia* can be used for those disorders with abnormally formed genitalia (severe penile hypospadias) to complete sex reversal (Smith-Lemli-Opitz syndrome). The most common etiology of isolated ambiguous genitalia is congenital adrenal hyperplasia (CAH), with masculinization of the female fetus (90% of cases). Other congenital abnormalities are present in up to 40% of infants with genital malformations. Additional etiologies of ambiguous genitalia, especially with associated malformations, are chromosomal abnormalities (trisomies 13 and 18, and triploidy) and over 50 genetic syndromes/associations, including Smith-Lemli Opitz syndrome, velocardiofacial syndrome, Prader-Willi syndrome, VACTERL (vertebral defects, anal atresia, cardiac defects, tracheoesophageal fistula, renal anomalies, limb abnormalities) association, CHARGE (coloboma, heart defect, atresia choanae, retarded growth, genital anomaly, ear abnormality) association, Fraser syndrome, and Cornelia de Lange syndrome.

**Inheritance Patterns** Congenital adrenal hyperplasia is autosomal recessive. Recurrence risks for other conditions are dependent on their specific inheritance patterns.

**Teratogens** Isotretinoin is teratogenic.

**Prognosis** Prognosis depends on the degree of genital malformation and the underlying etiology. The psychological and social implications of gender assignment in these infants require a multidisciplinary team approach.

## SONOGRAPHY

### FREQUENT FINDINGS

- Short phallus/clitoromegaly
- Bifid scrotum/fused labia
- Abnormal phallic shape
- Undescended testes in the third trimester
- Abnormal urinary stream
- Associated congenital anomalies
  - Urogenital
  - Extragenital

### LESS FREQUENT

- Discrepancy between the external and internal fetal gender
  - Presence or absence of the uterus
    - The presence of a uterus results in an increased distance between the bladder and rectum.

### KEY FINDINGS/PITFALLS

- Uncertain appearance of external genitalia should prompt a more detailed assessment.
  - Clitoris versus penis
  - Labia versus scrotum
- Late second- or third-trimester evaluation can look for testicular descent or the uterus.
  - Testicular descent is first noted at 25 weeks' gestation.
    - Testicular descent occurs in 62% of cases between 28 and 30 weeks' gestation; 93% of fetuses at 32 weeks' gestation have descended testes.
      - Visualization of the testes distinguishes XY and XX disorders of sexual development.
    - The presence of a uterus results in an increased distance between the bladder and rectum compared to normal male fetuses.
      - The term uterus measures 32 ± 5 mm in length and 20 mm transversely.
- Congenital adrenal hyperplasia
  - Hypertrophied adrenal glands
    - In the transverse plane, adrenals are enlarged and are circular rather than triangular.
    - They are first detected at 22 weeks' gestation.
- Hypospadias
  - Usually, hypospadias occurs (50%) on the distal penis (first degree).
  - With second-degree hypospadias (30%), the urethral opening is along the penile shaft.
  - In third-degree hypospadias (20%), the urethral opening is at the penoscrotal junction.
  - Third-degree hypospadias can be detected sonographically by the "tulip sign."
  - There is persistent angulation of the penile shaft due to chordee.
  - Bifid scrotum may be an associated finding.
  - Most often, hypospadias is an isolated finding.
  - First- and second-degree hypospadias are usually not detected prenatally, except when the external genitalia are carefully inspected in the context of other anomalies.
- Color Doppler can be used to distinguish the downward urinary stream of hypospadias.
- Three-dimensional (3-D) sonography can assist in the evaluation of the external genitalia.

### DIFFERENTIAL DIAGNOSIS

- Micropenis is a normally formed penis that is less than 2.5 standard deviations below the mean.

## PREGNANCY MANAGEMENT

**Investigations and Consultations Required** A complete ultrasound examination should be performed to determine whether this is an isolated abnormality. Fetal echocardiography should be done, as cardiac defects are associated with a number of the possible etiologic conditions. A careful history is essential to assess for congenital abnormalities in the parents or previous children. The history also should include information regarding consanguinity and any potential teratogen exposure. A fetal karyotype and microarray should be obtained. Consultation with a medical geneticist is essential to determine appropriate molecular testing, including for congenital adrenal hyperplasia, the most common cause for ambiguous genitalia in a female fetus. Other consultations obtained are based on the presumptive diagnosis and the need for neonatal, medical, or surgical therapy.

**Fetal Intervention** None is indicated. In cases of congenital adrenal hyperplasia, prevention of virilization of a female fetus using high-dose maternally administered corticosteroids has been studied. This therapy has no role once virilization has occurred but would be considered in an at-risk family for a subsequent pregnancy. This approach is controversial, as it is not entirely successful, carries substantial risks, and involves treating unaffected fetuses.

**Monitoring** Follow-up ultrasonographic examinations later in gestation may be performed to assess the maturation of the external genitalia and to reassess for associated anomalies that would affect the final diagnosis.

**Pregnancy Termination Issues** Unless a precise diagnosis has been established prenatally, the method of termination should provide an intact fetus for a complete morphologic and radiologic examination.

**Delivery** The complex nature of these multiple-malformation conditions requires that delivery and neonatal management occur in a tertiary center. Even if a diagnosis of congenital adrenal hyperplasia is made, the need for a multidisciplinary team for management makes delivery at a tertiary center mandatory.

## NEONATOLOGY

**Resuscitation** There are no special issues for delivery room management. If other associated anomalies exist, then management may need to be directed toward their related issues. Assignment of gender should be deferred until complete evaluation at a tertiary center.

**Transport** Referral to a tertiary perinatal center with multiple pediatric and surgical subspecialists is always indicated.

**Testing and confirmation** Careful physical examination and evaluation for associated congenital anomalies are essential. The initial laboratory evaluation should include chromosome analysis and assessment of gonadal and adrenal steroids. Additional laboratory values to be obtained include molecular genetic studies for the *SRY* gene (regulator of male sex determination); serum 17-OH progesterone measurement; serum DHEA (dehydroepiandrosterone), 17-hydroxyprenenolone, and 11-deoxycortisol levels; corticotropin (ACTH);

and serial serum and urine electrolytes. Abdominal and pelvic ultrasounds are performed to determine the presence of gonads, a uterus, or a vagina. Cystoscopy/vaginoscopy may be necessary to better delineate the anatomy.

**Nursery management** Evaluation should begin immediately at the time of birth as CAH due to 21-hydroxylase deficiency (salt wasting) may be life threatening if not diagnosed and treated. In the presence of electrolyte abnormalities suggestive of salt-wasting CAH, treatment with hydrocortisone is initiated pending the results of adrenal testing. If clinical symptoms of adrenal insufficiency develop, such as hypoglycemia, hyponatremia, hypovolemia, hyperkalemia, or vomiting and diarrhea, intravenous fluid therapy should be instituted immediately with dextrose and normal saline solution to restore electrolyte imbalance. Assignment of gender requires counseling with a multidisciplinary team consisting of individuals from pediatric genetics, endocrinology, surgery, urology, and neonatology specialties, in addition to professional counseling and psychosocial support for the family. Referral to a pediatric tertiary center that specializes in disorders of sexual development, is highly recommended.

## SUGGESTED READINGS


1. Achiron R, Pinhas-Hamiel O, Zalel Y, et al: Development of fetal male gender: prenatal sonographic measurement of the scrotum and evaluation of testicular descent. Ultrasound Obstet Gynecol 1998; 11:242-245.
2. American Academy of Pediatrics: Committee on Genetics: evaluation of the newborn with developmental anomalies of the external genitalia. Pediatrics 2000; 106:138-142.
3. Cafici D, Iglesias A: Prenatal diagnosis of severe hypospadias with two- and three-dimensional sonography. J Ultrasound Med 2002; 21:1423-1426.
4. Chitayat D, Glanc P: Diagnostic approach in prenatally detected genital abnormalities. Ultrasound Obstet Gynecol 2010; 35:637-646.
5. Hughes IA, Nihoul-Fekete C, Thomas B, Cohen-Kettenis PT: Consequences of the ESPE/LWPES guidelines for diagnosis and treatment of disorders of sex development. Best Prac Res Clin Endocrinol Metab 2007; 21:351-365.
6. Lee PA, Houk CP, Ahmed F, Hughes IA, in collaboration with the participants in the International Consensus Conference on Intersex organized by the Lawson Wilkins Pediatric Endocrine Society and the European Society for Paediatric Endocrinology: Consensus statement on management of intersex disorders. Pediatrics 2006; 118:e488-e500.
7. Meizner I, Mashiach R, Shalev J, et al: The "tulip sign": a sonographic clue for in-utero diagnosis of severe hypospadias. Ultrasound Obstet Gynecol 2002; 19:250-253.
8. Miller WL, Witchel SF: Prenatal treatment of congenital adrenal hyperplasia: risks outweigh benefits. Am J Obstet Gynecol 2013; 208:354-359.
9. Ocal G: Current concepts in disorders of sexual development. J Clin Res Pediatr Endocrinol 2011; 3:105-114.
10. Saada J, Grebille A-G, Aubry MC, et al: Sonography in prenatal diagnosis of congenital adrenal hyperplasia. Prenat Diagn 2004; 24:627-630.

11. Soriano D, Lipitz S, Seidman DS, et al: Development of the fetal uterus between 19 and 38 weeks of gestation: in-utero ultrasonographic measurements. Human Reprod 1998; 14:215-218.
12. Speiser PW, Azziz R, Baskin LS, et al: Congenital adrenal hyperplasia due to steroid 21-hydroxylase deficiency: an Endocrine Society clinical practice guideline. J Clin Endocrinol Metab 2010; 95:4133–4160.
13. Thyen U, Lanz K, Holterhus PM, Hiort O: Epidemiology and initial management of ambiguous genitalia at birth in Germany. Horm Res 2006: 66:195-203.

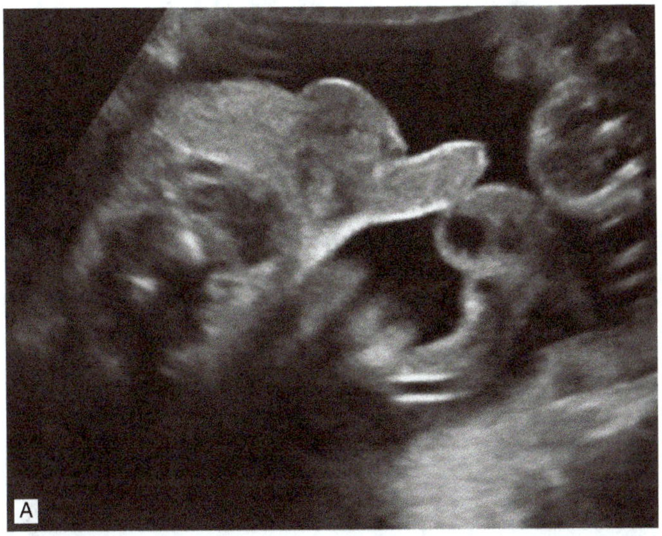


FIGURE 4.1A Normal male genitalia.

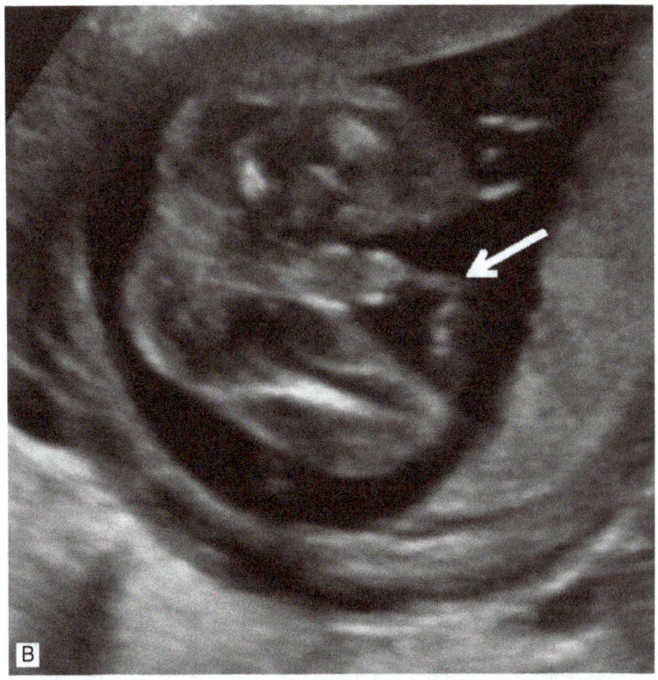


FIGURE 4.1B Normal male voiding (arrow).

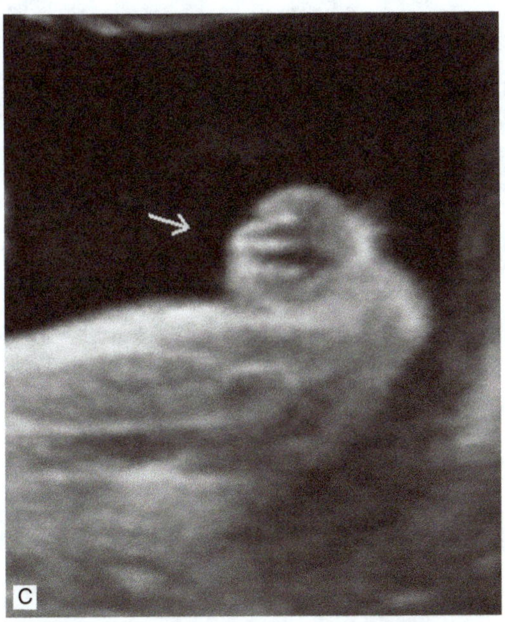


FIGURE 4.1C Normal female (31 weeks) (arrow).

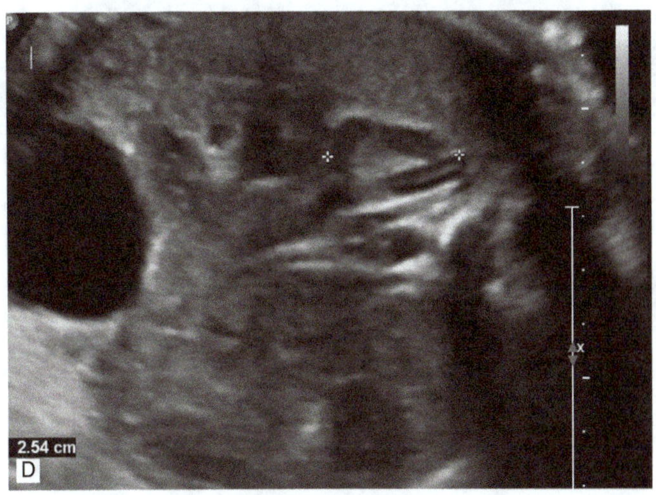


FIGURE 4.1D Normal fetal adrenal (+ … +).

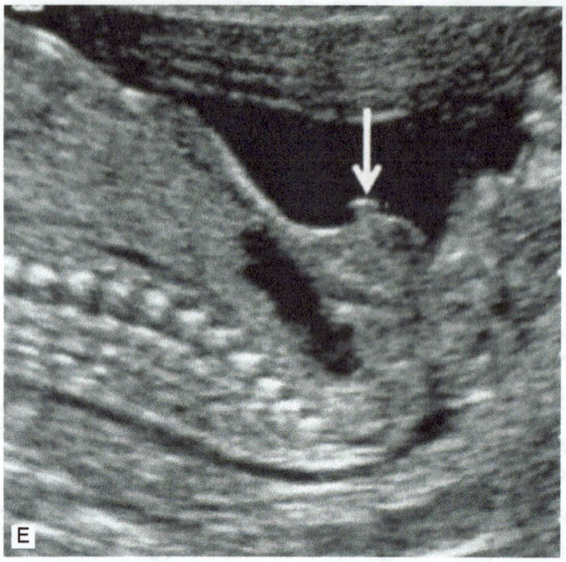

**FIGURE 4.1E** Micropenis (arrow).

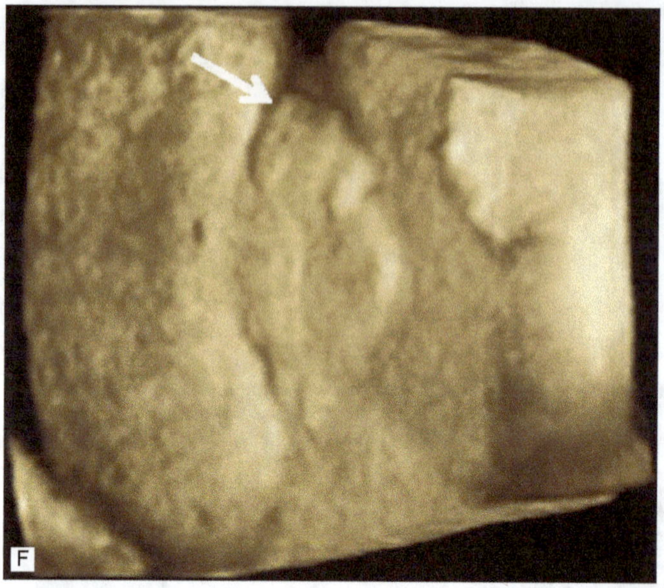

**FIGURE 4.1F** Three-dimensional image of fetus with hypospadias and the "tulip sign" (arrow).

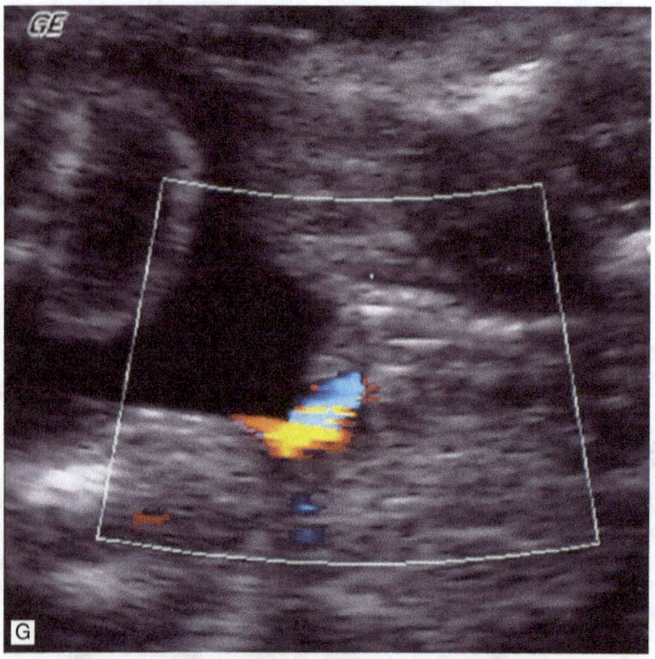

**FIGURE 4.1G** Fetus with hypospadias. Color Doppler indicates an abnormal urinary stream from the posterior aspect of the penis.

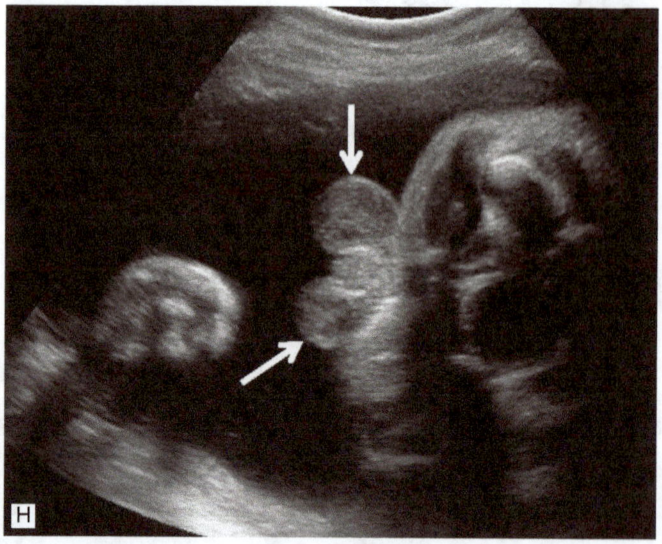

**FIGURE 4.1H** Severe hypospadias with a bifid scrotum (arrows).

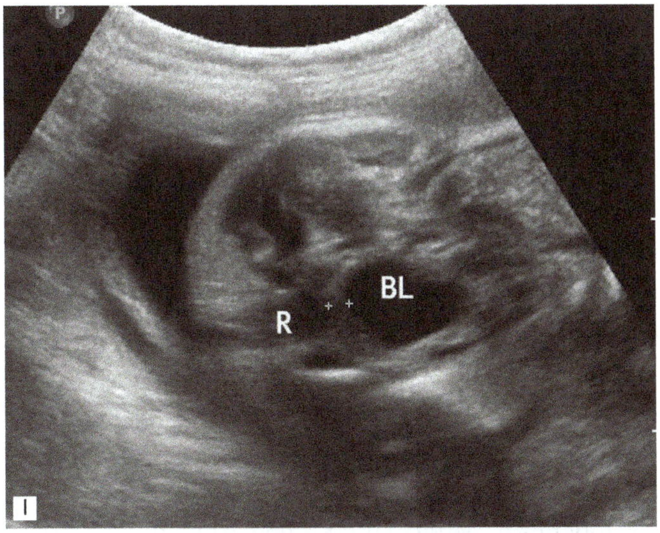


**FIGURE 4.1I** Narrow distance (+ … +) between rectum (R) and bladder (BL), indicating a male fetus.

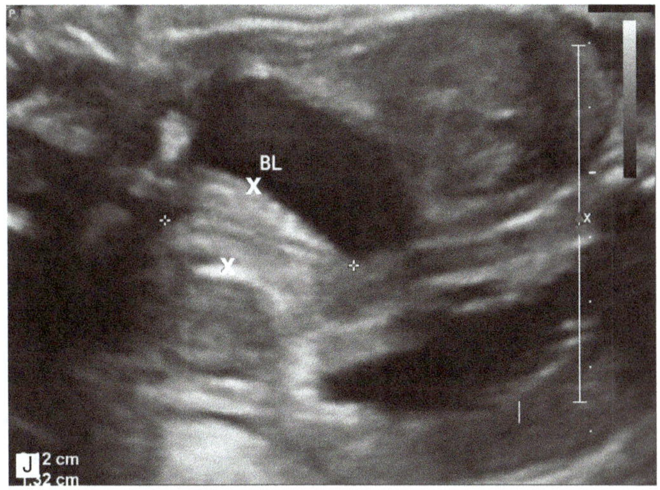


**FIGURE 4.1J** Normal uterus (+ … +; x … x). BL, bladder.)

# 4.2 BLADDER EXSTROPHY

## EPIDEMIOLOGY/GENETICS

**Definition** Bladder exstrophy is a failure of closure of the bladder, lower urinary tract, overlying symphysis pubis, rectus muscles, and skin. It is part of the exstrophy-epispadias complex that includes epispadias, exstrophy of the bladder, and cloacal exstrophy.

**Epidemiology** Occurrence is 1 per 10,000 to 50,000 births (M2:F1).

**Embryology** Bladder exstrophy is theorized to result from a disorder in the development of the cloacal membrane, preventing medial migration of mesenchyme, and early rupture of the membrane. The most commonly associated malformations involve the upper urinary tract (ureteropelvic junction [UPJ] obstruction, horseshoe kidney, ectopic kidney). Approximately 7% of patients will have a spinal abnormality, such as spina bifida occulta, scoliosis, or hemivertebrae.

**Inheritance Patterns** Most cases are likely the result of multifactorial inheritance, with a recurrence risk of approximately 1%. There are rare case reports of families that appear to have autosomal recessive or X-linked inheritance.

**Teratogens** None are known.

**Screening** Maternal serum α-fetoprotein is elevated in most cases of bladder exstrophy.

**Prognosis** Surgical correction is complicated, but approximately 80% of patients will eventually have continence; it is much lower with closure failures. With current surgical techniques, the majority of patients will have full continence, adequate sexual function, and normal psychosocial outcomes.

## SONOGRAPHY

### FREQUENT FINDINGS

- Absent fetal bladder
- Normal amniotic fluid volume
- Normal fetal kidneys
- Lower abdominal cauliflower mass (posterior wall of the bladder)
- Low umbilical cord insertion
- Laterally splayed iliac crests
- Ambiguous genitalia
  - Female: widely separated labia
  - Male: complete epispadias

### KEY FINDINGS/PITFALLS

- This may occur as an isolated congenital anomaly or as part of cloacal exstrophy or OEIS (omphalocele, exstrophy of the bladder, imperforate anus, and spinal defects, usually a meningomyelocele).
- In exstrophy, a persistent cloacal membrane prevents normal midline fusion. As a result, there is a shortened lower abdominal wall and a low cord insertion.
- Three-dimensional sonography can be utilized to better assess the lower abdominal mass and genitalia in cases of suspected bladder exstrophy.

## PREGNANCY MANAGEMENT

**Investigations and Consultations Required** Associated abnormalities other than of the spine or kidneys are rare in bladder exstrophy. In patients planning to continue the pregnancy, fetal echocardiography may be appropriate to exclude cardiac defects before deciding on the site for delivery. A pediatric urologist should be consulted to discuss management with the family. Although chromosome abnormalities are not associated with bladder exstrophy, confirmation of fetal sex may be useful in defining prognosis for surgical repair.

**Monitoring** No alteration in standard obstetric care is indicated.

**Pregnancy Course** No obstetric complications are associated with this disorder.

**Pregnancy Termination Issues** An intact fetus should be delivered to allow confirmation of the sonographic diagnosis.

**Delivery** There is no evidence that cesarean delivery improves prognosis. Delivery at a tertiary center is not required. It is more important that the infant be transferred to an institution with individuals experienced in the repair of this rare condition.

## NEONATOLOGY

**Resuscitation** Respiratory difficulty is not expected with this lesion.

**Transport** Referral to a tertiary center with a pediatric urologist experienced in the repair of exstrophy is essential for early surgical intervention.

**Testing and Confirmation** The bladder and lower urinary tract are open anteriorly from the urethral meatus to the umbilicus. There is wide separation of the pubic symphysis and rectus muscles. In males, the scrotum is broad with frequent undescended testes and a short broad penis without canalization. In females, the clitoris and labia are widely separated, with occasional vaginal stenosis. Upper tract anomalies are typically not associated with this lesion.

**Nursery Management** The exposed viscera should be covered with plastic film (Saran™ Wrap) to limit heat and evaporative water loss and contamination. Administration of antibiotics should be considered to reduce the risk of infection.

## SURGERY

**Preoperative Assessment** Complete physical examination; laboratory testing, including electrolytes and complete blood cell count; abdominal flat plate; renal ultrasound; and pelvic magnetic resonance imaging (MRI) should be performed.

**Types of Procedures** Two surgical approaches are currently used to correct bladder exstrophy: modern staged repair of bladder exstrophy (MSRE) and complete primary repair of bladder exstrophy (CPRE). In both, the bladder and posterior urethra are reapproximated to form a new bladder.

**Surgical Results/Prognosis** The prognosis is dependent on any associated renal anomalies, but there is a survival rate of more than 90%. Secondary surgical procedures are frequently required to achieve urinary continence and functioning genitalia. Possible short-term surgical complications include wound dehiscence and infection. Urinary continence, the primary goal of successful repair, is achieved in more than 70% of patients. Long-term follow-up is required to monitor bladder, renal, and sexual function and to address psychological issues that may result from poor body image.

## SUGGESTED READINGS

1. Baird AD, Nelson CP, Gearhart JP: Modern staged repair of bladder exstrophy: a contemporary series. J Pediatr Urol 2007; 3:311-315.
2. Barth RA, Filly RA, Sondheimer FK: Prenatal sonographic findings in bladder exstrophy: J Ultrasound Med 1990; 9:359-361.
3. Cacciari A, Pilu GL, Mordenti M, et al: Prenatal diagnosis of bladder exstropy: what counseling? J Urol 1999; 161:259-261.
4. Ebert A, Scheuering S, Schott G, Roesch WH: Psychosocial and psychosexual development in childhood and adolescence within the exstrophy-epispadias complex. J Urol 2005; 174:1094-1098.
5. Ebert AK, Reutter H, Ludwig M, Rosch WH: The exstrophy-epispadias complex. Orphanet J Rare Dis 2009; 4:23.
6. Evangelidis A, Murphy JP, Gatti JM: Prenatal diagnosis of bladder exstrophy by 3-dimensional ultrasound. J Urol 2004; 172:1111.
7. Gearhart JP, Ben-Chaim J, Jeffs RD, Sanders RC: Criteria for the prenatal diagnosis of classic bladder exstrophy. Obstet Gynecol 1995; 85:961-964.
8. Goldstein IK, Shalev E, Nisman D: The dilemma of prenatal diagnosis of bladder exstrophy: a case report and review of the literature. Ultrasound Obstet Gynecol 2001; 17:357-359.
9. Shaw MB, Rink RC, Kaefer M, et al: Continence and classic bladder exstrophy treated with staged repair. J Urol 2004; 172:1450-1453.
10. Wilcox DT, Chitty LS: Non-visualizations of the fetal bladder: aetiology and management. Prenat Diagn 2001; 21:977-983.

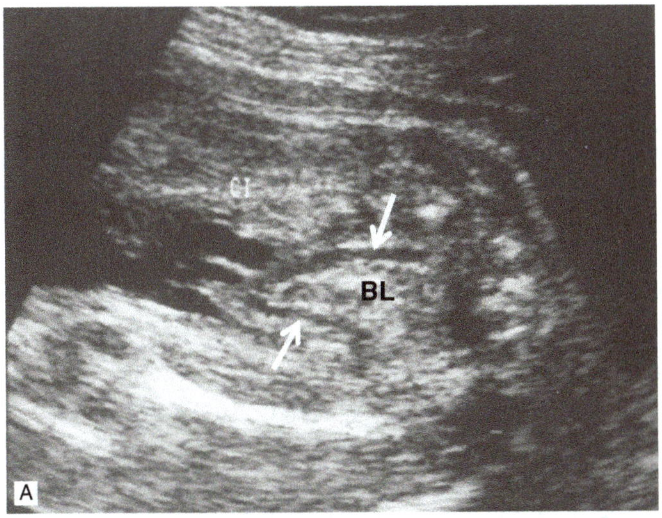


FIGURE 4.2A Fetus with bladder exstrophy showing apparent absent fetal bladder (BL); umbilical arteries (arrows).

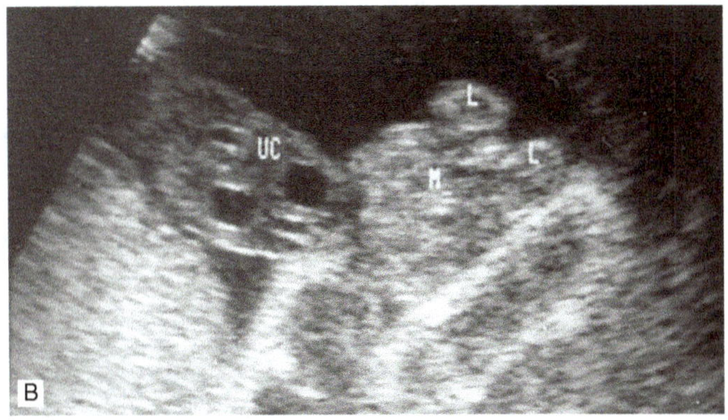


FIGURE 4.2B Bladder exstrophy (M) with widely splayed labia (L) and a low-lying umbilical cord insertion (UC).

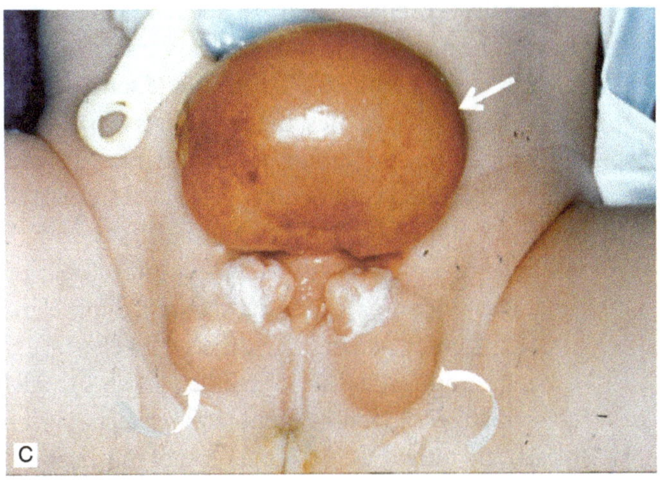


FIGURE 4.2C Infant with bladder exstrophy (straight arrow) and widely separated labia (curved arrows).

# 4.3 CLOACAL EXSTROPHY

## EPIDEMIOLOGY/GENETICS

**Definition** Cloacal exstrophy is an extensive lower abdominal wall defect that combines exstrophy of the bladder with intervening intestinal epithelium, imperforate anus, and wide separation of the anterior pubic arch.

**Epidemiology** Occurrence is 1 in 200,000 births. The sex ratio has been reported to be twice as common in males in some studies and more common in females in other studies. The incidence figures vary widely and likely reflect ascertainment biases, especially because of the high rate of pregnancy termination when detected prenatally. If stillborn and terminated fetuses are included, the incidence is more likely to be in the range of 1 in 30,000 pregnancies.

**Embryology** Exstrophies are theorized to result from a disorder in the development of the cloacal membrane, preventing medial migration of mesenchyme, and early rupture of the membrane. Cloacal exstrophy occurs if the rupture occurs before the urorectal septum divides the gastrointestinal from the genitourinary tracts. The bladder and lower urinary tract are open anteriorly from the urethral meatus to the umbilicus. There is wide separation of the pubic symphysis and rectus muscles. In males, the scrotum is broad with undescended testes, and there is a short, broad penis without canalization. In females, the clitoris and labia are widely separated with occasional vaginal stenosis. The upper urinary tract is malformed in approximately one-third of cases, with the common abnormalities being UPJ obstruction, horseshoe kidney, and ectopic kidney. In females, the uterus is frequently bicornuate, and the vagina is duplex, ending blindly near the bladder mucosa. Ninety percent of patients with cloacal exstrophy have an omphalocele or other gastrointestinal abnormalities, and nearly all have significant neurospinal abnormalities, including neural tube defects, vertebral anomalies, spinal myelodysplasia, and tethered cord. One form of the disorder is known as the OEIS complex.

**Inheritance Patterns** Inheritance is likely multifactorial. The overall risk of recurrence for disorders in the exstrophy-epispadias complex is approximately 1%. Only rare affected siblings have been described.

**Teratogens** None are known.

**Screening** Maternal serum α-fetoprotein is elevated in most cases.

**Prognosis** Surgical correction is complicated and requires a multidisciplinary team. Neonatal mortality in cloacal exstrophy is low in centers with experience in managing complex birth defects. Urinary and fecal continence are established in approximately 50% of cases. There are no data on sexual function and few on the quality of life. Intelligence in survivors is normal.

## SONOGRAPHY

### FREQUENT FINDINGS

- Absent fetal bladder
- Abnormally shaped cloaca in pelvis

- Midline infraumbilical septated cyst (cloacal membrane)
- Omphalocele
- Neural tube defect
- Ambiguous genitalia
- Pubic diastasis
- Didelphic uterus
- Single umbilical artery

### LESS FREQUENT

- Clubfeet
- Renal anomalies
  - Hydronephrosis
  - Pelvic kidney
  - Unilateral renal agenesis
  - Horseshoe kidney
  - Crossed renal ectopy
- Kyphoscoliosis
- Urinary ascites
- Ventriculomegaly
- First trimester
  - Increased nuchal translucency
  - Megacystis

### KEY FINDINGS/PITFALLS/DIFFERENTIAL DIAGNOSIS

- Visualization of normal external genitalia excludes cloacal exstrophy.
- If an evaluation of the lower pelvis detects an anal canal and rectum, cloacal exstrophy is excluded.
- The most common differential diagnosis is hydrocolpos with a distended, sometimes septated, vagina and lower urinary tract obstruction (LUTO).

## PREGNANCY MANAGEMENT

**Investigations and Consultations Required** Chromosomal studies, including microarray, and fetal echocardiography should be performed to exclude other malformations. Consultation with a pediatric urologist should be obtained.

**Fetal Intervention** None is indicated.

**Monitoring** Serial ultrasonographic studies should be done to monitor the urinary tract and possible associated anomalies.

**Pregnancy Course** No specific obstetric complications should be anticipated.

**Pregnancy Termination Issues** An intact fetus may be necessary to confirm the diagnosis and to exclude genetic syndromes that may have cloacal abnormalities as a component of the disorder.

**Delivery** In cases with an associated omphalocele or neural tube defect, delivery may be complicated. In general, no specific delivery issues are anticipated.

## NEONATOLOGY

**Resuscitation** Saline-soaked sterile dressings are applied to protect the exposed bowel and bladder mucosa and, if present, the accompanying omphalocele from surface contamination and trauma. Limitation of evaporative heat and water loss can be achieved by encasing the lower body in a sterile plastic bag (bowel bag).

**Transport** Transfer by an experienced neonatal transport team to a tertiary center with pediatric surgical subspecialists and diagnostic capabilities is indicated on an emergency basis.

**Testing and Confirmation** The assessment and determination of the exact spectrum and aberrant anatomy in these conditions require a coordinated multidisciplinary approach, often using the full range of imaging and endoscopic techniques. In cloacal exstrophy, there is a high association with cardiac, skeletal, and neurologic anomalies, necessitating diagnostic imaging of these organ systems as well. Chromosomal analysis for genetic gender identification is essential if it has not been obtained prenatally.

**Nursery Management** Initial management is directed toward providing fluid and electrolyte support and decompression of both the urinary and the intestinal systems, as indicated. The choice and staging of surgical procedures for palliation or correction will vary with the results of the diagnostic evaluation. Provision of social and emotional support and counseling for the parents is important in facilitating their adaptation to the long-term demands for the care of their child. Multiple surgeries will be required for complete management of all the abnormalities.

## SURGERY

**Preoperative Assessment** The major areas that require preoperative evaluation are the upper urinary tract anomalies, central nervous system abnormalities, musculoskeletal deformities, and gender. Ultrasonography is used to evaluate the spinal cord and genitourinary tract. Magnetic resonance imaging may be useful in assessing abdominal and central nervous system malformations.

**Operative Indications** All children with this anomaly require bladder reconstruction and omphalocele repair. If a myelomeningocele is present, repair will be needed. Diastasis of the pubic bones must also be repaired. The goal of reconstruction is to help the patient achieve adequate bowel and urinary control and satisfactory sexual function.

**Surgical Results/Prognosis** In the absence of lethal renal abnormalities, an excellent survival rate between 80% and 100% is expected.

### SUGGESTED READINGS

1. Austin PF, Homsy YL, Gearhart JP, et al: The prenatal diagnosis of cloacal exstrophy. J Urol 1998; 160:1179-1181.

2. Bianchi DW, Crombleholme TM, D'Alton ME. Cloacal exstrophy. In: Fetology: Diagnosis and Management of the Fetal Patient. New York: McGraw-Hill; 2000: 459.
3. Dhombres F, Jouannic JM, Brodaty G, et al: Contribution of prenatal imaging to the anatomical assessment of fetal hydrocolpos. Ultrasound Obstet Gynecol 2007; 30:101-104.
4. Ebert A-K, Reutter H, Ludwig M, Rosch WH: The exstrophy-epispadias complex. Orphanet J Rare Dis 2009; 4:23.
5. Fernando MA, Creighton SM, Wood D: The long-term management and outcomes of cloacal anomalies. Pediatr Nephrol 2015; 30:759-765.
6. Keppler-Noreuil K, Gorton S, Foo F, et al: Prenatal ascertainment of OEIS complex/cloacal exstrophy—15 new cases and literature review. Am J Med Genet A 2007; 143A:2122-2128.
7. Langer JC, Brennan B, Lappalainen RE, et al: Cloacal exstrophy: prenatal diagnosis before rupture of the cloacal membrane. J Pediatr Surg 1992; 27:1352-1355.
8. Lund DP, Hendren WH: Cloacal exstrophy: a 25-year experience with 50 cases. J Pediatr Surg 2001; 36:68-75.
9. Marshall VF, Muecke EC: Variations in exstrophy of the bladder. J Urol 1962; 88:766-796.
10. Matthews RI, Perlman E, Marsh DW, Gearhart JP: Gonadal morphology in cloacal exstrophy: implications in gender assignment. BJU Int 1999; 84:99-100.
11. Meizner I, Levy A, Barnhard Y: Cloacal exstrophy sequence: an exceptional ultrasound diagnosis. Obstet Gynecol 1995; 86:446-450.
12. Soffer SZ, Rosen NG, Hong AR, et al. Cloacal exstrophy: a unified management plan. J Pediatr Surg 2000; 35:932-937.
13. Taipale P, Heinonen K, Kainulainen S, et al: Cloacal anomaly simulating megalocystis in the first trimester. J Clin Ultrasound 2004; 32:419-422.
14. Warne S, Chitty LS, Wilcox DT: Prenatal diagnosis of cloacal anomalies. BJU Int 2002; 89:78-81.

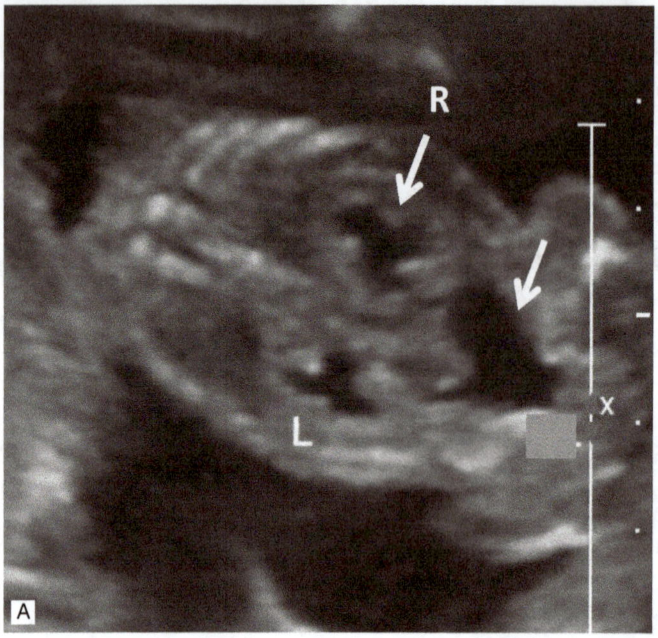


FIGURE 4.3A Cloaca (arrow) with bilateral pyelocaliectasis (L, R).

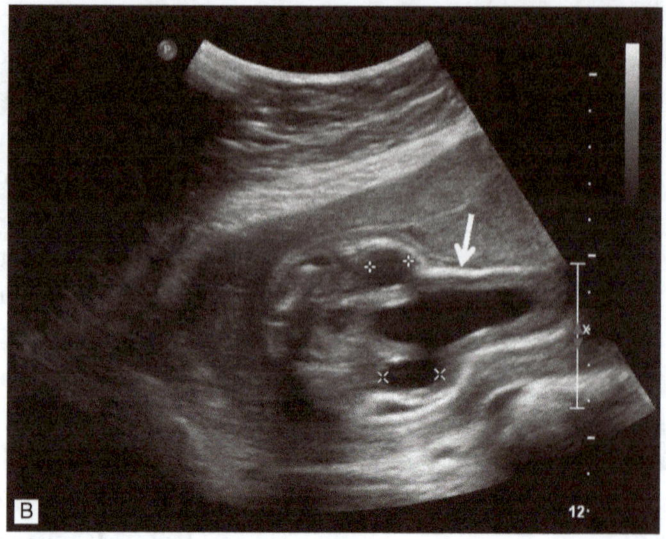


FIGURE 4.3B Fetus with cloacal exstrophy and hydrometrocolpos (arrow) and didelphic uterus (+..+; x..x).

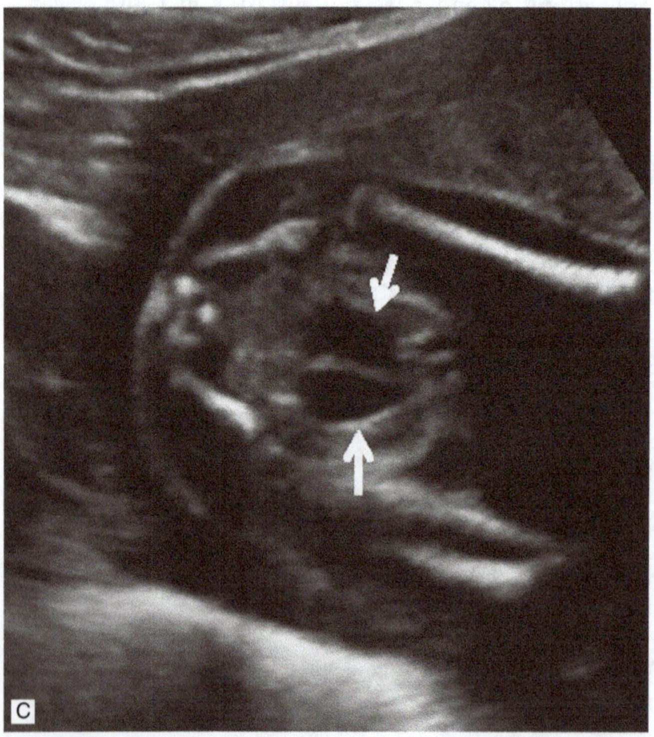


FIGURE 4.3C Septated vagina (arrows) in a fetus with cloacal exstrophy.

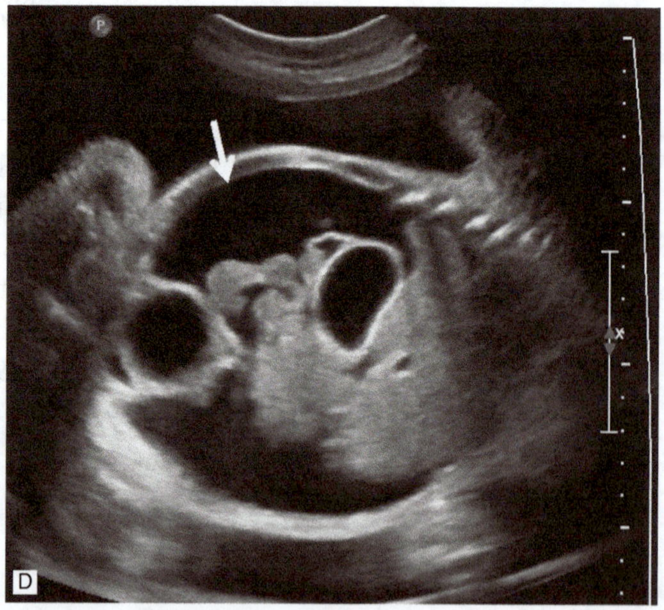


FIGURE 4.3D Urinary ascites (arrow).

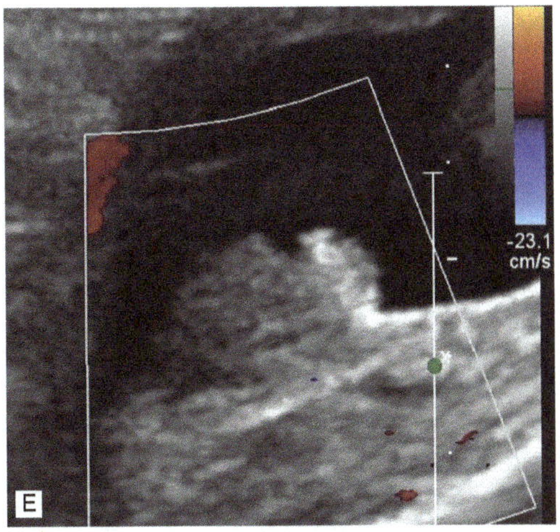


**FIGURE 4.3E** Severe hypospadias in fetus with cloacal exstrophy.

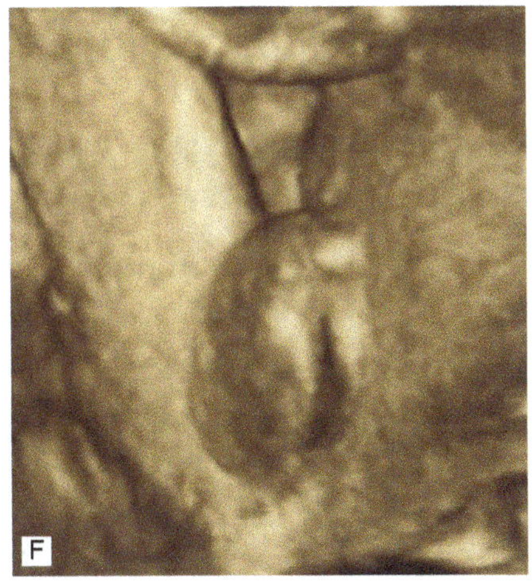


**FIGURE 4.3F** Three-dimensional view of severe hypospadias.

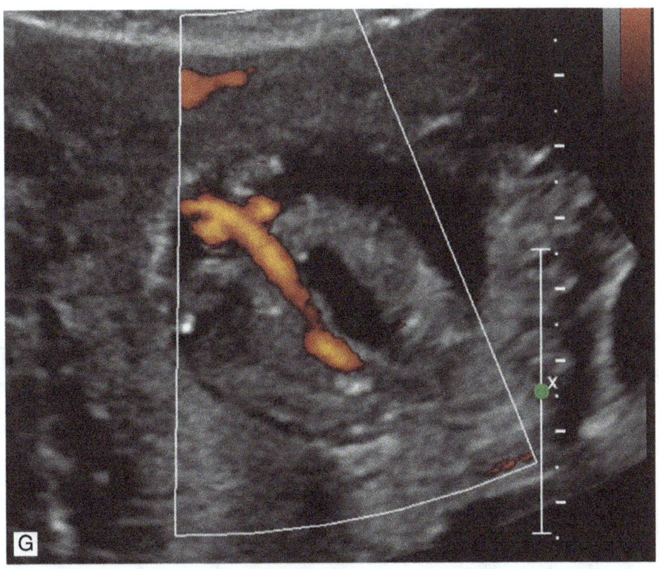


**FIGURE 4.3G** Power Doppler study illustrating a single umbilical artery.

# 4.4 DUPLEX COLLECTING SYSTEM/URETEROCELE

## EPIDEMIOLOGY/GENETICS

**Definition** A duplex collecting system is a single kidney that is drained by two pyelocaliceal systems. A ureterocele is a cystic dilatation of the terminal part of the ureter in the bladder.

**Epidemiology** A duplex collecting system is present in 1 in 125 in autopsy series, and antenatally, the incidence has been reported to be between 1:70 and 1:500 (M1:F2). Ureteroceles are found in 1 in 5000 neonates (M1:F3-5).

**Embryology** A duplex collecting system may drain into a single ureter, a bifid ureter, or two separate ureters. When there are two ureters,

- The lower pole drains cranially and laterally into the trigone.
  - The cranial position results in a shorter intramural tunnel and higher likelihood of reflux.
- The upper pole drains medially and caudally.
  - It usually ends in a ureterocele; it may also end in the urethra or vagina.
  - The upper pole may be dysplastic.
    - This may be confused with a suprarenal mass (i.e., a neuroblastoma).
- Weigert-Meyers law: The upper pole obstructs and the lower refluxes.

Approximately 10% to 20% of cases are bilateral. Renal dysplasia in a duplex kidney may be due to faulty embryogenesis or to obstruction. The faulty embryogenesis theory appears more likely based on embryologic and pathologic studies. Displacement of the orifices laterally or caudally results in abnormalities of the associated kidney segment. The further the ureter is displaced, the greater the abnormality will be; severe displacement results in renal dysplasia. Of duplex collecting systems, 70% have other congenital anomalies: Vesicoureteral reflux (VUR) is the most common abnormality. And, 80%-90% of ureteroceles are associated with a duplicated collecting system.

**Inheritance Patterns** Inheritance is sporadic in most cases. Rare families having dominant inheritance have been reported.

**Teratogens** None are known.

**Prognosis** The overall prognosis is excellent. The need for surgical intervention will depend on the degree of hydronephrosis and whether an obstructing ureterocele is present.

## SONOGRAPHY

### FREQUENT FINDINGS

- Two separate renal collecting systems
- Increased renal length
- Upper-/lower-pole hydronephrosis

- Cyst-like structure in the upper pole (i.e., second renal pelvis)
- Ureterocele

### LESS FREQUENT

- Hydroureter
- UPJ obstruction (4%)
- Renal dysplasia of the upper pole

### KEY FINDINGS/PITFALLS

- Of ureteroceles, 90% are associated with a duplex, two-ureter system.
- A ureterocele that is totally within the bladder is intravesical ("Foley catheter sign").
- A ureterocele partially within the bladder neck or urethra is ectopic.
  - Of ectopic ureteroceles, 80%-90% are associated with a duplex kidney.
- Bilateral ureteroceles may occur.

### DIFFERENTIAL DIAGNOSIS

- Hydronephrosis
- Polycystic kidneys
- Solitary renal cysts
- Ureteropelvic junction obstruction

## PREGNANCY MANAGEMENT

**Investigations and Consultations Required** In general, because this is an isolated anomaly, no other investigations are required. If the diagnosis is unclear, especially in the presence of significant hydronephrosis, detailed sonographic assessment is necessary to exclude other abnormalities. Pediatric urologic consultation should be obtained.

**Fetal Intervention** In general, no intervention is necessary, as these fetuses do well.

**Monitoring** No change in obstetric care is indicated. Serial ultrasonographic examinations monthly may be helpful in monitoring the kidneys for the degree of hydronephrosis and evidence of pathology in the contralateral kidney, as well as the rare case that develops oligohydramnios due to an obstructing ureterocele.

**Pregnancy Course** No obstetric complications should be expected.

**Pregnancy Termination Issues** In general, these cases do not usually result in pregnancy termination, but if that is chosen, an intact fetus, appropriate for confirming the anatomic findings on autopsy, is warranted.

**Delivery** In cases with significant obstruction, there may be a need for immediate neonatal evaluation to establish a diagnosis. Delivery in those cases should be in a tertiary center.

## NEONATOLOGY

**Resuscitation** In the absence of other conditions, resuscitative efforts are usually not required.

**Transport** In cases of an isolated duplex collecting system diagnosed antenatally, transfer to a tertiary center is not necessary. The evaluation can be performed as an outpatient at 1-2 weeks of age. In infants with suspected associated renal anomalies, hydroureter, bladder abnormalities, evidence of obstructive uropathy, or presence of a ureterocele, transfer to a tertiary center is indicated for evaluation and management.

**Testing and confirmation** Ultrasonography of the kidneys and bladder or voiding cystourethrogram (VCUG) are diagnostic. Timing of these studies is dependent on the severity of the associated congenital anomalies of the kidney and urinary tract, including obstructive uropathy, presence of a ureterocele, and VUR.

**Nursery Management** Depending on the severity of associated renal abnormalities and the presence of associated VUR or obstructive uropathy, antibiotic prophylaxis with amoxicillin (12-25 mg/kg orally daily) is recommended. While infants with an isolated duplex collecting system may be safely evaluated at an age older than 7 days, earlier evaluation in the immediate newborn period may help ease parental anxiety and concern. Follow-up with pediatric urology is indicated.

### SUGGESTED READINGS

1. Abuhamed AZ, Horton CE Jr, Horton SH, Evans AT: Renal duplication anomalies in the fetus: clues for prenatal diagnosis. Ultrasound Obstet Gynecol 1996; 7:174-177.
2. Bauer SP, Perlmutter AD, Retik AB: Anomalies of the upper urinary tract. In: Walsh PC, Retik AB, Stamey TA, et al, eds. Campbell's Urology. Philadelphia: Saunders; 1992: 1357-1442.
3. Bolduc S, Upadhyay J, Sherman C, et al: Histology of upper pole is unaffected by prenatal diagnosis in duplex system ureteroceles. J Urol 2002; 168:1123-1126.
4. Decter RM: Renal duplication and fusion anomalies. Pediatr Urol 1997; 44:1323-1341.
5. Ho DS, Jerkins GR, Williams M, Hoe HN: Ureteropelvic junction obstruction in upper and lower moiety of duplex systems. Urology 1995; 45:503-506.
6. Hulbert WC, Rabinowitz R: Prenatal diagnosis of duplex system hydronephrosis: effect on renal salvage. Urology 1998; 51(5A Suppl):23-26.
7. Mackie GG, Stephens D: Duplex kidneys: a correlation of renal dysplasia with position of the ureteral orifice. J Urol 1975; 114:274-280.
8. Sepulveda W, Campana C, Carstens E, Rodriguez J: Prenatal sonographic diagnosis of bilateral ureteroceles. The pseudoseptated fetal bladder. J Ultrasound Med 2003; 22:841-844.

9. Sherer DM, Menashe M, Lebensart P, et al: Sonographic diagnosis of unilateral fetal renal duplication with associated ectopic ureterocele. J Clin Ultrasound 1989; 17:371-373.

10. Siomou E, Papadopoulou F, Kollios KD, et al: Duplex collecting system diagnosed during the first 6 years of life after a first urinary tract infection: a study of 63 children. J Urol 2006; 175;678-682.

11. Whitten SM, McHoney M, Wilcox DT, et al: Accuracy of antenatal fetal ultrasound in the diagnosis of duplex kidneys. Ultrasound Obstet Gynecol 2003; 21:342-346.

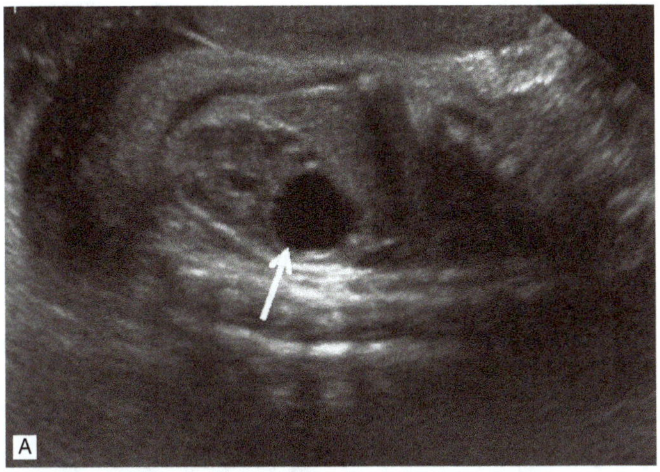


**FIGURE 4.4A** Duplex collecting system with normal kidney in lower pole and a cyst in upper pole (arrow).

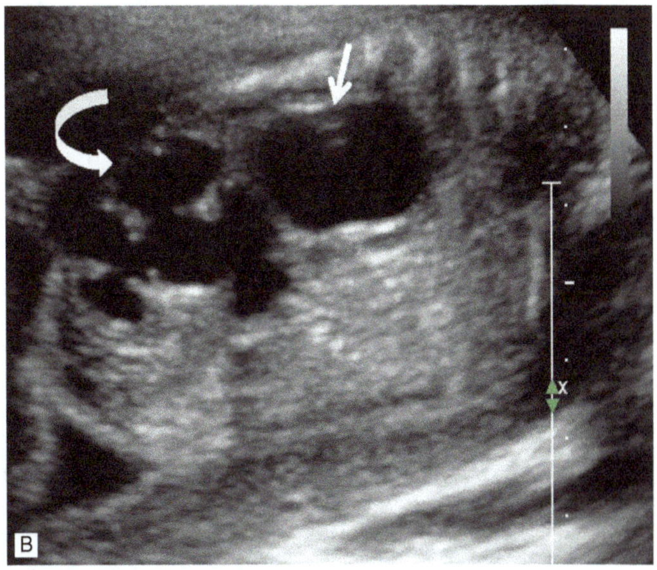


**FIGURE 4.4B** Duplex collecting system with cyst in the upper pole (straight arrow) and pyelocaliectasis in the lower pole (curved arrow).

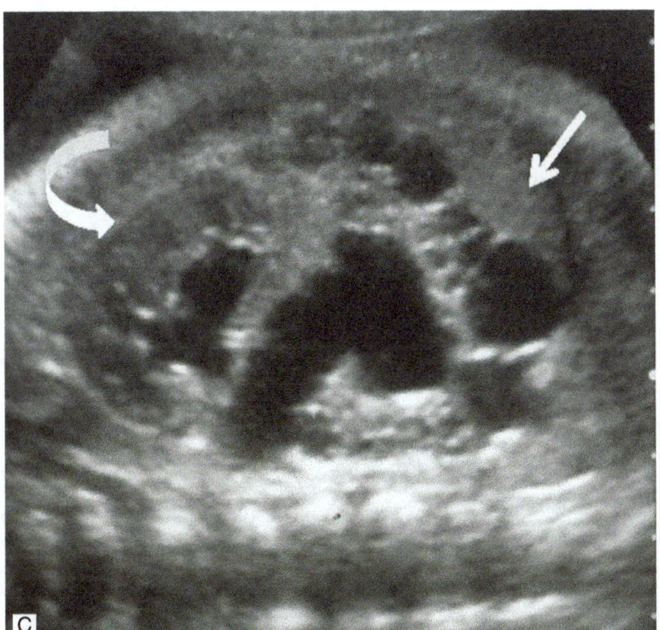


**FIGURE 4.4C** Duplex collecting system with a dysplastic upper pole (straight arrow) and pyelocaliectasis in the lower pole (curved arrow).

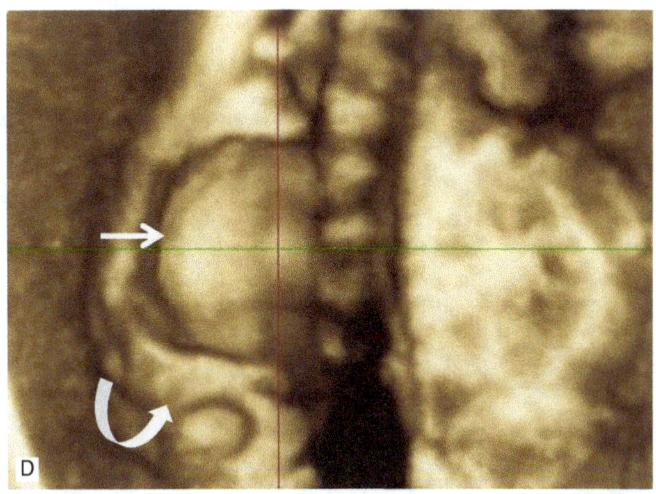


**FIGURE 4.4D** Three-dimensional image of a duplex collecting system with a cystic upper pole (straight arrow) and pyelectasis in the lower pole (curved arrow).

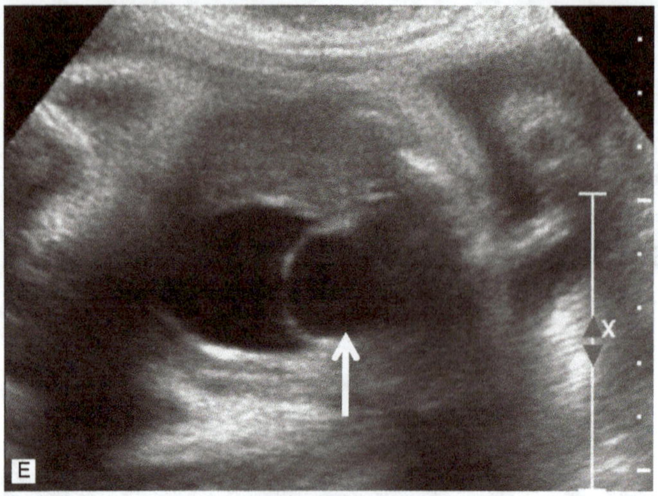


**FIGURE 4.4E** Ureterocele (arrow).

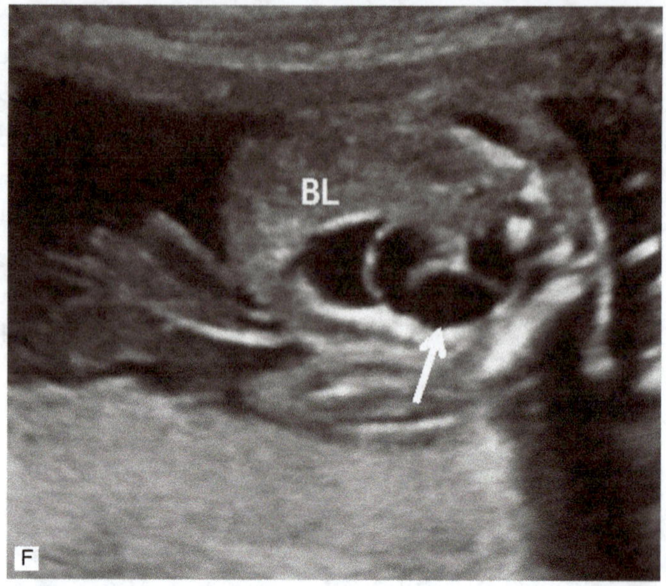


**FIGURE 4.4F** Bilateral ureteroceles (arrow). BL, bladder.

# 4.5 INFANTILE POLYCYSTIC KIDNEY DISEASE/ AUTOSOMAL RECESSIVE POLYCYSTIC KIDNEY DISEASE

## EPIDEMIOLOGY/GENETICS

**Definition** Infantile polycystic kidney disease/autosomal recessive polycystic kidney disease (ARPKD) is an autosomal recessive genetic disorder characterized by nonobstructive fusiform dilations of the renal collecting ducts, resulting in symmetric renal enlargement and renal failure. All patients have some degree of congenital hepatic fibrosis as well.

**Epidemiology** Occurrence is 1 in 20,000 births (M1:F1).

**Embryology** Autosomal recessive polycystic kidney disease causes both renal and hepatic disease. ARPKD is caused by numerous mutations in PKHD1 (polycystic kidney and hepatic disease 1). In general, the combination of mutations determines phenotypic presentation (i.e., the extent of renal and liver involvement), but there are no precise genotype-phenotype correlations. There is significant variation in the expression of ARPKD, resulting in renal manifestations occurring prenatally and neonatally, in infancy, and as a juvenile. There may be variable expression of ARPKD in one family.

**Inheritance Patterns** There is autosomal recessive inheritance. The gene for infantile polycystic kidney disease has been localized to chromosome 6p, and genetic diagnosis is available in involved families. In de novo cases, testing for a panel of causative genes is possible.

**Teratogens** None are known.

**Prognosis** The perinatal mortality rate is approximately 30% to 40% and is correlated with the presence of oligohydramnios prenatally. There is a 90% one-year survival rate. In survivors, the major morbidities are hypertension, renal failure requiring transplantation, and portal hypertension.

## SONOGRAPHY

### FREQUENT FINDINGS

- Kidneys retain reniform shape.
- Renal size is above the 95th centile.
- There are no detectable renal cysts.
- There is loss of corticomedullary differentiation.
- Kidneys are diffusely echogenic.
- Fetal bladder is absent.
- There is intrauterine growth restriction.

### KEY FINDINGS/PITFALLS

- The numerous tiny cysts are below the resolution of ultrasound equipment.
- The interface produced by the innumerable small cysts results in the increased echogenicity.
- Fetal kidneys are considered hyperechoic when they are more echogenic than adjacent spleen or liver.
- The earlier the presentation is, the worse the prognosis.
- It is first detected in the early second trimester.
- The kidneys may have a normal size and architectural pattern in the second trimester.
- Once the sonologist has made a presumptive diagnosis of ARPKD, serial ultrasound examinations every 2 to 3 weeks should be performed to assess renal size and amniotic fluid volume.
- Enlarged echogenic kidneys in a fetus are not diagnostic for polycystic kidney disease.
- Kidney size in ARPKD does not correlate with renal function.
- While ultrasound can diagnose severe prenatal disease, it cannot identify less-severe clinical types.

### DIFFERENTIAL DIAGNOSIS

- Meckel-Gruber syndrome (look for polydactyly and encephalocele): Renal cysts in this condition are usually visible.
- Benign glomerulosclerosis: There are large echogenic kidneys, but pyramids are echopenic and the amniotic fluid is normal or mildly increased.
- Adult polycystic kidney disease (autosomal dominant): There are large kidneys that may not be symmetrically enlarged. The kidneys are echogenic; cysts usually are seen in the fetus. A positive family history may be obtained.
- Trisomy 13: The kidneys may be slightly enlarged and are echogenic with or without cysts. Numerous other pathologic findings, such as holoprosencephaly, will be present.
- Beckwith-Wiedemann syndrome and Perlman syndrome: With both of these syndromes, the kidneys can be large and echogenic, but there is also macrosomia, and amniotic fluid volumes are normal. In the case of Beckwith-Wiedemann syndrome, omphalocele and macroglossia are often present.
- Fetal cytomegalovirus (CMV) infection typically infects the kidneys, resulting in increased renal echogenicity and oligohydramnios.

## PREGNANCY MANAGEMENT

**Investigations and Consultations Required** If there is no family history of ARPKD, the following investigations are appropriate:

- Chromosomal evaluation to include microarray.
- Fetal echocardiography to exclude other conditions that present with polycystic kidneys (trisomy 13 and Meckel-Gruber syndrome).

- Viral studies to exclude fetal CMV.
- Consultation with a pediatric nephrologist should be arranged to develop a management plan and to discuss the implications of this diagnosis with the family.

**Monitoring** Serial ultrasound examinations to monitor amniotic fluid volume and fetal abdominal circumference should be performed.

**Pregnancy Course** Most cases will develop oligohydramnios by the third trimester. Early-onset oligohydramnios is a poor prognostic sign. Intrauterine growth restriction is also common but does not affect prognosis.

**Pregnancy Termination Issues** A precise pathologic diagnosis is essential for counseling the family regarding the risk of recurrence. Unless the family is known to be at risk because of a previously affected pregnancy, an intact fetus should be delivered for complete external and internal examination.

**Delivery** Unless a precise diagnosis has been established prenatally, delivery should occur at a tertiary center, where an immediate evaluation can be performed to establish a diagnosis and to determine prognosis. Dystocia from extremely large abdominal circumference may be an indication for elective cesarean section in rare cases.

## NEONATOLOGY

**Resuscitation** If a lethal prognosis is certain because of past family history or the prenatal diagnosis of early-onset oligohydramnios, a decision to withhold resuscitation is appropriate. If limited renal function is possible, but not certain, initial support is indicated until the infant can be evaluated and the prognosis can be determined. Infants may present with respiratory distress at delivery, either from pulmonary hypoplasia as a result of long-standing oligohydramnios or from severe abdominal distension due to renal enlargement. Severely affected infants may present with clinical features of Potter's syndrome, including pulmonary hypoplasia, positional limb deformities, and facial dysmorphism secondary to oligohydramnios.

**Transport** Transport is indicated for full confirmation of the diagnosis and prognosis if an infant demonstrates survival potential initially.

**Testing and Confirmation** Ninety percent of patients with infantile polycystic kidney disease present with bilateral abdominal masses at birth. Careful, staged evaluation of renal function and structure by urine production, urinalysis, blood and urine chemistries, and ultrasonography is indicated. Subsequent procedures may be necessary to define renal function and survival potential.

**Nursery Management** Provide mechanical ventilation as necessary to maintain adequate gas exchange. Supportive care consists of management of hypertension; electrolyte imbalance, specifically hyponatremia requiring fluid restriction; and nutritional support. In severe cases, neonates with end-stage renal disease may require dialysis for survival. A multidisciplinary team consisting of neonatologists, nephrologists, hepatologists, and geneticists is required for the ongoing care of the infant.

**Prognosis** Currently, there is no cure for ARPKD. Long-term survival is dependent on the degree of renal and hepatic involvement. The mortality rate is 30% and is greatest in neonates who present with severe pulmonary hypoplasia and renal disease from the time of birth.

## SUGGESTED READINGS


1. Barth RA, Guillot AP, Capeless DL, Clemmons JJ: Prenatal diagnosis of autosomal recessive polycystic kidney disease: variable outcome with one family. Am J Obstet Gynecol 1992; 166:560-567.
2. Bergmann C, Senderek J, Windelen E, et al: Clinical consequences of PKHD1 mutations in 164 patients with autosomal-recessive polycystic kidney disease (ARPKD). Kidney Int 2005; 67:829-848.
3. Blyth H, Ochenden BG: Polycystic disease of kidneys and liver presenting in childhood. J Med Genet 1971; 8:257-284.
4. Bronstein M, Yoffe N, Brandes JM, Blumenfeld Z: First and early second trimester diagnosis of fetal urinary tract anomalies using transvaginal sonography. Prenat Diagn 1990; 10:653-666.
5. Choong KK, Gruenewald SM, Hodson EM: Echogenic fetal kidneys in cytomegalovirus infection. J Clin Ultrasound 1993; 21:128-132.
6. Guay-Woodford LM, Bissler JJ, Braun MC, et al: Consensus expert recommendations for the diagnosis and management of autosomal recessive polycystic kidney disease: report of an international conference. J Pediatr 2014; 165:611-617.
7. Guay-Woodford LM, Desmond RA: Autosomal recessive polycystic kidney disease: the clinical experience in North America. Pediatrics 2003; 111:1072-1080.
8. Guay-Woodford LM: Autosomal recessive polycystic kidney disease: the prototype of the hepato-renal fibrocystic diseases. J Pediatr Genet 2014; 3:89-101.
9. Romero R, Cullen M, Jeanty P, et al: The diagnosis of congenital renal anomalies with ultrasound. II. Infantile polycystic kidney disease. Am J Obstet Gynecol 1984; 150:259-262.
10. Rossetti S, Harris PC: Genotype-phenotype correlation in autosomal dominant and autosomal recessive polycystic kidney disease. J Am Soc Nephrol 2007; 18:1374-1380.
11. Zerres K, Hansmann M, Mallmann R, Gembruch U: Autosomal recessive polycystic kidney disease. Problems of prenatal diagnosis. Prenat Diagn 1988; 8:215-229.

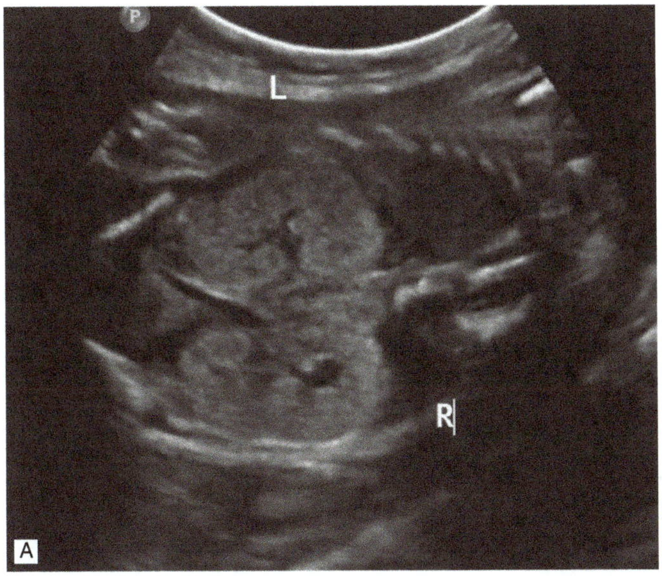


**FIGURE 4.5A** Fetus with autosomal recessive infantile polycystic renal disease at 25 wks : left (L) and right (R) kidney.

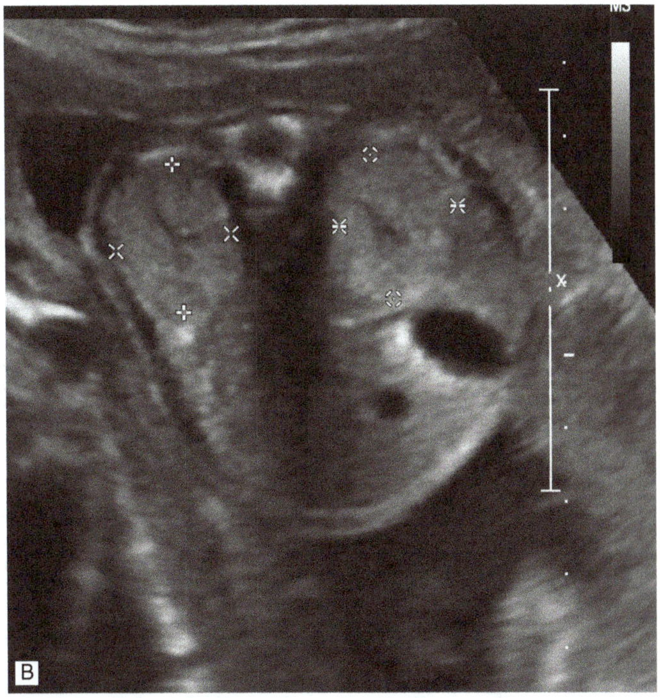


**FIGURE 4.5B** Transverse view of kidneys in autosomal recessive infantile polycystic renal disease (+. . .+; x. . .x).

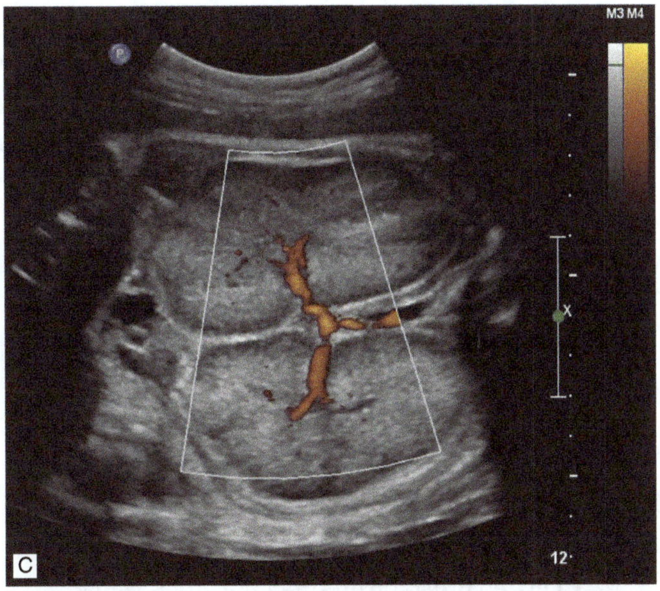


**FIGURE 4.5C** Autosomal recessive infantile polycystic kidneys. Enlarged echogenic kidneys with loss of cortico-medullary differentiation. Power Doppler of the renal arteries.

# 4.6 LOWER URINARY TRACT OBSTRUCTION (POSTERIOR URETHRAL VALVES, URETHRAL ATRESIA, URETHRAL STENOSIS)

## EPIDEMIOLOGY/GENETICS

**Definition** In general, the disorders designated as lower urinary tract obstruction (LUTO) have a blockage at the level of the urethra. In the case of posterior urethral valves (PUVs), the prostatic urethra is obstructed.

**Epidemiology** The incidence of LUTO is 2.2 per 10,000 live births. PUV occurs only in males, with an incidence of 1 in 4000 to 1 in 7500 infants. At least 60% of LUTO are on the basis of PUVs.

**Embryology** Posterior urethral valves are structures that normally develop in the prostatic urethra between 6 and 8 weeks of gestation. Hypertrophy of these valves causes proximal urethral distention, a thick-walled distended bladder, reflux, and hydronephrosis. Chromosome abnormalities, including trisomies 21, 13, and 18, have been reported in up to 20% of cases. Urethral atresia or stenosis is much more commonly associated with chromosome abnormalities, especially trisomies 13 and 18.

**Inheritance Patterns** Inheritance is sporadic. There are rare reports of familial recurrence.

**Teratogens** None are known.

**Prognosis** The prognosis is dependent on renal function. The overall mortality rate for antenatally diagnosed cases is 50%, but the mortality rate is 95% for those cases with oligohydramnios. Fifty percent of neonatal survivors develop chronic renal failure.

## SONOGRAPHY

### FREQUENT FINDINGS: POSTERIOR URETHRAL VALVES

- Male fetus
- Distended bladder
- Thickened bladder wall in a contracted state
- Bilateral pyelocaliectasis
- Dilated prostatic urethra ("keyhole" sign)
- Hydroureter

### LESS FREQUENT

- Urinoma
- Urinary ascites
- Renal cortical cysts
- Increased renal echogenicity
- Oligohydramnios

### KEY FINDINGS/PITFALLS

- Fetal bladder outlet obstruction has been diagnosed at 11 weeks' gestation.
- Dilatation of the proximal urethra anterior to the bladder is a characteristic sonographic finding with severe lower tract obstruction.
- Spontaneous remission of fetal urinary tract obstruction from PUVs may occur due to rupture of the urethral valves.
- The triad of increased renal echogenicity, cortical cysts, and oligohydramnios is highly predictive of renal damage.
  - Cortical cysts correlate with interstitial fibrosis and a decreased number of glomeruli.
  - Cortical cysts predict dysplasia. However, the absence of cortical cysts does not exclude dysplasia.
  - Increased renal echogenicity is a subjective assessment and is less predictive of renal dysplasia than cortical cysts.
- Bladder wall thickness changes with the degree of bladder distention.
  - Thickness is best assessed when the bladder is contracted.
- In the presence of early (18-24 weeks' gestation) oligohydramnios, there is a high risk of pulmonary hypoplasia; normal amniotic fluid does not guarantee normal postnatal renal function.
- Urethral obstruction with a massively enlarged bladder or urinary ascites may result in a "prune-belly" abdomen (i.e., abdominal muscle deficiency).
- Urinary ascites is first detected at 23 weeks' gestation.
  - Urine extravasation into the peritoneal cavity occurs too late to protect fetal renal function.
- The detection rate of PUVs is 50% at 18-22 weeks' gestation and 80% at 28 weeks' gestation.

### DIFFERENTIAL DIAGNOSIS

- The most common diagnosis in false-positive cases of PUVs is severe VUR.
  - Of cases suspected of having PUVs, 5% actually have severe reflux.
- Megacystis-microcolon-intestinal hypoperistalsis syndrome
  - The bladder wall is not thickened.
  - Ureters are generally not dilated.
  - Amniotic fluid volume is most commonly normal.

## PREGNANCY MANAGEMENT

**Investigations and Consultations Required** Chromosome abnormalities are found in up to 20% of cases. Therefore, fetal karyotyping and microarray are essential. Fetal echocardiography should be performed to exclude associated heart defects, although these are uncommon associated anomalies. Pediatric urologic consultation is recommended to plan postnatal management. Consultation with pediatric nephrology may be beneficial, especially when in utero intervention is being entertained, to provide parents information on the long-term consequences of chronic renal insufficiency.

**Fetal Intervention** LUTO has long been proposed as a diagnosis for which in utero fetal intervention may be helpful and is achievable. The main goal of fetal intervention for LUTO is to prevent pulmonary hypoplasia due to anhydramnios during the canalicular phase of lung development (16-24 weeks' gestation). For this reason, LUTO fetuses with normal amniotic fluid volume are not candidates for in utero intervention. A secondary, and more elusive, goal is the preservation of renal function. The majority of survivors of LUTO have some degree of renal insufficiency, and the need for dialysis is frequent. Renal transplant is complicated by a high incidence of failure to thrive among survivors.

Ultrasound has not been proven to be useful in predicting long-term renal function in survivors. Although cortical thinning, echogenicity, and cyst formation are indicative of renal dysplasia and a poor prognosis, their absence is not indicative of a good outcome. Serial vesicocentesis to assess for the preservation of renal concentrating capacity can better discriminate patients with "good prognosis" from "bad prognosis" after 20 weeks' gestation. This information may be useful when considering in utero intervention.

Options for in utero intervention include vesicoamniotic shunt placement, fetoscopic antegrade cystoscopy with laser fulguration, and fetal vesicostomy by hysterotomy. Vesicoamniotic shunt placement is the least invasive but is associated with a high rate of shunt-related complications, such as clogging and migration. Vesicostomy reliably drains urine, but at the cost of maternal morbidity and prematurity. Fetoscopic laser fulguration has demonstrated limited success. In utero intervention should be performed in centers with expertise in such procedures.

**Monitoring** Pregnancies suspected of developing LUTO should be monitored every 2 weeks for evidence of progression, especially during the canalicular phase of lung development and when intervention is being considered. Patients who have undergone in utero intervention will require increased sonographic surveillance to assess for evidence of ongoing urinary decompression and normalization of amniotic fluid volume.

**Pregnancy Course** LUTO has a broad spectrum of presentation, from high-grade obstruction in the first trimester to mild obstruction in the third. Patients with early high-grade obstruction and sonographic markers for poor renal function should be offered pregnancy termination. Serial vesicocentesis can be performed to prove poor function if necessary. Alternatively, the pregnancy can be continued with comfort measures only, avoiding interventions on behalf of the fetus that would expose the mother to risk. Patients presenting in the midtrimester can be offered intervention versus expectant management depending on sonographic findings and patient wishes. Patients presenting after 32 weeks may benefit from early delivery and postnatal treatment.

**Pregnancy Termination Issues** There is no clear advantage to labor induction over dilation and evacuation, as the sonographic diagnosis is usually clear.

**Delivery** The potential for respiratory complications in cases with oligohydramnios and the need for immediate neonatal and urologic evaluation and treatment require that delivery occur in a tertiary center.

## NEONATOLOGY

**Resuscitation** If there was significant oligohydramnios, infants usually present with respiratory distress secondary to pulmonary hypoplasia. Onset of effective respiration may be impeded from abdominal distension secondary to bladder enlargement or renal enlargement.

**Transport** If the infant demonstrates survival potential, transfer to a tertiary center with neonatology, pediatric urology, and nephrology is indicated for full confirmation of diagnosis and prognosis.

**Testing and Confirmation** Neonatal presentation depends on the severity and timing of the urethral obstruction. Severe obstruction early in gestation causes an oligohydramnios sequence with pulmonary hypoplasia and increased risk of morbidity and mortality. Severe, early obstruction that is later relieved may cause a prune belly. Milder or later obstruction is compatible with survival to birth. Presentations in the newborn period and early infancy include decreased urinary stream, distended bladder, urinary infection, abdominal distention, renal failure, palpable kidneys, and failure to thrive. VUR and bladder dysfunction are often seen in infants with PUV. Evaluation at birth includes careful evaluation of renal function, measurement of urine production, urinalysis, and blood and urine chemistry.

Voiding cystourethrogram is diagnostic, and a renal and bladder ultrasound should be obtained to identify characteristic abnormalities associated with PUV. A renal DMSA (dimercaptosulfasuccinic acid) radionuclide scan is useful to detect renal parenchymal abnormalities and to assess the degree of obstruction. Based on VCUG findings, a cystoscopy is performed to confirm the diagnosis and ablate the PUV.

**Nursery Management** Support respiration as necessary to maintain adequate gas exchange. Provide intravenous fluid support and closely monitor renal function.

## SURGERY

**Preoperative Assessment** Dysplastic changes in the kidneys are assessed by a postdelivery sonogram and a DMSA scan. A VCUG is obtained to be certain that the dilated bladder, ureters, and renal pelvis are not caused by reflux.

**Operative Indications** Surgical management is based on decompression of the chronically obstructed, bilateral upper urinary tracts and bladder. If the urethra is patent, early temporary catheter drainage is feasible. Surgical repair is required to achieve bladder and upper tract decompression and prevent further renal parenchymal damage.

**Types of Procedures** Drainage is best accomplished by vesicostomy, temporary loop cutaneous ureterostomies, or a pyelostomy. These procedures are usually planned dependent on the degree of lung hypoplasia and potential for pulmonary function. Milder forms of PUVs can be successfully treated by transurethral or open vesicostomy repair of the lesion with resection of the PUVs.

**Surgical Results/Prognosis** The degree of renal function is difficult to determine by radiographic contrast examination and is best assessed by nuclear renal scan technique. Potential renal function may appear to be insufficient, but early poor function can improve significantly after adequate decompression. Some patients have borderline renal function that becomes insufficient with subsequent skeletal growth, and the need for dialysis and/or renal transplantation becomes apparent. Urethral bladder dysfunction, associated with PUVs, can have an adverse effect on the success of renal transplantation. PUVs can be associated with prune-belly syndrome with marginal early renal function. Incontinence occurs in approximately 14% to 38% of surviving patients. Over the long term, there is often impaired sexual function, with a much higher incidence of undescended testes and impaired ejaculatory mechanism.

## SUGGESTED READINGS


1. Ethun CG, Zamora IJ, Roth DR, et al: Outcomes of fetuses with lower urinary tract obstruction treated with vesicoamniotic shunt: a single institution experience. J Pediatr Surg 2013; 48:956-962.
2. Hecher K, Henning K, Spernol R, Szaley S: Spontaneous remission of urinary tract obstruction and ascites in a fetus with posterior urethral valves. Ultrasound Obstet Gynecol 1991; 1:426-430.
3. Hodges SJ, Patel B, McLorie G, Atala A: Posterior urethral valves. Sci World J TSW Urol 2009; 9:1119–1126.
4. Kaefer M, Peers CA, Retik AB, Benacerraf BB: Increased renal echogenicity: a sonographic sign for differentiating between obstructive and nonobstructive etiologies of in utero bladder distension. J Urol 1997; 158:1026-1029.
5. Kibar Y, Ashley RA, Roth CC, et al: Timing of posterior urethral valve diagnosis and its impact on clinical outcome. J Pediatr Urol 2011; 7:538-542.
6. Malin G, Tonks AM, Morris RK, et al: Congenital lower urinary tract obstruction: a population based epidemiological study. Br J Obstet Gynaecol 2012; 119:1455-1464.
7. Morris RK, Malin GL, Khan KS, Kilby MD: Antenatal ultrasound to predict postnatal renal function in congenital lower urinary tract obstruction: systemic review of test accuracy. Br J Obstet Gynaecol 2009; 116:1290-1299.
8. Morris RK, Malin GL, Khan KS, Kilby MD: Systemic review of the effectiveness of antenatal intervention for the treatment of congenital lower urinary tract obstruction. Br J Obstet Gynaecol 2010; 117:382-390.
9. Morris RK, Ruano R, Kilby MD: Effectiveness of fetal cystoscopy as a diagnostic and therapeutic intervention for lower urinary tract obstruction: a systematic review. Ultrasound Obstet Gynecol 2011; 37:629-637.
10. Pagon RA, Smith DW, Shepard TH: Urethral obstruction malformation complex: a cause of abdominal muscle deficiency and the "prune belly." J Pediatr 1979; 94:900-906.
11. Spaggiari E, Dreux S, Czerkiewicz I, et al: Fetal obstructive uropathy complicated by urinary ascites: outcome and prognostic value of fetal serum B-2-microglobulin. Ultrasound Obstet Gynecol 2013; 41:185-189.
12. Stiller RJ: Early ultrasonic appearance of fetal bladder outlet obstruction. Am J Obstet Gynecol 1989; 160:584-585.

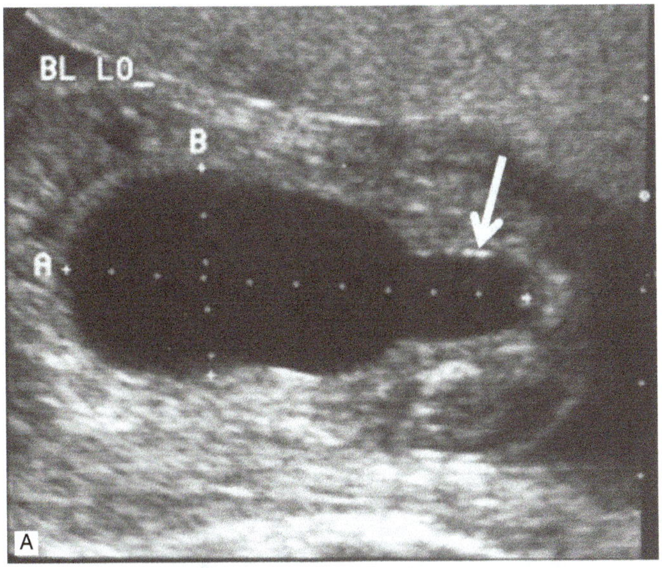


**FIGURE 4.6A** Posterior urethral valves illustrating the "keyhole bladder" resulting in a dilated urethra (arrow).

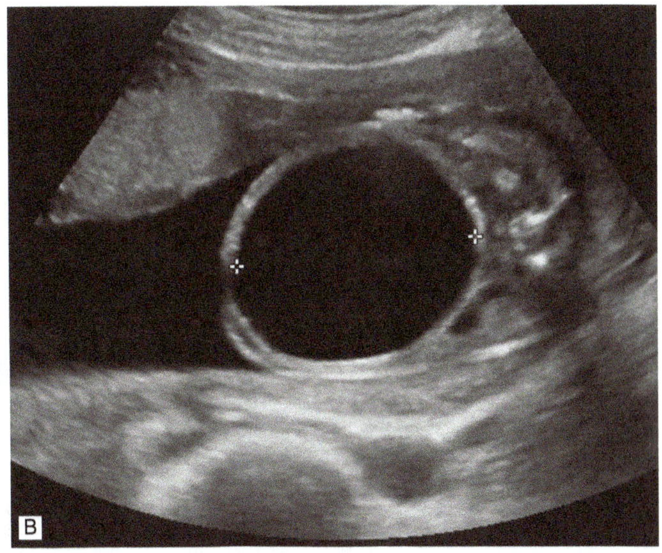

**FIGURE 4.6B** Posterior urethral valves with enlarged fetal bladder (+ … +).

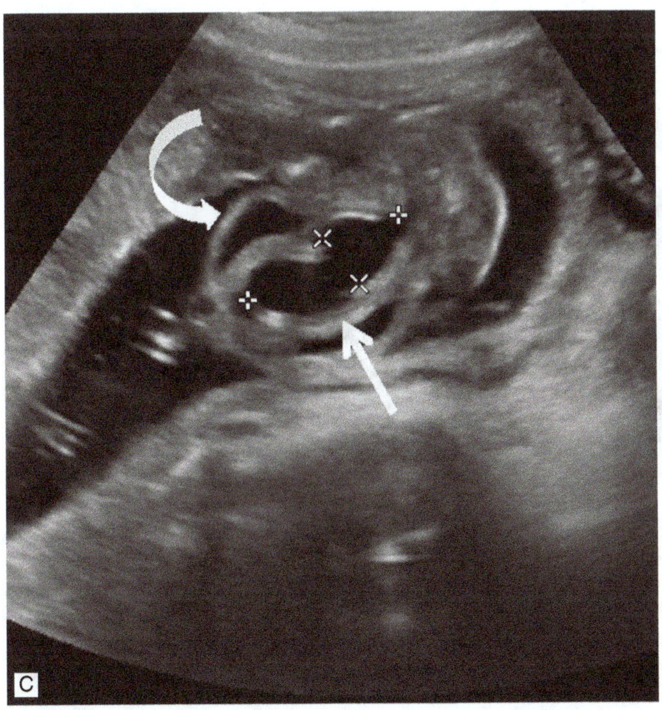

**FIGURE 4.6C** Posterior urethral valves following a bladder tap. Residual urine with thick bladder wall (straight arrow) and urinary ascites (curved arrow).

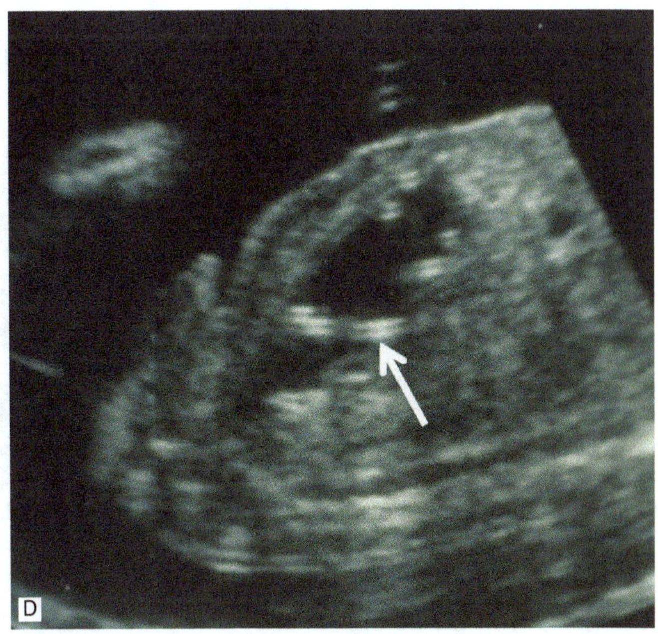

**FIGURE 4.6D** Image showing a vesicoamniotic shunt (arrow).

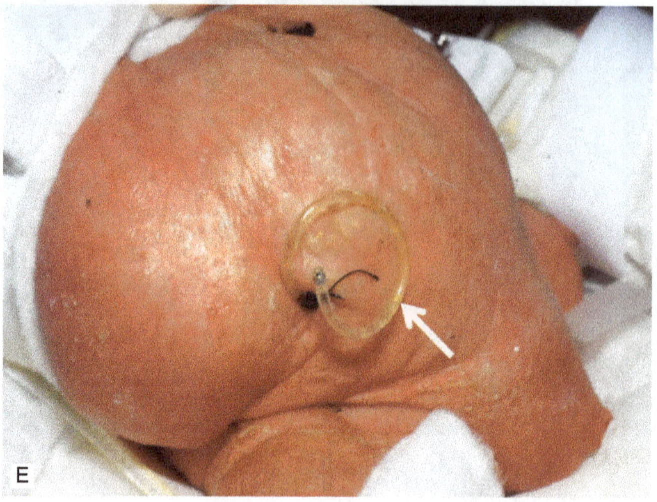


**FIGURE 4.6E** Infant with vesicoamniotic shunt (arrow). Note the "prune-belly" abdomen.

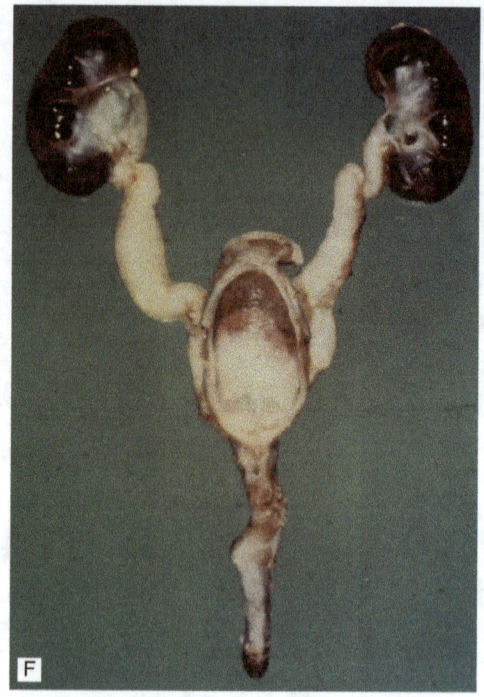


**FIGURE 4.6F** Pathologic specimen from a fetus with posterior urethral valves and bilateral hydroureters.

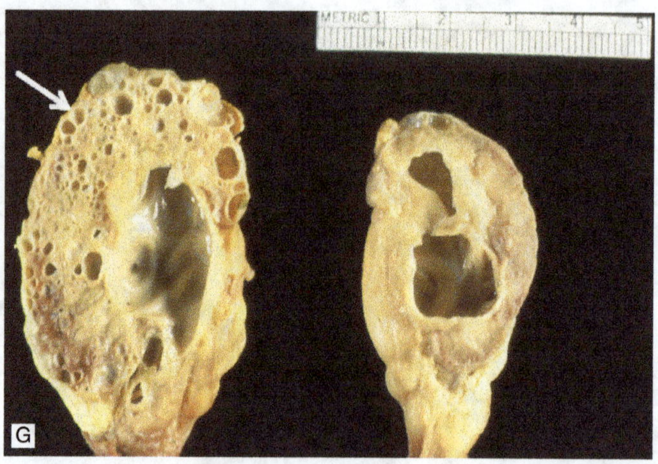


**FIGURE 4.6G** Kidneys from a fetus with posterior urethral valves illustrating cortical dysplasia (arrow).

# 4.7 MESOBLASTIC NEPHROMA, CONGENITAL

## EPIDEMIOLOGY/GENETICS

**Definition** Congenital mesoblastic nephroma (CMN) is a massive, firm, infiltrative, solitary renal tumor, grossly and microscopically resembling a leiomyoma or a low-grade leiomyosarcoma with trapped nephrons.

**Epidemiology** CMN is rare (M1.5:F1). CMN accounts for 3% to 10% of renal masses in childhood and 50% during the neonatal period.

**Embryology** Generally, this is a benign hamartomatous congenital renal tumor. There are three pathological variants: classic CMN, the more aggressive cellular CMN, and the mixed variant. The cellular type is associated with the potential for malignancy.

**Inheritance Patterns** Sporadic inheritance is reported.

**Teratogens** None are known.

**Prognosis** The tumor is generally benign, but prognosis depends on histologic findings and on prematurity induced by the associated polyhydramnios. Most recurrences are local and result from incomplete resection. Rare cases of metastatic disease to lungs and brain have been reported.

## SONOGRAPHY

### FREQUENT FINDINGS

- Homogeneous solid mass in the renal fossa
  - May have an echogenic peripheral rim
- Increased abdominal circumference
- Vascularization
  - Intratumoral perfusion
  - Vascular “ring” sign around part of the nephroma
  - No vascular flow detected
- Polyhydramnios

### LESS FREQUENT

- Hydrops

### KEY FINDINGS/PITFALLS

- Two-thirds of fetal abdominal masses are renal in origin.
- CMN tends to develop in the late third trimester.
- Sonographic detection of CMN has occurred in the second trimester.
- A normal kidney on a second-trimester ultrasound examination does not exclude the subsequent development of CMN.
- CMN is almost always unilateral.
- CMN is well demarcated from renal tissue. Bands of tumor infiltrate the kidney.

- Development of hydrops is associated with a high risk of intrauterine demise.
- Three-dimensional ultrasound provides a volume estimation of a CMN. Multiplanar imaging will sometimes detect the normal component of the kidney on the side of the mesoblastic nephroma.

### DIFFERENTIAL DIAGNOSIS

- Neuroblastoma: This arises from the adrenal gland and is usually echogenic or contains calcifications. There is no direct invasion of normal renal parenchyma.
- Wilms tumor: The prenatal detection of a Wilms tumor is rare. There are no distinguishing characteristics that differentiate it from mesoblastic nephroma.

## PREGNANCY MANAGEMENT

**Investigations and Consultations Required** Because of the similarity of sonographic features between mesoblastic nephroma and Wilms tumor, an evaluation should be done to exclude other syndromes that are associated with Wilms tumor. Amniocentesis should be performed and fluorescent in situ hybridization done to exclude the chromosome 11 deletion seen in the WAGR (Wilms tumor, aniridia, genital abnormalities, mental retardation) syndrome. A consultation with a pediatric urologist should be obtained.

**Fetal Intervention** None is indicated.

**Monitoring** Pregnancies complicated by fetal mesoblastic nephroma usually have associated polyhydramnios. Serial sonograms should be performed to assess fluid volume and growth of the mass.

**Pregnancy Course** Polyhydramnios and preterm labor may be a complication. Tocolytic agents may be required to prolong the pregnancy.

**Pregnancy Termination Issues** Generally, termination issues are not applicable, as these nephromas are usually detected in the third trimester.

**Delivery** Although immediate neonatal complications from mesoblastic nephroma are rare, delivery in a tertiary center allows for thorough evaluation and confirmation of the diagnosis.

## NEONATOLOGY

**Resuscitation** Infants with mesoblastic nephroma have a high incidence of polyhydramnios and preterm delivery. Hydrops fetalis has been reported, as has dystocia and rupture of the mass in the perinatal period. Respiratory distress secondary to either prematurity or mechanical compromise from the abdominal distension is also possible. The approach to resuscitation is dictated by the presence of any of these complicating factors. Establishing adequate ventilation by the gentlest means possible, with avoidance of undue pressure on the abdomen, is essential.

**Transport** Transfer to a tertiary center with pediatric surgical and diagnostic imaging capabilities is indicated.

**Testing and Confirmation** Diagnostic imaging of the tumor mass with MRI is indicated. Differentiation from other solid renal tumors requires histopathologic examination.

**Nursery Management** The definitive treatment is surgical excision of the tumor. Some CMNs are associated with paraneoplastic syndromes, such as hypertension, due to hyperreninemia and hypercalcemia resulting from tumor prostaglandin secretion.

## SURGERY

**Preoperative Assessment** Magnetic resonance imaging is used to assess the extent of the tumor and to ensure that local invasion has not taken place.

**Operative Indications** Nephrectomy is performed as soon as the infant is stable. Chemotherapy and radiotherapy are not generally required unless there is an intraperitoneal tumor spill or incomplete tumor removal. There are two predominant subtypes of CMN. The typical type is the more common, is benign, and has a better prognosis. The second type is the atypical cellular tumor and tumors of mixed histologic type, which can behave more aggressively.

**Surgical Results/Prognosis** A 100% survival rate is reported, provided there are no postoperative complications.

### SUGGESTED READINGS

1. Chen WY, Lin CN, Chao CS, et al: Prenatal diagnosis of congenital mesoblastic nephroma in mid-second trimester by sonography and magnetic resonance imaging. Prenat Diagn 2003; 23:927-931.
2. Fuchs IB, Henrich W, Brauer M, et al: Prenatal diagnosis of congenital mesoblastic nephroma in 2 siblings. J Ultrasound Med 2003; 22:823-827.
3. Garble SH, Crombleholme TM, Semple JP, Bhan I: Prenatal diagnosis and management of fetal tumors. Semin Perinatol 1994; 18:350-365.
4. Giulian BB: Prenatal ultrasonographic diagnosis of fetal renal tumors. Radiology 1984; 152:69-70.
5. Haddad B, Haziza J, Touboul C, et al: The congenital mesoblastic nephroma: a case report of prenatal diagnosis. Fetal Diagn Ther 1996; 11:61-66.
6. Heidelberger KP, Ritchey ML, Dauser RC, et al: Congenital mesoblastic nephroma metastasis to the brain. Cancer 1993; 72:2499-2502.
7. Howell CG, Otherson HB, Kiviat NE, et al: Therapy and outcome in 51 children with mesoblastic congenital nephroma: a report of the National Wilms Tumor Study. Pediatr Surg 1982; 17:826-831.
8. Irsutti M, Puget C, Baunin C, et al: Mesoblastic nephroma: prenatal ultrasonographic and MRI features. Pediatr Radiol 2000; 30:147-150.
9. Liu YC, Mai YL, Chang CC, et al: The presence of hydrops fetalis in a fetus with congenital mesoblastic nephroma. Prenat Diagn 1996; 16:363-365.

10. Schild RL, Plath H, Hofstaetter C, Hansmann M: Diagnosis of a fetal mesoblastic nephroma by 3-D ultrasound. Ultrasound Obstet Gyneol 2000; 15:533-536.
11. Suresh I, Suresh S, Arumugam R, et al: Antenatal diagnosis of Wilms tumor. J Ultrasound Med 1997; 16:69-72.
12. Wang ZP, Li K, Dong KR, Zheng S: Congenital mesoblastic nephroma: clinical analysis of eight cases and review of the literature. Oncol Letters 2014; 8:2007-2011.

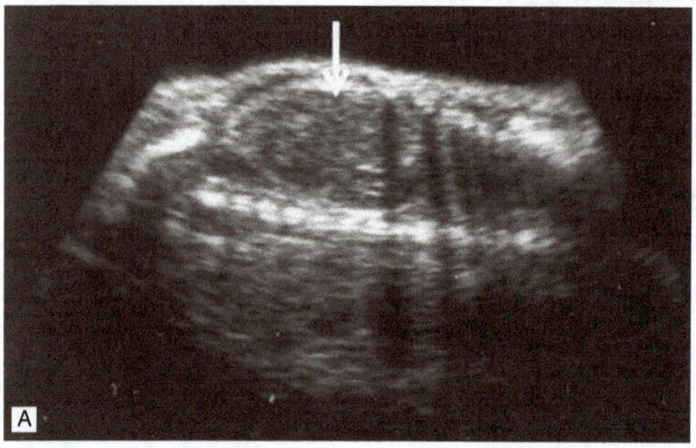

FIGURE 4.7A Mesoblastic nephroma (arrow).

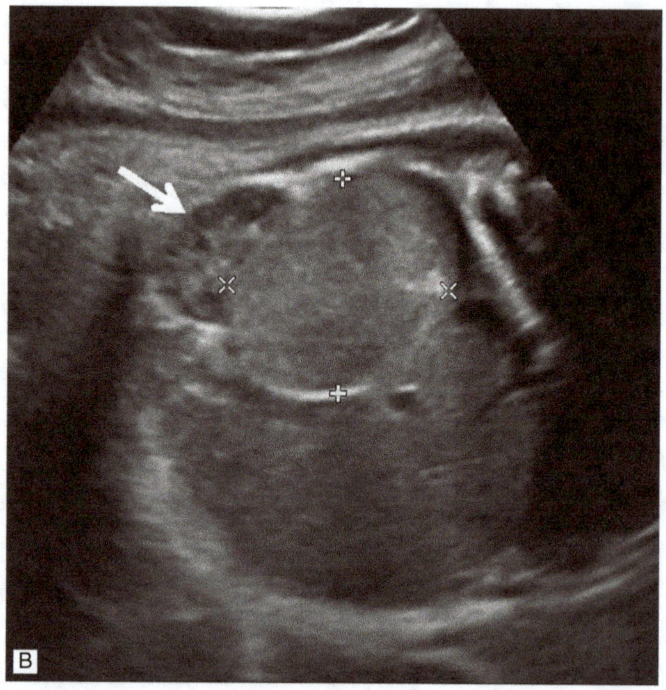

FIGURE 4.7B Mesoblastic nephroma (markers) adjacent to kidney (arrow).

# 4.8 MULTICYSTIC DYSPLASTIC KIDNEY

## EPIDEMIOLOGY/GENETICS

**Definition** Multicystic dysplastic kidney (MCDK) is a congenital dysplasia of the kidneys that is characterized by large, nonhomogeneous dilations of the collecting tubules. It may occur unilaterally or bilaterally.

**Epidemiology** Occurrence is 1 in 1000 to 5000 births (M > F). This is the most common cystic renal abnormality noted in the newborn.

**Embryology** This is likely due to an abnormal ureteral bud-metanephric mesenchymal induction. The cortex, pyramids, and calyces are absent, and the nephron ends blindly at the distal convoluted tubule. The ureter is dysplastic or absent. The kidney characteristically does not function. Several genes (*PAX2, GATA3, TCF2*) have been identified that play an important role in the development of renal dysplasia. It may be unilateral, bilateral, or segmental, with most segmental MCDKs occurring in the upper pole of a duplex kidney. Most cases are sporadic. However, there are many associated nonrenal malformations, including anencephaly, hydrocephalus, spina bifida, cleft palate, microphthalmia, duodenal stenosis, tracheoesophageal fistula, and imperforate anus. More than 35 genetic, chromosomal, and sporadic syndromes have been described with dysplastic kidneys.

**Inheritance Patterns** As an isolated abnormality, it is usually sporadic, but families with autosomal dominant inheritance have been described whose defects range from bilateral renal agenesis (BRA) to double ureter, renal cysts, or hydronephrosis. It can occur as part of the Meckel-Gruber syndrome (autosomal recessive), short-rib polydactyly syndromes (autosomal recessive), Zellweger syndrome (autosomal recessive), Roberts syndrome (autosomal recessive), Fryns syndrome (autosomal recessive), Smith-Lemli-Opitz syndrome (autosomal recessive), Apert syndrome (autosomal dominant), and brachio-oto-renal syndrome (autosomal dominant).

**Teratogens** Maternal diabetes is teratogenic.

**Prognosis** Unilateral and isolated abnormalities may be asymptomatic and go undetected. Unilateral multicystic kidney disease spontaneously regresses with time, and by age 2 the mass has disappeared in about one-third of the cases. Alternatively, the kidney may lose its characteristic shape and consist of multiple noncontiguous cysts of different sizes. Bilateral severe defects are lethal. Partial dysplastic involvement of both kidneys leads eventually to renal function impairment. UPJ obstruction may occur in the contralateral kidney, and up to 20% of children may have reflux in the contralateral kidney.

## SONOGRAPHY

### FREQUENT FINDINGS

- Nonreniform shape
- Multiple renal cysts of various sizes

- Kidney size variable based on the size of renal cysts
- Echogenic renal parenchyma
- Contralateral renal hypertrophy may be detected in the third trimester
- Lack of communication between cysts
- Absent fetal bladder when bilateral

### KEY FINDINGS/PITFALLS

- Resorption of fluid results in a decrease in overall renal size.
- Some of these kidneys will completely involute over time.
- Overall rate of anomalies in the contralateral kidney is approximately 40%.
- Contralateral reflux exists in 25% of cases.

## PREGNANCY MANAGEMENT

**Investigations and Consultations Required** An extended ultrasound examination to exclude associated anomalies is indicated; fetal echocardiography should be performed to rule out an associated heart defect. A pediatric urologist should be consulted to discuss the neonatal evaluation and management of unilateral MCDK with the family. The presence of bilateral MCDK is a lethal condition, and a neonatologist should be consulted to assist in the development of a noninterventional perinatal management plan.

**Fetal Intervention** No intervention is indicated for isolated unilateral or bilateral MCDK. Because there is an increased incidence of contralateral renal malformation when unilateral MCDK is present, there may be rare cases in which an obstructive uropathy is present. Early delivery or in utero placement of a shunt may be necessary if oligohydramnios develops.

**Monitoring** No changes in obstetric management should be necessary for unilateral MCDK. Monthly ultrasonographic examinations should be performed to monitor the status of the normal kidney and the size of the affected kidney. In bilateral MCDK, no intervention for fetal indications should be performed. Electronic fetal monitoring in labor is contraindicated once this diagnosis has been established.

**Pregnancy Course** No specific obstetric complications are to be expected.

**Pregnancy Termination Issues** Pathologic confirmation is essential because of the similar sonographic appearance of MCDK and other forms of renal dysplasia. Termination should be by a nondestructive procedure unless performed in an institution with special expertise in suction evacuation and retrieval of the fetal organs.

**Delivery** For unilateral disease, no special considerations for delivery are necessary. In cases of bilateral MCDK, the site should be one where the staff is comfortable with a noninterventional approach to labor management.

## NEONATOLOGY

**Resuscitation** Infants with bilateral MCDK and an antenatal history of significant oligohydramnios often present with respiratory distress secondary to pulmonary hypoplasia. Positive-pressure ventilation should be used cautiously when pulmonary hypoplasia is suspected because of the high risk for pneumothorax. Onset of effective respiration may be impeded by abdominal distension from renal enlargement, particularly with bilateral involvement. When a prenatal diagnosis of a lethal prognosis is certain, as with bilateral involvement and severe oligohydramnios, a decision to withhold resuscitation may be considered. If limited renal function is possible but not certain, initial support is indicated until the prognosis can be determined.

Infants with a unilateral MCDK do not typically present with respiratory distress at the time of delivery.

**Transport** If the infant with bilateral disease demonstrates survival potential after resuscitation, transfer to a tertiary center is indicated for full confirmation of diagnosis and assessment of prognosis. Infants with isolated unilateral lesions and normal renal function, as indicated by serum creatinine and serum urea nitrogen levels, can be referred for outpatient evaluation and management in the immediate newborn period.

**Testing and Confirmation** In the presence of both bilateral and unilateral MCDK, staged evaluation of renal function and structure by urine production, urinalysis, blood and urine chemistries, renal sonogram, and often VCUG are recommended.

**Nursery Management** In infants with bilateral MCDK, support respiration as necessary to maintain adequate gas exchange and provide judicious fluid and electrolyte support. Infants with bilateral lesions who have limited function at birth but adequate upper tract development (ureters) may be candidates for renal transplantation in early childhood. In infants with unilateral MCDK, involution of the affected kidney and compensatory hypertrophy of the normal contralateral kidney occurs in 60% of MCDK kidneys within the first 3 years of life. Approximately 25% of patients will demonstrate VUR in the contralateral kidney. Long-term follow-up of these children includes serial renal ultrasounds, monitoring of blood pressure, serial urinalysis, and renal function studies.

## SUGGESTED READINGS

1. Aslam M, Watson AR: Unilateral multicystic dysplastic kidney: long term outcomes. Arch Dis Child 2006; 91:820-823.
2. Bonsib SM: The classification of renal cystic diseases and other congenital malformations of the kidney and urinary tract. Arch Pathol Lab Med 2010; 134:554-568.
3. Cambio AJ, Evans CP, Kurzrock EA: Non-surgical management of multicystic dysplastic kidney. BJU Int 2008; 101:804-808.
4. D'Alton M, Romero R, Grannum P, et al: Antenatal diagnosis of renal anomalies with ultrasound. IV. Bilateral multicystic kidney disease. Am J Obstet Gynecol 1986; 154:532-537.

5. Hashimoto B, Filly RA, Callen PW: Multicystic dysplastic kidney in utero: changing appearance on US. Radiology 1986; 159:107-109.
6. Hill LM, Nowak A, Hartle R, Tush B: Fetal compensatory renal hypertrophy with a unilateral non-functioning kidney. Ultrasound Obstet Gynecol 2000; 15:191-193.
7. Hitchcock R, Burge DM: Renal agenesis: an acquired condition? J Pediatr Surg 1994; 29:454-455.
8. Kleiner B, Filly RA, Mack L, Callen PW: Multicystic dysplastic kidney: observations of contralateral disease in the fetal population. Radiology 1986; 161:27-29.
9. Lazebnik N, Bellinger MF, Ferguson JE, et al: Insights into the pathogenesis and natural history of fetuses with multicystic dysplastic kidney disease. Prenat Diagn 1999; 19:418-423.
10. Lin CC, Tsai JD, Sheu JC, et al: Segmental multicystic dysplastic kidney in children: clinical presentation, image finding, management, and outcome. J Pediatr Surg 2010; 45:1856-1862.
11. Mandell J, Paltiel HJ, Peters CA, Benacerraf BR: Prenatal findings associated with a unilateral nonfunctioning or absent kidney. J Urol 1994; 152:176-178.
12. Mansoor O, Chandar J, Rodriguez MM, et al. Long-term risk of chronic kidney disease in unilateral multicystic dysplastic kidney. Pediatr Nephrol 2011; 26:597-603.
13. Nagata M, Shibata S, Shu Y: Pathogenesis of dysplastic kidney associated with urinary tract obstruction in utero. Nephrol Dial Transplant 2002; 17:37-38.
14. Osathanondh V, Potter EL: Pathogenesis of polycystic kidneys. Type 2 due to inhibition of ampullary activity. Arch Pathol 1964; 77:474-484.
15. Schreuder M, Westland R, van Wijk JA: Unilateral multicystic dysplastic kidney: a meta-analysis of observational studies on the incidence, associated urinary tract malformations, and the contralateral kidney. Nephrol Dial Transplant 2009; 24:1810-1818.
16. Van Eijk L, Cohen-Overbeek TE, Den Hollander NS, et al: Unilateral multicystic dysplastic kidney: a combined pre- and postnatal assessment. Ultrasound Obstet Gynecol 2002; 19:180-183.

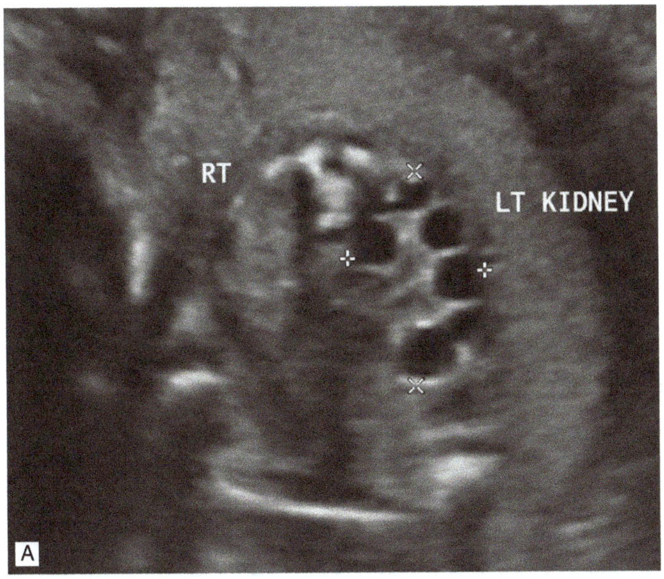


FIGURE 4.8A Left multicystic dysplastic kidney (+ … +; x … x).

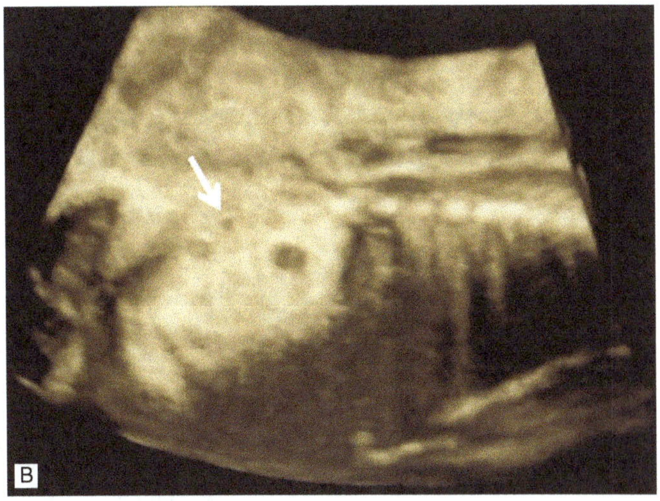


FIGURE 4.8B Three-dimensional image of a multicystic dysplastic kidney at 25 weeks (arrow).

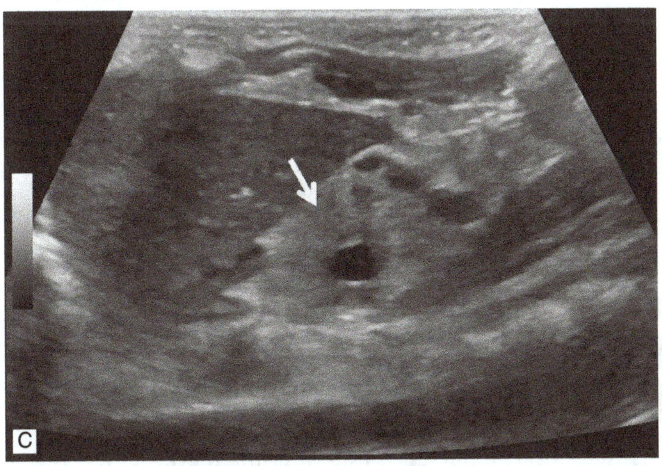


FIGURE 4.8C Neonatal ultrasound showing a dysplastic kidney (arrow).

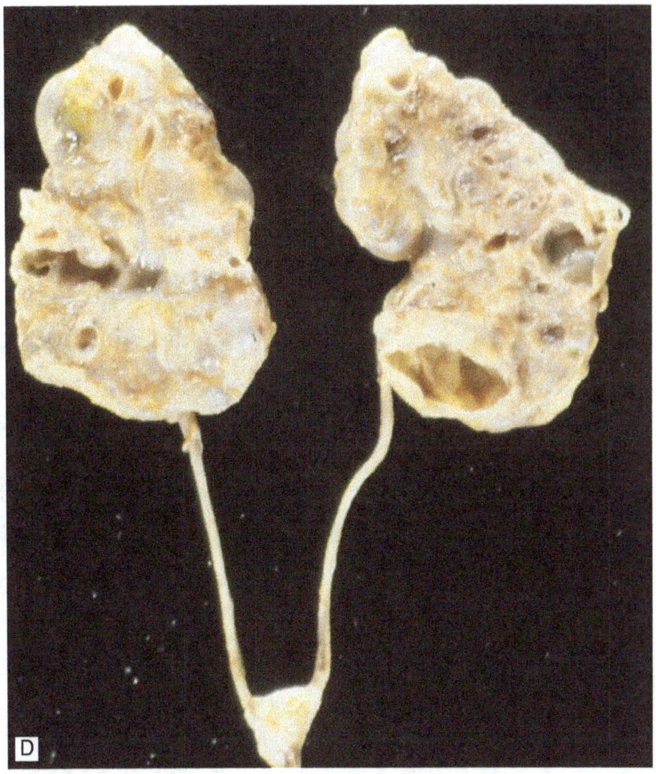


FIGURE 4.8D Pathologic specimen of bilateral multicystic dysplastic kidneys.

# 4.9 NEUROBLASTOMA

## EPIDEMIOLOGY/GENETICS

**Definition** Neuroblastoma is the most frequently diagnosed neoplasm in infants and the most common extracranial solid tumor of childhood.

**Epidemiology** Incidence is 1 in 40 in autopsies, but 10 per million in children under the age of 15 years (1.1:1; M > F). It is slightly more common in whites.

**Embryology** The tumor originates in neural crest cells of the sympathetic nervous system and can develop anywhere from the posterior cranial fossa to the coccyx. About 60%-70% of the tumors arise in the abdomen (50% in the adrenal gland), and another 20% arise in the posterior mediastinum. The familial form is thought to support the Knudson two-mutation model for a "tumor suppressor gene." This model presumes an inherited first mutation, followed by a somatic second mutation resulting in the tumor. Sporadic cases presumably require two somatic mutations. Neuroblastoma in situ is a common autopsy finding in newborn adrenal glands. Most tumors presumably spontaneously regress.

**Inheritance Patterns** Both familial and sporadic cases occur. Familial cases are rare (1%-2% of cases) and show autosomal dominant inheritance. One of the common mutations associated with the familial form of the disease is in the *ALK* receptor tyrosine kinase gene. Sporadic neuroblastomas show complex genetic inheritance, with multiple mutations having been associated with the disease.

**Teratogens** The condition has been reported in association with fetal Dilantin and fetal alcohol exposure, but this is most likely coincidental.

**Additional Investigations** Elevated catecholamine metabolites are seen in 95% of cases and may cause antenatal symptoms in the mother. Affected pregnancies may have maternal tachycardia and nausea and vomiting during the third trimester. Maternal hypertension and preeclampsia may also be seen.

**Prognosis** Prior to 3 months of age, neuroblastomas frequently undergo spontaneous regression. Survival rates of infants with low-stage disease exceed 90%. Perinatally detected neuroblastomas have favorable biologic features that result in a 4-year survival of more than 95%. Of those diagnosed perinatally, 90% are stage I or II. Infants with high-risk disease have a 4-year event-free survival of approximately 60%. Genomic amplification of the *N-myc* oncogene is an indicator of a poor prognosis.

## SONOGRAPHY

### FREQUENT FINDINGS

- Mass superior to the upper pole of the kidney
  - Solid/isoechoic (50%)
  - Cystic
  - Complex cystic/solid

### LESS FREQUENT

- Suprarenal mass with a rim of calcification
- Paraspinal mass
- Hydrops
- Metastatic lesions
  - Liver
  - Placenta
- Hepatomegaly
- Congenital heart defects
- Doppler waveform pattern with a low impedance within a suprarenal mass
- Polyhydramnios

### KEY FINDINGS/PITFALLS

- The normal fetal adrenal has a V shape on a longitudinal view.
  - The central fetal zone is echogenic.
  - The peripheral cortex is hypoechoic.
- Neuroblastomas are usually detected in the third trimester; earliest diagnosis is at 20 weeks.
- Small neuroblastomas may regress.
- Two-thirds of neuroblastomas are on the right.
- Calcifications may be detected in a neuroblastoma.
- Hydrops associated with a neuroblastoma indicates metastatic disease.
- There are no reports of fetal neuroblastomas metastasizing to the mother.
- Large tumors may compress the fetal bowel, resulting in polyhydramnios.
- MRI can be used as an adjunct to ultrasound in the assessment of a fetal suprarenal mass.
- The most common liver tumors in the fetal/neonatal period are metastatic neuroblastoma and hepatoblastoma.

### DIFFERENTIAL DIAGNOSIS

- Adrenal hemorrhage
  - Incidence: 1.9 in 1000 live births
  - Three to four times as many cases on the right
  - Initial sonographic appearance is hypoechoic; subsequently, internal echoes and increased internal echogenicity develop. Calcifications are occasionally present.
- Pulmonary sequestration
  - Characteristically, an echogenic left-side mass is detected in the second trimester.
  - Neuroblastomas are right sided and first identified in the third trimester.
  - There is one pulmonary sequestration for every 2.5 neuroblastomas.
  - Of pulmonary sequestrations, 60% have other significant congenital anomalies, most commonly a diaphragmatic hernia.
  - If there is a normal second-trimester scan that is followed by a third-trimester suprarenal mass, the positive predictive value for neuroblastoma approaches 100%.

- Mesoblastic nephroma
  - A solid renal mass, characteristically associated with third-trimester polyhydramnios

## PREGNANCY MANAGEMENT

**Investigations and Consultations Required** If the diagnosis is relatively certain based on sonographic findings, no additional diagnostic evaluations are needed. A consultation should be obtained with a pediatric oncologist and a pediatric surgeon to discuss neonatal management.

**Fetal Intervention** Early delivery may be indicated if there is evidence of fetal compromise, particularly hydrops.

**Monitoring** Serial ultrasound examinations are indicated to monitor the growth of the mass. This may also be helpful in the early detection of fetal hydrops or polyhydramnios.

**Pregnancy Course** This may be uncomplicated, but in cases with metastatic disease in the liver, polyhydramnios and hydrops may complicate the pregnancy.

**Pregnancy Termination Issues** If the pregnancy is terminated, careful histologic evaluation should be done to confirm the diagnosis. An intact fetus is essential to obtain appropriate organ samples.

**Delivery** Delivery in a tertiary center should be planned to allow management of these potentially unstable neonates. No special interventions in labor are necessary.

## NEONATOLOGY

**Resuscitation** The presence of hydrops prior to delivery or evidence of metastatic disease should serve as an alert for aggressive respiratory support from birth. Otherwise, the need for intervention for cardiorespiratory adaptation following delivery is unlikely.

**Transport** Transfer to a tertiary center with pediatric oncology and surgery subspecialty capabilities is indicated.

**Testing and Confirmation** Careful diagnostic imaging with computed tomography (CT) or MRI coupled with bone marrow aspiration, assay of catecholamine excretory by-products, and identification of tumor oncogenes are the key components for diagnosis and staging.

**Nursery Management** Most infants require only general supportive care while the diagnostic evaluation is completed. Recent advances in understanding the biology and genetics of neuroblastomas have allowed classification into low-, intermediate-, and high-risk groups. This allows the most appropriate intensity of therapy to be selected, ranging from observation alone to aggressive, multimodality therapy. Asymptomatic infants who present with low-risk disease often demonstrate spontaneous tumor regression. Recent research has shown that infants with small, local adrenal masses may be observed expectantly with serial ultrasound and catecholamine measurements. Infants in both the intermediate- and high-risk group require aggressive management with surgical intervention, chemotherapy, or radiation therapy. The need for, and timing of, surgery is based on tumor staging at the time of diagnosis.

## SUGGESTED READINGS

1. Brodeur GM, Bagatell R: Mechanisms of neuroblastoma regression. Nat Rev Clin Oncol 2014; 11:704-713.
2. Cheung NK, Dyer MA: Neuroblastoma: developmental biology, cancer genomics, and immunotherapy. Nat Rev Cancer 2013; 13:397-411.
3. Curtis MR, Mooney DP, Vaccaro TJ, et al: Prenatal ultrasound characterization of the suprarenal mass: distinction between neuroblastoma and subdiaphragmatic extralobar pulmonary sequestration. J Ultrasound Med 1997; 16:75-83.
4. George RE, Lipshultz SF, Lipsitz SR, et al: Association between congenital cardiovascular malformations and neuroblatomas. J Pediatr 2004; 144:444-448.
5. Goldstein I, Gomez K, Copel J: The real time color Doppler appearance of adrenal neuroblastomas in a third trimester fetus. Obstet Gynecol 1994; 83:854-856.
6. Jaffa AJ, Many A, Hartoov J, et al: Prenatal sonographic diagnosis of metastatic neuroblastoma: report of a case and review of the literature. Prenat Diagn 1993; 13:73-77.
7. Lanning M, Lanning P: Prenatal ultrasonic diagnosis of cystic adrenal mass with postnatal hemorrhage and in situ neuroblastoma. Pediatr Surg Int 1992; 7:396-399.
8. Lin JN, Lin GJ, Jung IJ, Hsueh C: Prenatally detected tumor mass in the adrenal gland. J Pediatr Surg 1999; 34:1620-1623.
9. Louis CU, Shohet JM: Neuroblastoma: molecular pathogenesis and therapy. Annu Rev Med 2015; 66:49-63.
10. Maki E, Oh K, Rogers S, Sohaey R: Imaging and differential diagnosis of suprarenal masses in the fetus. J Ultrasound Med 2014; 33:895-904.
11. Maris JM, Kyemba SM, Rebbeck TR, et al: Familial predisposition to neuroblastoma does not map to chromosome band 1p36. Cancer Res 1996; 56:3421-3425.
12. Shen MR, Lin YS, Huang SC, Chou CY: Rapid growth of a fetal abdominal mass: a case report of congenital neuroblastoma. J Clin Ultrasound 1997; 25:39-42.
13. Tomá P, Lucigrai G, Marzoli A, Lituania M: Prenatal diagnosis of metastatic adrenal neuroblastoma with sonography and MR imaging. Am J Roentgenol 1994; 162:1183-1184.

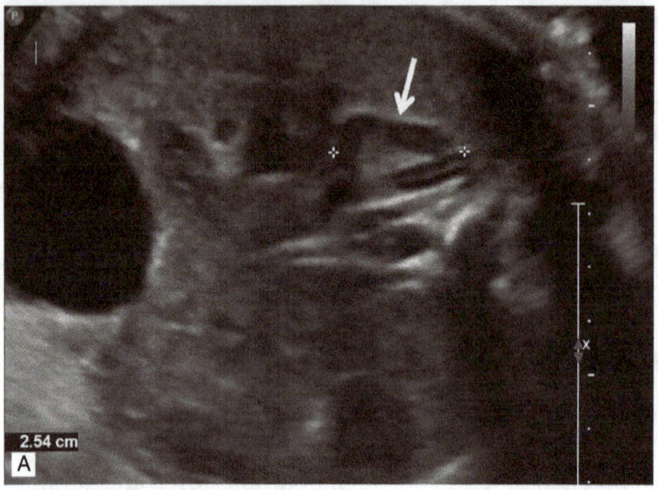


FIGURE 4.9A Normal fetal adrenal cortex (arrow). Note the central zone.

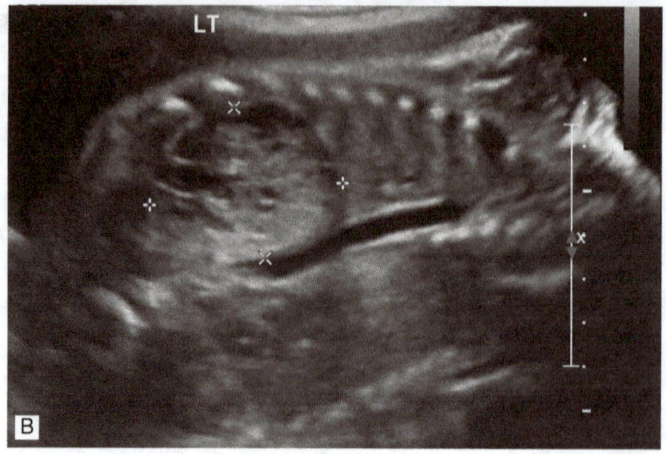


FIGURE 4.9B Left (LT) adrenal neuroblastoma (+ … +; x … x).

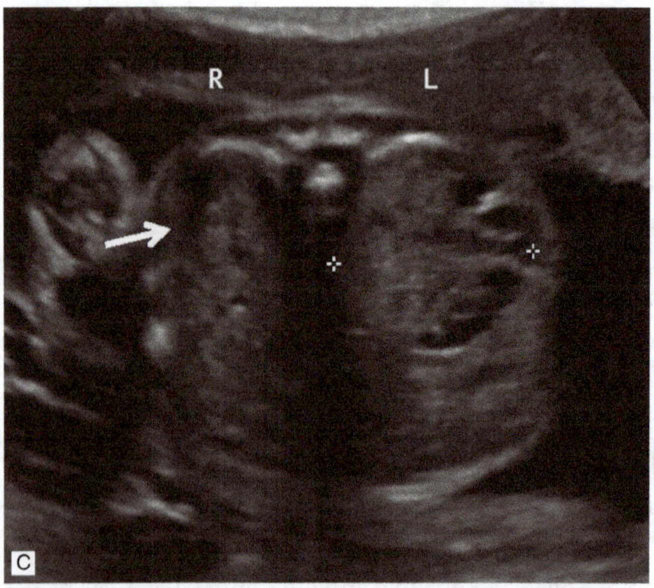


FIGURE 4.9C Transverse view showing left (L) adrenal neuroblastoma (+ … +); right (R) kidney (arrow).

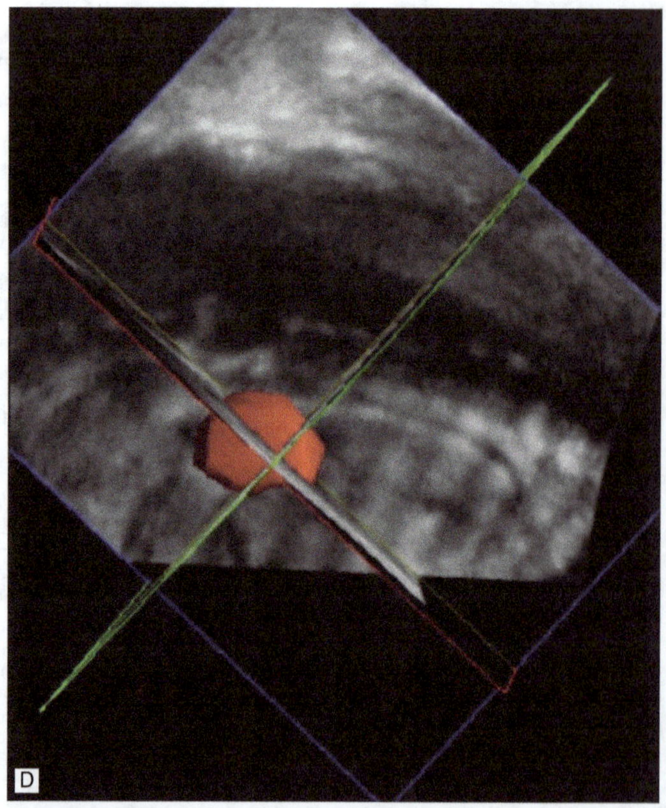


FIGURE 4.9D Three-dimensional volume of adrenal neuroblastoma.

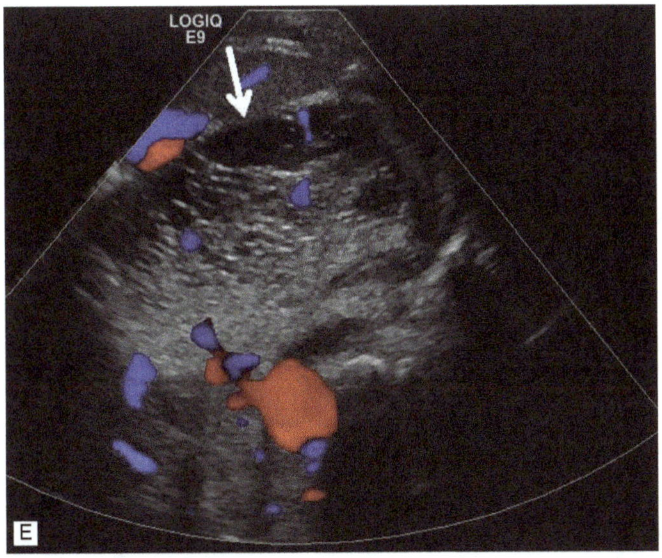


**FIGURE 4.9E** Adrenal neuroblastoma (arrow).

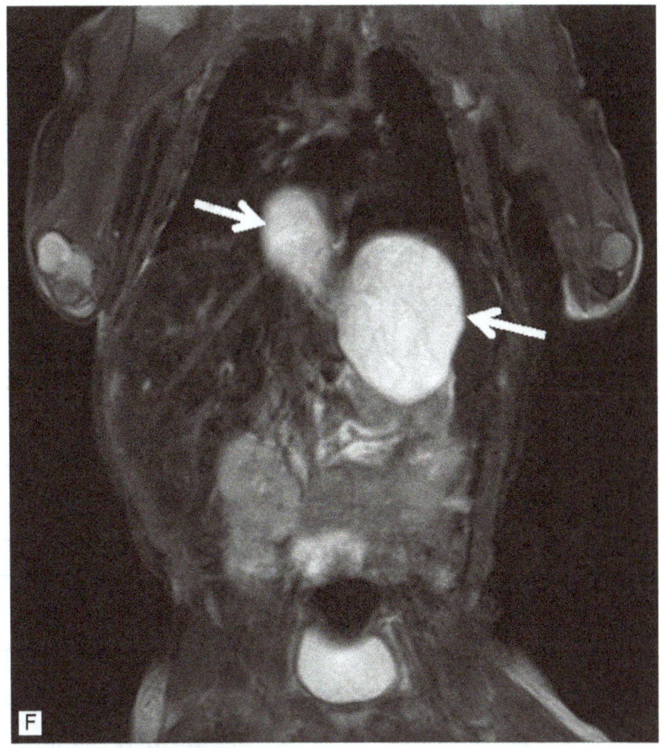


**FIGURE 4.9F** Neonatal MRI showing a paraspinal neuroblastoma (arrows).

# 4.10 FETAL OVARIAN CYSTS

## EPIDEMIOLOGY/GENETICS

**Definition** Ovarian cysts are fluid-filled ovarian tumors.

**Epidemiology** The incidence is 1 in 2600 pregnancies. In infants, the incidence is unknown because they are rarely diagnosed unless they have been detected prenatally.

**Embryology** The etiology is controversial but is most likely linked to maternal estrogens or placental human chorionic gonadotropin (hCG). Cysts are usually follicular or theca-lutein in origin. Of stillbirths, 34% have mature follicles, ranging in size from 1 to 20 mm. An ovarian cyst should therefore have a diameter greater than 20 mm.

**Inheritance Patterns** Most cases are sporadic, except for very rare genetic syndromes, such as the McKusick-Kaufman syndrome (autosomal recessive) with congenital heart disease, polydactyly, and hydrometrocolpos.

**Teratogens** None are known.

**Prognosis** Generally, prognosis is excellent. Most spontaneously resolve without postnatal treatment. In the postnatal period, larger cysts may cause complications, such as ovarian torsion.

## SONOGRAPHY

### FREQUENT FINDINGS

- Female fetus
- Thin-walled cyst above and distinct from bladder
  - May contain septations and debris

### LESS FREQUENT

- Polyhydramnios
- Ascites

### KEY FINDINGS/PITFALLS

- The frequency of ovarian cysts increases with gestational age.
- The diagnosis of ovarian cysts is usually made between 27 and 41 weeks' gestation.
  - Diagnosis in the second trimester has been reported.
- Simple fetal ovarian cysts are unilocular, clear, and thin walled.
- Complicated ovarian cysts may be heterogeneous, contain debris, or have intracystic septations.
- An internal daughter cyst virtually excludes other etiologies for a fetal abdominal cyst.
- There are isolated case reports of ovarian mucinous and serous cystadenomas, teratomas, and granulosa cell tumors.

- Three-dimensional volume rendering may help to assess the anatomic relationship between the ovarian cyst and other abdominal structures.
- The size of most ovarian cysts remains stable through the third trimester; an equal number either increase or decrease in size.
- Torsion is the main complication of fetal ovarian cysts (30%-50%).
  - Sonographic characteristics of torsion include fluid/debris interface, solid components, and septations.
    - Complex fetal adnexal masses without venous or arterial flow are consistent with torsion.
  - Cyst size does not correlate with the possibility of torsion.
  - Fetal tachycardia due to peritoneal irritation is a sign of torsion.
  - Torsion may lead to autoamputation and ovarian loss.
- Fetal ascites is derived from ovarian cyst transudate.
- Fetal ovarian cysts may occasionally rupture.
- Polyhydramnios occurs with a mean ovarian cyst size of 67 × 90 mm, secondary to partial gastrointestinal tract obstruction.

### DIFFERENTIAL DIAGNOSIS

- Mesenteric or omental cysts
  - Incidence: 1 in 20,000 pediatric hospital admissions
  - Derived from abnormally dilated lymphatic channels
  - Usually multilocular, and thin walled, without peristalsis
    - The thin wall differentiates them from enteric duplication cysts.
  - Most commonly occur in the small bowel mesentery
  - An omental cyst is, by definition, within the greater or lesser omentum.
- Enteric duplication cyst
  - Arises from any segment of the gastrointestinal tract
  - Characteristically elongated and thick walled
    - An inner mucosa-submucosa layer is surrounded by an outer layer of smooth muscle (double wall or "muscular rim" sign).
  - Peristalsis may be detected.
- Urachal cyst
  - This is due to abnormal persistence of the urachus.
  - There is a midline cyst adjacent to the bladder that is surrounded by the umbilical arteries.
- Choledochal cyst
  - This is a cystic dilatation of the extrahepatic or intrahepatic bile duct.
  - The presence of a narrow "neck" on an abdominal cyst, located below the liver, indicates a choledochal cyst.
  - This is more common in females (4:1).
  - It is first detected sonographically at 15 weeks' gestation.

## PREGNANCY MANAGEMENT

**Investigations and Consultations Required** In general, ovarian cysts are a diagnosis of exclusion, and an extended examination is the only evaluation required. Occasionally, the diagnosis may be in question, and a further evaluation, including chromosomal studies, microarray, or fetal echocardiography, may be appropriate. Pediatric surgical consultations prenatally are generally not necessary but may be useful for large cysts in the event that neonatal complications require surgical intervention.

**Fetal Intervention** Aspiration of the cysts is contraindicated because of the high incidence of spontaneous resolution, the significant risk of misdiagnosis, and the theoretical concerns of spillage of an irritant (contents of a dermoid cyst) or malignant cells into the peritoneal cavity.

**Monitoring** No alterations in obstetric care are necessary. Those cases complicated by polyhydramnios should be monitored for evidence of preterm labor. Follow-up sonograms at monthly intervals to check ovarian cyst size and to look for polyhydramnios and intestinal dilatation are helpful.

**Pregnancy Course** Polyhydramnios may develop secondary to extrinsic bowel obstruction, but this is rare.

**Pregnancy Termination Issues** Termination of pregnancy is generally not applicable as these are often third-trimester diagnoses.

**Delivery** Labor management should not be affected, and delivery at a tertiary center is not required. In cases of large cysts that could result in significant abdominal distention with dystocia in labor or neonatal respiratory distress, cesarean section may be indicated, and delivery at a tertiary center may be prudent.

## NEONATOLOGY

**Resuscitation** Rarely is there need for resuscitative interventions. However, large cysts may create severe abdominal distension, which inhibits efficient breathing and may necessitate intubation and respiratory support at birth.

**Transport** Neonatal transport to a tertiary facility with neonatology and pediatric surgery is indicated for infants symptomatic at the time of birth. The majority of neonates will be asymptomatic and can be evaluated with a follow-up ultrasound as an outpatient.

**Testing and Confirmation** Obtain an abdominal sonogram to confirm the prenatal diagnosis. Additional contrast studies of the gastrointestinal and urinary tracts may be necessary for a large mass.

**Nursery Management** Provide mechanical ventilator support if abdominal distension is severe and impedes adequate gas exchange. As most fetal ovarian cysts spontaneously regress by 4 to 6 months, expectant management with serial ultrasounds is indicated until the cyst resolves. Surgical intervention is required for cysts that continue to enlarge, become symptomatic, or persist for more than 4 to 6 months.

## SURGERY

**Preoperative Assessment** An abdominal ultrasound is sufficient to confirm the diagnosis.

**Operative Indications** There is little support for antenatal intervention for the majority of fetal ovarian cysts. Most ovarian cysts can also be managed conservatively in the neonatal period and followed by serial ultrasounds. In general, conservative management may result in improved ovarian salvage.

**Types of Procedures** For cysts that are persistent or increasing in size, a laparoscopic approach to cystectomy or cyst fenestration with preservation of ovarian tissue may be considered. Oophorectomy is rarely required but may be necessary in the case of antenatal torsion with necrosis of the ovary. Surgery is not mandatory in the setting of presumed antenatal torsion, and in many cases, the complex cyst will resolve over time. Although concern over the risk of postnatal torsion is often the motivation for surgery on larger antenatally identified ovarian cysts, there are limited data supporting a significant risk of torsion.

**Surgical Results and Prognosis** Surgery is rarely required because the outcomes are excellent with conservative management.

## SUGGESTED READINGS

1. Bagolan P, Giorlandino C, Nahom A, et al: The management of fetal ovarian cysts. J Pediatr Surg 2002; 37:25-30.
2. Ben-Ami I, Kogan A, Fuchs N, et al: Long-term follow-up of children with ovarian cysts diagnosed prenatally. Prenat Diagn 2010; 30:342-347.
3. Campbell BA, Gary RS, Garg K, et al: Perinatal ovarian cyst: a non-surgical approach. J Pediatr Surg 1992; 27:1618-1619.
4. Cheng G, Soboleski D, Daneman A, et al: Sonographic pitfalls in the diagnosis of enteric duplication cysts. Am J Roentgenol 2005; 184:521-525.
5. Giolandino C, Bilancioni E, Bagolan P, et al: Antenatal ultrasonic diagnosis and management of foetal ovarian cysts. Int J Gynecol Obstet 1993; 44:27-31.
6. Hata T, Mori N, Tenkumo C, et al: Three-dimensional volume rendered imaging of normal and abnormal fetal fluid-filled structures using inversion mode. J Obstet Gynaecol 2011; 37:1748-1754.
7. Kirkinen P, Joupplia P: Perinatal aspects of pregnancy complicated by fetal ovarian cyst. J Perinat Med 1985; 13:245-251.
8. Papic JC, Billmire DF, Rescorla FJ, et al: Management of neonatal ovarian cysts and its effect on ovarian preservation. J Pediatr Surg 2014; 49:990-993.
9. Perrotin F, Potin J, Haddad G, et al: Fetal ovarian cysts: a report of three cases managed by intrauterine aspiration. Ultrasound Obstet Gynecol 2000; 16:655-659.
10. Quarello E, Gorincour G, Merrot T, et al: The "daughter cyst sign": a sonographic clue to the diagnosis of fetal ovarian cyst. Ultrasound Obstet Gynecol 2003; 22:431-436.
11. Sakala EP, Leon ZA, Rouse GA: Management of antenatally diagnosed fetal ovarian cysts. Obstet Gynecol Surv 1991; 46:407-414.
12. Schroeder D, Smith L, Prain HC: Antenatal diagnosis of choledochal cyst at 15 weeks' gestation: etiologic implications and management. J Pediatr Surg 1989; 24:936-938.

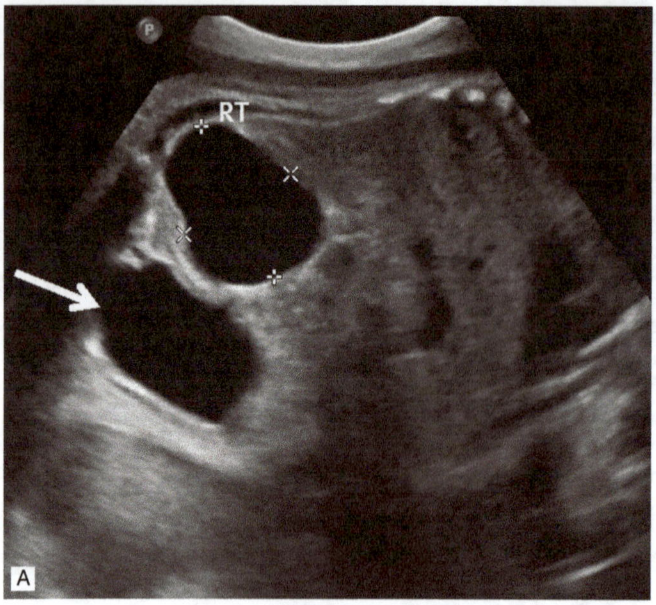


**FIGURE 4.10A** Fetal ovarian cyst (RT; + … +; x … x) anterior to the bladder (arrow).

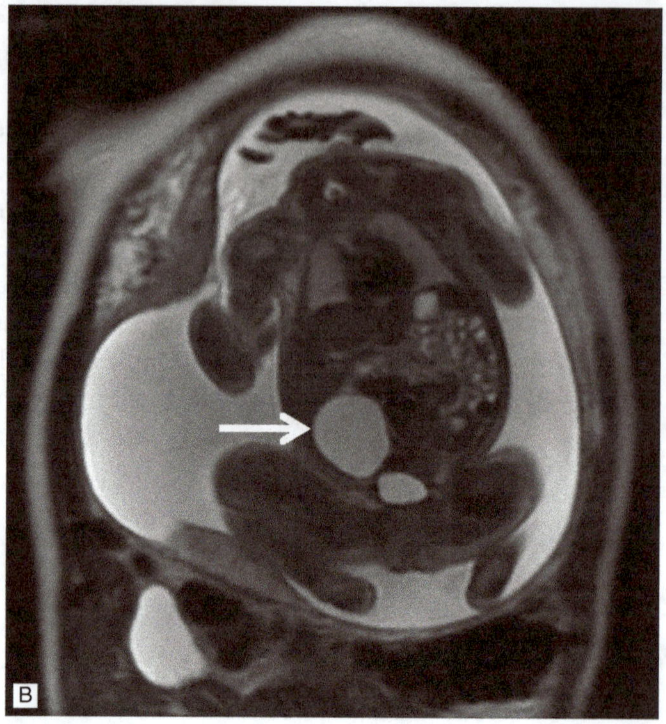


**FIGURE 4.10B** Magnetic resonance image of a fetal ovarian cyst (arrow).

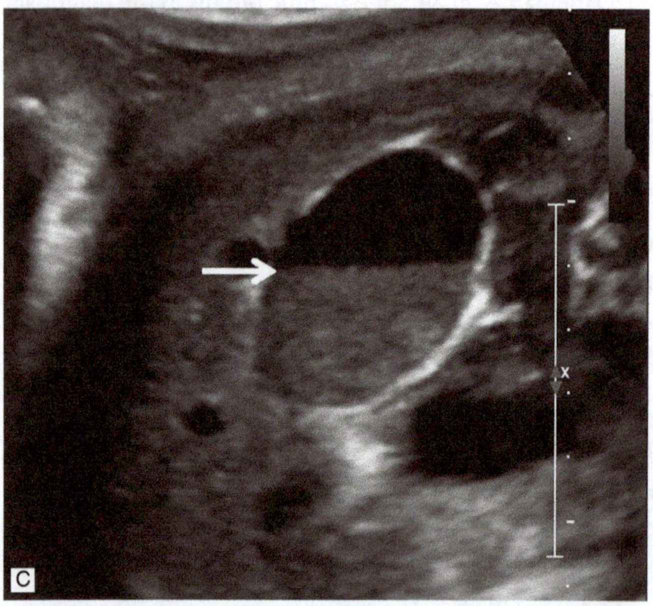


**FIGURE 4.10C** Fetal ovarian cyst with a fluid/debris interface (arrow) consistent with torsion.

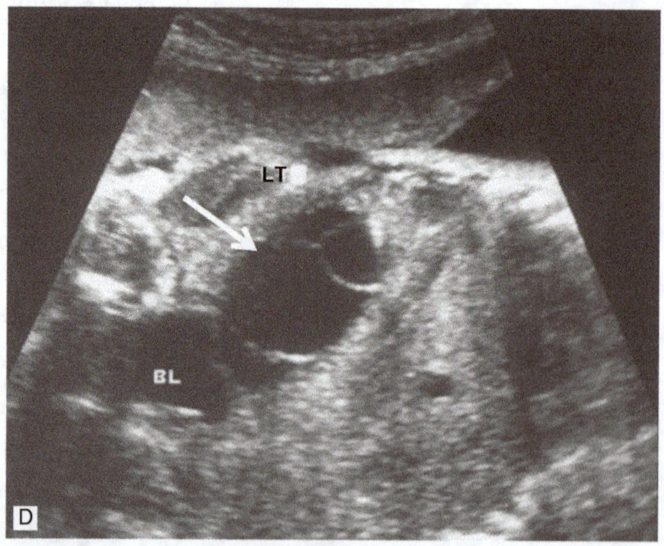


**FIGURE 4.10D** Septated left (LT) fetal ovarian cyst (arrow). BL, bladder.

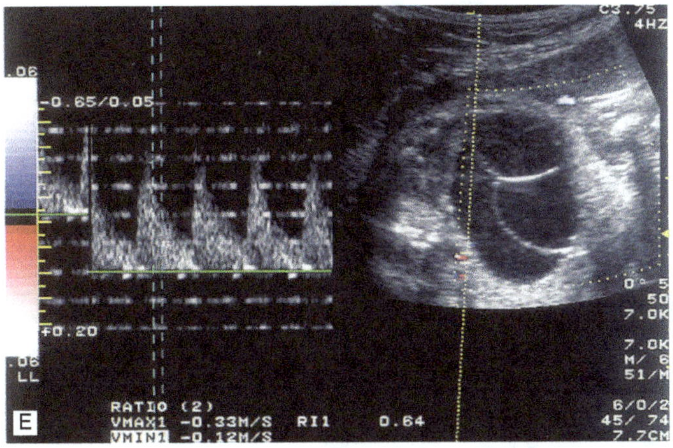


**FIGURE 4.10E** Vascular flow around fetal ovarian cyst.

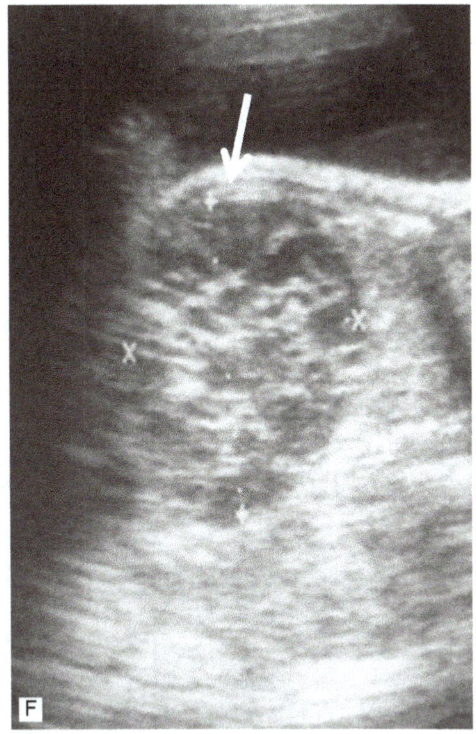


**FIGURE 4.10F** Fetal germ cell tumor (arrow, + … +; x … x).

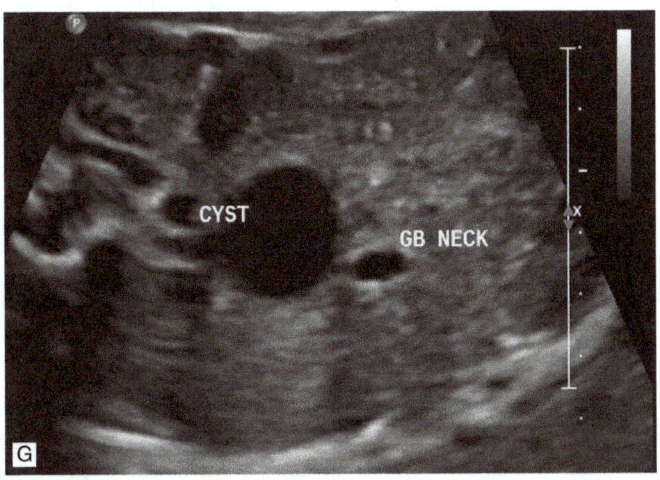


**FIGURE 4.10G** Choledochal cyst. GB NECK, gallbladder neck.

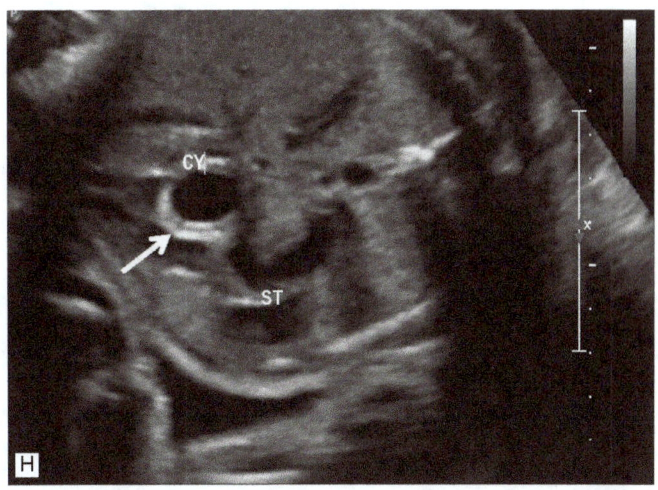


**FIGURE 4.10H** Enteric duplication cyst (CY). Note the double wall or "muscular rim" sign (arrow). ST, stomach.

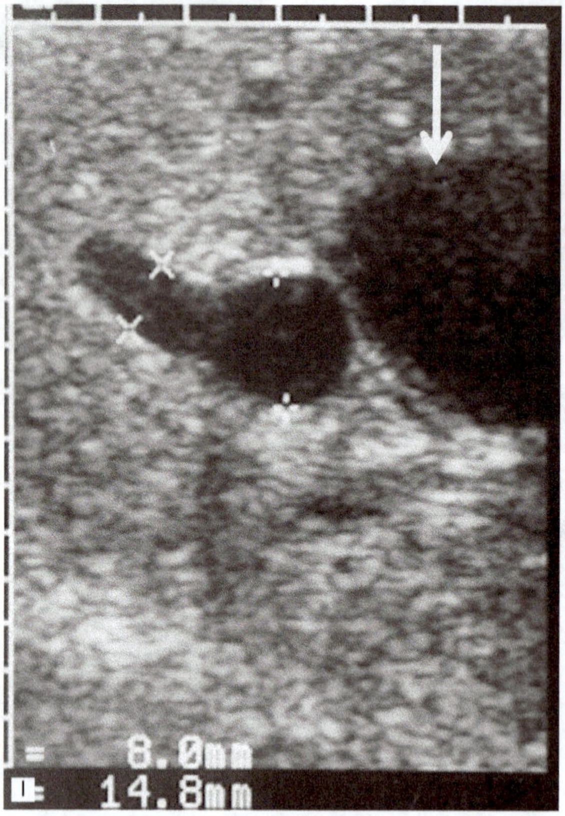


**FIGURE 4.10I** Midline urachal cyst (x…x; +…+) adjacent bladder (arrow).

# 4.11 PYELECTASIS

## EPIDEMIOLOGY/GENETICS

**Definition** Pyelectasis refers to a sonographic finding of an increased anterior-posterior (AP) diameter of the fetal renal pelvis; it is also called pelviectasis.

**Epidemiology** Occurrence is in 0.5% to 4.5% of fetuses (M2:F1).

**Embryology** Most commonly, it represents a transient, physiologic state in the fetus. Only about 10%-15% will have postnatal pathology, and most will have vesicoureteral reflux (VUR). A duplicated kidney with a ureterocele is one of the more common anatomic causes. Second-trimester pyelectasis has a weak association with karyotypic abnormalities, specifically trisomy 21.

**Inheritance Patterns** Most cases are sporadic.

**Teratogens** None are known.

**Prognosis** The majority of antenatally diagnosed cases of pyelectasis will resolve prior to birth or in the neonatal period. Approximately 5% will require surgical intervention, and another 5%-10% will have some degree of VUR.

## SONOGRAPHY

### FREQUENT FINDINGS

- Low-risk prenatal intervention
  - AP renal pelvis
    - 4.0-6.9 mm at 16-27 weeks
    - 7.0-9.9 mm at 28 weeks or more
  - May have central but not peripheral calyceal dilatation
  - Normal renal parenchyma
  - Bladder and ureter normal
- High-risk prenatal intervention
  - AP renal pelvis
    - 7 mm or greater at 16-27 weeks
    - 10.0 mm or greater at 28 weeks or more
  - Peripheral calyceal dilatation
  - Thin renal parenchyma
  - Possible hydroureters
  - Thickened bladder wall
  - Enlarged bladder volume
  - Oligohydramnios from a genitourinary cause

**TABLE 4.1** Definition of Antenatal Pyelectasis

| | GESTATIONAL AGE | |
|---|---|---|
| | 16-27[a] weeks | >28 weeks |
| Mild | >4.0 mm | >7.0 mm |
| Moderate | >7.0 mm | >9.0 mm |
| Severe | >10.0 mm | >15.0 mm |

[a] *Sources*: Adapted from Nguyen HT, et al. J Pediatr Urol 2010; 6:212; Nguyen HT, et al. J Pediatr Urol 2014; 10:982.

### KEY FINDINGS/PITFALLS

- Gestational age, degree of fetal bladder distention, and maternal hydration affect renal pelvis diameter.
- Renal pelvic diameters progress along a continuum. Hence, there is not a single threshold that separates normal from abnormal (Table 4.1).
- The likelihood of pathology increases with renal pelvis dilation.
  - A lower cutoff improves sensitivity but increases the false-positive rate for detecting renal pathology.
- Pyelectasis that resolves, or improves, from the second to the third trimester is usually not associated with significant neonatal pathology.
- Renal pyelectasis that worsens in the third trimester correlates with a higher likelihood of significant pathology.
- When there is second-trimester pyelectasis, a follow-up ultrasound examination in the third trimester is recommended.

## PREGNANCY MANAGEMENT

**Investigations and Consultations Required** Pyelectasis is a relatively common finding on a second-trimester anatomic survey. The bladder and amniotic fluid volume should be examined and appear normal. The ureters should not be identified, and the kidneys should otherwise appear normal. If these criteria are not met, another more complex diagnosis should be considered, and further evaluation may be warranted. If isolated, pyelectasis found in the second trimester often resolves; therefore, a follow-up examination at 32 weeks is suggested. Recommendations for further evaluation are made if the degree of renal pelvis dilatation has increased. If there is persistent renal pelvis dilatation, consultation with pediatric urology and plans to deliver at a tertiary center are the only necessary antenatal interventions.

As pyelectasis is also a soft marker for fetal Down syndrome, this finding in the second trimester should also trigger reevaluation of the patient's Down syndrome risk. In the presence of an otherwise-normal extended fetal anatomic survey, a normal first-trimester genetic screen, second-trimester multiple-marker screen, or noninvasive prenatal test, pyelectasis is not an indication for fetal chromosomal analysis.

**Fetal Intervention** In general, no intervention is necessary, as these fetuses do well.

**Monitoring** No change in obstetric care is indicated.

**Pregnancy Course** No obstetric complications should be expected.

**Pregnancy Termination Issues** In general, these cases do not usually result in pregnancy termination, but if that is chosen, an intact fetus appropriate for confirming the anatomic findings on autopsy is warranted.

**Delivery** In cases with significant obstruction, there may be a need for immediate neonatal evaluation to establish a diagnosis, and delivery in those cases should be in a tertiary center.

## NEONATOLOGY

**Resuscitation** In the absence of other conditions, resuscitative efforts are usually not required.

**Transport** In cases of mild pyelectasis diagnosed antenatally, transfer to a tertiary center is not necessary, as evaluation can be performed as an outpatient at 1-2 weeks of age. In infants with significant bilateral pyelectasis, severe unilateral pyelectasis, or associated renal anomalies, transfer to a tertiary center is indicated for evaluation and management.

**Testing and confirmation** Physical exam can detect congenital abnormalities that are associated with significant pyelectasis. These include ear abnormalities, a two-vessel umbilical cord, palpable kidney or bladder, or abnormalities of the lower extremities. Ultrasonography of the kidneys and bladder or VCUG is diagnostic. Timing of these studies is dependent on the severity of the antenatally diagnosed pyelectasis and presence of suspected associated congenital anomalies of the kidney and urinary tract, including obstructive uropathy and VUR.

**Nursery Management** Depending on the severity of pyelectasis and presence of associated VUR or obstructive uropathy, antibiotic prophylaxis with amoxicillin (12-25 mg/kg orally daily) is recommended. While infants with mild-to-moderate unilateral pyelectasis may be safely evaluated at more than 7 days of age, earlier evaluation in the immediate newborn period may help to ease parental anxiety and concern. Follow-up with pediatric urology is indicated.

A suggested algorithm for the postnatal management of infants with antenatal pyelectasis delivered at a tertiary center with pediatric urology and radiology is as follows: (Note APD =anterior-posterior diameter of the renal pelvis, and SFU=Society for Fetal Urology).

**Normal Low Risk–Normal renal parenchyma ureter and no oligohydramnios**

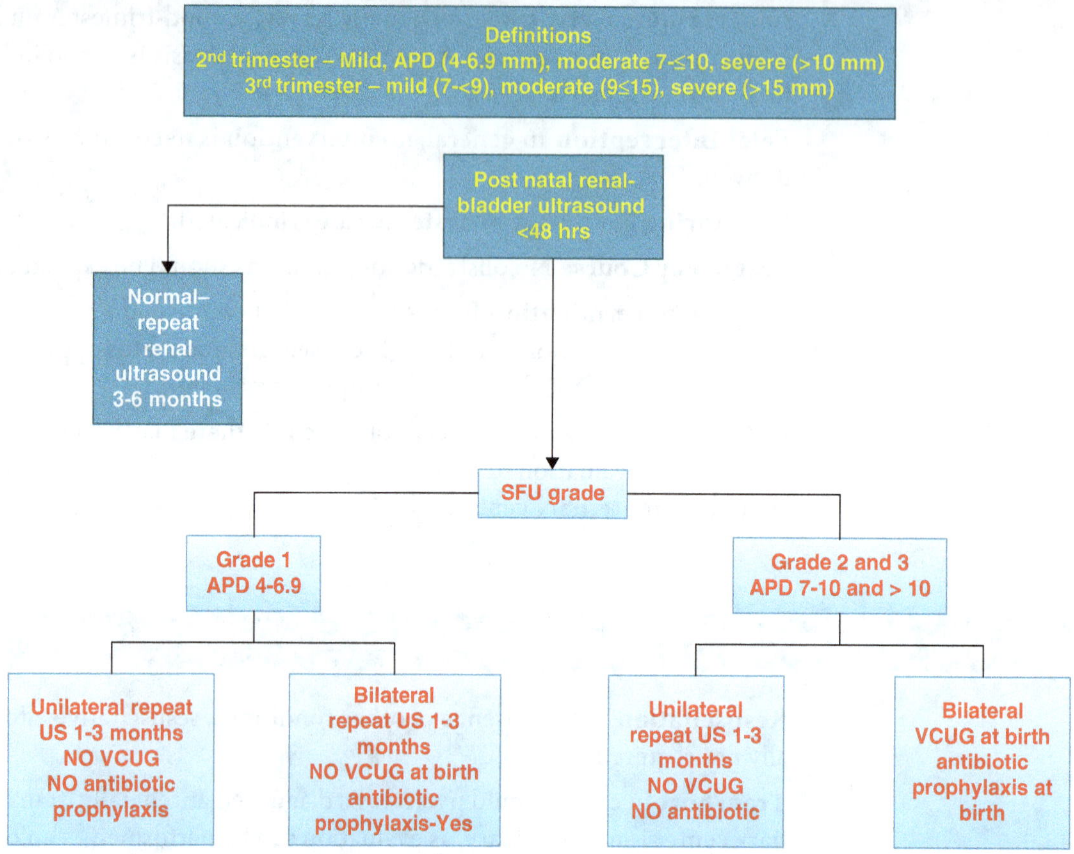


## SUGGESTED READINGS


1. Babcook CJ, Silvera M, Drake C, Levine D: Effect of maternal hydration on mild fetal pyelectasis. J Ultrasound Med 1998; 17:539-544.
2. Carbone JF, Tuuli G, Dicke JM, et al: Revisiting the risk for aneuploidy in fetuses with isolated pyelectasis. Prenat Diagn 2011; 31:566-570.
3. Corteville JE, Gray DL, Crane JP: Congenital hydronephrosis: correlation of fetal ultrasonographic findings with infant outcome. Am J Obstet Gynecol 1991; 165:384-388.
4. Damen-Elias HA, Luijnenburg SE, Visser GH, et al: Mild pyelectasis diagnosed by prenatal ultrasound is not a predictor of urinary tract morbidity in childhood. Prenat Diagn 2005; 25:1239-1247.
5. Ismaili K, Hall M, Donner C, et al: Results of systemic screening for minor degrees of fetal renal pelvis dilatation in an unselected population. Am J Obstet Gynecol 2003; 188:242-246.
6. Lee RS, Cendron M, Kinnamon DD, Nguyen HT: Antenatal hydronephrosis as a predictor of postnatal outcome: a meta-analysis. Pediatrics 2006; 118:586-593.

7. Nguyen HT, Benson CB, Bromley B, et al: Multidisciplinary consensus on the classification of prenatal and postnatal urinary tract dilation (UTD classification system). J Pediatr Urol 2014; 10:982-999.

8. Nguyen HT, Herndon CDA, Cooper C, et al: The Society for Fetal Urology consensus statement on the evaluation and management of antenatal hydronephrosis. J Pediatr Urol 2010; 6:212-231.

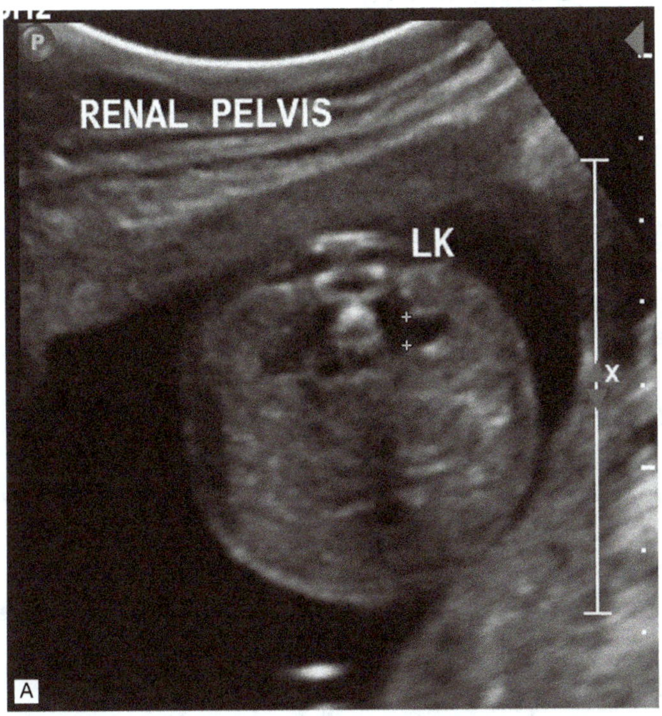


**FIGURE 4.11A** Normal second-trimester renal pelvis (3 mm). LK, left kidney.

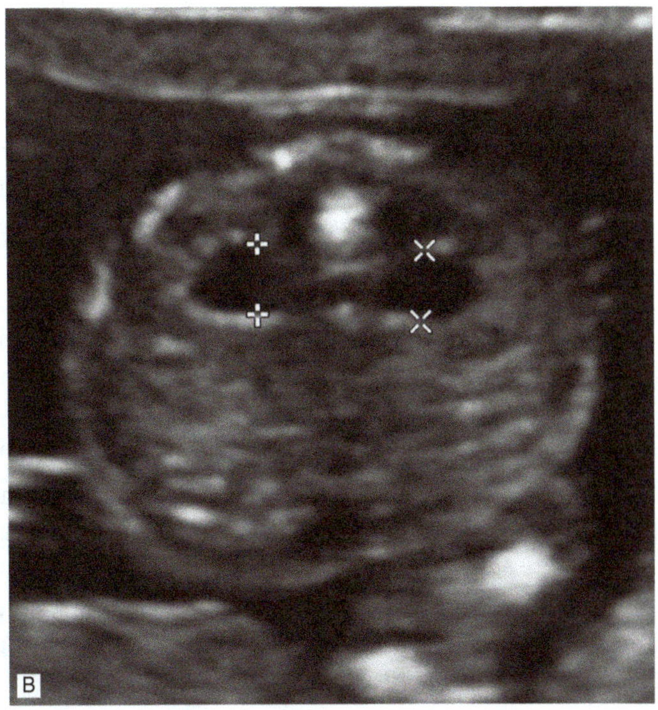


**FIGURE 4.11B** Second-trimester bilateral renal pyelectasis measuring 5 mm (+ … +; x … x).

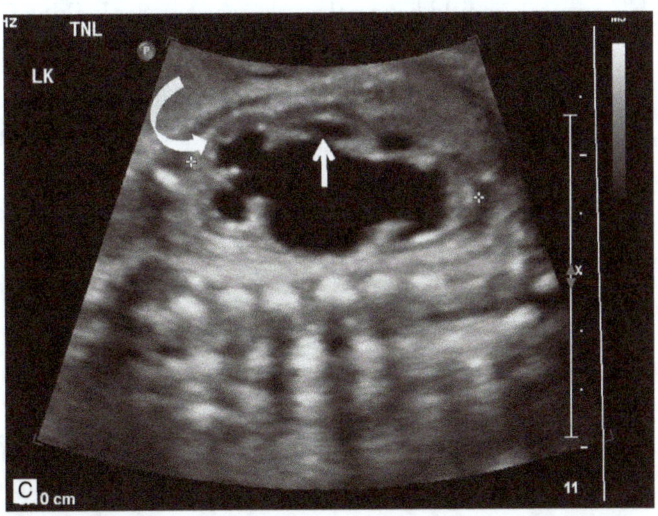


**FIGURE 4.11C** Severe pyelectasis at 29 weeks with dilatation of major (straight arrow) and minor (curved arrow) calices.

# 4.12 RENAL AGENESIS

## EPIDEMIOLOGY/GENETICS

**Definition** Renal agenesis is bilateral or unilateral absence of the kidneys.

**Epidemiology** Unilateral renal agenesis occurs in 1 in 1000 births (M1:F1), and BRA occurs in 1 in 4000 births (M2.5:F1). Incidence of BRA on prenatal ultrasound is 1 in 4000 to 1 in 7000. The incidence of unilateral disease is 1 in 1500 second-trimester ultrasound examinations.

**Embryology** The pathophysiology of this abnormality is unknown. The group of disorders that are part of the renal hypodysplasia complex include renal agenesis, renal hypoplasia, and cystic and noncystic dysplasia. In bilateral disease, the clinical findings include pulmonary hypoplasia, oligohydramnios, limb contractures, and characteristic facies (Potter sequence). Renal agenesis is associated with other genitourinary (50%), gastrointestinal, and cardiac abnormalities and is part of more than 50 multiple-malformation syndromes. Two birth defect associations, the VACTERL association and the MURCS (mullerian, renal, cervicothoracic somite abnormality) association, have a high incidence of renal abnormalities, including renal agenesis.

**Inheritance Patterns** Generally, inheritance is sporadic. Some cases may represent a highly variable autosomal dominant gene. Parents and siblings should have renal ultrasounds to look for unilateral renal agenesis or other renal abnormalities that may suggest autosomal dominant inheritance. In the case of dominantly inherited renal agenesis, the recurrence in future pregnancies can be normal kidneys, unilateral agenesis, or bilateral agenesis. The empiric risk for recurrence with isolated renal agenesis is 2%-5%.

**Teratogens** Maternal diabetes mellitus is teratogenic.

**Prognosis** Up to 40% of infants with BRA may be stillborn, and the remainder die shortly after birth from pulmonary hypoplasia. Unilateral renal agenesis may be asymptomatic and compatible with a normal life span. Girls with unilateral renal agenesis should have pelvic ultrasonograms looking for müllerian abnormalities.

## SONOGRAPHY

### FREQUENT FINDINGS: BILATERAL RENAL AGENESIS (BRA)

- Failure to visualize the kidneys
- Bladder not visualized
- Second- and third-trimester oligohydramnios
- "Lying down" adrenal
- Failure to identify the renal arteries with color Doppler
- Decreased chest circumference secondary to pulmonary hypoplasia
- Intrauterine growth restriction
- Associated congenital anomalies
  - Congenital heart defects

  - Neural tube defects
  - Tracheoesophageal fistula
  - Sirenomelia
  - Chromosome abnormalities
  - VACTERL syndrome
  - Müllerian anomalies

### KEY FINDINGS/PITFALLS

- Adrenals with BRA have an ovoid shape.
  - The renal pelvis should be identified to confirm the presence of a kidney.
- Transvaginal ultrasound can be utilized to more accurately assess the renal fossae and the bladder region in fetuses in breech presentation.
- The sensitivity of ultrasound in the diagnosis of BRA is 78%-91% at a median gestational age of 21 weeks.
- In the second trimester, a urachal cyst may mimic a normal bladder.

### DIFFERENTIAL DIAGNOSIS

- Sirenomelia: In both BRA and sirenomelia, the renal arteries are not visualized with power Doppler. An aortic bifurcation into two iliac arteries is present with BRA and absent with sirenomelia.

### FREQUENT FINDINGS: UNILATERAL RENAL AGENESIS

- Failure to visualize one kidney
  - Absence of pelvic kidney
- Third-trimester compensatory renal hypertrophy of the remaining kidney
- Normal fetal bladder
- Normal amniotic fluid volume
- Associated anomalies
  - Vesicoureteral reflux
  - UPJ obstruction
  - Ureterovesical junction obstruction
  - Congenital heart defects
  - Esophageal atresia
  - Müllerian abnormalities

## PREGNANCY MANAGEMENT

**Investigations and Consultations Required** Isolated renal agenesis, unilateral or bilateral, is not likely to be a marker for chromosome abnormalities. Fetal echocardiography should be performed to exclude associated congenital heart disease. In cases with either unilateral renal agenesis or BRA, evaluation of parents' kidneys should be done to detect those families with autosomal dominant inheritance.

**Fetal Intervention** Although the diagnosis is often straightforward, oligohydramnios may obscure visualization. In these cases, an amnioinfusion procedure may be helpful in establishing the diagnosis. Injection of 150 to 250 mL of saline into the amniotic space will improve fetal visualization. Concomitant injection of indigo carmine may allow detection of premature rupture of membranes, which may also be in the differential diagnosis.

**Monitoring** No change in obstetric care is indicated for unilateral renal agenesis. For the pregnancy in which the fetus has BRA, no further fetal assessment or monitoring is appropriate. Supportive care of the family should be provided and plans made for comfort care after delivery.

**Pregnancy Course** No specific obstetric complications are to be expected with unilateral lesions. The same is true of bilateral lesions, although an increase in stillbirth rate is expected.

**Pregnancy Termination Issues** Bilateral renal agenesis may be a component of multiple-malformation syndromes. Therefore, a complete evaluation of an intact fetus should be done.

**Delivery** No special precautions are necessary for the fetus with unilateral disease. For BRA, vaginal delivery without electronic fetal monitoring in labor is appropriate.

## NEONATOLOGY

**Resuscitation** The majority of newborns with BRA manifest severe respiratory distress from birth secondary to associated severe pulmonary hypoplasia. Positive pressure should be used cautiously, as the risk for pneumothorax is high. Early cessation of resuscitative efforts should be discussed with the parents prior to delivery, as this is a uniformly lethal condition.

**Transport** In the presence of a confirmed antenatal diagnosis, transport is not indicated, as survival time is usually limited to hours, even with ventilator support. In the occasional infant with mixed agenesis/dysplasia in whom respiratory insufficiency initially may be adequately controlled with ventilatory assistance, transport is indicated for confirmation of diagnosis and prognosis.

**Testing and Confirmation** A postnatal renal sonogram will confirm the absence of kidneys.

**Nursery Management** Continuing ventilatory support, even with severe respiratory failure, is appropriate until diagnostic confirmation, determination of associated abnormalities, and parental counseling is completed. At present, there is no palliative or curative treatment for complete renal agenesis. Prolonged renal dialysis has not been successful.

### SUGGESTED READINGS

1. Bronshtein M, Amit A, Achiron R, Blumenfeld Z: The early prenatal sonographic diagnosis of renal agenesis: techniques and possible pitfalls. Prenat Diagn 1994; 14:291-297.
2. Cascio S, Paran S, Puri P: Associated urological anomalies in children with unilateral renal agenesis. J Urol 1999; 162:1081-1083.
3. DeVore G: The value of color Doppler sonography in the diagnosis of renal agenesis. J Ultrasound Med 1995; 14:443-449.

4. Garne E, Luane M, Dolk H, et al: Prenatal diagnosis of severe structural congenital malformations in Europe. Ultrasound Obstet Gynecol 2005; 25:6-11.
5. Hill LM, Rivello D: Role of transvaginal sonography in the diagnosis of bilateral renal agenesis. Am J Perinatol 1991;8:395-397.
6. Hoffman CK, Filly RA, Callen PW: The "lying down" adrenal sign: a sonographic indicator of renal agenesis or ectopia in fetuses and neonates. J Ultrasound Med 1992; 11:533-536.
7. Potter EL: Bilateral absence of ureters and kidneys: a report of 50 cases. Obstet Gynecol 1965; 25:3-12.
8. Rodriguez MM: Congenital anomalies of the kidney and the urinary tract (CAKUT). Fetal Pediatr Pathol 2014; 33:293-320
9. Romero R, Cullen M, Grannum P, et al: Antenatal diagnosis of renal anomalies with ultrasound. III. Bilateral renal agenesis. Am J Obstet Gynecol 1985; 151:38-43.
10. Sepulveda W, Corral E, Sanchez J, et al: Sirenomelia sequence versus renal agenesis: prenatal differentiation with power Doppler ultrasound. Ultrasound Obstet Gynecol 1998; 11:445-449.
11. Wiesel A, Queisser-Luft A, Clementi M, et al: EUROSCAN Study Group: prenatal detection of congenital renal malformations by fetal ultrasonographic examination: an analysis of 709,030 births in 12 European countries. Eur J Med Genet 2005; 48:131-144.

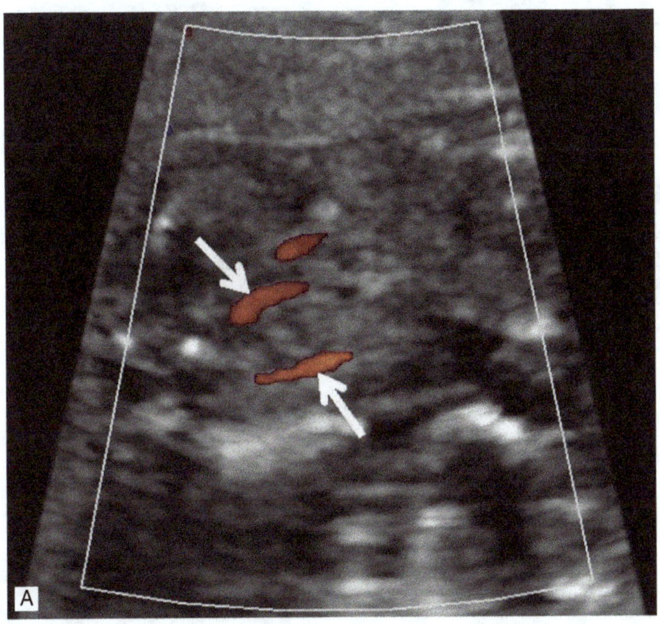


**FIGURE 4.12A** Fetus with bilateral renal agenesis and absent fetal bladder. Note the umbilical arteries (arrows).

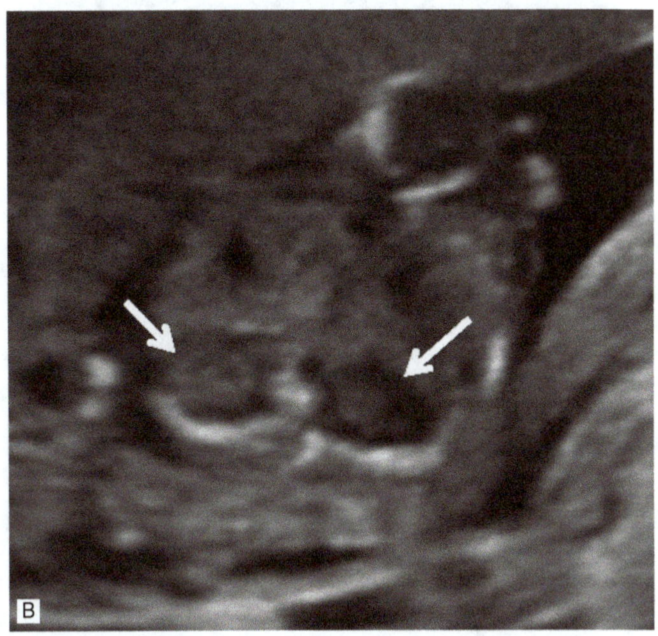


**FIGURE 4.12B** Bilateral renal agenesis illustrating the normal adrenals (arrows), which can be mistaken for kidneys.

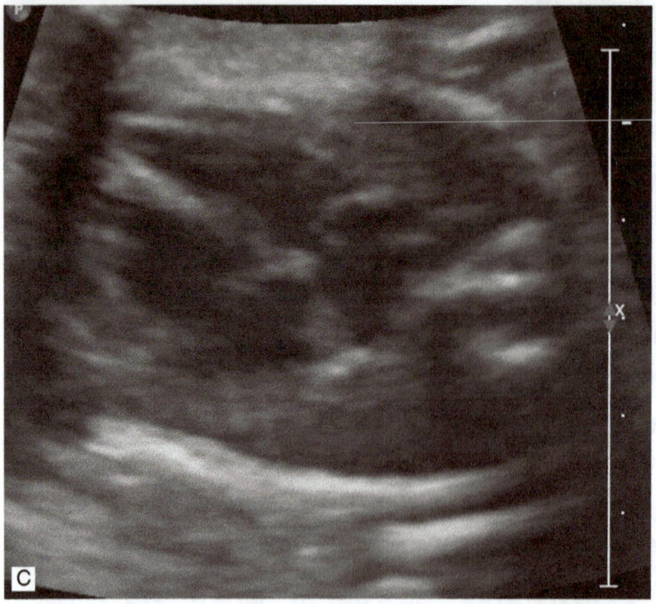


**FIGURE 4.12C** Bilateral renal agenesis illustrating pulmonary hypoplasia. The heart takes up more than 50% of the chest.

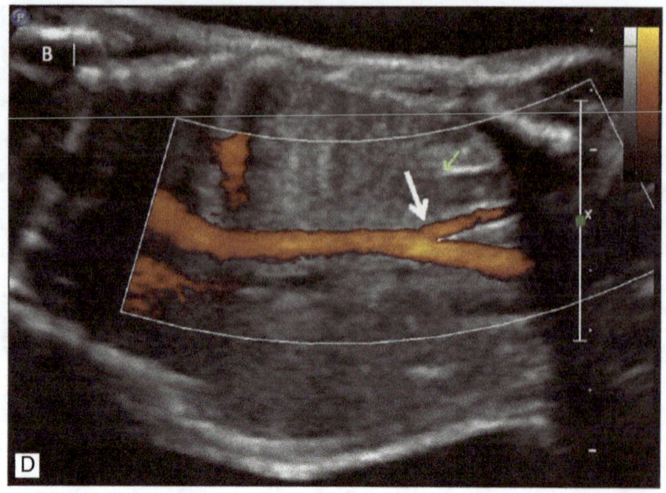


**FIGURE 4.12D** Power Doppler illustrating absent renal arteries. Note the iliac bifurcation (white arrow).

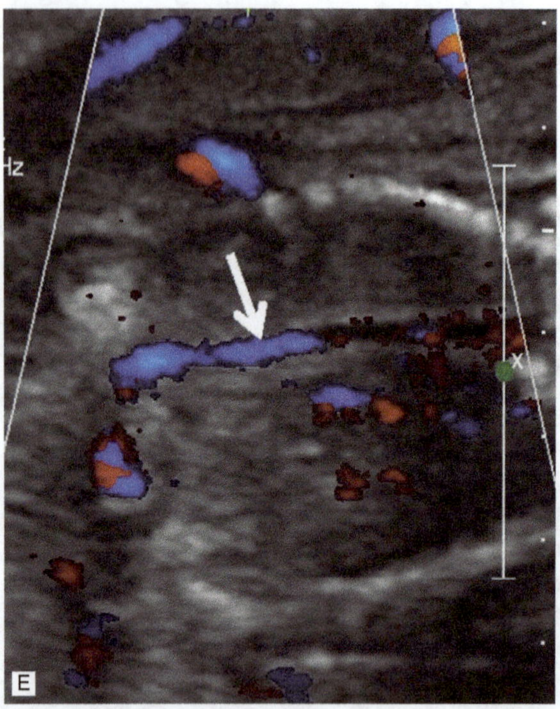


**FIGURE 4.12E** Fetus with sirenomelia. Note the aorta (arrow) does not bifurcate.

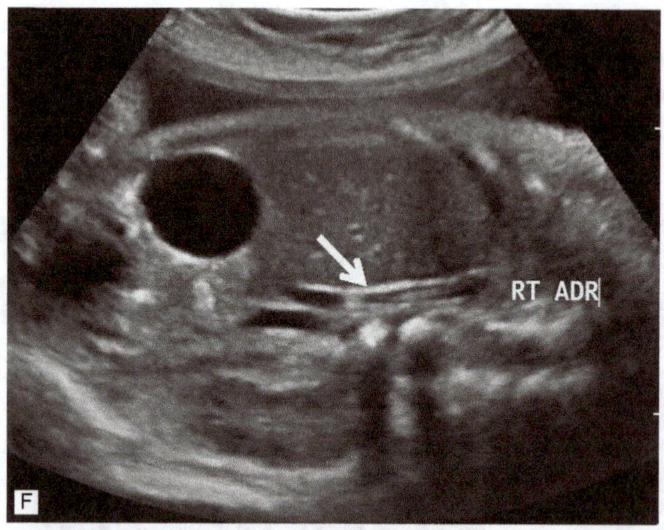


**FIGURE 4.12F** Unilateral renal agenesis illustrating the lying down adrenal (RT ADR) (arrow).

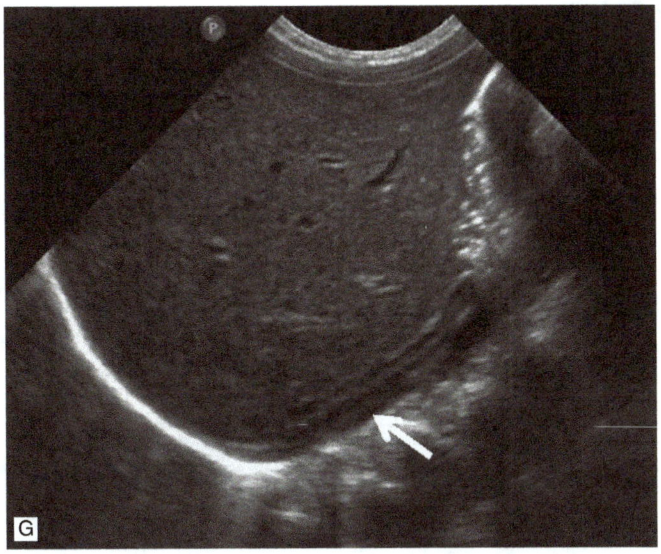


FIGURE 4.12G Neonatal ultrasound showing a lying down adrenal (arrow).

# 4.13 SACROCOCCYGEAL TERATOMA

## EPIDEMIOLOGY/GENETICS

**Definition** Teratomas are tumors that are derived from totipotent cells and include embryonic ectodermal, endodermal, and mesodermal tissue derivatives. Sacrococcygeal teratomas (SCTs) are derived from the pleuripotential cells of Hensen's node, anterior to the coccyx.

- Classification based on location:

| Type | Description |
|---|---|
| I | Predominantly external |
| II | Predominantly external with an internal component |
| III | Predominantly intrapelvic with an exterior extension |
| IV | Entirely intrapelvic |

**Epidemiology** Occurrence is 1 in 40,000 births (M1:F4); it is the most common tumor of the fetus.

**Embryology** Teratomas occur most often in a para-axial, gonadal, or midline location from the brain to the sacral area. Primary sites in infants and children include the sacrococcyx (60%), gonads (20%), and chest/abdomen (15%). SCTs are the most common tumors presenting at birth. Forty-seven percent of the tumors are external, 34% are external with a significant presacral component, and 19% are predominantly, or completely, presacral. Additional malformations occur in approximately 15% of cases and include imperforate anus, sacral bone defects, uterine or vaginal abnormalities, and spina bifida.

**Inheritance Patterns** Generally, inheritance is sporadic. Rare families with autosomal dominant presacral teratomas and sacral dysgenesis have been reported.

**Teratogens** None are known.

**Prognosis** Diagnosis at an earlier gestational age, development of hydrops, and premature delivery predict a poor outcome, with approximately 10% survival for cases diagnosed before 30 weeks' gestation. Cases diagnosed later have a reported 75% survival rate. The natural history for prenatally diagnosed and postnatally diagnosed SCTs differs; malignant degeneration is rare with prenatal diagnosis.

## SONOGRAPHY

### FREQUENT FINDINGS

- Presacral cystic/solid mass
- Polyhydramnios

### LESS FREQUENT

- Hydrops
  - Cardiomegaly
  - Pericardial effusion
  - Pleural effusion
  - Anasarca
  - Ascites
  - Placentomegaly
  - Increased inferior vena cava diameter
- Bladder obstruction
- Bladder displacement
- Pyelocaliectasis
- Urinary ascites
- Renal dysplasia
- Hydroureters

### KEY FINDINGS/PITFALLS

- The size of SCTs has been defined as small (20-50 mm), moderate (50-100 mm), and large (>100 mm).
- Rapidly growing SCTs are predominantly solid.
- Solid tumors may have significant arteriovenous shunting.
- Solid vascular SCTs that are highly vascularized are more likely to develop hydrops. Predominantly cystic avascular SCTs have a more favorable prognosis.
- An SCT with hydrops is generally considered lethal. However, preterm delivery and prompt neonatal surgery have resulted in survivors.
- Rapid growth of an SCT is associated with increased perinatal mortality and preterm labor.
- Sacrococcygeal teratomas that develop fetal hydrops may be associated with the "mirror syndrome," which is manifest by maternal edema. The pathophysiology of the mirror syndrome is unknown, but maternal hypertension and proteinuria are seen in over 40% of the cases, suggesting a relationship with preeclampsia. The maternal symptoms resolve after delivery or in some cases with successful treatment of the fetal hydrops.
- The diagnosis has been made as early as the first trimester.
- Three-dimensional ultrasound can improve visualization, surveillance of volume changes, and staging.
- MRI can more accurately evaluate the intrapelvic extension of an SCT than ultrasound.

## PREGNANCY MANAGEMENT

**Investigations and Consultations Required** No specific associated abnormalities are known, but the high likelihood that intervention may be necessary mandates that other life-threatening abnormalities be excluded. Chromosome analysis, with microarray, and fetal echocardiography should be performed. It should be noted that the amniotic fluid α-fetoprotein level may be elevated, and acetylcholinesterase may be present in cases of SCT. Amniotic fluid analysis will, therefore, not help differentiate SCT from myelomeningocele. MRI may be useful in defining fetal anatomy and the extent of the tumor. As with most significant fetal anomalies, a multidisciplinary team approach to diagnosis and management is necessary, especially when in utero intervention is being considered.

**Fetal Intervention** In cases diagnosed prior to 32 weeks' gestation in which hydrops develops, prognosis is dismal. This small subset of fetuses (less than 20% of cases) should be referred to a treatment center with expertise in open fetal surgery, which has been successful in a limited number of cases to date. Due to the morbidity of hysterotomy, minimally invasive approaches to management are under investigation, such as interstitial laser photocoagulation, radio-frequency ablation, and microembolization of the dominant feeding vessels. Fetuses at 32 weeks or beyond who develop hydrops should be delivered for ex utero therapy.

**Monitoring** Serial sonograms should be performed every 1 to 2 weeks to assess for (1) the size of the mass, which may grow rapidly; (2) evidence of obstructive uropathy; (3) evidence of bowel obstruction; (4) polyhydramnios; and (5) early signs of hydrops. Large lesions with predominantly solid components are associated with an increased risk for polyhydramnios, fetal hydrops, and mirror syndrome.

**Pregnancy Course** The patient should be monitored for early signs of mirror syndrome. Development of mirror syndrome requires prompt delivery, despite gestational age or fetal status. The presence of polyhydramnios may increase the risk of preterm labor, and regular assessment is necessary.

**Pregnancy Termination Issues** The procedure for termination should provide an intact fetus for a complete autopsy.

**Delivery** The significant risk of maternal and neonatal complications necessitates delivery in a tertiary center. Moderate-size (50 mm or larger) lesions should prompt cesarean delivery to avoid dystocia. Because of the significant risk of neonatal hemorrhage, large masses will require adequate surgical exposure to avoid trauma at the time of delivery and may include a vertical (classical) uterine incision, which will have implications in future pregnancies.

## NEONATOLOGY

**Resuscitation** Assistance with onset of respiration is usually not required unless the infant is premature or fetal hydrops is present. Extreme care must be taken with the tumor mass, as tears of surface vessels can result in life-threatening hemorrhage. If there is a "stalk," the mass should be supported to avoid torsion. When the surface of an SCT is thin and membranous, the mass should be covered with a warm, moist sterile dressing to minimize heat and water loss.

**Transport** Transfer to a tertiary care center is always indicated. Extreme care must be taken to avoid trauma to the mass, insensible water loss, and surface contamination. Reliable venous access should be established and adequate blood pressure documented before beginning transport.

**Testing and Confirmation** Postnatally, elevated serum α-fetoprotein level and β-hCG levels are highly correlated with malignancy. Diagnostic evaluation should include CT or MRI of the primary site to assess the extent of the internal tumor. Staging should include CT of the chest and bone scan. The majority of SCTs are benign.

**Nursery Management** Provide cardiopulmonary support and monitor hemodynamic status closely. Maintain thermal balance and perfusion with volume expanders, packed red blood cells, and fluid and electrolytes. If the mass involves the distal gastrointestinal tract or the course is complicated, parenteral nutrition may be required for a protracted period of time. Systemic antibiotics may be indicated preoperatively and throughout the early recovery period.

## SURGERY

**Preoperative Assessment** Acute management includes evaluation of the extent of the intraperitoneal presacral portion of the tumor. Diagnostic studies should include serum levels of α-fetoprotein and β-hCG to determine if there is a possible malignant component and sonography to determine the degree of presacral and intraperitoneal extension. A decision is then made about whether to use an abdominal approach to obtain control of the primary feeding vessels of the tumor, the middle sacral arteries, before attempting a perineal excision.

The acute preoperative complications of a large SCT are cardiac failure due to arteriovenous shunting in the tumor, renal failure due to bilateral ureteral obstruction, and hemorrhage secondary to intraperitoneal, retroperitoneal, or surface necrotic tumor with bleeding.

If high-output failure is not present, there is no urgency to resect the tumor. Attention initially should focus on the treatment of respiratory distress and correction of anemia. The delayed excision of a necrotic SCT can predispose the neonate to sepsis. If a hyperdynamic state exists with elevated cardiac output, attention should focus on supporting the newborn heart with inotropic agents and urgent resection of the SCT. The goal of this resection is reversal of the high-output state, and this can usually be accomplished by resection of the exophytic portion of the tumor. Aortic occlusion by vessel loop may be used to minimize hemorrhage when resecting an SCT in a severely premature infant. If residual pelvic tumor remains, the urgency of resection can be guided by the pathologic lesion. The presence of malignant yolk sac differentiation within a residual SCT would necessitate earlier resection. In the absence of yolk sac differentiation, however, several months of growth of the infant can facilitate subsequent resection of the coccyx and the intrapelvic portion of the tumor.

**Operative Indications** Unless serious hemorrhaging is present, surgical excision can be delayed to permit completion of the diagnostic evaluation.

**Types of Procedures** Most tumors can be excised from the perineal approach, but blood loss can be great, and preparations for adequate replacement are essential. Careful dissection and preservation of the thinned gluteal muscles over the tumor, excision of the coccyx, and reconstruction of the levator sling are important to a good functional outcome.

**Surgical Results/Prognosis** Survival after successful excision is excellent. Intraoperative mortality can approach 5% to 10%, depending on tumor and patient size. A malignancy occurs in approximately 10% of the newborn infants with SCTs and can be totally excised in most patients. If a total coccygectomy is performed, secondary operations for retained benign teratoma are uncommon. The malignant germ cell tumors that commonly occur in SCTs are usually responsive to platinum-based chemotherapy modalities. A major long-term disability is stool and urinary incontinence in patients who have had neurologic impairment due to the pressure of very large SCTs. The incidence of this condition is as high as 25% in some series.

## SUGGESTED READINGS


1. Altman RP, Randolph JG, Lilly JR: Sacrococcygeal teratoma. American Academy of Pediatrics Surgical Section Survey. J Pediatr Surg 1973; 9:389-398.
2. Braun T, Brauer M, Fuchs I, et al: Mirror syndrome: a systematic review of fetal associated conditions, maternal presentation and perinatal outcome. Fetal Diagn Ther 2010; 27:191-203.
3. Carney JA, Thompson DP, Johnson CL: Teratromas in children: clinical and pathologic aspects. J Pediatr Surg 1972; 7:271-286.
4. Danzer E, Hubbard AM, Hedrick HL, et al: Diagnosis and characterization of fetal sacrococcygeal teratoma with prenatal MRI. Am J Roentgenol 2006; 187:W350-W356.
5. Hedrick HL, Flake AW, Crombleholme TM, et al: Sacrococcygeal teratoma: prenatal assessment, fetal intervention, and outcome. J Pediatr Surg 2004; 39:430-438.
6. Nakayama DK, Killian A, Hill LM, et al: The newborn with hydrops and sacrococcygeal teratoma. J Pediatr Surg 1991; 26:1435-1438.
7. Roman AS, Montegeagudo AM, Timor-Tritsch I, Rebarber A: First-trimester diagnosis of sacrococcygeal teratoma: the role of three-dimensional ultrasound. Ultrasound Obstet Gynecol 2004; 23:612-614.
8. Schneider DT, Calaminus G, Gobel U: Diagnostic value of alpha-fetoprotein and beta-human chorionic gonadotropin in infancy and childhood. Pediatr Hematol Oncol 2001; 18:11–26.
9. Sheth S, Nussbaum AR, Sanders RC, et al: Prenatal diagnosis of sacrococcygeal teratoma: sonographic-pathologic correlation. Radiology 1988; 169:131-136.
10. Srivastava A, Jaiswal AK, Jain K, Behari S: Sacrococcygeal teratoma. J Pediatr Neurosci 2010; 5:30-31.
11. Tuladhar R, Patole SK, Whitehall JS: Sacrococcygeal teratoma in the perinatal period. Postgrad Med J 2000; 76:754-759.

12. Westerberg B, Feldstein VA, Sandberg PL, et al: Sonographic prognostic factors in fetuses with sacrococcygeal teratoma. J Pediatr Surg 2000; 35:322-326.

13. Wilson RD, Hedrick H, Flake AW, et al: Sacrococcygeal teratomas: prenatal surveillance, growth, and pregnancy outcome. Fetal Diagn Ther 2009; 25:15-20.

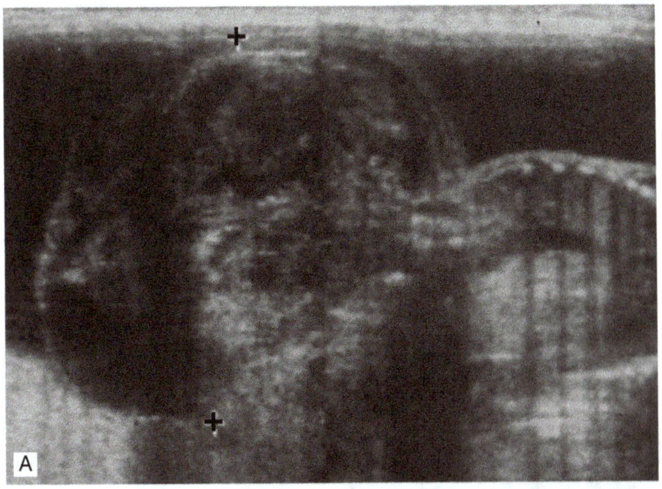


**FIGURE 4.13A** Solid external (type I) sacrococcygeal teratoma (+ … +).

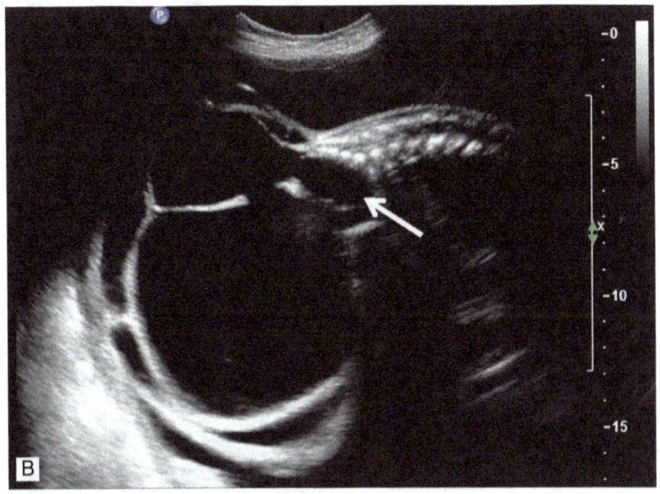


**FIGURE 4.13B** Cystic sacrococcygeal teratoma (type II) that is predominantly external with internal component (arrow).

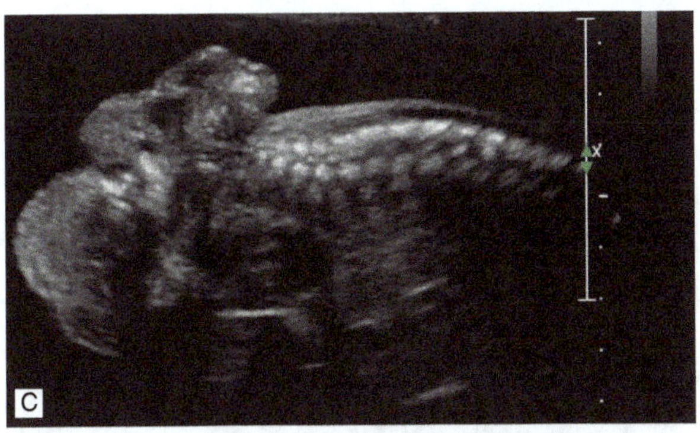


**FIGURE 4.13C** Two-dimensional image of sacrococcygeal teratoma at 23 weeks.

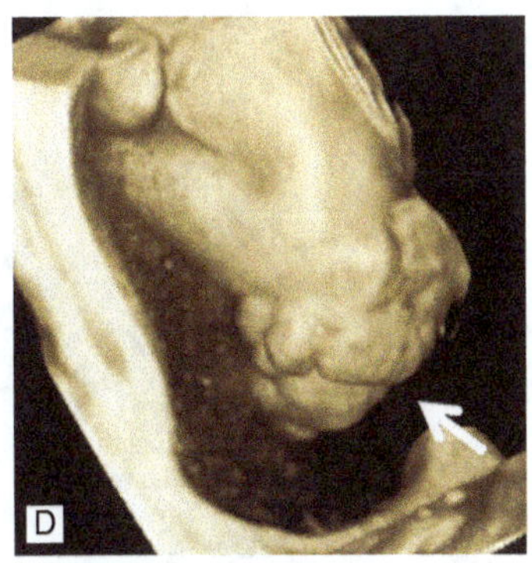


**FIGURE 4.13D** Three-dimensional image of sacrococcygeal teratoma (arrow).

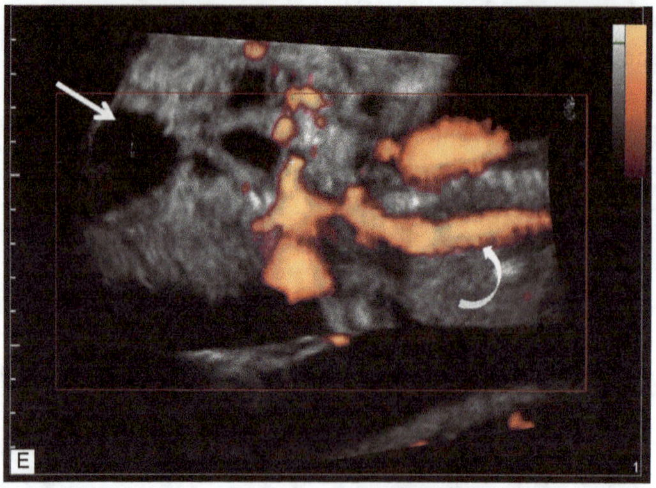


**FIGURE 4.13E** Three-dimensional power Doppler of a sacrococcygeal teratoma (straight arrow) with a dilated inferior vena cava (curved arrow).

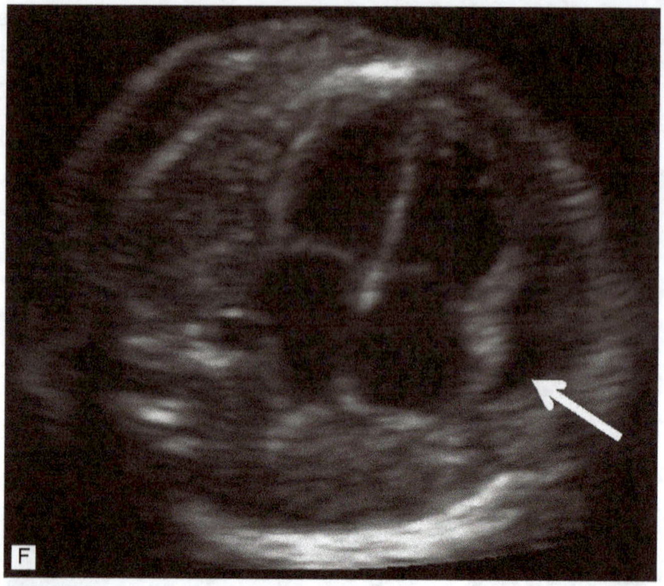


**FIGURE 4.13F** Hydrops in a fetus with a sacrococcygeal teratoma. Note the cardiomegaly and pericardial effusion (arrow).

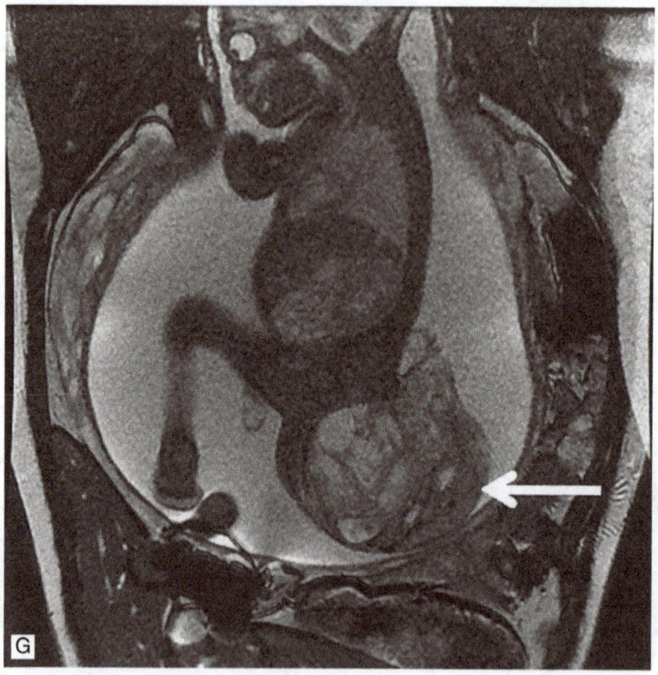


**FIGURE 4.13G** Fetal MRI of a sacrococcygeal teratoma (arrow).

# 4.14 SIRENOMELIA

## EPIDEMIOLOGY/GENETICS

**Definition** Sirenomelia is a partial or complete fusion and/or severe deformity of the lower extremities frequently associated with renal agenesis, oligohydramnios, and anogenital anomalies.

**Epidemiology** Occurrence is 1 to 4 in 100,000 (M3:F1).

**Embryology** The pathogenesis is probably heterogeneous. Some cases may represent the severe end of the caudal regression spectrum, while a more recent theory has suggested a vascular pathogenesis, resulting from a vitelline arterial steal, which diverts blood flow from caudal structures.

**Inheritance Patterns** All cases have been sporadic. The incidence in monozygotic twins is increased 100 to 150 times.

**Teratogens** Thalidomide and maternal diabetes are teratogenic, although the association with diabetes is much weaker than with caudal dysplasia.

**Prognosis** Essentially, sirenomelia is lethal in all cases. There are rare reports of mild cases in infants with good renal function who have survived the newborn period.

## SONOGRAPHY

### FREQUENT FINDINGS

- Oligohydramnios
- Bilateral renal agenesis
- Absent bladder
- Single umbilical artery
- Single lower extremity or femurs lying side by side that do not change position with time

### LESS FREQUENT

- Absent fibulas
- Scoliosis
- Hypoplastic pelvis
- Ambiguous genitalia
- Absent radius and ulna
- Imperforate anus
- Abnormal distal abdominal aorta
- Congenital heart defects
- Ventriculomegaly
- Renal dysplasia

### KEY FINDINGS/PITFALLS

- Categories of sirenomelia are based on the feet:
  - One femur, one tibia, no feet (most common)
  - Two femurs, tibia and fibula; one foot
  - Two fused legs; two feet
- Earliest detection: first trimester.
- 100 times more frequent in monozygotic twins
- Lower extremity fusion and single pelvic bone can be documented on 3-D ultrasound.
- Oligohydramnios hinders a thorough second- and third-trimester ultrasound examination.
- The presence of two umbilical arteries is consistent with caudal regression syndrome rather than sirenomelia.

## PREGNANCY MANAGEMENT

**Investigations and Consultations Required** The mother should have glucose tolerance testing to exclude diabetes mellitus, although it is considered to be a rare cause of true sirenomelia. Fetal echocardiography should be performed, as cardiac defects are common.

**Fetal Intervention** Fetal intervention is not appropriate in this lethal condition.

**Monitoring** Maternal status should be monitored in standard fashion. Fetal evaluation is not appropriate because intervention for fetal indications is not indicated. Repeat ultrasound examinations may be considered, particularly as the initial examination may have been suboptimal due to the oligohydramnios.

**Pregnancy Course** Oligohydramnios is seen in all cases.

**Pregnancy Termination Issues** Oligohydramnios may make a precise diagnosis difficult. In many cases, delivery of an intact fetus may be necessary to ensure that correct counseling information can be given for subsequent pregnancies.

**Delivery** Electronic fetal monitoring and cesarean section are contraindicated given the lethal nature of this condition.

## NEONATOLOGY

**Resuscitation** Given a uniformly lethal prognosis, resuscitation is not indicated.

**Transport** This is not a consideration given the prognosis.

**Testing and Confirmation** Careful physical examination, complemented by detailed postmortem examination, will confirm the spectrum of abnormalities.

**Nursery Management** In the rare circumstance of fetal survival beyond delivery, comfort measures only are indicated. Support for parental grieving and genetic counseling for future pregnancies are essential.

## SUGGESTED READINGS

1. Cavaliere A, Dinatale A, Cardinale G, et al: A prenatally diagnosed case of sirenomelia with dextrocardia and omphalocele. J Perinatal Med 2009; 3:42-43.
2. Garrido-Allepuz C, Haro E, Gonzalex-Lamuno, et al: A clinical and experimental overview of sirenomelia: insight into the mechanisms of congenital limb malformations. Dis Model Mech 2011; 4:289-299.
3. Monteagudo A, Mayberry P, Rebanker A, et al: Sirenomelia sequence: first-trimester diagnosis with both two- and three-dimensional sonography. J Ultrasound Med 2002; 21:915-920.
4. Patel S, Suchet I: The role of color and power Doppler ultrasound in the prenatal diagnosis of sirenomelia. Ultrasound Obstet Gynecol 2004; 24:684-691.
5. Sintori M, Ghidini A, Romero R, Hobbins JC: Prenatal diagnosis of sirenomelia. J Ultrasound Med 1989; 8:83-83.
6. Stocker JT, Heifetz SA: Sirenomelia. A morphological study of 33 cases and review of the literature. Perspect Pediatr Pathol 1987; 10:7-50.
7. Valenzano M, Paoletti R, Rossi A, et al: Sirenomelia. Pathological features, antenatal ultrasonographic clues, and a review of current embryogenic theories. Hum Reprod Update 1995; 5:82-86.
8. Vijayaraghavan SB, Amudha AP: High-resolution sonographic diagnosis of sirenomelia. J Ultrasound Med 2006; 25:555-557.

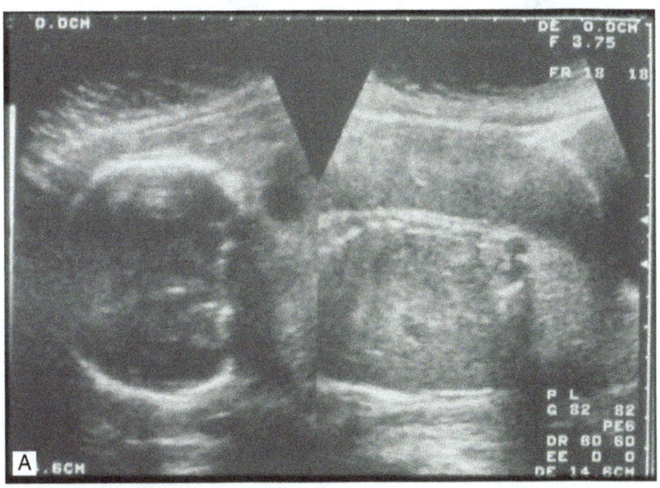


**FIGURE 4.14A** Oligohydramnios in fetus with sirenomelia.

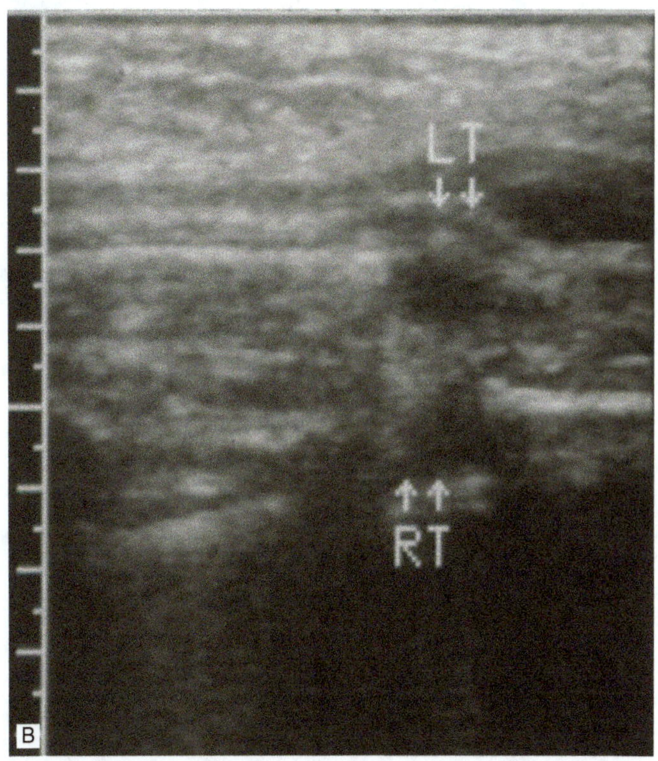


**FIGURE 4.14B** Parallel fixed femurs and tibias; left (LT) and right (RT) knee.

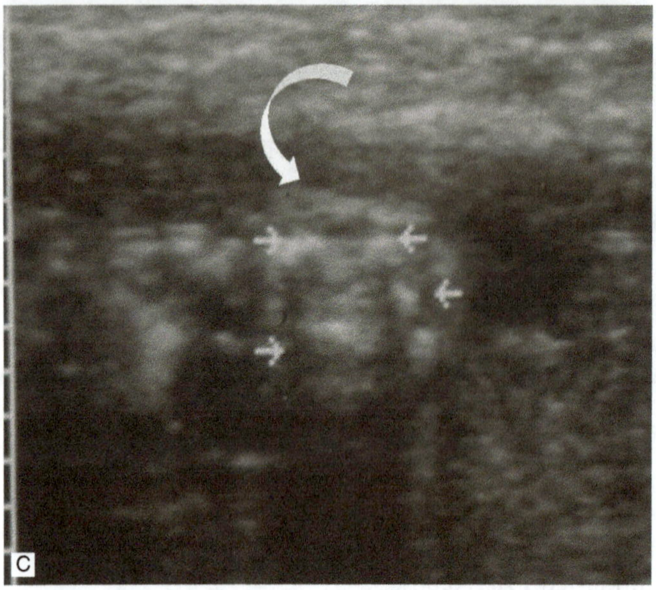

**FIGURE 4.14C** Transverse scan through lower leg showing two tibias and two femurs (straight arrows) with continuous surrounding skin (curved arrow).

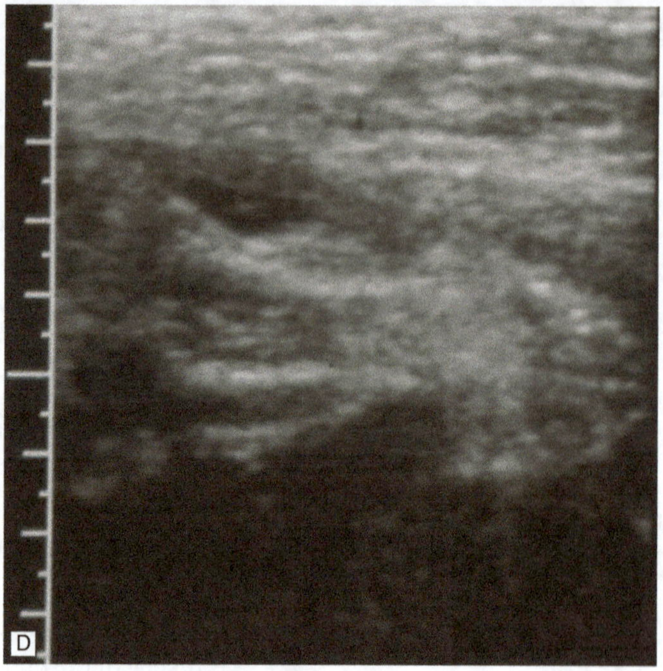

**FIGURE 4.14D** Parallel fixed tibias and fused feet.

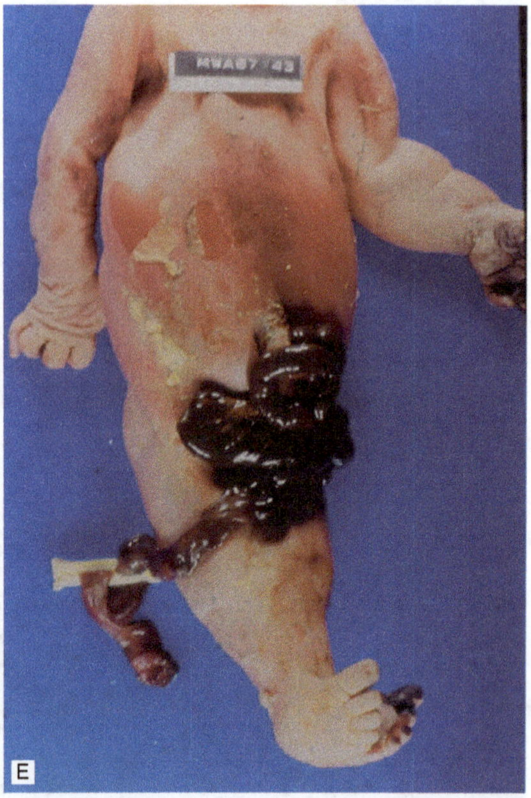

**FIGURE 4.14E** Fetus with two fused legs and two feet.

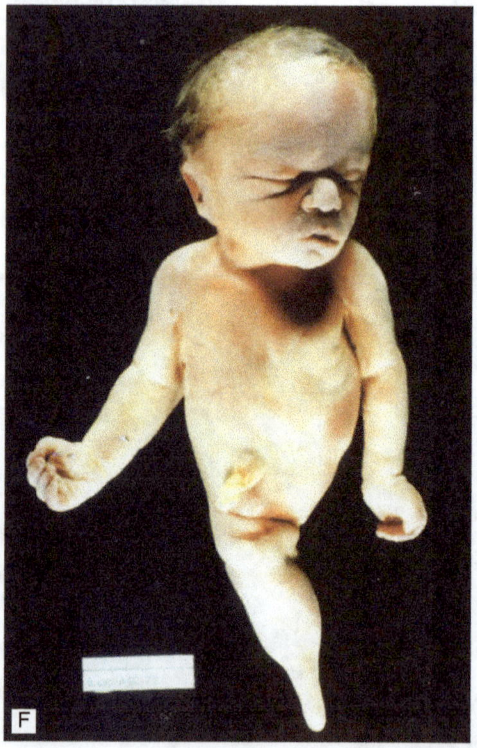

**FIGURE 4.14F** Fetus with one femur, one tibia, and no feet.

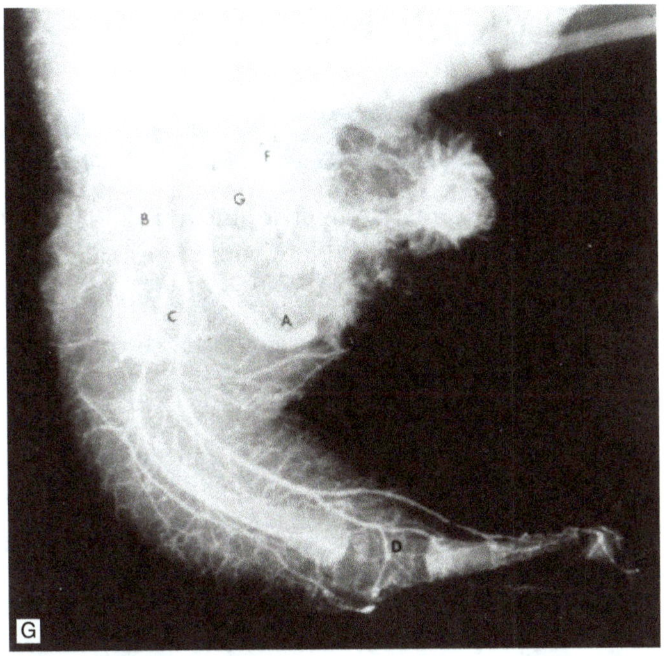


**FIGURE 4.14G** Note the abnormal distal abdominal aorta (A) and the absence of iliac and femoral arteries.

# 4.15 URETEROPELVIC JUNCTION OBSTRUCTION

## EPIDEMIOLOGY/GENETICS

**Definition** Ureteropelvic junction (UPJ) obstruction is distention of the pelvis and calyces of the kidney with urine as a result of ureteral obstruction.

**Epidemiology** Incidence is 1 in 1500 births (M3:F1).

**Embryology** Ureteropelvic junction obstruction is the most common cause of obstructive uropathy; it is unilateral in 70% of cases. Of cases, 30%-50% have associated urinary tract abnormalities, and 20% of cases have extrarenal abnormalities. In most cases, UPJ obstruction is "functional" or "physiologic." It is due to abnormalities in the maturation of the smooth muscle innervation of the renal pelvis ureteral transition or to mild narrowing that resolves with growth of the ureter. Because there is no true structural obstruction, maturation of the innervation process or the structure of the UP junction results in an alleviation of the "obstruction." Anatomic causes of true UPJ obstruction include ureteral stricture, anomalous crossing vessel to the lower pole of the kidney, and an abnormally rotated kidney.

**Inheritance Patterns** There is sporadic inheritance unless part of a recognizable syndrome, such as the urofacial syndrome (autosomal recessive), which combines a distinctive grimacing face with bilateral hydronephrosis.

**Teratogens** Thalidomide, maternal diabetes, and cocaine are teratogenic.

**Prognosis** The majority of antenatally diagnosed cases of pyelectasis are "functional" and will resolve prior to birth or in the neonatal period. Less than 10% ultimately require surgical treatment. Of infants with true UPJ, only 20%-25% will require surgery. Most patients with UPJ who require surgical correction will have good renal function.

## SONOGRAPHY

### FREQUENT FINDINGS

- Pyelectasis

| AP Renal Pelvis | Gestational Age (Weeks) |
|---|---|
| >4.0 mm | 16-27 |
| >7.0 mm | ≥ 28 |

- Caliectasis
- Caudal end of the renal pelvis
  - Blunted
  - Rounded

### LESS FREQUENT

- Paranephric cyst secondary to calyceal rupture
- Polyhydramnios

### KEY FINDINGS/PITFALLS

- Concurrent renal malformations (50%) include
  - Renal agenesis
  - Multicystic dysplastic kidney
  - Duplex collecting system
  - Ectopic kidney
  - Horseshoe kidney
  - Vesicoureteral reflux (VUR)
- The sonographic manifestations of UPJ are dependent on the severity of obstruction.
- Scoring system for upper urinary tract dilatation (Society for Fetal Urology):

| Grade | Description |
|---|---|
| 0 | No dilatation |
| I | Renal pelvis dilation |
| II | Renal pelvis dilation; calyces visible |
| III | Renal pelvis dilation; calyces dilated |
| IV | Grade III with parenchymal thinning |

- Because of its poor sensitivity and specificity, a single renal pelvis diameter at any gestational age is a poor predictor of postnatal pathology.
- Severe UPJ obstruction may result in a single large abdominal cyst.
- Even severe pyelocaliectasis does not necessarily equate with significant obstruction and long-term renal functional damage.
- Three-dimensional ultrasound can be used to accurately assess renal pelvis volume and might assist in predicting whether surgery is required.

### DIFFERENTIAL DIAGNOSIS

- Multicystic kidneys: The cysts associated with multicystic kidneys do not communicate; the calyces of UPJ obstruction can always be connected.
- Severe VUR: The ureters are usually dilated along with the renal pelvis.

## PREGNANCY MANAGEMENT

**Investigations and Consultations Required** The diagnosis of UPJ is often not certain, particularly in milder cases, which present as pyelectasis. An extended ultrasound examination is indicated, particularly specifically looking for other urinary tract abnormalities. Revisiting the patient's risk for trisomy 21 is indicated, as pyelectasis is a soft marker for fetal Down syndrome. However, in the absence of other findings or an elevated a priori Down syndrome risk, no other diagnostic evaluation is necessary. If the renal pelvis dilatation is marked in the second trimester, or mild but persistent into the third trimester, consultation with a pediatric urologist is necessary to develop a postnatal management plan and determine site of delivery.

**Fetal Intervention** In general, no fetal intervention is necessary. In cases with bilateral disease and decreasing amniotic fluid volume, closer monitoring should be instituted. Early delivery may be considered at gestational ages over 32 weeks if oligohydramnios is present and renal functional studies appear normal. Prior to 32 weeks, intervention by catheter placement can be considered if amniotic fluid is decreasing. The same assessment as outlined in cases of lower urinary tract obstruction (LUTO) should be performed. The need for in utero intervention in UPJ obstruction is unusual.

**Monitoring** Mild degrees of renal pelvis dilation should be assessed by a follow-up sonogram at 32 to 34 weeks' gestation. More significant dilation at any gestational age should be followed with sonographic evaluation every 3 to 4 weeks.

**Pregnancy Course** No specific obstetric complications should be expected, although either oligohydramnios or polyhydramnios may develop in rare cases.

**Pregnancy Termination Issues** The method of termination should provide an intact fetus for pathologic confirmation of the sonographic diagnosis.

**Delivery** When there is severe obstruction, the need for neonatal evaluation and treatment requires that delivery occur in a tertiary center with a pediatric urologist available. No change in standard obstetric care is necessary.

## NEONATOLOGY

**Resuscitation** Resuscitation is usually not an issue. Occasionally, onset of effective respiration may be impeded by abdominal distension secondary to renal enlargement, and intubation and ventilation may be required at least initially.

**Transport** Transport is indicated with bilateral lesions for full confirmation of diagnosis and establishment of care plan, including surgical intervention. Infants with isolated unilateral lesions and normal renal function, as indicated by serum urea nitrogen and creatinine, can be referred for outpatient evaluation and management.

**Testing and Confirmation** Renal ultrasonography, diuretic renography, and VCUG will confirm the diagnosis. In the presence of an enlarged obstructed kidney, an abdominal mass may be palpable on initial physical exam.

**Nursery Management** Support respiration as necessary to maintain adequate gas exchange. Subsequent procedures will be contingent on the specific lesion identified.

## SURGERY

**Preoperative Assessment** If the obstruction is considered to be of a severity that may warrant surgery, careful staged evaluation of renal function and structure by urine production, urinalysis, blood and urine chemistries, and an abdominal sonogram is appropriate. If the infant is minimally symptomatic and immediate relief of obstruction is not necessary, imaging can be delayed for several days for better visualization. If the anatomy is not clearly defined prenatally or immediate relief of obstruction is required, ultrasonographic imaging should be performed immediately. Subsequent procedures will be needed to further delineate the site of obstruction, status of reflux, and renal function, including cystogram and renal scan with diuretic stimulation, which should be done after 2 weeks of age when the glomerular filtration rate has increased.

**Operative Indications** The surgical goal is to perform any needed decompression or pyeloplasty procedure prior to hypertrophy of the contralateral kidney. Poor renal function can frequently be improved by a decompression pyelostomy or ureterostomy. After 2 to 3 months of decompression, the renal scintigraphic study is repeated. If the kidney demonstrates at least 10% of total renal function, a pyeloplasty is indicated.

**Types of Procedures** Decompression versus primary repair is dependent on the amount of ipsilateral renal function. Early neonatal pyeloplasty is very successful, with a low recurrence rate.

**Surgical Results/Prognosis** Ultimate prognosis is dependent on the amount of remaining renal function and the degree of associated lung hypoplasia. It is excellent for unilateral or mild bilateral hydronephrosis. Repeat pyeloplasties are uncommon, even when the initial procedure is done in early infancy (1.5%).

## SUGGESTED READINGS


1. Alberti C: Congenital ureteropelvic junction obstruction: physiopathology, decoupling of tout court pelvic dilatation—obstruction semantic connection, biomarkers to predict renal damage evolution. Eur Rev Med Pharmacol Sci 2012; 16:213-219.
2. Barbosa JA, Chow JS, Benson CB, et al: Postnatal longitudinal evaluation of children diagnosed with prenatal hydronephrosis: insights in natural history and referral pattern. Prenat Diagn 2012; 32:142-1249.
3. Corteville JE, Gray DL, Crane JP: Congenital hydronephrosis: correlation of fetal ultrasonographic findings with infant outcome. Am J Obstet Gynecol 1991; 165:384-388.
4. Duin LK, Willekes C, Vossen M, et al: Reproducibility of fetal renal pelvic volume measurement using three-dimensional ultrasound. Ultrasound Obstet Gynecol 2008; 35:657-661.
5. Fernbach SK, Maizels M, Conway JJ: Ultrasound grading of hydronephrosis: introduction of the system used by the Society for Fetal Urology. Pediatr Radiol 1993; 23:478-480.
6. Ghidini A, Sintori M, Vergani P, et al: Ureteropelvic junction obstruction in utero and ex utero. Obstet Gynecol 1990; 75:805-808.
7. Jaffe R, Abramowicz J, Fejgin M, Ben-Aderet N: Giant fetal abdominal cyst. Ultrasonic diagnosis and management. J Ultrasound Med 1987; 6:45-47.
8. Lee RS, Cendron MD, Kinnamon MS, Nguyen HT: Antenatal hydronephrosis as a predictor of postnatal outcome: a meta-analysis. Pediatrics 2006; 118:586-593.
9. Nguyen HT, Benson CB, Bromley B, et al: Multidisciplinary consensus on the classification of prenatal and postnatal urinary tract dilation (UTD classification system). J Pediatr Urol 2014; 10:982-999.

10. Rosen S, Peters CA, Chevalier RL, Huang WY: The kidney in congenital ureteropelvic junction obstruction: a spectrum from normal to nephrectomy. J Urol 2008; 179:1257-1263.

11. Thornburg LL, Pressman EK, Chedamkuri S, et al: Third trimester ultrasound of fetal pyelectasis: predictor for postnatal surgery. J Pediatr Urol 2008; 4:51-54.

12. Yamamura Y, Swartout JP, Anderson EA, et al: Management of mild fetal pyelectasis: a comparative analysis. J Ultrasound Med 2007; 26:1539-1543.

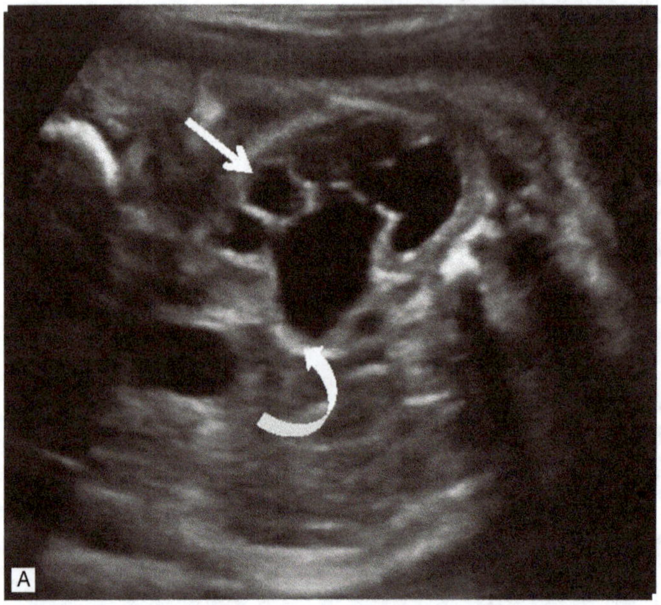


**FIGURE 4.15A** Ureteropelvic junction obstruction illustrating dilated calyces (straight arrow) and rounded caudal end of renal pelvis (curved arrow).

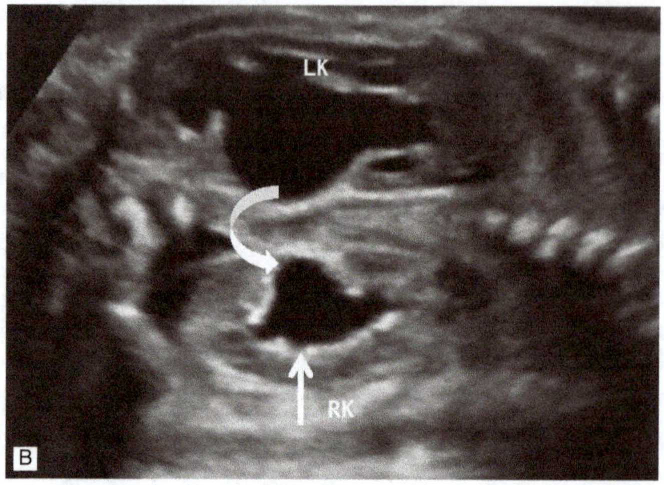


**FIGURE 4.15B** Bilateral UPJ obstruction showing loss of calyces (straight arrow) and blunted caudal end of renal pelvis (curved arrow). LK, left kidney; RK, right kidney.

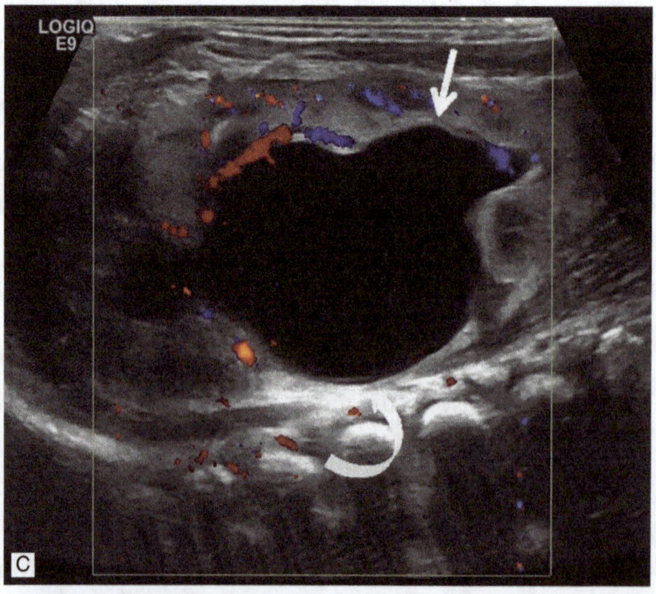


**FIGURE 4.15C** Ureteropelvic junction obstruction with loss of calyces (straight arrow) and blunted end of renal pelvis (curved arrow).

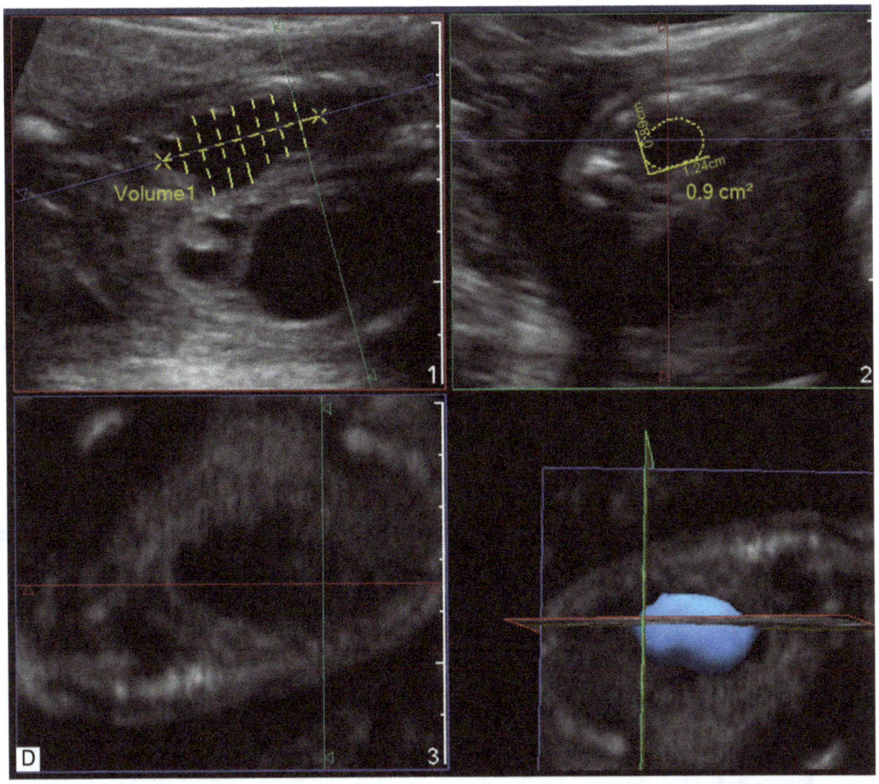


**FIGURE 4.15D** Multiplanar imaging and 3-D volume of UPJ obstruction.

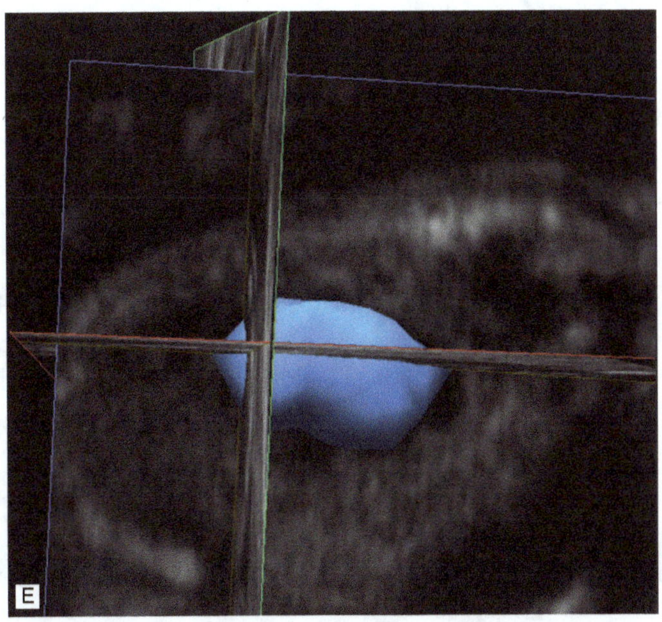


**FIGURE 4.15E** Three-dimensional volume of UPJ obstruction.

# 4.16 VESICOURETERAL REFLUX

## EPIDEMIOLOGY/GENETICS

**Definition** Vesicoureteral reflux (VUR) is the reverse flow of urine from the bladder into the ureters or kidneys with micturition.

**Epidemiology** The prevalence in children is 0.2%-6% (M3:F1). VUR accounts for approximately 10% of antenatally diagnosed "hydronephrosis."

**Embryology** Vesicoureteral reflux is a common cause of renal pelvocalyceal dilation, particularly in males. Effective valve function requires coordinated ureteric peristalsis; muscular function of the trigone; and appropriate length of the submucosal ureter and width of the ureteric opening. VUR likely results from abnormalities involving a combination of the factors rather than a single cause in each case. VUR is graded based on the following criteria:

- Grades of VUR:

I. Ureter only
II. Extends to the renal pelvis
III. Dilatation of ureter, renal pelvis, and calyces
IV. Moderate dilatation/tortuosity of ureter; moderate dilatation of renal pelvis and calyces
V. Severe dilatation/tortuosity of the ureter; significant dilatation of the renal pelvis with loss of calyces

**Inheritance Patterns** Multifactorial inheritance is most likely, given the higher occurrence within families. In some families, autosomal dominant or X-linked inheritance has been proposed.

**Teratogens**. None are reported.

**Prognosis** The outcome for most children with VUR is excellent. However, renal impairment associated with severe fetal reflux may be due to congenital dysplasia; that is, it is present at birth and not secondary to neonatal/infant infection. Lesser degrees of VUR are rarely associated with renal impairment and usually resolve by 6 years of age.

## SONOGRAPHY

### FREQUENT FINDINGS

- Unilateral or bilateral pyelectasis
  - Gestational age
    - 16-27 weeks: renal pelvis diameter greater than 4.0 mm
    - 28 weeks: renal pelvis diameter greater than 7.0 mm

### LESS FREQUENT

- Caliectasis
- Continually full bladder
  - Urine refluxes up the lower ureters and rapidly refills the bladder after voiding.
- Megacystis
- Thickened bladder wall
- Hydroureter

### KEY FINDINGS/PITFALLS

- Posterior urethral valve-like syndrome in VUR is likely due to uncoordinated fetal voiding.
- VUR may be unilateral or bilateral.
- In the same patient, the severity of VUR may vary on the right and left.
- Variable ureteric and renal pelvic size over the course of the examination suggests the presence of reflux.
- VUR is associated with other renal anomalies, such as unilateral renal agenesis and multicystic dysplastic kidney.

## PREGNANCY MANAGEMENT

**Investigations and Consultations Required** The diagnosis of VUR is often not certain, particularly in milder cases, which may present as pyelectasis, without marked ureteral dilatation. An extended ultrasound examination is indicated, looking specifically for other urinary tract abnormalities. Revisiting the patient's risk for trisomy 21 is indicated, as pyelectasis is a soft marker for fetal Down syndrome. However, in the absence of other findings or an elevated a priori Down syndrome risk, no other diagnostic evaluation is necessary. If hydroureter is seen or if the renal pelvis dilatation is marked in the second trimester or mild but persistent into the third trimester, consultation with a pediatric urologist is necessary to develop a postnatal management plan and determine site of delivery.

**Fetal Intervention** Intervention is not indicated.

**Monitoring** Mild degrees of renal pelvis dilation should be assessed by a follow-up sonogram at 32 to 34 weeks' gestation. More significant dilation at any gestational age should be followed with sonographic evaluation every 4 weeks.

**Pregnancy Course** No specific obstetric complications should be expected.

**Pregnancy Termination Issues** The method of termination should provide an intact fetus for pathologic confirmation of the sonographic diagnosis.

**Delivery** When there is severe disease, the potential need for neonatal evaluation and treatment requires that delivery occur in a tertiary center with a pediatric urologist available. No change in standard obstetric care is necessary.

## NEONATOLOGY

**Resuscitation** Resuscitation is usually not an issue. Occasionally, the onset of effective respiration may be impeded by abdominal distension secondary to renal enlargement, and intubation and ventilation may be required at least initially.

**Transport** Transport is indicated with bilateral lesions for full confirmation of diagnosis and establishment of a care plan, including surgical intervention. Infants with isolated unilateral lesions and normal renal function, as indicated by serum urea nitrogen and creatinine, can be referred for outpatient evaluation and management.

**Testing and Confirmation** All infants with suspected VUR and hydronephrosis detected on antenatal ultrasound should have a renal ultrasound. Renal ultrasonography, diuretic renography, and VCUG will confirm the diagnosis.

**Nursery Management** Support respiration as necessary to maintain adequate gas exchange. Subsequent procedures will be contingent on the specific lesion suspected or discovered. Referral to pediatric urology is indicated for evaluation. In the presence of low-grade VUR (grades I-III), the parents can be reassured that there is often spontaneous resolution.

### SUGGESTED READINGS

1. Anderson PA, Rickwood AM: Features of primary vesicoureteric reflux detected by prenatal sonography. Br J Urol 1991; 67:267-271.
2. Connolly LP, Traves ST, Connolly SA, et al: Vesicoureteral reflux in children: incidence and severity in siblings. J Urol 1997; 157:2287-2290.
3. Fägerquist M, Sillén U, Blomberg SG: Postnatal vesico-ureteral reflux in a boy with urinary bladder dysfunction as the only prenatal sonographic sign. Ultrasound Obstet Gynecol 1997; 9:64-66.
4. Lebowitz RL, Olbing H, Parkkulainne KV, et al: International system of radiographic grading of vesioureteric reflux. Pediatr Radiol 1985; 15:105-109.
5. Marra G, Barbieri G, Moioli C, et al: Mild fetal hydronephrosis indicating vesicoureteric reflux. Arch Dis Child Fetal Neonatal Ed 1994; 70:F147-F150.
6. Najmaidin A, Burge DM, Atwell JD: Reflux nephropathy secondary to intrauterine vesicoureteric reflux. J Ped Surg 1990; 25:387-390.
7. Nguyen HT, Benson CB, Bromley B, et al: Multidisciplinary consensus on the classification of prenatal and postnatal urinary tract dilation (UTD classification system). J Pediatr Urol 2014; 10:982-999.
8. Reuter KL, Lebowitz RL: Massive vesicoureteral reflux mimicking posterior urethral valves in a fetus. J Clin Ultrasound 1985; 13:584-587.
9. Stock JA, Wilson D, Hanna MK: Congenital reflux nephropathy and severe unilateral fetal reflux. J Urol 1998; 160:1017-1018.
10. Williams G, Fletcher JT, Alexander SI, Craig JC: Vesicoureteral reflux. J Am Soc Nephrol 2008; 19:847-862.

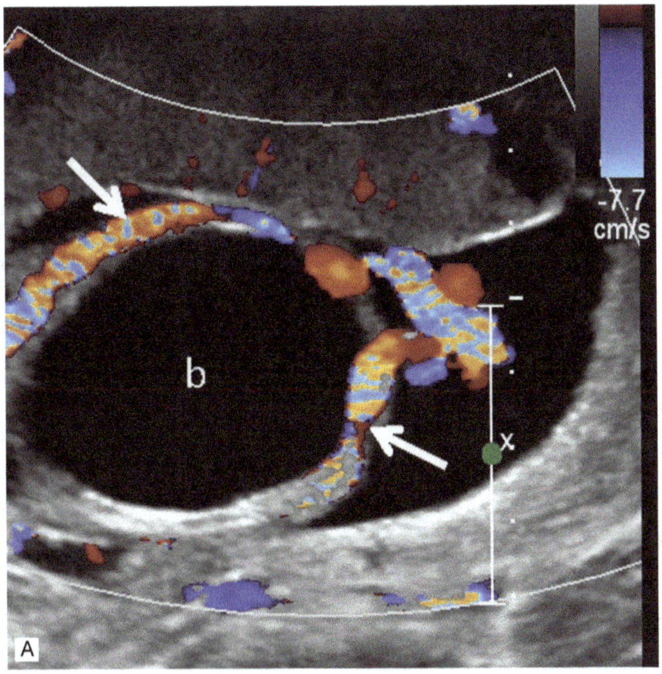


FIGURE 4.16A Vesicoureteral reflux with an enlarged bladder (b). Note the umbilical arteries (arrows).

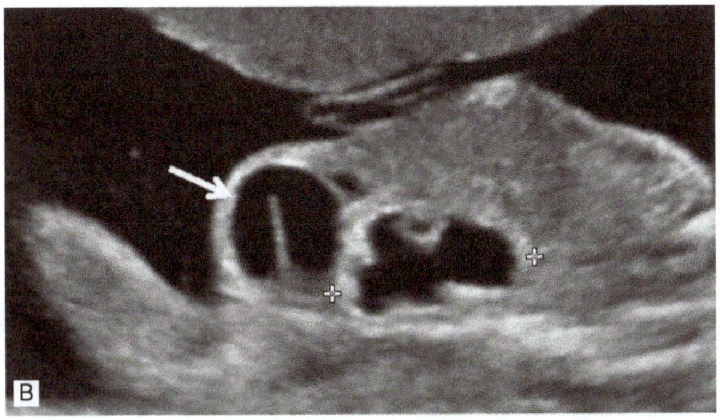


FIGURE 4.16B Severe pyelocaliectasis (+ … +) and hydroureter (arrow) associated with severe vesicoureteral reflux.

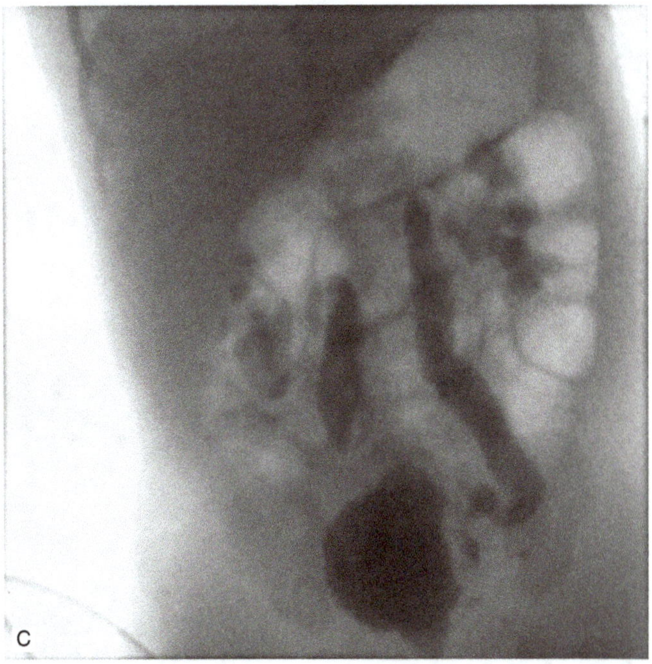


FIGURE 4.16C Imaging of grade 4 reflux in a neonate.

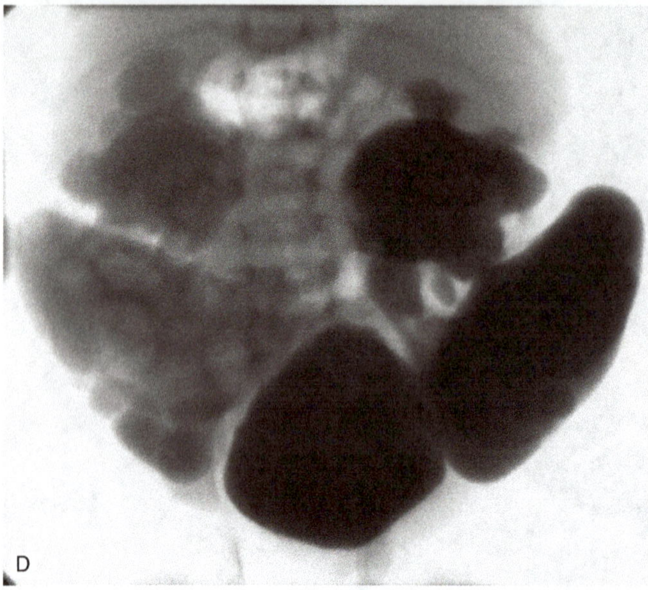


FIGURE 4.16D Imaging of grade 5 reflux in a neonate.

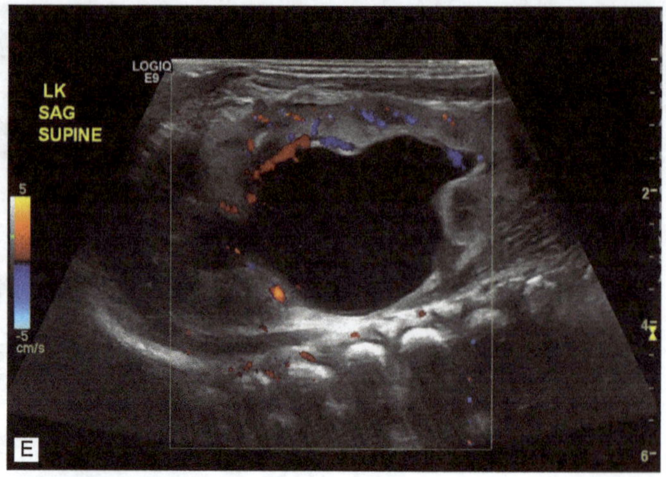


FIGURE 4.16E Ultrasound of grade 5 reflux in a neonate.

# CHAPTER 5

# THE CHEST

# 5.0 OVERVIEW: CONGENITAL LUNG LESIONS

There are multiple echogenic lung lesions that must await neonatal assessment to determine a specific diagnosis. The generic term *congenital lung lesion* (CLL) should be used, instead of trying to make a histologic diagnosis based on specific sonographic criteria.

There has been a rise in the number of CLLs over the past 20 years to the current rate of 4.15 cases per 10,000 births. This appears to be a true rise in incidence rather than increased antenatal recognition because of the prevalence of second- and third-trimester ultrasound examinations.

Fetal assessment/management should be based on the sonographic criteria that can be evaluated on serial examinations: gestational age at first detection, the size of the mass, mediastinal deviation, eversion of the diaphragm, cystic and solid components, detection of a feeding vessel to the mass, and signs of hydrops.

## SUGGESTED READINGS

1. Demos N, Teresi A: Congenital lung malformations: a unified concept and a case report. J Thorac Cardiovasc Surg 1975; 70:260-264.
2. Puligandia PS, Laberge J-M: Congenital lung lesions. Clin Perinatol 2012; 39:331-347.
3. Stocker LJ, Wellesley DG, Stanton MP, et al: The increasing incidence of foetal echogenic congenital lung malformations: an observational study. Prenat Diagn 2015; 35:148-153.

# 5.1 CONGENITAL HIGH AIRWAY OBSTRUCTION SYNDROME

## EPIDEMIOLOGY/GENETICS

**Definition** Laryngeal atresia is the most common etiology of congenital high airway obstruction syndrome (CHAOS). Other etiologies of CHAOS include tracheal agenesis, tracheal atresia, subglottic stenosis, laryngeal web, tracheal membrane, and laryngeal cyst.

**Epidemiology** True incidence is unknown.

**Embryology** Tracheal or laryngeal atresia is thought to result from failure of recanalization of the upper airway. CHAOS occurs with Fraser syndrome (autosomal recessive), which has laryngeal atresia, urogenital abnormalities, and syndactyly. Fetal hydrops or polyhydramnios may occur. It has also been reported with cri du chat (5p-) syndrome, short-rib polydactyly syndrome, and the velocardiofacial syndrome.

**Inheritance Patterns** Inheritance is sporadic in most cases and autosomal recessive in the case of Fraser syndrome. One case of autosomal dominant inheritance has been reported with an affected father and two children.

**Teratogens** None are described.

**Prognosis** The absence of hydrops is associated with survival but with significant morbidity. Respiratory function is rarely normal due to long-term exposure to high airway pressure. The presence of other anomalies worsens the prognosis with CHAOS.

## SONOGRAPHY

### FREQUENT FINDINGS

- Large diffusely echogenic lungs
- Dilated airways distended with fluid
- Inverted diaphragms
- Heart compression from lung expansion
- Splaying of the ribs due to enlarged fetal lungs
- Ascites

### LESS FREQUENT

- Hydrops
  - Pericardial effusion
  - Pleural effusion
  - Anasarca
  - Placentomegaly

- Polyhydramnios
- Mirror syndrome
  - Preeclampsia in the mother

### KEY FINDINGS/PITFALLS/DIFFERENTIAL DIAGNOSIS

- Main stem bronchial atresia results in unilateral CHAOS. Other than an enlarged unilateral hyperechoic lung, the sonographic findings and outcome are similar to laryngeal atresia.
- CHAOS is most frequently assumed to represent type III congenital cystic pulmonary airway malformation.
- The subtype of CHAOS with a pharyngotracheal or laryngotracheal communication is less severe; ultrasound findings may resolve. The fistula allows decompression of the obstructed tracheal bronchial tree.
- Sonographic findings associated with CHAOS have been reported as early as 16 weeks' gestation.
- Two-dimensional (2-D) ultrasound permits an anatomic and functional evaluation of the larynx and pharynx.
- Color Doppler can be used to show an absence of flow through the larynx with fetal breathing movements. The larynx is occupied by nonstructured tissue.
- With a unilateral hyperechoic lung mass, three-dimensional (3-D) power Doppler can be used to look for the feeding vessel associated with bronchopulmonary sequestration (PS).
- Three-dimensional multiplanar imaging can evaluate an enlarged echogenic lung lesion for the anechoic nonvascular, tubular image of a bronchus or bronchi.
- Three-dimensional assessment of the larynx and pharynx, with multiplanar reconstruction, permits an assessment of basic anatomic relationships and helps in the differentiation of laryngeal atresia from a tracheal membrane.

## PREGNANCY MANAGEMENT

**Investigations and Consultations Required** Most cases are isolated and sporadic. In those cases with sonographically detected abnormalities, chromosome studies, including microarray, should be done. Fetal echocardiography can assess both cardiac structure and function. Fetal magnetic resonance imaging (MRI) may be helpful in defining the obstructing lesion (ranging from a laryngeal web to tracheal agenesis). Consultations with a pediatric surgeon and a neonatologist are essential for planning delivery management.

**Pregnancy Course** Without intervention, many will progress to fetal hydrops and fetal demise. The presence of hydrops is an ominous sign.

**Fetal Intervention** When short-segment tracheal lesions, or webs, are demonstrated on fetal MRI, fetal bronchoscopy and tracheoplasty may be options if done by experienced interventionists at specialized centers. Successful in utero intervention has been reported.

**Monitoring** In the limited number of cases reported to date, there has been a high incidence of in utero deaths. There are no studies on which to base treatment recommendations. However, once the fetus has reached sufficient size that ex utero tracheotomy could be performed, weekly assessment of fetal status will help to determine the most appropriate time for delivery.

**Pregnancy Termination Issues** Given the poor prognosis despite interventions, pregnancy termination should be presented as an option. For counseling regarding future pregnancies, an intact fetus is necessary to determine whether the airway obstruction is isolated or part of a syndrome.

**Delivery** In those cases where ultrasound and MRI suggest lesions amenable to postnatal repair, early EXIT (ex utero intrapartum treatment) should be considered. Delivery must occur in a center where a multidisciplinary team is skilled in the EXIT procedure. In this procedure, only the head and shoulders are delivered through the uterine incision. A saline infusion is used to maintain uterine volume and to prevent umbilical cord compression. Uterine relaxation is maintained by a high concentration of inhalation anesthetics and tocolytic agents, if necessary. If the fetal airway cannot be established by direct laryngoscopy or bronchoscopy, tracheostomy is performed. Only after the airway is established is the infant delivered and the umbilical cord clamped.

## NEONATOLOGY

**Resuscitation** Emergent airway management is enhanced if there has been prenatal diagnosis. Few infants establish spontaneous ventilation following delivery. Given the severity of the prognosis, a prenatal discussion with the parents of management options is indicated. If the decision is for full resuscitative efforts, the EXIT procedure offers the potential for survival in this otherwise-lethal condition. Delivery should be arranged to facilitate rapid surgical establishment of an airway, if needed, and with full pediatric subspecialty diagnostic and intensive care capabilities available. The postnatal course of CHAOS is dependent on whether the airway obstruction is complete. In the absence of a prenatal diagnosis, emergent airway management consists of tracheoesophageal intubation or emergent tracheostomy.

**Transport** If the diagnosis is made antenatally and temporary stabilization of the airway is achieved at the time of delivery, emergency transport with a skilled neonatal team to a tertiary center with full pediatric and surgical subspecialty capabilities is indicated.

**Testing and Confirmation** Flexible endoscopy will confirm the blind tracheal pouch and in some cases identify the communication, or communications, between the esophagus and the distal airway or airways. Contrast studies or MRI may be needed to elucidate the structural anatomy of the communications in planning for surgical intervention. Evaluation for additional malformations is indicated. Multiple organ system anomalies have been documented in reported cases, including pulmonary, genitourinary, musculoskeletal, and cardiovascular malformations.

**Nursery Management** The first priority is a stable and functional airway, which is achievable only with skilled surgical intervention. The next focus is complete evaluation, as multiple organ system anomalies occur in many of these infants. The exact diagnostic and therapeutic management, beyond full life support, is dictated by the associated anomalies.

## SUGGESTED READINGS


1. Abitayeh G, Ruano R, Martinovic J, et al: Prenatal diagnosis of main stem bronchial atresia using 3-dimensional ultrasonographic technologies. J Ultrasound Med 2010; 29:633-638.
2. Joshi P, Satija L, George RA, et al: Congenital high airway obstruction syndrome-antenatal diagnosis of a rare case of airway obstruction using multimodality imaging. Med J Armed Forces India 2012; 68:78-80.
3. Kuwahima S, Kitajima K, Kaji Y, et al: MR imaging appearance of laryngeal atresia (congenital high airway obstruction syndrome): unique course in a fetus. Pediatr Radiol 2008; 38:344-347.
4. Liberty G, Boldes R, Shen O, et al: The fetal larynx and pharynx: structure and development on two- and three-dimensional ultrasound. Ultrasound Obstet Gynecol 2013; 42:140-148.
5. Lim FY, Crombleholme TM, Hedrick HL, et al: Congenital high airway obstruction syndrome: natural history and management. J Pediatr Surg 2003; 38:940-945.
6. Martínez JM, Castañón M, Gómez O, et al: Evaluation of fetal vocal cords to select candidates for successful fetoscopic treatment of congenital high airway obstruction syndrome: preliminary case series. Fetal Diagn Ther 2013; 34:77-84.
7. Martínez JM, Prat J, Gómez O, et al: Decompression through tracheobronchial endoscopy of brachial atresia presenting as massive pulmonary tumor: a new indication for fetoscopic surgery. Fetal Diagn Ther 2013; 33:69-74.
8. Oepkes D, Teunissen AKK, Van de Velde M, et al: Congenital high airway obstruction syndrome successfully managed with ex utero intrapartum treatment. Ultrasound Obstet Gynecol 2003; 22:437-439.
9. Roybal JL, Liechty KW, Hedrick HL, et al: Predicting the severity of congenital high airway obstruction syndrome. J Pediatr Surg 2010; 45:1633-1639.
10. Saadi P, Jelin EB, Nijagal A, et al: Long-term outcomes after fetal therapy for congenital high airway obstruction syndrome. J Pediatr Surg 2012; 47:1095-1100.
11. Vidaeff AC, Szmuk P, Mastrobattista JM, et al: More or less CHAOS: case report and literature review suggesting the existence of a distinct subtype of congenital high airway obstruction syndrome. Ultrasound Obstet Gynecol 2007; 30:114-117.

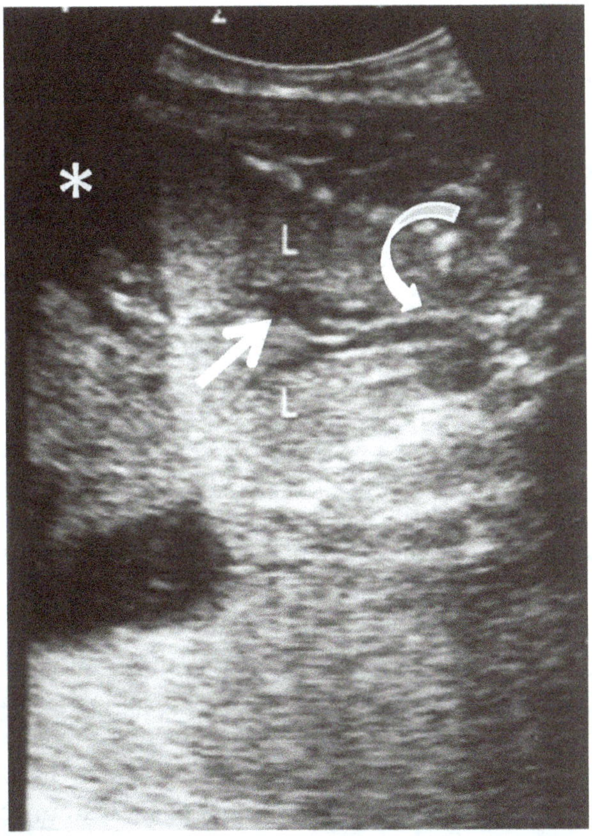


**FIGURE 5.1A** CHAOS with ascites (*), echogenic lung fields (L) with everted diaphragm and dilated, fluid-filled trachea (curved arrow) and main stem bronchi (straight arrow).

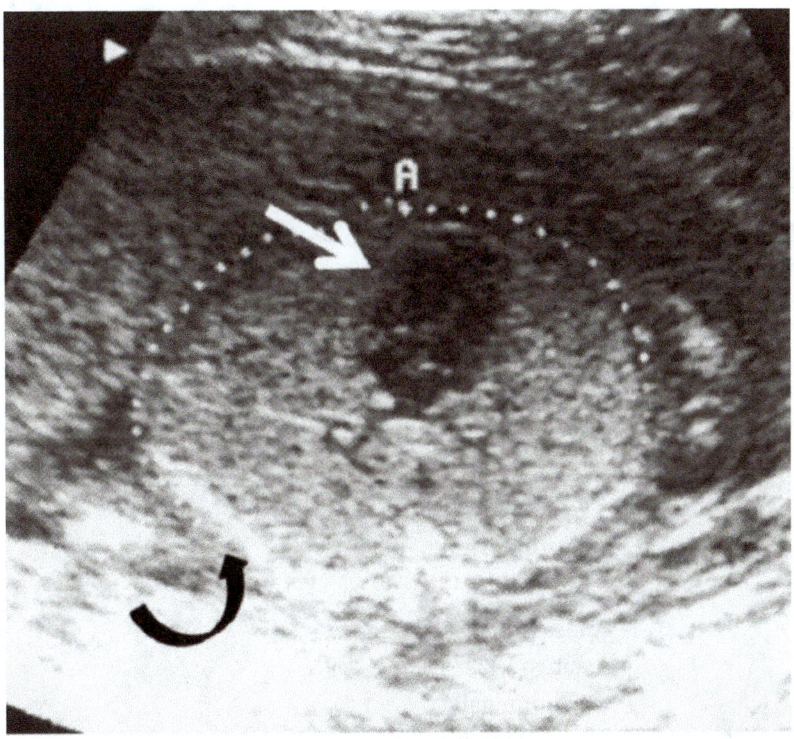


**FIGURE 5.1B** CHAOS with bilateral echgenic lung fields. The heart is compressed in the midline (straight arrow) and the ribs splayed apart (curved arrow).

# 5.2 CONGENITAL PULMONARY AIRWAY MALFORMATION

## EPIDEMIOLOGY/GENETICS

**Definition** Congenital pulmonary airway malformations (CPAMs; previously called congenital cystic adenomatoid malformations) are benign hamartomatous, or dysplastic, lung tumors characterized by overgrowth of terminal bronchioles.

**Epidemiology** Occurrence is 1 in 25,000 to 35,000 live births (M1:F1).

**Embryology** CPAMs develop during the first 6 weeks of gestation. CPAM is theorized to be induced by localized overexpression of fibroblast growth factor 10. They are generally unilateral and classified into macrocystic (type I), mixed (type II), or microcystic (type III) forms. This Stocker three-stage classification of CPAM is based on clinical, radiological, and pathologic criteria in the postnatal period. Stocker subsequently expanded the classification by adding acinar dysplasia or agenesis (type 0) and large thin-walled peripheral cysts (type IV). The last two categories have been questioned, resulting in the development of other classification systems. There is a 26% incidence of associated malformations, including reports of pectus excavatum, renal agenesis, pulmonary sequestration (PS), congenital heart defects, and imperforate anus. Trisomy 18 has also been seen in association with CPAM.

**Inheritance Patterns** Inheritance is sporadic.

**Teratogens** There are no known teratogens.

**Prognosis** The majority of patients with CPAM detected antenatally have a good outcome. Many cases appear to regress or resolve in utero. Others can be successfully resected with normal outcomes. Early hydrops may be associated with a lethal prognosis.

## SONOGRAPHY

### FREQUENT FINDINGS

- Echogenic lung mass
- Multicystic lung mass

### LESS FREQUENT

- Mediastinal shift
- Hydrops
  - Anasarca
  - Ascites
  - Cardiomegaly
  - Pleural effusion
  - Pericardial effusion
- Inverted diaphragm

- Increased thoracic diameter
- Polyhydramnios

### KEY FINDINGS/PITFALLS

- Antenatal sonography can only distinguish between macrocystic (one or more visible cysts) and microcystic (echogenic cysts < 5 mm) CPAM.
- CPAM is usually in one pulmonary lobe (80%-95% of cases).
  - Multilobar or bilateral CPAM is rare.
- CPAMs are evenly distributed between the right and left lung.
- Microcystic CPAM with a coexisting pulmonary sequestration (PS) is frequently missed, even when a feeding vessel to the mass is specifically sought with color Doppler.
- Karyotyping should be considered if additional congenital anomalies are detected.
  - The risk of a karyotypic abnormality is not increased with an isolated CPAM.
- Rapid growth of microcystic CPAMs occurs between 20 and 26 weeks' gestation.
  - At 26 weeks' gestation, growth patterns of microcystic CPAMs begin to regress.
  - Macrocystic lesions generally do not regress.
- In the third trimester, microcystic CPAM becomes isoechoic with normal lung parenchyma, resulting in their apparent "disappearance."
- Weekly ultrasound examinations should be performed to look for hydrops when a microcystic CPAM has a mediastinal shift, a mass-to-thoracic ratio of 0.56 or greater, and diaphragmatic eversion.
  - After 28 weeks, ultrasound surveillance can be individualized based on the lesion's size.
- In the presence of macrocystic CPAM, serial ultrasound examinations until delivery are required.
- The cysts in macrocystic CPAM have intracystic communication.
- Compression of the contralateral lung by a large CPAM can result in pulmonary hypoplasia.
- A CPAM volume ratio (CVR) has been used to predict survival.
  - CVR volume: Length × Height × Width × 0.52 of the CPAM divided by the head circumference.
  - A CVR of 1.6 or less predicts a 97% survival if a dominant cyst is not present. This is in contrast to a survival of 56% with a CVR of 1.6 or greater.
  - CVR measurements extend along a continuum; the cutoff selected (1.4, 1.6, or 2.0) determines its sensitivity and specificity for the development of fetal hydrops.
- Accurate predictors of outcome are as follows:
  - Decrease in size of the lung mass over serial ultrasound examinations predicts survival.
  - The presence of hydrops is strongly associated with demise.
- Regression of a microcystic CPAM lesion occurs in 50% of cases, even in the presence of associated hydrops.

### DIFFERENTIAL DIAGNOSIS

- Pulmonary sequestration may resemble microcystic CPAM and can only be differentiated by the detection of a feeding vessel to a PS.
- Congenital lobar emphysema is an intrinsic obstruction due to a mucous plug or defective bronchial cartilage. A mucous plus obstructing a bronchus can create an echogenic lung lesion. If the obstruction is relieved, the echogenic lung lesion resolves.
- Lobar bronchial atresia resembles microcystic CPAM. A fluid-filled bronchus distal to an obstruction will assist in the diagnosis. There is an associated mediastinal shift and eversion of the diaphragm. Severe cases are associated with ascites and polyhydramnios.
- Bronchogenic cysts. A simple or septated bronchogenic cyst may have the same appearance as a macrocystic CPAM. A bronchogenic cyst is derived from the foregut and therefore originates in the midline. As its size increases, a bronchogenic cyst becomes more difficult to distinguish from a CPAM. Three-dimensional multiplanar imaging can help to distinguish between a bronchogenic cyst compressing surrounding lung and a CPAM.

## PREGNANCY MANAGEMENT

**Investigations and Consultations Required** An extended ultrasound examination is indicated to exclude other anomalies and possible coexisting bronchopulmonary sequestration (BPS). Invasive testing is not indicated if a precise diagnosis can be made by ultrasonography and other anomalies are not present. Cardiac status should be assessed by fetal echocardiography. Early consultation with a neonatologist or pediatric surgeon is warranted to establish a perinatal management plan.

**Fetal Intervention** Most of these masses are stable, and many regress during pregnancy. Fetal intervention would only be considered in cases without associated anomalies in which there is rapid growth of the lesion or hydrops is present or develops. In microcystic lesions with rapid growth early in gestation, one or two courses of betamethasone may arrest the growth of the CPAM lesion. In macrocystic lesions with rapid growth, mediastinal shift, or hydrops development early in gestation, aspiration of the cyst may be therapeutic. If the cyst reaccumulates, a cyst-amniotic shunt may be placed. Multicystic lesions are generally not appropriate for shunt placement.

**Monitoring** Ultrasonographic examinations every 4 weeks are appropriate to monitor the size of the mass and to detect early evidence of hydrops.

**Pregnancy Course** Polyhydramnios may develop in some cases and may result in preterm labor. However, many lesions regress or disappear during pregnancy.

**Pregnancy Termination Issues** Unless a clear diagnosis is made by ultrasound, a nondestructive procedure that provides both anatomic and microscopic evaluation is appropriate.

**Delivery** In the absence of fetal hydrops, delivery should be at term. After 32 weeks' gestation, any evidence of fetal compromise should prompt steroid administration to enhance fetal lung maturity and early delivery. If hydrops is present after 32 weeks, consideration should be given to delivery via an EXIT procedure. Because immediate resuscitation may be necessary in any infant with CPAM, delivery should occur in a tertiary center.

## NEONATOLOGY

**Resuscitation** The management of newborns with CPAM depends on whether the infant presents with signs of respiratory distress. Approximately half of infants diagnosed prenatally with CPAM are asymptomatic at birth. Infants with symptomatic CPAM typically present with early-onset respiratory distress and may require intubation following delivery and assisted ventilation.

**Transport** Symptomatic patients require transfer to a tertiary center with the availability of pediatric surgery. Mechanical ventilator support may be required, and the infant should be positioned with the involved side dependent in an attempt to avoid overdistension.

**Testing and Confirmation** Asymptomatic infants with a prenatal diagnosis of CPAM require a chest radiograph at the time of delivery. If the infant is stable, subsequent evaluation with a chest computerized tomographic (CT) scan or MRI at 3-6 months should performed. Elective surgical resection at a future date is recommended. In symptomatic patients, a CT scan or MRI are recommended, and prompt surgical resection is often indicated in the immediate newborn period. Classification of the type of CPAM is made based most definitively on the characteristics of the lesion as assessed by the pathologist after excision. This may be different from the classification assigned antenatally by ultrasound criteria.

**Nursery Management** Larger and more extensive CPAM lesions are associated with an increased incidence, and severity, of respiratory distress. Type 0 CPAM is the rarest form and is lethal. Infants with types 1, 2, and 4 CPAM may require respiratory support depending on the size of the cyst(s) and presence of respiratory distress at birth. Infants with type 3 CPAM typically present with severe respiratory distress and may require prolonged mechanical ventilation. Infants with a large CPAM who present with hydrops often require mechanical ventilation and additional pharmacologic support. Asymptomatic patients may be seen as outpatients by pediatric surgery for further evaluation and management

## SURGERY

**Preoperative Assessment** The newborn should be evaluated in the nursery to confirm the prenatal diagnosis and exclude other associated anomalies. Most neonates will be hemodynamically stable, without signs of respiratory distress. A chest x-ray should be obtained to assess for the CPAM or mediastinal shift. In the setting of a stable infant without significant findings on chest x-ray, further evaluation may be deferred until later in infancy, allowing the neonate to be discharged home with his or her family. Even in the setting of a normal chest x-ray, further evaluation with either a CT scan or an MRI should be completed within the next several months of age. Many CPAM lesions will not be evident on chest x-ray but will be identified on more definitive 3-D imaging.

**Operative Indications** CPAM is usually confined to a single lobe. Rare cases have been reported of multilobar involvement of one lung or bilateral lesions. Complete resection of the CPAM, usually by lobectomy, is the treatment of choice. In cases of extensive involvement of nearly the entire lung, resection of multiple lobes, or pneumonectomy, may rarely be necessary. There should be consideration of the infant's stability and the long-term risk of the lesion prior to proceeding with extensive pulmonary resection. The need for urgent surgery is determined by the presence of respiratory distress requiring ventilatory support. In a minority of patients, and particularly those with an early intrauterine diagnosis, the pulmonary symptoms are severe and unresponsive to standard respiratory support.

The newborn with a CPAM detected antenatally that subsequently regressed needs postnatal evaluation. Often, subtle abnormalities will be evident on chest radiograph, but chest CT or MRI may be necessary to detect residual CPAM. Several authors have recommended that, as long as these lesions are asymptomatic, they be observed closely and managed without resection. The argument against this approach includes the reported cases of myxosarcoma, embryonal rhabdomyosarcoma, and bronchoalveolar carcinoma arising in CPAMs. Although primary lung tumors are rare in the first two decades of life, 4% of those reported were associated with congenital cystic lesions of the lung, including CPAM. A more common concern is the risk of secondary infection of the CPAM, with the potential for the development of an abscess or difficult-to-eradicate infection, confusion with recurrent pneumonia that results in multiple courses of antibiotics, and technical difficulty at the time of resection.

**Types of Procedures** CPAMs may be approached by either thoracoscopy or thoracotomy. The advantage of deferring surgical excision until later in infancy is the greater likelihood of success via a thoracoscopic approach in the older, larger infant, as compared to the neonate. Most commonly, the CPAM is removed via lobectomy, but smaller lesions may be resected with a nonanatomic approach.

**Surgical Results/Prognosis** The long-term outcome of infants with CPAM following resection is excellent. If residual CPAM is left behind or the mass is not resected, the child will be at risk for complications. These complications include infection and malignancy arising within the CPAM. The infants usually have remarkable compensatory growth of the residual lung following resection, with continued alveolarization for several years. These children appear to have no excessive limitations and are no more at risk for respiratory infections than other children. The small number of children who have survived open fetal surgery for CPAMs associated with hydrops are doing well several years after their procedure.

## SUGGESTED READINGS

1. Achiron R, Strauss S, Sediman DS, et al: Fetal lung hyperechogenicity: prenatal ultrasonographic diagnosis, natural history and neonatal outcome. Ultrasound Obstet Gynecol 1995; 6:40-42.

2. Adzick NS, Harrison MR, Crombleholme TM, et al: Fetal lung lesions: management and outcome. Am J Obstet Gynecol 1998; 179:884-889.
3. Adzick NS, Harrison MR, Glick PL, et al: Fetal cystic adenomatoid malformation: prenatal diagnosis and natural history. J Pediatr Surg 1985; 20:483-488.
4. Bonnefoy C, Blanc P, Coste K, et al: Prenatal diagnosis of lobar bronchial atresia. Ultrasound Obstet Gynecol 2011; 37:110-112.
5. Cass DL, Olutoye OU, Cassidy CI, et al: Prenatal diagnosis and outcome of fetal lung masses. J Pediatr Surg 2011; 46:292-298.
6. Crombleholme TM, Coleman B, Hedrick H, et al: Cystic adenomatoid malformation volume ratio predicts outcome in prenatally diagnosed cystic adenomatoid malformation of the lung. J Pediatr Surg 2002; 37:331-338.
7. Curran PF, Jelin EB, Rand L, et al: Prenatal steroids for microcystic congenital cystic adenomatoid malformations. J Pediatr Surg 2010; 45:145-150.
8. Gonzaga S, Henriques-Coelho T, Davey M, et al: Cystic adenomatoid malformations are induced by localized FGF10 overexpression in fetal rat lung. Am J Respir Cell Mol Biol 2008; 39:346-355.
9. Kunisaki SM, Barnewolt CE, Estroff JA, et al: Large fetal cystic adenomatoid malformations: growth trends and pediatric survival. J Pediatr Surg 2007; 42:404-410.
10. Laberge JM, Flageole H, Pugash D, et al: Outcome of the prenatally diagnosed congenital cystic adenomatoid lung malformation: a Canadian experience. Fetal Diagn Ther 2001; 16:178-186.
11. Langston C: New concepts in the pathology of congenital lung malformations. Semin Pediatr Surg 2003; 12:17-37.
12. Lo AY, Jones S: Lack of consensus among Canadian pediatric surgeons regarding the management of congenital cystic adenomatoid malformation of the lung. J Pediatr Surg 2008; 43:797-799.
13. Miller JA, Corteville JE, Langer JC: Congenital cystic adenomatoid malformation in the fetus: natural history and predictors of outcome. J Pediatr Surg 1996; 31:805-808.
14. Sauvat F, Michel JL, Benachi A, et al: Management of asymptomatic neonatal cystic adenomatoid malformations. J Pediatr Surg 2003; 38:548-552.
15. Schrey S, Kelly EN, Langer JC, et al: Fetal thoracoamniotic shunting for large macrocystic congenital cystic adenomatoid malformation of the lung. Ultrasound Obstet Gynecol 2012; 39:515-520.
16. Stocker JT: Congenital pulmonary airway malformation: a new name for and an expanded classification of cystic adenomatoid malformation of the lung. Histopathology 2002; 41:424-431.
17. Vu L, Tsao K, Lee H, et al: Characteristics of congenital cystic adenomatoid malformations associated with nonimmune hydrops and outcome. J Pediatr Surg 2007; 42:1351-1356.

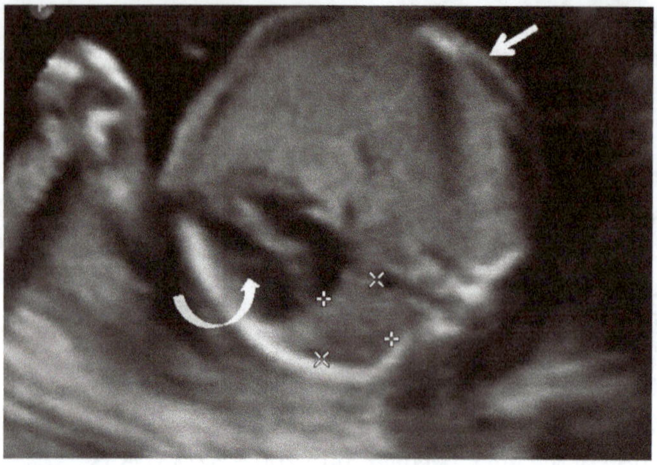

**FIGURE 5.2A** Left microcystic CPAM (straight arrow) with the heart in dextroposition (curved arrow) and a compressed left lung (+ … +).

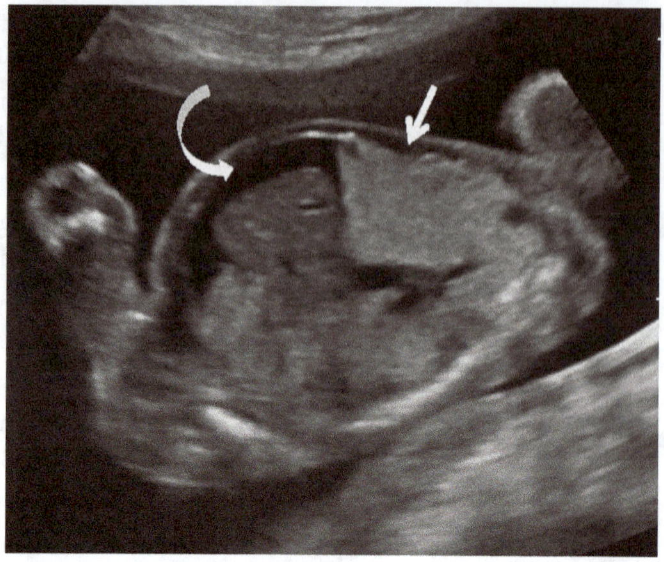

**FIGURE 5.2B** Microcystic CPAM (straight arrow) with hydrops. Note the ascites (curved arrow).

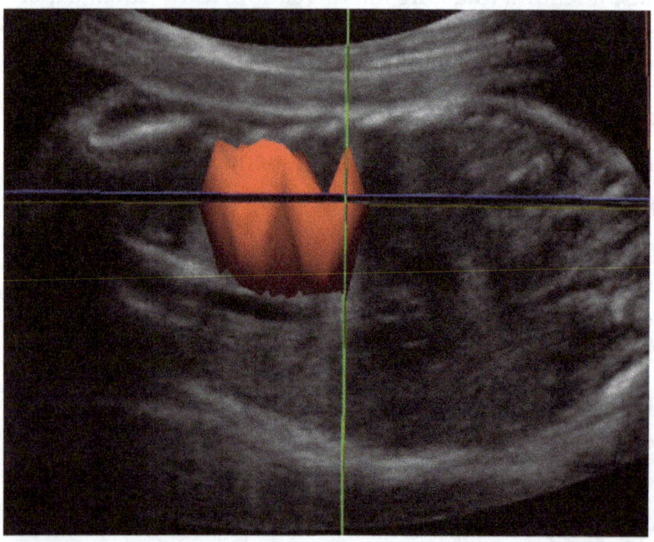

**FIGURE 5.2C** Three-dimensional image of a microcystic CPAM.

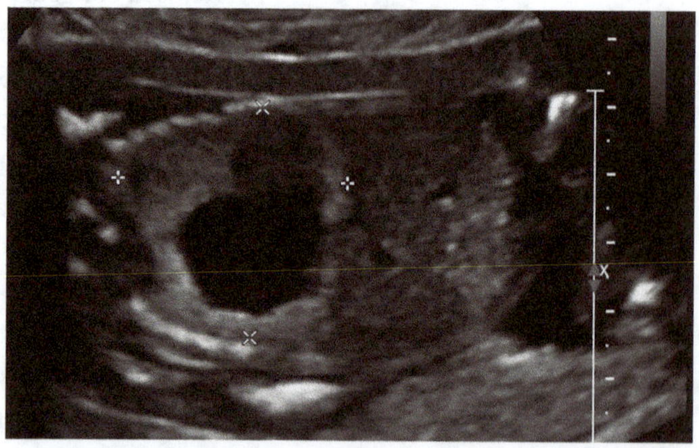

**FIGURE 5.2D** Macrocystic CPAM (+ … +).

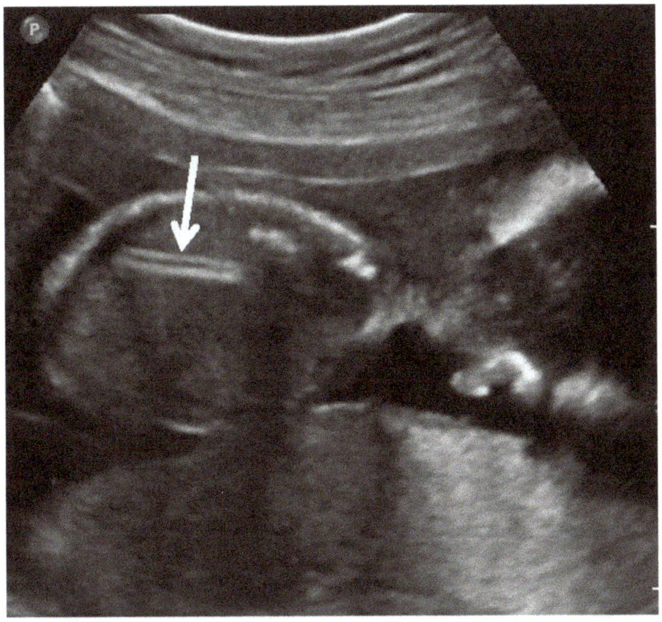


FIGURE 5.2E Shunt (arrow) placed for macrocystic CPAM with hydrops.

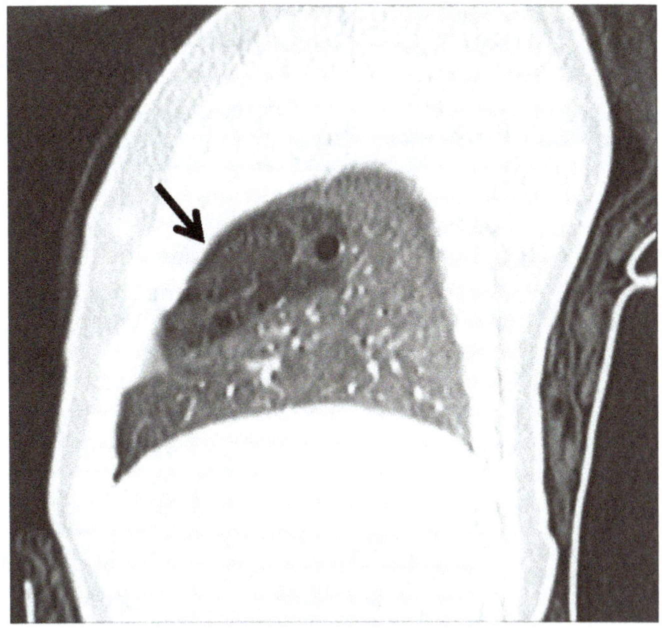

FIGURE 5.2F CT in a neonate with CPAM (arrow).

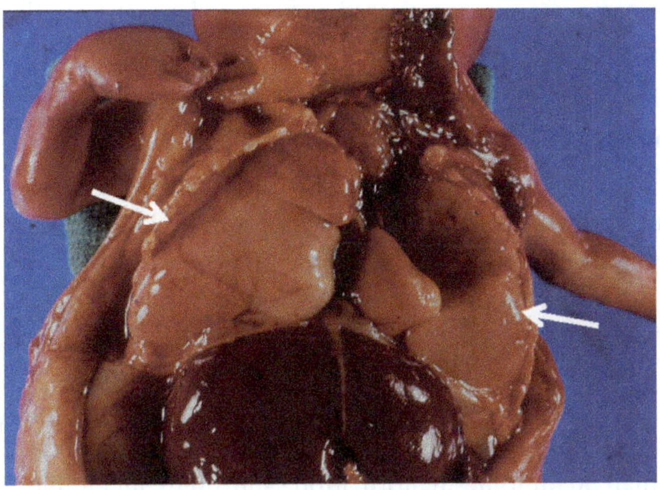

FIGURE 5.2G Fetal lungs with bilateral CPAM (arrows).

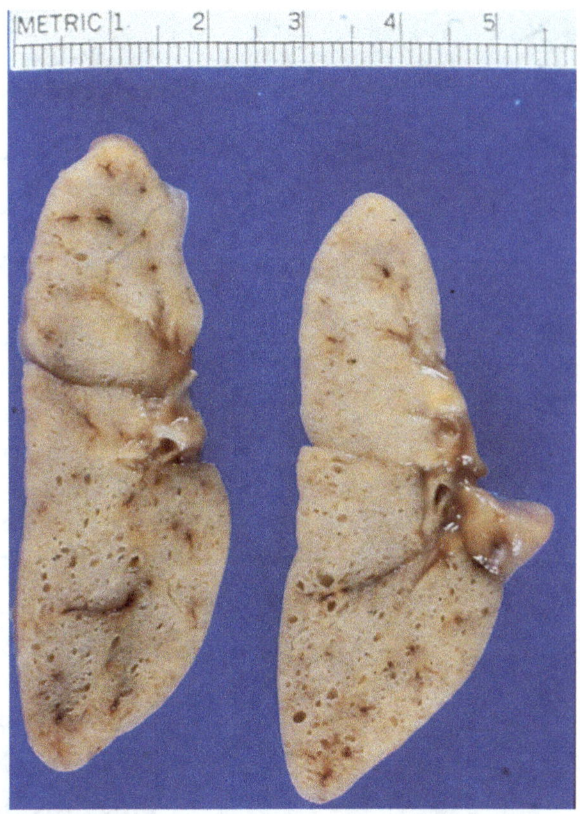


FIGURE 5.2H Gross pathology of lungs with bilateral CPAM.

# 5.3 CONGENITAL DIAPHRAGMATIC HERNIA

## EPIDEMIOLOGY/GENETICS

**Definition** Congenital diaphragmatic hernias (CDHs) involve a group of diaphragmatic defects in which some portion of the abdominal contents protrudes into the chest cavity. This occurs most frequently through a posterolateral (foramen of Bochdalek hernia) or retrosternal (foramen of Morgagni hernia) defect.

- CDH may be considered intrapleural or ventral.
  - Intrapleural
    - Types
      - Left-sided posterolateral defect (Bochdalek): 80%
      - Right-sided defect: 10%
      - Bilateral: 4%
        - Midline positioned heart with abdominal contents on both sides of the chest
        - Associated with severe pulmonary hypoplasia
  - Anterior (Morgagni): 6%
    - Small hernia.
    - Generally, these do not cause pulmonary hypoplasia.
    - Liver or spleen may herniate.
    - If the diaphragm and pericardium are affected, the viscera herniate into the pericardial cavity.
      - A large pericardial effusion may be present.

**Epidemiology** Prevalence is 1 in 3000 to 5000 births (M > F).

**Embryology** Diaphragmatic hernias probably develop between the sixth and the tenth week of gestation, when the gut is returning from the yolk sac and the diaphragm is developing. One mechanism of formation proposes an imbalance in timing of these events, with thoracic migration of the gut, resulting in failure of diaphragmatic closure. Frequently associated abnormalities include cardiac malformations (20% of cases) and central nervous system malformations (30% of cases). Less common are renal anomalies, vertebral defects, pulmonary hypoplasia, and facial clefts. Chromosome abnormalities, such as trisomies 18 and 21, as well as more than 30 multiple-malformation syndromes, including Fryns and Cornelia de Lange syndromes, have been described with diaphragmatic hernias.

**Inheritance Patterns** Generally, inheritance is sporadic. There is less than 2% recurrence risk in siblings for isolated defects. Rare families have shown dominant, X-linked, and recessive inheritance for isolated diaphragmatic hernias. Cases with bilateral defects are more likely to be familial.

**Teratogens** No teratogens are known.

**Prognosis** The two primary factors determining survival are the degree of pulmonary hypoplasia and the coexistence of other abnormalities. The severity of the pulmonary hypoplasia correlates with the volume and content of visceral herniation and is principally related to herniation of the fetal liver. The most sensitive prognostic tool is the measurement of the lung-to-head ratio (volume of contralateral lung divided by the head circumference). Fetuses with a lung-to-head ratio of greater than 1.4 have a good prognosis, and those with a lung-to-head ratio of less than 0.6 are not likely to survive without in utero therapy. There is increasing evidence that MRI data on total fetal lung volume (TFLV) may be even more sensitive in determining survival.

In live-born infants, survival potential has been correlated with age at presentation and severity of gas exchange problems as markers for the degree of pulmonary hypoplasia. Mortality rates of less than 5% are reported for those who are minimally affected to asymptomatic in the first 6 hours with near-normal blood gases. Approximately 30% in the group who are symptomatic early but who can achieve normal blood gases with ventilatory support will die. The mortality is 100% in the most severe group, who are symptomatic from birth and, despite maximal support, do not achieve normal blood gas values. Long-term sequelae, including lower (15 IQ points) cognitive function, have been reported. It should be noted that neonatal survival figures are biased in a positive fashion because of several factors including the following: (1) Survivors may also have late herniation of viscera into the chest or smaller hernias, with lack of prenatal detection. (2) Fetuses with multiple abnormalities may be excluded from the data. (3) Some prenatally diagnosed cases are terminated or have a fetal demise.

## SONOGRAPHY

### FREQUENT FINDINGS

- Herniated abdominal viscera
- Stomach within the chest
- Displaced heart
  - Dextroposition
  - Levoposition
- Paradoxical fetal breathing

### LESS FREQUENT

- Fluid in the chest
- Hydrops
- Polyhydramnios
- Spleen within the chest
- Kidney within the chest
- Superior mesenteric artery deviating into the chest
- Right-sided CDH specific
  - Horizontal orientation of the fetal stomach in the abdomen
  - Marked bowing of the umbilical segment of the portal vein to the left
  - Deviation of the umbilical vein on a transverse image
    - A ratio of the distance from the umbilical vein to the inner left and right rib margin of less than 0.4 is associated with liver herniation.
  - Portal blood flow extending into the chest
  - Gallbladder within the chest

### KEY FINDINGS/PITFALLS

- A normal ultrasound examination at 20 weeks' gestation does not exclude the subsequent development of CDH.
- There is paradoxical fetal breathing—that is, with diaphragmatic movement, the abdominal contents enter the chest on the side of the defect; the diaphragm on the intact side descends appropriately.
- Preferential ductus venosus and inferior vena cava streaming toward the right heart in some cases of left-sided CDH hemodynamically explain the underdevelopment of the left ventricle.
- Assessment of survival with an isolated CDH
  - Currently, liver position is considered a categorical variable (i.e., "up" or "down").
    - MRI or 3-D sonography can assess the volume of liver within the chest.
      - The volume of herniated liver is an independent predictor of postnatal survival.
  - Impaired lung development in CDH has been evaluated with a ratio of the remaining visible lung volume–to–head circumference (lung-head ratio [LHR]).
    - The head circumference is measured in millimeters.
    - The longest two perpendicular transverse diameters of the contralateral lung to the defect (in millimeters) are used to calculate lung area.
    - The predictive accuracy of this ratio has been variable and inconsistent.
  - When fetal MRI is available, an observed to expected TFLV can be obtained in CDH.
    - A value less than 0.35 is associated with a higher neonatal mortality.
  - There is a lower survival rate with antenatally detected cases in contrast to undetected cases.

### DIFFERENTIAL DIAGNOSIS

- Pulmonary sequestration. While there may be a chest mass with dextroposition, the stomach is normally located within the abdomen. A feeding vessel may be identified from the aorta to the intrathoracic mass.
- Hiatal hernias pass through the esophageal hiatus, contain stomach, and therefore are located centrally and posteriorly.

## PREGNANCY MANAGEMENT

**Investigations and Consultations Required** Prenatal diagnosis of CDH requires prompt referral to a tertiary center for consultation with a multidisciplinary team, including neonatology, pediatric surgery, maternal fetal medicine, and genetics. Prenatal assessment to determine the likelihood of survival should include fetal MRI and antenatal ultrasound to assess the severity of pulmonary hypoplasia and the position of the liver; perinatal echocardiography to evaluate for cardiac anomalies; and fetal chromosomal studies, including microarray. Chromosomal studies on fetal blood will miss the chromosome abnormality (isochromosome 12p) seen in Pallister-Killian syndrome, a rare, but lethal, cause of diaphragmatic hernia. Uncultured amniocytes are the best source for fluorescence in situ hybridization (FISH) or microarray assessment to detect isochromosome 12p. Morbidity and mortality are increased in the presence of a right-sided defect, herniation of the liver, lower fetal lung volume, lower LHR, abnormal microarray, and presence of other severe associated congenital anomalies.

**Fetal Intervention** In utero repair of diaphragmatic hernia has been proposed in several forms for a number of years. Open repair of CDH by either fetal thoracotomy or tracheal occlusion has largely been abandoned due to inherent maternal morbidity and prematurity. A minimally invasive approach involving fetoscopic tracheal occlusion with an inflatable balloon is under investigation and holds some promise of improved survival in severe cases. However, technical difficulties are significant, including the need for 24/7 access to a surgical team capable of removing the balloon in the event of preterm birth.

**Monitoring** Patients should undergo repeat ultrasound evaluations every 4 weeks. These examinations should monitor fetal growth and also reexamine the fetus for possible associated anomalies. In addition, the size, position, and content of the defect; the chest structures and their positions; and the liver and the lung volumes should be assessed. Ultrasound (LHR) and MRI (total lung volume) measurements can be used to refine the neonatal prognosis, allowing for more realistic parental expectations of neonatal response to resuscitation. If cardiac structure or precordial vasculature appear compromised, serial fetal echocardiograms may be helpful in assessing cardiac anatomy and function. The development of polyhydramnios is common.

**Pregnancy Course** Polyhydramnios is a common complicating factor and may result in preterm labor. The presence of polyhydramnios is correlated with pulmonary hypoplasia and therefore a worse prognosis. Prematurity markedly worsens outcome.

**Pregnancy Termination Issues** Diaphragmatic hernia is a component of a number of genetic syndromes. To provide appropriate counseling regarding recurrence, a complete external and internal pathologic examination of an intact fetus is required.

**Delivery** There are no fetal indications for early delivery or delivery by cesarean section. Immediate resuscitation is necessary at delivery; therefore, delivery should be in a tertiary center unless the family has opted for comfort care and no intervention.

## NEONATOLOGY

**Resuscitation** At the time of delivery, immediate elective intubation and assisted ventilation is indicated. A repogle tube is placed to decompress the bowel and is maintained at continuous suction. Preductal oxygen saturations are monitored in the delivery room to assess oxygenation with the goal of obtaining preductal oxygen saturations greater than 85%. Umbilical catheters are placed to achieve central access, and maintenance intravenous fluids are started. Volume and inotropic support may be necessary for significant hypotension, poor perfusion, metabolic acidosis, or persistent hypoxemia. Surfactant may be administered to infants less than 34 weeks' gestation.

**Transport** Transfer to a tertiary center with pediatric surgeons, neonatologists, and extracorporeal membrane oxygenation (ECMO) capability is mandatory.

**Testing and Confirmation** Chest radiographs and echocardiography are performed to confirm the presence the diaphragmatic hernia, pulmonary hypertension, or cardiac abnormalities. Because associated anomalies are seen in approximately 50% of cases, chromosomal analysis and microarray should be sent if not obtained antenatally.

**Nursery Management** The objective of respiratory management is to minimize ventilator and oxygen-induced lung injury utilizing a strategy of "gentle ventilation and permissive hypercapnea." Minimizing lung trauma is essential, as barotrauma to the hypoplastic lungs is felt to be a contributing factor for morbidity and mortality. For worsening oxygenation, a trial of inhaled nitric oxide (iNO) starting at 20 ppm may be instituted. High-frequency oscillatory ventilation (HFOV) may be required for infants with persistent hypoxia and hypercarbia refractory to conventional ventilation. Consider gentle sedation, but avoid paralysis if possible. Infants who fail to respond to either conventional ventilation or HFOV may be candidates for ECMO. ECMO is provided as a temporary measure to support the infant until the pulmonary hypertension improves and the infant can be transitioned to conventional ventilation. Care is redirected to comfort measures only in those infants who fail to respond to supportive therapy, including ECMO. Infants who are less than 34 weeks' gestation, have a a birth weight of less than 2 kg, or have been diagnosed with chromosomal anomalies are not candidates for ECMO. Timing of surgical intervention is based on the infant's respiratory status, specifically the severity of pulmonary hypoplasia, pulmonary hypertension, and response to medical management.

## SURGERY

**Preoperative Assessment** The acute pathophysiology of a CDH postnatally results from the combination of pulmonary hypoplasia and pulmonary vascular hypertension. The hypoxemia is therefore the result of pulmonary hypoplasia plus associated pulmonary hypertension, neither of which will be ameliorated by surgical intervention. Surgery is therefore delayed until the infant's respiratory status is stable.

**Operative Indications and Techniques** The operative goals are reduction of the viscera from the thoracic cavity and closure of the diaphragmatic defect.

Surgical options include abdominal versus thoracic repair and open versus a minimally invasive approach. Left posterior-lateral diaphragmatic lesions occur 75% to 80% of the time, and most surgeons prefer an abdominal approach to accomplish the goals mentioned. If a minimally invasive approach is preferred, most surgeons will choose a thoracoscopic approach, and the limited insufflation into the thoracic cavity will help decompress the hernia. Some surgeons may choose a thoracic approach, particularly for the less-frequent right posterior lateral CDH. This defect is associated with a higher incidence of hepatic herniation into the chest and may result in abnormal angulation of the suprahepatic inferior vena cava, with more difficulty in reducing the liver back into the abdomen without occluding the lower body venous return. An abdominal approach for this problem is possible, but a thoracic approach improves surgical exposure and manipulation of the vessels. Rare anterior retrosternal CDH is repaired via the abdominal approach. Posterior lateral CDH is frequently associated with insufficient remaining diaphragmatic musculature and will not allow closure of the defect with native tissue. Tailored nonabsorbable woven plastic prosthetic sheets are used to cover this defect and are attached to the surrounding musculature or chest wall. Unfortunately, there is a significant risk of recurrent hernia in the setting of patch repair, likely due to growth of the infant/child without growth of the patch. The ipsilateral chest is not drained by a chest tube with applied suction because this tends to acutely shift the mobile infant mediastinum and produce hemodynamic instability.

Extracorporeal membrane oxygenation can be used as preoperative therapy to stabilize the neonate with significant pulmonary hypertension. Most commonly, efforts are made to wean and discontinue ECMO support prior to operative repair of the CDH to minimize bleeding complications at the time of surgery. It is critical that the family and the care team recognize that surgical repair of the CDH will not acutely improve oxygenation. Therefore, there is no reason to push forward with repair while on ECMO. ECMO is not applicable in small premature infants because of the need for anticoagulation or in patients who have complex, noncorrectable cardiac defects. There are potential acute, and chronic, complications of ECMO, including the risk of bleeding, renal dysfunction, and neurologic sequelae.

**Surgical Results/Prognosis** The overall survival rate is 65% to 75%. This rate has improved with the use of ECMO and more careful and gentle ventilation. A prenatal diagnosis made before 24 weeks' gestation is associated with poorer long-term results. Morbidity can be related to the congenital defects but can also be iatrogenic. Chronic respiratory insufficiency can occur in survivors and may be related to barotrauma induced by the need for prolonged oxygenation and ventilation. These children have an increased incidence of pathologic gastroesophageal reflux that is frequently unresponsive to standard medical therapy and increases their respiratory and nutritional complications. Long-term problems include failure to thrive and sensorineural hearing loss due to the prolonged need for antibiotics or diuretics. Seizures and developmental delay are seen in 20% to 30% of patients. Scoliosis and pectus excavatum occur in a minority of children.

## SUGGESTED READINGS

1. Ba'ath ME, Jesudason EC, Losty PD: How useful is the lung-to-head ratio in predicting outcomes in the fetus with congenital diaphragmatic hernia? A systematic review and meta-analysis. Ultrasound Obstet Gynecol 2007; 30:897-906.
2. Bootstaylor BS, Filly RA, Harrison MR, Adzick S: Prenatal sonographic predictors of liver herniation in congenital diaphragmatic hernia. J Ultrasound Med 1995; 14:515-520.
3. Bronshtein M, Lewit N, Sujov PO, et al: Prenatal diagnosis of congenital diaphragmatic hernia: timing of visceral herniation and outcome. Prenat Diagn 1995; 15:695-698.

4. Cannie M, Jani J, Chaffiotte P, et al: Quantification of intrathoracic liver herniation by magnetic resonance imaging and prediction of postnatal survival in fetuses with congenital diaphragmatic hernia. Ultrasound Obstet Gynecol 2008; 32:627-632.
5. Conturso R, Giorgetta F, Bellussi F, et al: Horizontal stomach: a new sonographic clue to the antenatal diagnosis of right-sided congenital diaphragmatic hernia (Letter to the editor). Ultrasound Obstet Gynecol 2013; 41:340-342.
6. Gallot D, Boda C, Ughettos S, et al: Prenatal detection and outcome of congenital diaphragmatic hernia: a French registry-based study. Ultrasound Obstet Gynecol 2007; 29:276-283.
7. Getti L, Mari G, Ferguson JE: Color Doppler ultrasonography of the superior mesenteric artery for prenatal ultrasonographic diagnosis of a left-sided congenital diaphragmatic hernia. J Ultrasound Med 2001; 20:689-692.
8. Graf JL, Gibbs DL, Adzick NS, Harrison MR: Fetal hydrops after in utero tracheal occlusion. J Pediatr Surg 1997; 32:214-216.
9. Hedrick HL, Crombleholme TM, Flake AW, et al: Right congenital diaphragmatic hernia: prenatal assessment and outcome. J Pediatr Surg 2004; 39:319-323.
10. Jani J, Keller RL, Benachi A, et al on behalf of the Antenatal-CDH-Registry Group: Prenatal prediction of survival in isolated left-sided diaphragmatic hernia. Ultrasound Obstet Gynecol 2006; 27:18-22.
11. Mehollin-Ray AR, Cassady CI, Cass DL, Olutoye OO: Fetal MR imaging of congenital diaphragmatic hernia. RadioGraphics 2012; 32:1067-1084.
12. Richards DS, Kays DM: Fetal umbilical vein deviation in congenital diaphragmatic hernia. J Ultrasound Med 2013; 32:263-268.
13. Robnett-Filly B, Goldstein RB, Sampior D, Hom M: Morgagni hernia: a rare form of congenital diaphragmatic hernia. J Ultrasound Med 2003; 22:537-539.
14. Ruano R, Benachi A, Joubin L, et al: Three-dimensional ultrasonographic assessment of fetal lung volume as prognostic factor in isolated congenital diaphragmatic hernia. Br J Obstet Gynaecol 2004; 111:423-429.
15. Ruano R, da Silva MM, Campos JA, et al: Fetal pulmonary response after fetoscopic tracheal occlusion for severe isolated congenital diaphragmatic hernia. Obstet Gynecol 2012; 119:93-101.
16. Sista AK, Filly RA: Paradoxical movement of abdominal contents. A real time sonographic finding indicating a congenital diaphragmatic hernia. J Ultrasound Med 2007; 26:1617-1619.

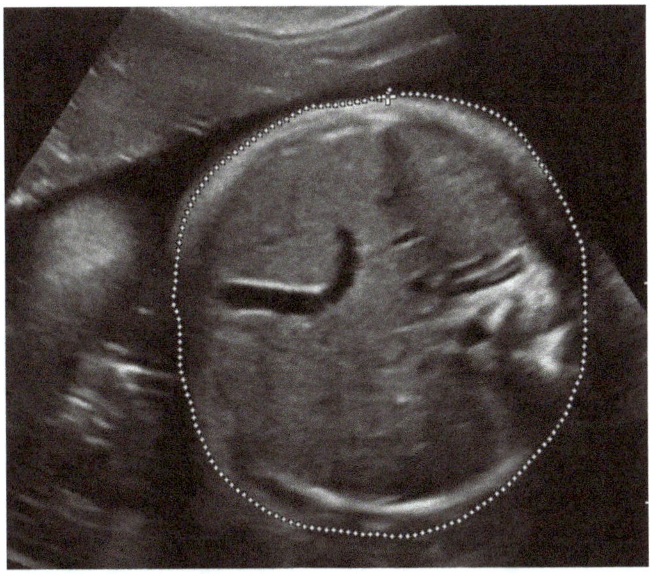

**FIGURE 5.3A** Congenital diaphragmatic hernia. The stomach is not visible in the abdomen.

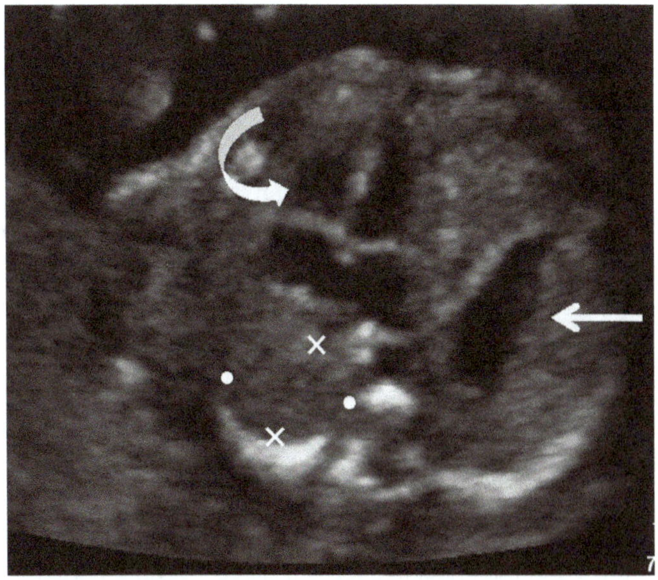

**FIGURE 5.3B** Stomach in the left chest (straight arrow) with cardiac dextroposition (curved arrow) and the ipsilateral lung (∘ … ∘; x … x) visualized.

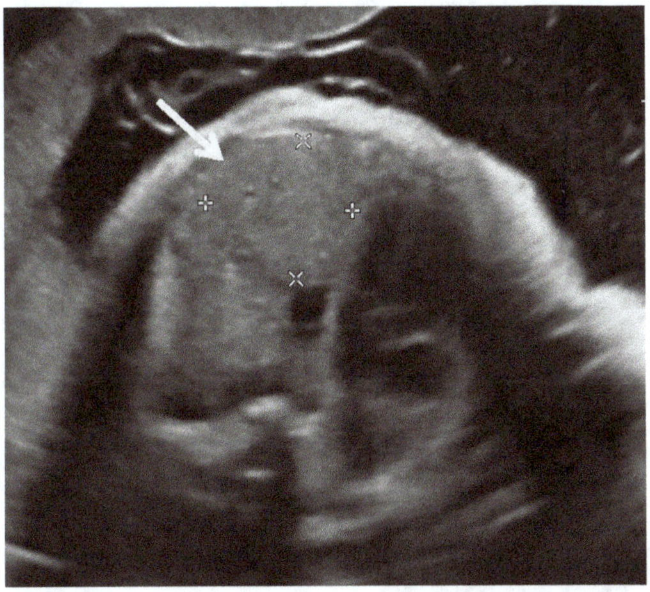

**FIGURE 5.3C** Right-sided diaphragmatic hernia with liver in chest (straight arrow) (+ … +; x … x).

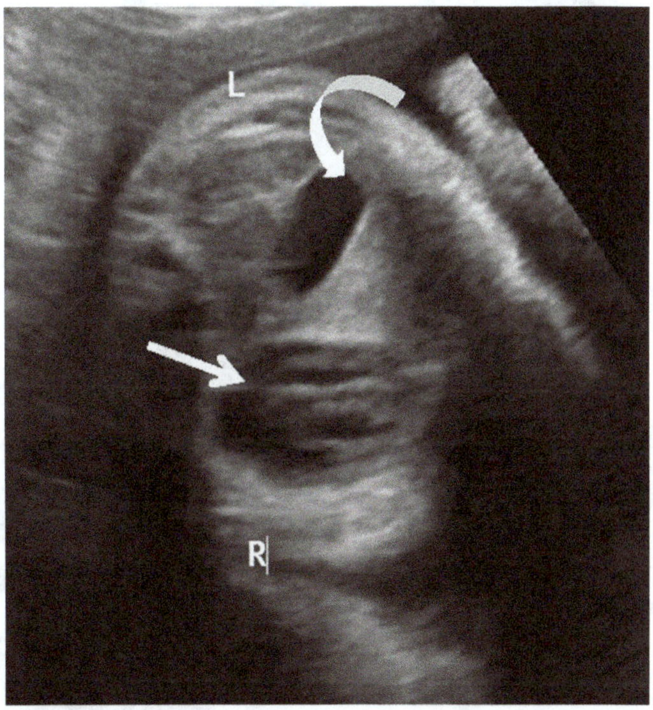


**FIGURE 5.3D** Left-sided congenital diaphragmatic hernia. Left heart underdeveloped (straight arrow), and the stomach (curved arrow) is in the left chest.

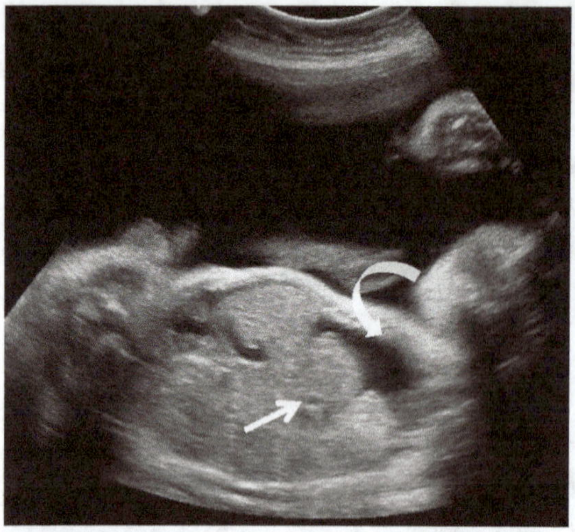

FIGURE 5.3E Right-sided congenital diaphragmatic hernia. Liver (straight arrow) and fluid within the chest (curved arrow). Note the polyhydramnios.

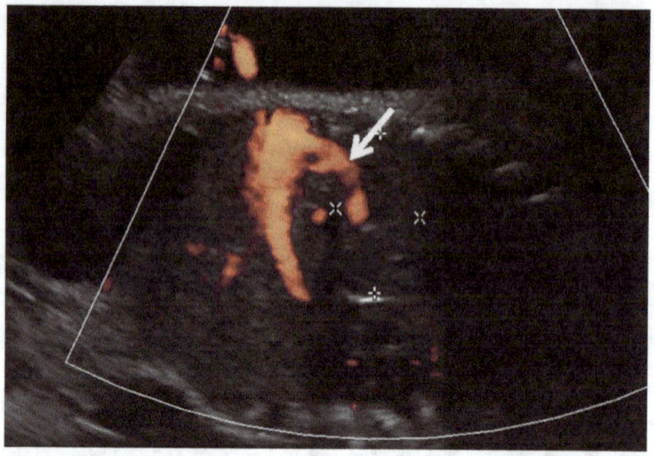

FIGURE 5.3F Liver up congenital diaphragmatic hernia. The portal branch to the left hepatic lobe (arrow) is above the diaphragm. Liver (+ … +; x … x).

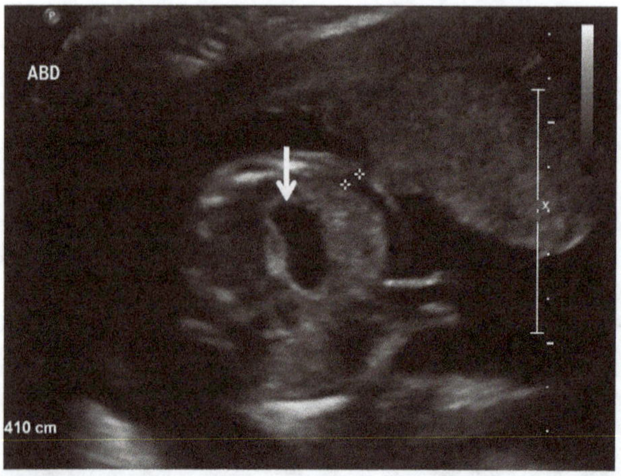


FIGURE 5.3G Horizontal orientation of stomach (arrow) with right-sided CDH.

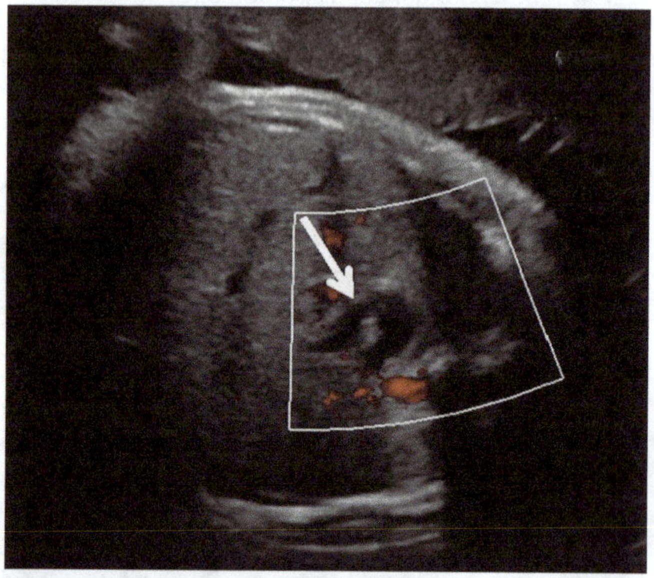

FIGURE 5.3H Hiatal hernia (arrow).

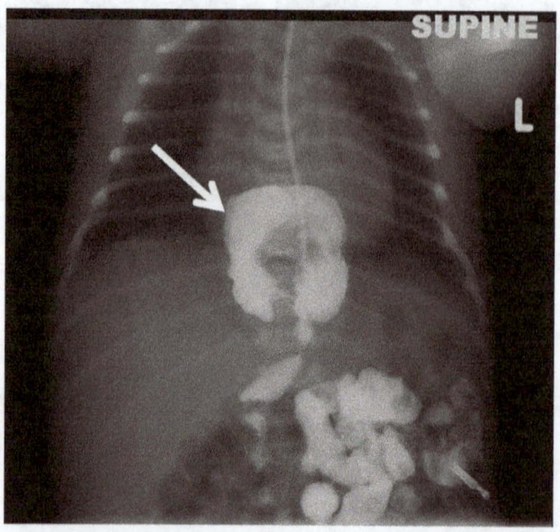


FIGURE 5.3I Neonatal gastrointestinal series of a hiatal hernia (arrow).

# 5.4 HYDROTHORAX

## EPIDEMIOLOGY/GENETICS

**Definition** A pleural effusion is an accumulation of fluid in the pleural space. In the neonate, effusions can be either chylous or clear (hydrothorax), with most primary congenital effusions chylous and occurring on the right. In the fetus, all effusions are clear because the fetus has not ingested protein that is essential to the production of a chylous effusion.

**Epidemiology** This involves 1 in 10,000 to 15,000 births (M2:F1).

**Embryology** The cause of pleural effusions is not known, but they may result from either overproduction of lymph or impaired reabsorption. Pleural effusions may be

- Primary: derived from aberrant lymphatic drainage
- Secondary: multiple pathologic etiologies including karyotypic abnormalities (10%), congenital infection, congenital anomalies (20%), isoimmunization, and maternal fetal hemorrhage
  - Nonimmune hydrops is most commonly associated with the secondary causes of pleural effusions.

More than 50 genetic, chromosome, and sporadic syndromes have been reported that include pleural effusion.

**Inheritance Patterns** A number of genetic syndromes, including Caffey cortical hyperostosis (autosomal dominant) and the Opitz-Frias hypertelorism-hypospadias syndrome (autosomal dominant), have been reported with pleural effusions, hydrops, or chylothorax. The recurrence risk will depend on establishing a precise diagnosis.

**Teratogens** No teratogens are known.

**Prognosis** Overall mortality for pleural effusions presenting in the neonatal period is 25%, ranging from less than 10% for isolated effusions to 95% for those with associated hydrops. Overall mortality for antenatally diagnosed cases is approximately 50%. Mortality is related to hydrops, pulmonary hypoplasia, and prematurity.

## SONOGRAPHY

### FREQUENT FINDINGS

- Fluid within one or both pleural cavities
- Decreased lung volume
- Mediastinal shift
- Diaphragmatic inversion

### LESS FREQUENT

- Hydrops
  - Anasarca
  - Pleural effusion

  - Pericardial effusion
  - Placental thickening
  - Ascites
- Cardiac effect
  - E wave greater than A wave at the mitral valve due to external cardiac compression
- Polyhydramnios

### KEY FINDINGS/PITFALLS

- Spontaneous resolution of primary hydrothorax may occur.
- The risk of a chromosomal abnormality is significantly increased with the first-trimester detection of hydrothorax.
- Earliest diagnosis of bilateral hydrothorax is 8.5 weeks' gestation.
- Overall mortality (50%) is due to pulmonary hypoplasia, prematurity, or hydrops.
- The development of pulmonary hypoplasia is determined by gestational age at onset, the length of time that the effusion persists, and the severity of the effusions.

## PREGNANCY MANAGEMENT

**Investigations and Consultations Required** An extended ultrasound examination should be performed to determine whether the hydrothorax is primary or secondary and whether hydrops is present. Further studies to determine etiology are indicated, including a fetal karyotype and microarray. Maternal viral serology and viral studies of amniotic fluid are indicated to exclude cytomegalovirus (CMV), parvovirus, and other viral etiologies. The significant incidence of congenital heart disease requires fetal echocardiographic evaluation of the fetus. Consultation with a neonatologist is essential to plan perinatal management. Further consultations may be indicated depending on the results of the studies listed and the presumed etiology.

**Fetal Intervention** Fetal intervention is reserved for cases in which the hydrothorax is considered primary, as defined previously. Unless the effusion is large or hydrops is present, the patient can initially be managed expectantly with follow-up examinations. Once hydrops develops or there is significantly abnormal lung volume, fetal treatment should be initiated. Intervention should not be performed until other fetal anomalies have been excluded and chromosome and viral studies are completed and are normal. Those with fetal pleural effusions that are part of nonimmune hydrops from other causes or fetal nonimmune hydrops of unknown etiology are not candidates for intervention.

Initially, a thoracentesis should be performed. Although the fluid will reaccumulate in 75% of patients, it is less invasive than shunt placement. In addition, a failure of the lung to reexpand after thoracentesis suggests that pulmonary hypoplasia has developed and may aid in further treatment planning. If the fluid reaccumulates, a thoracoamniotic shunt may be placed to continuously drain the thorax. Placement of a thoracoamniotic shunt may reverse the hydrops, if present, and result in a good outcome. Prognosis is poor if a significant effusion is diagnosed prior to 32 weeks' gestation, with a reported survival rate of 40% to 45%. However, isolated effusions that are treated with shunting have a more favorable prognosis.

**Monitoring** Persistent effusions require that management be coordinated at a tertiary center. Ultrasonographic examinations should be performed every 1 to 2 weeks to detect progression or development of fetal hydrops. If fetal therapy has been undertaken, the follow-up may be more frequent until the fetal condition stabilizes.

**Pregnancy Course** The pregnancy course may be affected by polyhydramnios and preterm labor.

**Pregnancy Termination Issues** If an accurate diagnosis cannot be made prior to delivery, a nondestructive method of termination should be performed to allow complete fetal evaluation.

**Delivery** Delivery should occur at a tertiary perinatal center. In cases with lung compression from a large effusion and anticipated difficulty with neonatal resuscitation, immediate predelivery thoracentesis or delivery via an EXIT procedure may be useful.

## NEONATOLOGY

**Resuscitation** Preparations should be made for intubation, assisted ventilation, and immediate postdelivery thoracentesis. Term infants who have had drainage of the fluid collections within 24 hours of delivery and infants with small effusions may not require assistance with the onset of respiration.

**Transport** Delivery at a tertiary center is preferable. Transfer after delivery is indicated if bilateral effusions are present, if the fluid reaccumulates after initial drainage, or if the infant requires respiratory support.

**Testing and Confirmation** A chest radiograph will show the extent of the pleural effusion. Further diagnostic evaluation is required to determine the etiology of the pleural effusion. Aspirated pleural fluid is obtained and sent for analysis to determine its classification as transudate, exudate, or chylous fluid.

**Nursery Management** Facilitation of normal cardiorespiratory adaptation is the primary goal. Respiratory distress syndrome may complicate the course if the infant is delivered prematurely, in which case surfactant replacement therapy is indicated. Placement of a thoracotomy tube with continuing pleural drainage for several days may be required.

### SUGGESTED READINGS

1. Cadkin A, Pargament E: Bilateral pleural effusion at 8.5 weeks gestation with Down syndrome and Turner syndrome (Letter to the editor). Prenat Diagn 1993; 13:659-660.
2. Longacker MT, Laberge JM, Danserveau J, et al: Primary fetal hydrothorax: Natural history and management. J Pediatr Surg 1989; 24:573-576.

3. Petersen S, Kaur R, Thomas JT, et al: The outcome of isolated primary fetal hydrothorax: a 10-year review from a tertiary center. Fetal Diagn Ther 2013; 34:69-76.

4. Rodeck CH, Fisk NM, Fraser DI, Nicolini U: Long-term in utero drainage of fetal hydrothorax. N Engl J Med 1985; 319:1135-1138.

5. Rustico MA, Lanna M, Coviello D, et al: Fetal pleural effusion. Prenat Diagn 2007; 27:793-799.

6. Sherer DM, Abromowicz JS, Eggers PC, Woods JR Jr: Transient severe unilateral and subsequent bilateral primary fetal hydrothorax with spontaneous resolution at 34 weeks' gestation associated with normal neonatal outcome. Am J Obstet Gynecol 1992; 166:169-170.

7. Waller K, Chaithongwongwatthana S, Yamasmit W, Donnenfeld AE: Chromosomal abnormalities among 246 fetuses with pleural effusions detected on prenatal ultrasound examination: factors associated with an increased risk of aneuploidy. Genet Med 2005; 7:417-421.

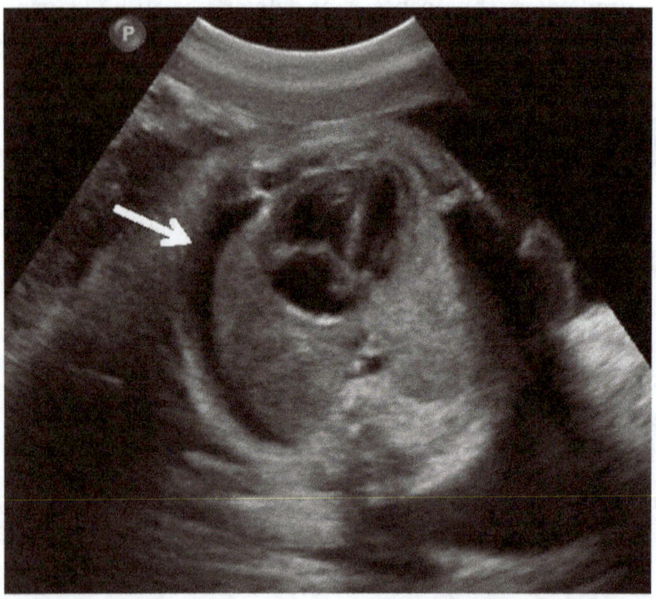

FIGURE 5.4A Unilateral right pleural effusion (arrow).

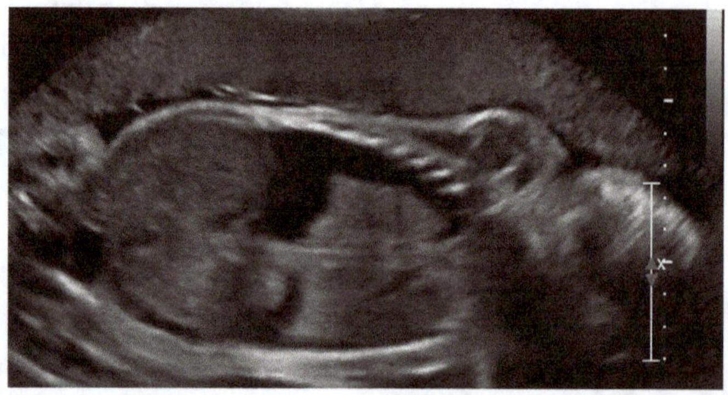

FIGURE 5.4B Bilateral pleural effusions without lung compression.

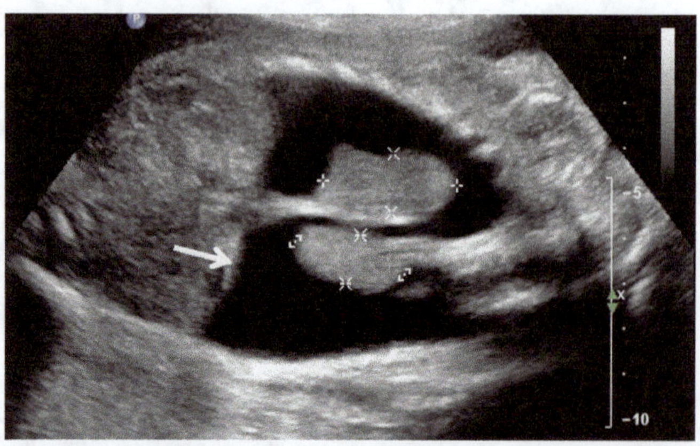



FIGURE 5.4C Bilateral pleural effusions with lung compression (markers). Flattened diaphragm (arrow).

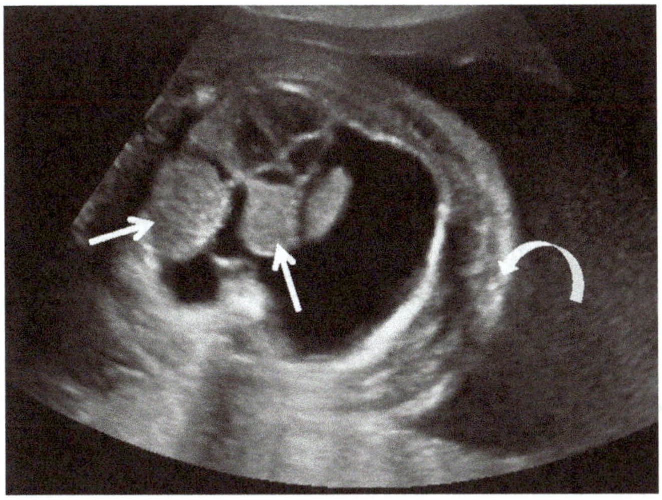

FIGURE 5.4D Bilateral hydrothorax, pulmonary hypoplasia (straight arrows), and anasarca (curved arrow).

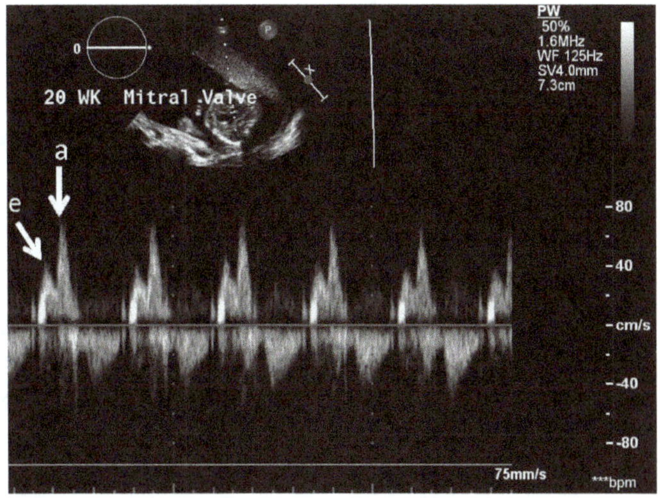


FIGURE 5.4E Normal mitral valve e/a ratio (arrows) at 20 weeks.

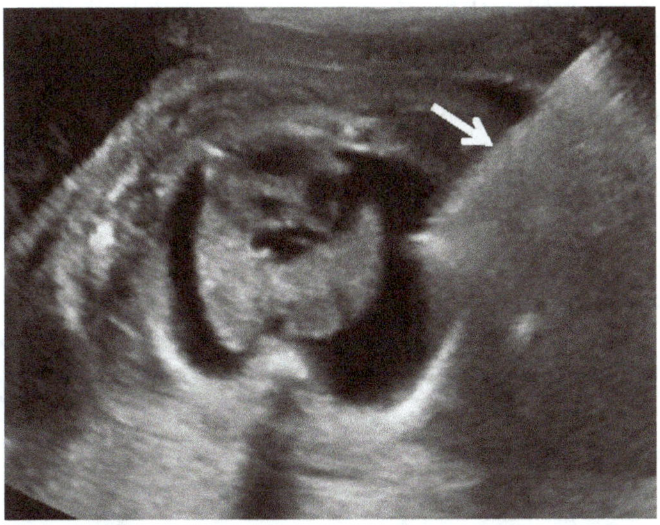

FIGURE 5.4F Thoracentesis for unilateral pleural effusion. Arrow marks the needle.

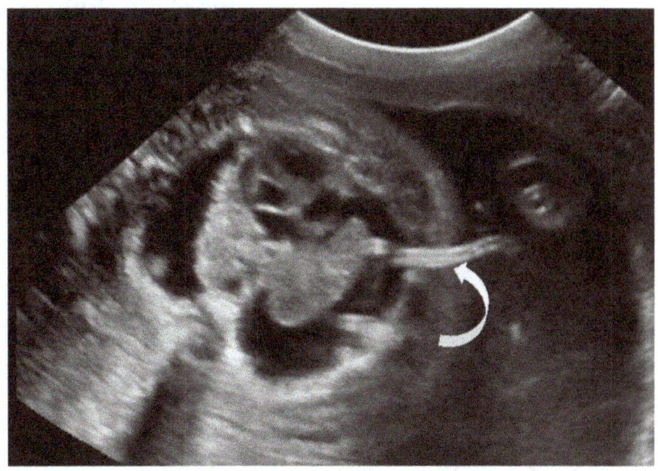

FIGURE 5.4G Pleuro-amniotic shunt (curved arrow).

# 5.5 PULMONARY SEQUESTRATION

## EPIDEMIOLOGY/GENETICS

**Definition** Pulmonary sequestrations (PSs) are intralobar (ILS) and extralobar (ELS) masses of benign pulmonary tissue lacking tracheobronchial communication and having their own vascular supply that usually arises from the thoracic or abdominal aorta. Extralobar PS is anatomic separation from normal lung with a distinct pleural covering. ILS is a lung mass contiguous with normal lung and shares the visceral pleural covering with normal lung parenchyma.

**Epidemiology** Occurrence is 1 in 1000 births (intralobar, M1:F1; extralobar, M1:F4).

**Embryology** Most investigators believe that sequestrations are ectopic pulmonary buds, with the timing of the budding determining the type of sequestration. Early ectopic budding results in ILS, whereas later budding results in the less-common ELS (25%) with its own pleural covering. Ten percent of ELSs lie below the diaphragm. Eighty percent of ELSs are on the left side. Ten percent of ILSs and 50% of ELSs have associated abnormalities, including diaphragmatic hernias, tracheoesophageal fistulas, foregut duplications, congenital heart disease, and renal abnormalities. The incidence of chromosomal abnormalities is not increased with isolated PS. The risk of a chromosomal abnormality does increase with the presence of other anomalies or nonimmune hydrops. Fetuses and newborns with significant vascular shunts can present with congestive heart failure and hydrops. Older children most commonly present with recurrent pulmonary symptoms. One-half of postnatal cases are diagnosed in adults.

**Inheritance Patterns** There is sporadic inheritance.

**Teratogens** None are described.

**Prognosis** In the absence of hydrops or a severe mediastinal shift, there is an 80% to 90% survival rate. Significant, or complete, regression may occur antenatally and is likely due to vascular occlusion or torsion of the feeding vessel. With modern surgical resection, cases with residual tumor at birth have an excellent outcome.

## SONOGRAPHY

### FREQUENT FINDINGS

- Triangular or spherical echogenic mass within the lower chest/suprarenal region
  - Cysts may be present within the mass, especially in hybrid lesions with CPAM.
- Left lung most frequently affected (80%)
- Systemic feeding artery
- Ipsilateral pleural effusion (10%)

### LESS FREQUENT

- Mediastinal shift
- Pulmonary hypoplasia
- Associated congenital anomalies
- Hydrops
- Polyhydramnios

### KEY FEATURES/PITFALLS

- Extralobar sequestration
  - Arterial supply: usually the aorta; other sites include the splenic or gastric artery
  - Venous drainage into the azygous, inferior vena cava, or pulmonary veins
- Intralobar sequestration
  - Arterial supply: aorta
  - Venous drainage: 95% to the pulmonary veins
- The only distinguishing sonographic feature between ILS and ELS is the venous drainage pattern.
- Of ELSs, 80% are on the left; ILS shows no preference for side.
- Most prenatally diagnosed sequestrations are extralobar.
- In some cases of ELS, fluid transudate results in a tension hydrothorax that is due to venous obstruction within the mass.
- Up to 50% of PSs are atypical.
  - Hybrid lesions can have characteristics of PS, as well as CPAM (i.e., histologic features of CPAM with an anomalous aortic vessel).
  - Congenital bronchopulmonary foregut malformations (CBPFMs) have a communication between PS and the gastrointestinal tract. CBPFM, esophageal atresia, and tracheoesophageal atresia are part of a spectrum due to defective budding and separation of the primitive foregut.
- Ultrasound examinations in the first and second trimester may be normal with PS.
- The earliest diagnosis of PS has been at 16 weeks' gestation.
- The antenatal evolution of PS is highly variable.
  - Once an echogenic lung lesion is diagnosed, serial ultrasound examinations are required to monitor the subsequent course of the mass.
  - Over time, a PS may become isoechoic with normal lung.
  - The presence of a midline shift or hydrops indicates a persistent effect from PS, even if its borders cannot be adequately assessed.
- Three-dimensional power Doppler can be used to help identify the feeding vessel of a PS.

### DIFFERENTIAL DIAGNOSIS

- Neuroblastoma
  - Neuroblastomas are usually detected in the third trimester and grow over time. A PS is usually identified in the second trimester and tends to regress over serial ultrasound examinations.

- When there is a normal second-trimester ultrasound examination followed by the detection of a left suprarenal mass in the third trimester, a neuroblastoma is the most likely diagnosis.
- An extralobar PS is usually in the left suprarenal area.

- Congenital lobar emphysema (congenital lobar hyperinflation)
  - There is an echogenic lung mass with normal pulmonary blood flow.
  - An aberrant feeding vessel is not identified.
  - The presence of normal pulmonary blood flow excludes the diagnosis of PS.
- Congenital diaphragmatic hernia
  - Bowel loops within the chest may mimic an echogenic cystic lung mass.
  - A stomach bubble within the abdomen is not identified; the stomach is within the chest.
  - When the liver is in the thoracic cavity, power Doppler can visualize the hepatic vessels extending from the abdomen into the chest.
- Adrenal hemorrhage
  - The changing appearance over time distinguishes an adrenal hemorrhage from ELS.
  - Calcifications may develop within an adrenal hemorrhage.
  - ELS has a systemic feeding vessel.

## PREGNANCY MANAGEMENT

**Investigations and Consultations Required** An extended ultrasound examination should be performed and the diagnosis clearly established. Associated anomalies should be excluded or, if present, may warrant further testing. Fetal echocardiogram is not always necessary but should be performed if hydrops or a pleural effusion is present. Consultation with neonatology or a pediatric surgeon is warranted to establish a fetal management plan.

**Fetal Intervention** In most cases, no intervention is required. If hydrops or a pleural effusion with a mediastinal shift occurs, early delivery or fetal intervention may be indicated, depending on gestational age. Occlusion of the feeding vessel may be considered, although success has been mixed. The poor prognosis in these cases warrants referral to a fetal surgery center for consideration of this option.

**Fetal Monitoring** Fetuses should have monthly ultrasonographic evaluations to monitor the size of the mass. A significant number of lesions will resolve over the course of the pregnancy. However, seeming resolution may be misleading, as the lesion may still be present, because its echotexture is isoechoic with normal lung. Continued monitoring is therefore recommended in cases of apparent resolution. If complications such as hydrops develop, more frequent monitoring is necessary.

**Pregnancy Course** In the absence of fetal hydrops, no specific pregnancy complications are to be expected.

**Pregnancy Termination Issues** If termination is chosen, a nondestructive method is necessary to establish a precise diagnosis.

**Delivery** In the absence of fetal hydrops, delivery should be at term in a tertiary center. The development of hydrops after 32 weeks should prompt steroid administration to enhance fetal lung maturity, and delivery should be accomplished.

## NEONATOLOGY

**Resuscitation** The prenatal presentation and course determine the immediate postdelivery management. The clinical presentation is variable and depends on the type, size, and location of the lesion. Three distinct antenatal courses have been identified: (1) progressive enlargement with compression of thoracic viscera, pleural effusion, or hydrops (a rare outcome in PS); (2) involution of the mass prior to delivery; and (3) persistent mass without associated complications. Infants presenting with hydrops are at increased risk for morbidity and mortality. In the presence of respiratory distress, intubation and mechanical ventilation may be required.

**Transport** Transfer to a tertiary center with pediatric medical and surgical subspecialists is always indicated in infants with symptomatic PS. An experienced neonatal transport team is essential to maintain cardiorespiratory function during the transfer.

**Testing and Confirmation** The distinguishing diagnostic finding for sequestration, compared to other chest masses, is the presence of an aberrant vasculature, which may be demonstrated by ultrasonography with Doppler color flow, CT, or MRI. On chest radiograph, an opaque mass usually is seen.

**Nursery Management** Initially, support of adequate pulmonary gas exchange and cardiac output is the principal focus of care. Timing of surgery is based on the clinical course, the presence of other anomalies, the degree of respiratory distress, and other complicating factors.

## SURGERY

**Preoperative Assessment** Acute management includes evaluation of the degree of respiratory insufficiency and identification of major associated anomalies, most notably cardiac defects.

**Operative Indications** The newborn with intra-abdominal BPS usually has no respiratory compromise and can undergo elective resection. The management of the newborn infant with an intrathoracic BPS is determined by the severity of pulmonary hypoplasia. Therapeutic needs may vary from minimal (not requiring ventilatory support) to severe (requiring ventilatory and vasopressor support, alkalinization, HFOV, or ECMO). Overall, it is relatively rare to have significant respiratory compromise. Large pleural effusions should be treated immediately by tube thoracostomy. In the infant with pulmonary hypoplasia secondary to BPS, thoracotomy should be deferred until it is clear that the infant has stabilized. The infant's condition often deteriorates after surgery because of changes in chest wall compliance and pulmonary vascular resistance, superimposed on pulmonary hypoplasia.

In the case of the prenatally diagnosed BPS that appears to regress, postnatal imaging studies should be performed. If the lesion is evident on plain chest radiograph, surgical resection should be planned. If the chest radiograph does not demonstrate the malformation, CT or MRI should be performed, but deferred until several months of age. Even though these lesions are asymptomatic, postnatal resection should be performed because of the risk of infection, hemorrhage, and malignant transformation.

**Types of Procedures** A posterolateral thoracotomy, or more commonly thoracoscopy, with resection of the involved lobe is the standard therapy used. Intra-abdominal sequestrations are treated by resection. The surgical approach to BPS is straightforward, with the exception of the management of anomalous blood supply. These vessels are often huge, thin walled, and elastic rather than muscular arteries. In 20% of cases, these vessels are subdiaphragmatic in origin, and in 15%, more than one vessel is present. Subdiaphragmatic origin of anomalous vessels is more common with right-sided lesions. These vessels can retract into the mediastinum or diaphragm and continue to bleed. Intraoperative death due to hemorrhage from unrecognized anomalous vessels has been reported. Of note, one series reported that 60% of right-sided ILSs had anomalous venous return compatible with the scimitar syndrome. The importance of preoperative assessment of venous drainage, as well as arterial supply, is underscored by the reports of postoperative fatalities due to ligation of anomalous veins that constituted the sole or major venous drainage of the entire ipsilateral lung. Occlusion of the supplying vessel by angiographic techniques is an alternative approach.

**Surgical Results/Prognosis** Most children with uncomplicated cases of intrathoracic or intra-abdominal sequestration have an excellent prognosis. Those cases with a higher incidence of associated anomalies or fetal hydrops have a much lower survival rate and poorer long-term outcome, with chronic respiratory insufficiency the major complication. The presence of fetal hydrops is ominous, with few survivors expected if in utero therapy is not instituted.

## SUGGESTED READINGS


1. Adzick NS: Management of fetal lung lesions. Clin Perinatol 2003; 30:481-492.
2. Azizkhan RG, Crombleholme TM: Congenital cystic lung disease: contemporary antennal and postnatal management. Pediatr Surg Int 2008; 24:643-657.
3. Bratu I, Flageole H, Chen MF, et al: The multiple facets of pulmonary sequestration. J Pediatr Surg 2001; 36:784-790.
4. Cass DL, Crombleholme TM, Howell LJ, et al: Cystic lung lesions with systemic arterial blood supply: a hybrid of congenital cystic adenomatoid malformation and bronchopulmonary sequestration. J Pediatr Surg 1997; 32:986-990.
5. Curtis MR, Mooney DP, Vaccaro TJ, et al: Prenatal ultrasound characterization of the suprarenal mass: distinction between neuroblastoma and subdiaphragmatic extralobar pulmonary sequestration. J Ultrasound Med 1997; 16:75-83.

6. Dhingsa R, Coakley F, Albanese CT, et al: Prenatal sonography and MRI imaging of pulmonary sequestration. Am J Roentgenol 2003; 180:433-437.
7. Gomez L, Robert JA, Sepulveda W: Fetal retroperitoneal pulmonary sequestrataion with an atypical vascular pattern. Prenat Diagn 2009; 29:290-291.
8. Kitano Y, Matsuoka K, Honna T, et al: Venous anterialization in extralobar pulmonary sequestration associated with fetal hydrops. J Pediatr Surg 2006; 41:490-494.
9. Puligandla P, Laberge JM: Congenital lung lesions. Clin Perinatol 2012; 39:331-347.
10. Ruano R, Benachi A, Aubry M-C, et al: Prenatal diagnosis of pulmonary sequestration using three-dimensional power Doppler ultrasound. Ultrasound Obstet Gynecol 2005; 25:128-133.
11. Ruano R, de A Pimenta EJ, da Silva MM, et al: Percutaneous intrauterine laser ablation of the abnormal vessel in pulmonary sequestration with hydrops at 29 weeks' gestation. J Ultrasound Med 2007; 26:1235-1241.
12. Smulian JC, Guzman ER, Ranzini AC, et al: Color and duplex Doppler sonographic investigation of in utero spontaneous regression of pulmonary sequestration. J Ultrasound Med 1996; 15:789-792.
13. Vijayaraghaven SB, Rao PS, Selvarasu CD, Rao TM: Prenatal sonographic features of intralobar bronchopulmonary sequestration. J Ultrasound Med 2003; 22:541-544.
14. Zeidan S, Gorincour G, Potier A, et al: Congenital lung malformation: evaluation of prenatal and postnatal radiological findings. Respirology 2009; 14:1005-1011.

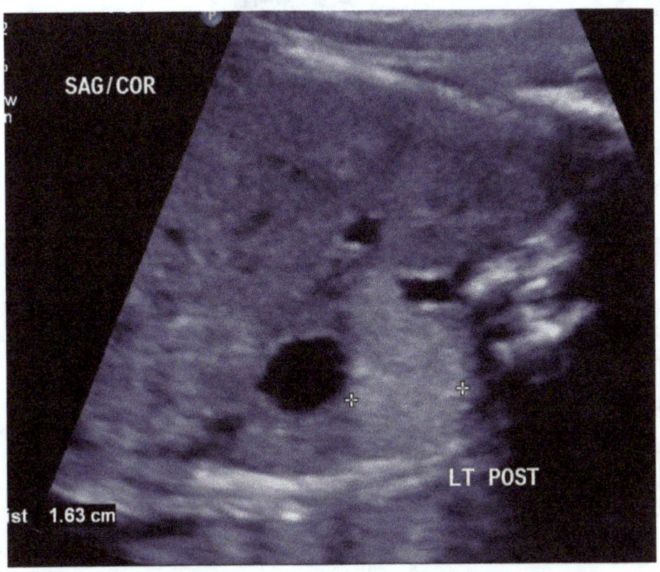


**FIGURE 5.5A** Extrapulmonary sequestration (+ … +).

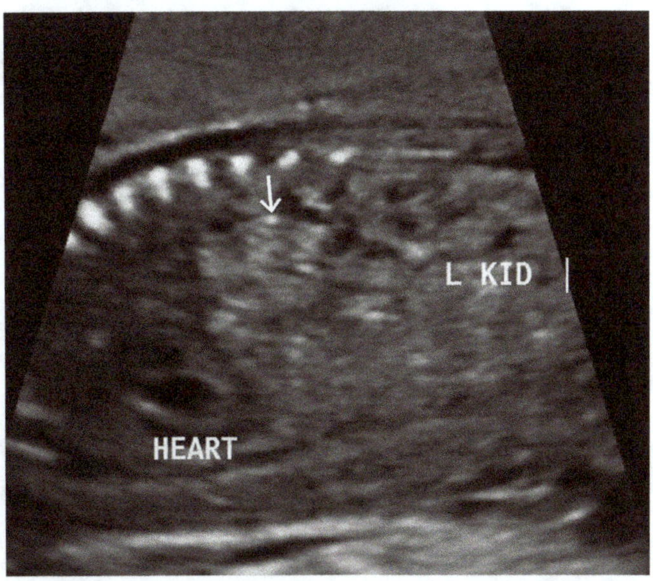


**FIGURE 5.5B** Left subdiaphragmatic extrapulmonary sequestration (arrow) adjacent to the left kidney (L KID).

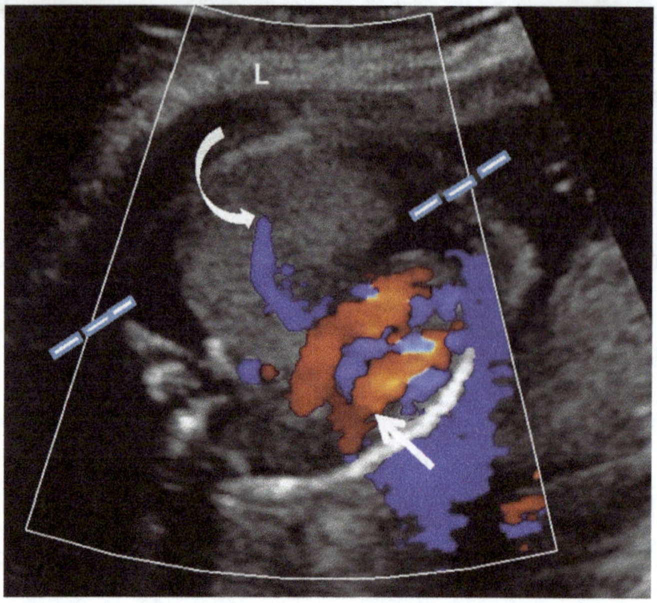


**FIGURE 5.5C** Extrapulmonary sequestration with the heart in dextroposition (straight arrow). Note the feeding vessel (curved arrow) and pleural effusion (– – –).

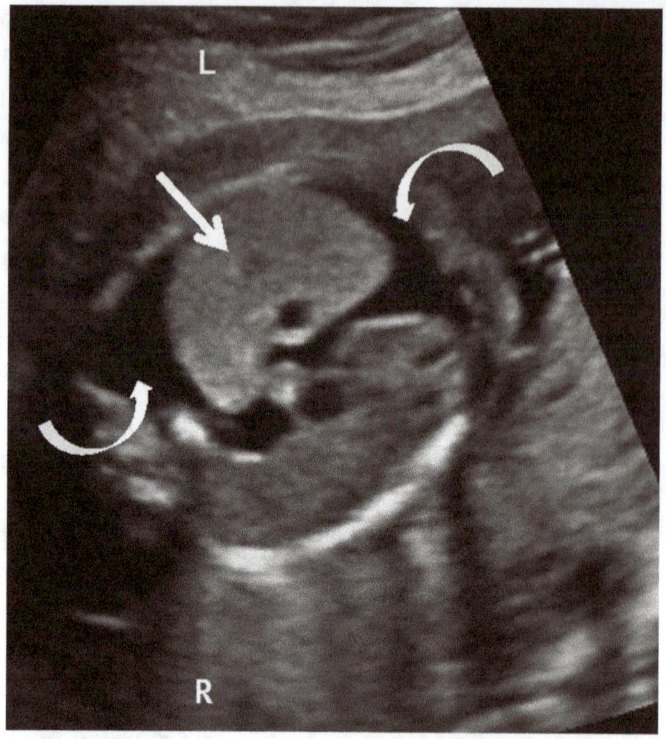


**FIGURE 5.5D** Hybrid extrapulmonary sequestration and congenital pulmonary airway malformation (straight arrow) with a pleural effusion (curved arrows).

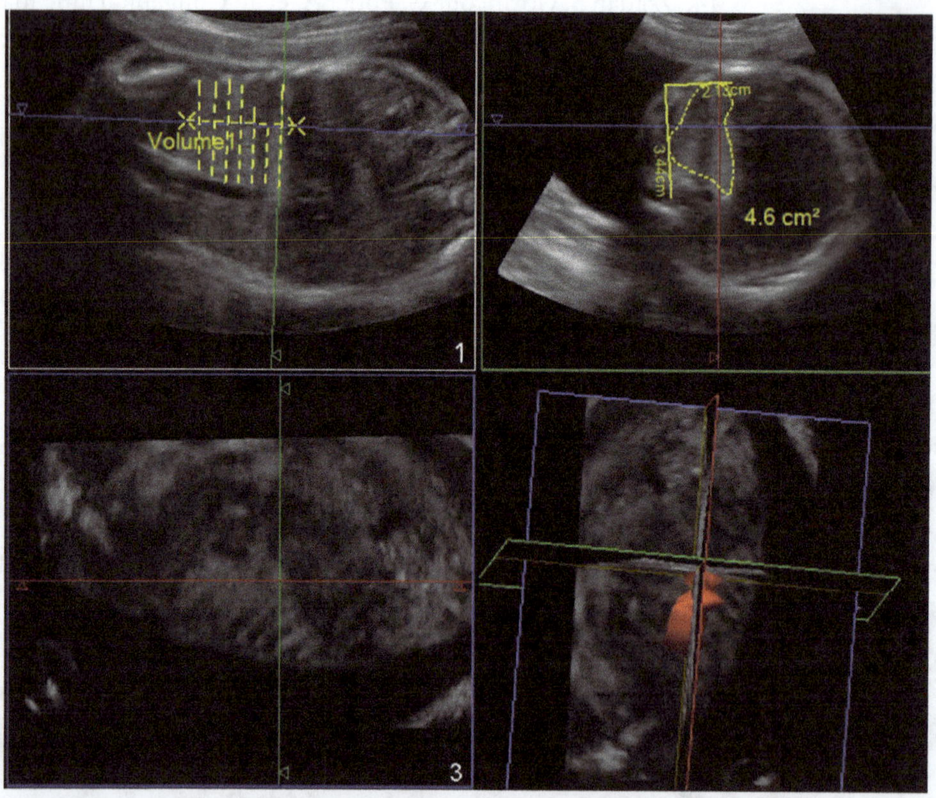


**FIGURE 5.5E** Three-dimensional multiplanar imaging and volume of PS.

# CHAPTER 6

# THE GASTROINTESTINAL SYSTEM

# 6.1 ANAL ATRESIA

## EPIDEMIOLOGY/GENETICS

**Definition** Anal atresia is the congenital absence of an anal opening.

**Epidemiology** Occurrence is 1 5000 births (M3:F2).

**Embryology** Anal atresia results from an arrest in the division of the cloaca into the urogenital sinus and rectum that occurs during the ninth week of fetal development. There are two types: (1) high anal atresia, which is above the levator sling and is associated with urinary tract fistula in males or complex cloacal anomalies in the female; and (2) low anal atresia, which is below levator sling and is not associated with urinary fistula in males or the vagina in females. More than 80 genetic, chromosomal, and sporadic syndromes have been reported with anal atresia. Associated abnormalities occur in 85% of cases and include spinal/skeletal abnormalities, genitourinary abnormalities (50%), tracheoesophageal abnormalities, and cardiac malformations. The VACTERL (vertebral defects, anal atresia, cardiac defects, tracheoesophageal fistula [TEF], renal anomalies, limb abnormalities) association should be considered in these cases. Caudal regression and the OEIS (omphalocele, exstrophy of the bladder, imperforate anus, and spinal defects) sequence also may have anal atresia as a feature. Trisomies 18 and 21 both have been reported in cases of anal atresia.

**Inheritance Patterns** Inheritance is sporadic, with a 3% to 4% recurrence risk in first-degree relatives. However, the genetic syndromes with anal atresia as a feature include ones that are autosomal recessive, autosomal dominant, and multifactorial.

**Teratogens** Alcohol, thalidomide, and maternal diabetes are teratogenic.

**Prognosis** Prognosis is dependent on associated malformations and the nature of the anal atresia. Of isolated cases, 80% to 90% will have successful functional repair.

## SONOGRAPHY

### FREQUENT FINDINGS

- Absence of an "anal dimple"
- Dilated colon/rectum (15% to 40%)
- Associated anomalies (85%)
  - Urogenital anomalies (54%)
    - Bilateral renal agenesis
    - Urethral atresia
    - Cloacal anomaly

### LESS FREQUENT

- Calcified meconium due to vesicocolic fistula

### KEY FINDINGS/PITFALLS

- There is a low prenatal detection rate: sensitivity (8%); positive predictive value (15%).
- First-trimester prenatal diagnosis has been reported.
  - Early bowel dilatation may resolve.
- Primary diagnostic clue: enterolithiasis: Coprolites form in the intestine in the presence of urine.
- A V- or U-shape segment of dilated bowel in the lower pelvis suggests anorectal atresia.
- The absence of the fetal anal sphincter can be used to diagnose an imperforate anus.
  - A transverse image of the anus has a "bull's-eye" appearance.
- Associated anomalies allow prenatal diagnosis.
  - Most frequently, it is diagnosed as part of VACTERL.
- Anal atresia is associated with complete or partial urorectal septal malformation (URSM).
  - In complete URSM, there is an absence of the perineal and anal opening.
    - Usually, this is lethal due to pulmonary hypoplasia from oligohydramnios.
  - In partial URSM, there is a single outlet for urine and feces.
- Dilated bowel may not be apparent until the third trimester.
  - Bowel dilatation may be transient in the second or third trimester.

### DIFFERENTIAL DIAGNOSIS

- Hirschsprung disease
  - There is congenital absence of ganglion cells of the mysenteric plexus.
  - There is a dilated loop of distal bowel.
  - Haustral markings are present.
  - There is an absence of peristalsis.
  - Bowel involvement:
    - Entire colon: 10%
    - Rectosigmoid: 74%
    - Distal-to-splenic flexure: 90%
  - Ten percent have associated meconium peritonitis.

## PREGNANCY MANAGEMENT

**Investigations and Consultations Required** Fetal echocardiography should be performed to diagnose associated cardiovascular anomalies. Amniocentesis should be performed for chromosomal analysis and chromosomal microarray, especially if other anomalies are present. Fetal magnetic resonance imaging (MRI) may be helpful in defining the type of lesion and presence of associated anomalies. Consultation with a pediatric surgeon is indicated.

**Monitoring** Standard obstetric care is appropriate.

**Pregnancy Course** No specific obstetric complications are to be expected.

**Pregnancy Termination Issues** The late clinical presentation of this malformation generally will preclude the option of pregnancy termination.

**Delivery** The high association with other abnormalities makes delivery at a tertiary center with multiple pediatric and surgical subspecialists the best option. A pediatric geneticist should be available to evaluate the neonate for a possible genetic syndrome.

## NEONATOLOGY

**Resuscitation** There are no special issues for delivery room management with isolated anal atresia. If other associated anomalies exist, then management may need to be directed toward their related issues.

**Transport** Transfer to a tertiary center having a pediatric surgeon is always indicated. Beyond orogastric decompression, there are no special precautions during transfer.

**Testing and Confirmation** This should be obvious on newborn examination. Postnatal radiologic studies will define the defect. The newborn should undergo plain films of the lumbar-sacral segments to assess for completeness, as this will have a significant impact on the long-term prognosis regarding continence. In addition, a spinal ultrasound should be completed for assessment of a tethered cord, a commonly associated finding. Renal ultrasound and cardiac echocardiogram are done to complete the workup and assess for other anomalies.

**Nursery Management** Once the lack of patency of the anus has been established, all enteral intake is contraindicated. Maintenance intravenous fluids should be administered. Nasogastric decompression should be maintained.

### SUGGESTED READINGS


1. Berlin B, Corteville JE, Langer JC: How accurate is prenatal sonography for the diagnosis of imperforate anus and Hirschsprung's disease? Pediatr Surg Int 1995; 10:30-32.
2. Brantberg A, Blaas H-GK, Haugen SE, et al: Imperforate anus: a relatively common anomaly rarely diagnosed prenatally. Ultrasound Obstet Gynecol 2006; 28:904-910.
3. Eliyahu S, Yanai N, Blondheim O, et al: Sonographic presentation of Hirschsprung's disease. A case of an entirely aganglionic colon and ileum. Prenat Diagn 1994; 14:1170-1172.
4. Kaponis A, Paschopoulos M, Paraskevaidis E, Makrydimas G: Fetal anal atresia presenting as transient bowel dilatation at 16 weeks' of gestation. Fetal Diagn Ther 2006; 21:383-385.
5. Lubusky M, Prochazka M, Dhaifalah I, et al: Fetal enterolithiasis: prenatal sonographic and MRI diagnosis in two cases of ureorectal septum malformation (URSM) sequence. Prenat Diagn 2006; 26:345-349.
6. Moon MH, Cho JY, Kim JH, et al: In-utero development of the fetal anal sphincter. Ultrasound Obstet Gynecol 2010; 35:556-559.

7. Pohl-Schickinger A, Henrich W, Degenhardt P, et al: Echogenic foci in the dilated fetal colon may be associated with the presence of a recto-urinary fistula. Ultrasound Obstet Gynecol 2006; 28:341-344.
8. Taipale P, Rovamo L, Hilesmaa V: First-trimester diagnosis of imperforate anus. Ultrasound Obstet Gynecol 2005; 25:187-188.
9. Vijayaraghavan SB, Prema AS, Suganyadevi P: Sonographic depiction of the fetal anus and its utility in the diagnosis of anorectal malformations. J Ultrasound Med 2011; 30:37-45.
10. Wheeler PG, Weaver DD: Partial urorectal septum malformation sequence. Am J Med Genet 2001; 103:99-105.

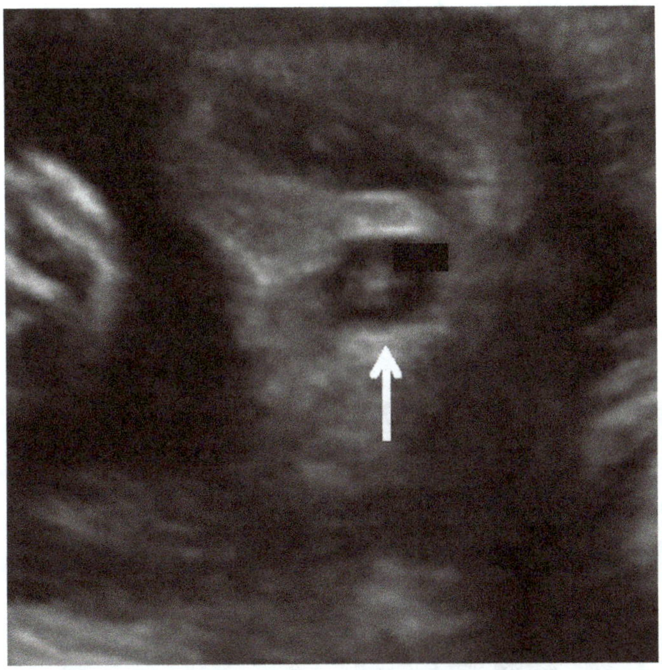

FIGURE 6.1A Perianal muscular complex illustrating the normal anus (arrow).

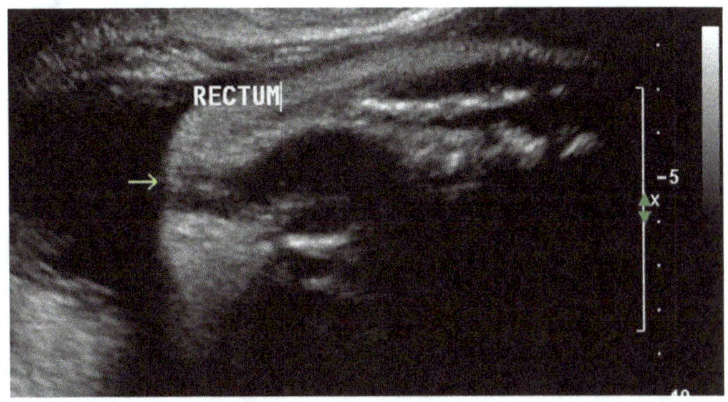


FIGURE 6.1B Normal rectum (arrow).

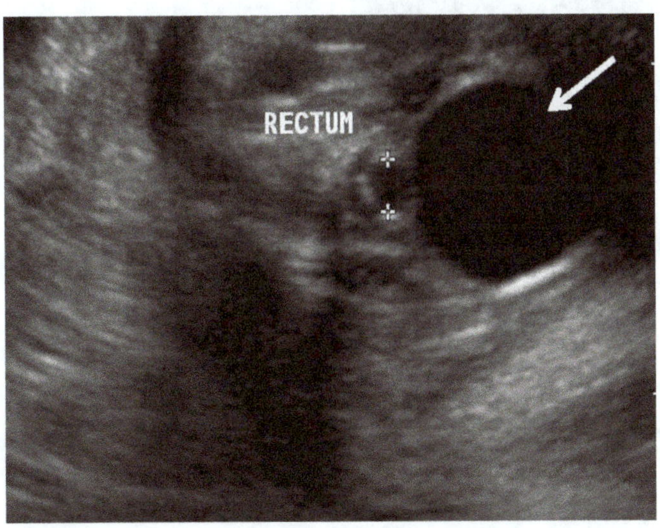


FIGURE 6.1C Rectum (+ … +) and adjacent bladder (arrow).

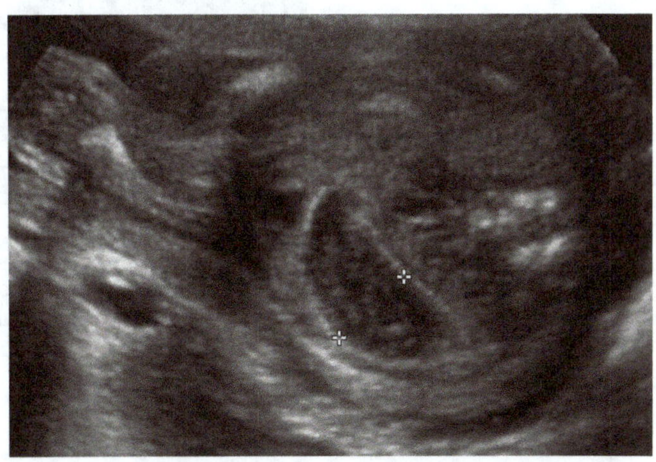

FIGURE 6.1D Anal atresia: dilated loop of colon (+ … +).

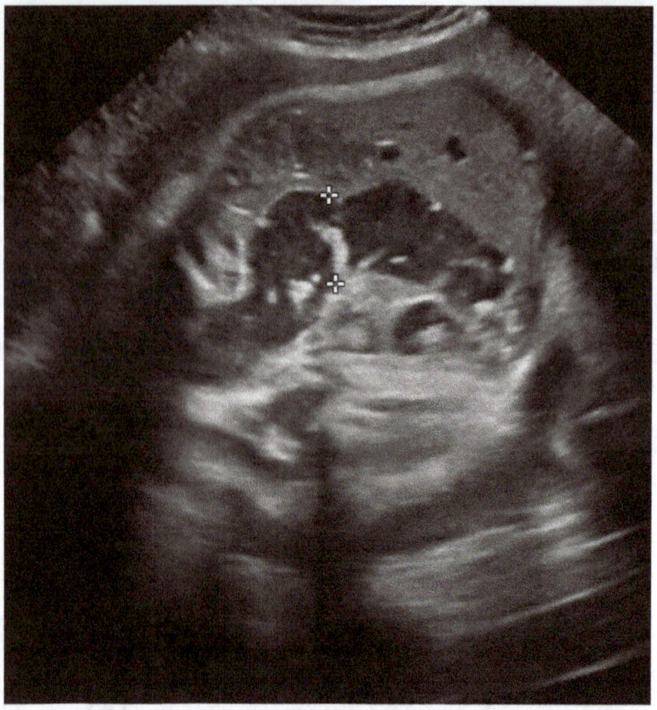

FIGURE 6.1E Imperforate anus with dilated colon (+ … +).

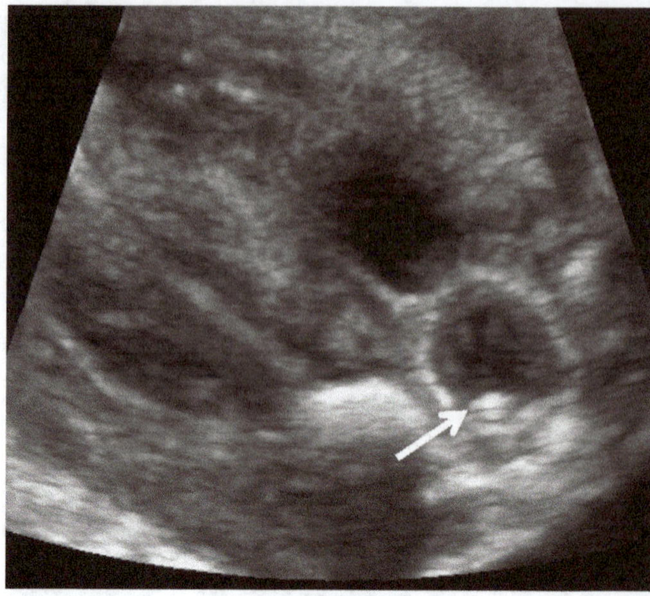

FIGURE 6.1F Anal atresia illustrating urolithiasis (arrow).

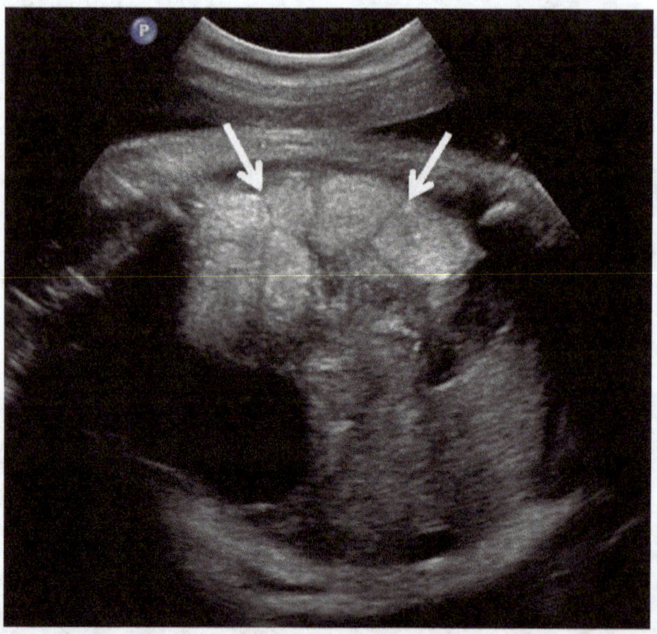

FIGURE 6.1G Third-trimester normal large bowel containing meconium. Haustral markings (arrow) are well delineated.

# 6.2 DUODENAL ATRESIA

## EPIDEMIOLOGY/GENETICS

**Definition** Duodenal atresia is characterized by complete obliteration of the lumen of the duodenum and is the most common type of congenital small bowel atresia.

**Epidemiology** Incidence is 1 in 6000 to 1 in 10,000 births or 1 in 3500 in the second trimester.

**Embryology** At 6 weeks of embryonic life, the lumen of the duodenum is obliterated by proliferating epithelium. Patency is usually restored by the 11th week. Failure of this recanalization results in duodenal atresia. Another anatomical mechanism causing duodenal obstruction is an annular pancreas. An annular pancreas most likely results from a failure of completion of pancreatic rotation, and as a result, there is pancreatic tissue present circumferentially around the duodenum. Associated abnormalities occur in 50% of patients, with trisomy 21 occurring in 30% to 40% of cases. Additional abnormalities include skeletal defects (vertebral, rib, sacral agenesis, radial anomalies, and clubfoot); gastrointestinal abnormalities (annular pancreas, esophageal atresia [EA], TEF, intestinal malrotation, Meckel's diverticulum, and anal atresia); cardiac malformations; and renal defects. More than 15 genetic, chromosome, and sporadic syndromes have been reported with duodenal atresia.

**Inheritance Patterns** Generally, inheritance is sporadic, with rare reports of autosomal dominant inheritance.

**Teratogens** Maternal diabetes is teratogenic.

**Prognosis** Mortality is due to associated abnormalities or preterm labor (50% of cases). With current neonatal and surgical management, mortality and morbidity are only about 5%.

## SONOGRAPHY

### FREQUENT FINDINGS

- Distended stomach
- Distended duodenum
- Continuity between a distended stomach and duodenum
- Associated congenital anomalies
  - Trisomy 21
  - Cardiac
  - Tracheoesophageal fistula
  - Renal anomalies
  - Bowel atresias
  - Vertebral anomalies
- Late second- and third-trimester polyhydramnios

### KEY POINTS/PITFALLS/DIFFERENTIAL DIAGNOSIS

- Duodenal duplication cyst:
  - There is lack of communication between a dilated stomach and the duplication cyst.
- Earliest diagnosis of duodenal atresia is at 14 weeks.
  - Usually, it is identified after 24 weeks' gestation.
  - Gastric motility and emptying increase significantly after 24 weeks' gestation.
- Duodenal atresia is occasionally associated with EA, resulting in a "C-shaped" upper abdominal cystic mass. The combination of EA with TEF and duodenal atresia may result in surgical urgency or emergency due to the increasing distension of the obstructed stomach.

## PREGNANCY MANAGEMENT

**Investigations and Consultation Required** An extended ultrasound examination to search for any anomalies in other organ systems should be undertaken. A fetal echocardiogram is warranted to exclude fetal heart defects, as these are relatively common. A fetal karyotype and microarray should be performed. Consultation with neonatology and a pediatric surgeon is indicated for the family to discuss neonatal management.

**Fetal Intervention** No intervention is warranted.

**Monitoring** The diagnosis is usually made in the third trimester. Follow-up ultrasound examinations to monitor the degree of polyhydramnios should be scheduled monthly, depending on maternal symptoms. As preterm labor is common, prenatal visits should also be scheduled at intervals to detect this and the patient educated on signs and symptoms.

**Pregnancy Course** The major obstetric complication of this disorder is severe polyhydramnios with a high incidence of preterm labor. In cases of polyhydramnios with severe maternal discomfort or respiratory compromise, a therapeutic amniocentesis is indicated. Whether it also abates preterm labor is less certain. As the fluid will reaccumulate rapidly, this procedure may need to be repeated.

**Pregnancy Termination Issues** Pregnancy termination is rarely an issue as the options for termination are limited by the late clinical presentation of duodenal atresia.

**Delivery** The site for delivery should be one capable of managing a preterm infant and one where appropriate personnel are available for surgical repair.

## NEONATOLOGY

**Resuscitation** With high obstruction, amniotic fluid may be green stained from regurgitated bilious secretions, giving the erroneous impression that there has been meconium passage in utero. Aspiration of bilious material into the lungs may be damaging, and every effort should be made to prevent its occurrence. If there are indications of respiratory distress, it is safer to assume that aspiration may have occurred, and laryngoscopy and tracheal suction are indicated before the onset of respiration. In the absence of other markers of fetal distress, and if the fluid is thin and without particulate matter, airway instrumentation is probably not indicated. If positive-pressure ventilation is required because of respiratory depression, bag and mask ventilation should be avoided to reduce the likelihood of gaseous distension of the stomach and duodenum.

A nasogastric tube should be placed and the stomach emptied prior to transfer of the infant from the delivery room to reduce the risk of regurgitation and aspiration.

**Transport** Transfer to a tertiary center where there is a pediatric surgeon is always indicated. Orogastric decompression and maintenance of intravenous fluid infusion in transit are essential.

**Testing and Confirmation** Confirmation of the diagnosis is best established by abdominal radiographs or abdominal ultrasound. The classic radiograph shows the double bubble of an air-filled stomach and proximal duodenum. Air is an excellent and safe contrast medium for suspected upper tract obstruction. Contrast studies may be indicated if the patient is stable and other causes of duodenal obstruction are suspected, such as malrotation with volvulus. Although duodenal atresia may be an isolated finding, it can be associated with other anatomic malformations or chromosomal anomalies. Additional diagnostic evaluation for associated cardiac, gastrointestinal, renal, and vertebral anomalies should be obtained, as indicated. If trisomy 21 is suspected or diagnosed antenatally, confirmatory chromosomal analysis should be obtained at the time of delivery.

**Nursery Management** If cardiorespiratory resuscitation has been required, the first priority is to facilitate cardiorespiratory adaptation with oxygen, fluids, and ventilatory support as needed. Intravenous access should be established and fluid and electrolyte support instituted.

Nasogastric decompression should be maintained to minimize the risk of aspiration and respiratory complication. Parenteral nutrition is often required in the postoperative period, as there is usually a significant interval before adequate enteral intake is established.

## SURGERY

**Preoperative Assessment** Most neonates present with an antenatal diagnosis of duodenal atresia, allowing for a thoughtful preoperative evaluation and elective scheduling of the operative repair. The most critical aspect of preoperative evaluation is the assessment for the presence of complex congenital heart disease. An echocardiogram should be completed preoperatively and findings of significant congenital heart disease discussed with cardiology and anesthesia to achieve consensus regarding a safe operative plan. Surgery may be deferred in the neonate born prematurely to allow for adequate weight and overall maturation prior to operative intervention. It is critical that the neonate has had adequate fluid and electrolyte resuscitation prior to surgical repair.

**Operative Indications** The surgical management of the duodenal atresia is relatively elective. That is, the operation can be safely delayed while possible associated anomalies are evaluated and the patient is stabilized. The exception to this is the neonate with both tracheoesophageal fistula and esophageal atresia (TEF/EA) and duodenal atresia. In this situation, the stomach may rapidly become distended, and even perforate, due to the distal obstruction. Depending on the neonate's hemodynamic stability and respiratory status, a staged operative approach may be needed to allow adequate decompression of the obstructed stomach with eventual repair of all associated anomalies. When the neonate's status allows, repair of the TEF/EA, allowing nasogastric decompression of the stomach prior to repair of the duodenal atresia, is generally optimal.

**Types of Procedures** Nasogastric decompression is immediately instituted, as well as intravenous fluid management. The defect usually occurs at the level of the second to third portion of the duodenum and frequently is in close association with the ampulla and the sphincter of Oddi. Most commonly, the obstruction is proximal, or cephalad, to the ampulla, resulting in nonbilious nasogastric drainage. The operation of choice is a duodenoduodenostomy, with careful evaluation at the time of laparotomy, or laparoscopy, to assess for intestinal malrotation or other sites of bowel atresia. The dilated proximal duodenum can have poor peristalsis with slow emptying across the anastomotic site, making delayed enteral nutrition a possibility. Total parenteral nutrition via a central venous line may be required, or a transanastomotic feeding nasojejunal tube may be used for earlier enteral nutrition. In neonates with Down syndrome, delay in return of gastrointestinal function should prompt an evaluation for Hirschsprung disease.

**Surgical Results/Prognosis** A major associated, and potentially lethal, problem is the presence of a cardiac defect in 20% of patients, which accounts for high mortality and chronic complication rates. Uncomplicated duodenal atresia has an excellent prognosis, with a greater than 95% survival rate.

## SUGGESTED READINGS

1. Brantberg A, Blaas H-GK, Salvesen KÅ, et al: Fetal duodenal obstructions: increased risk of prenatal sudden death. Ultrasound Obstet Gynecol 2002; 20:439-446.
2. Choudhry MS, Rahman N, Boyd P, Lakhoo K: Duodenal atresia: associated anomalies, prenatal diagnosis and outcome. Pediatr Surg Int 2009; 25:727-730.
3. Cragun JD, Martin ML, Moore CA, Khoury MJ: Descriptive epidemiology of small intestinal atresia, Atlanta, Georgia. Teratology 1993; 48:441–450.
4. Estroff JA, Parad RB, Share JC, Benacerraf BR: Second trimester prenatal findings in duodenal and esophageal atresia without tracheoesophageal fistula. J Ultrasound Med 1994; 13:375-379.
5. Fonkalsrud EW, deLorimer AA, Hays DM: Congenital atresia and stenosis of the duodenum. A review compiled from members of the Surgical Section of the American Academy of Pediatrics. Pediatrics 1969; 43:79-83.
6. Nelson LH, Clark CE, Fishburne JI, et al: Value of serial sonography in the in utero detection of duodenal atresia. Obstet Gynecol 1982; 59:657-660.
7. Petrikovsky BM: First trimester diagnosis of duodenal atresia. Am J Obstet Gynecol 1994; 171:569-570.

8. Sase M, Nakata M, Tashima R, Kato H: Development of gastric emptying in the human fetus. Ultrasound Obstet Gynecol 2000; 16:56-59.

9. Tsukèrman GL, Krapiva GA, Kirillova IA: First-trimester diagnosis of duodenal stenosis associated with oesophageal atresia. Prenat Diagn 1993; 13:371-376.

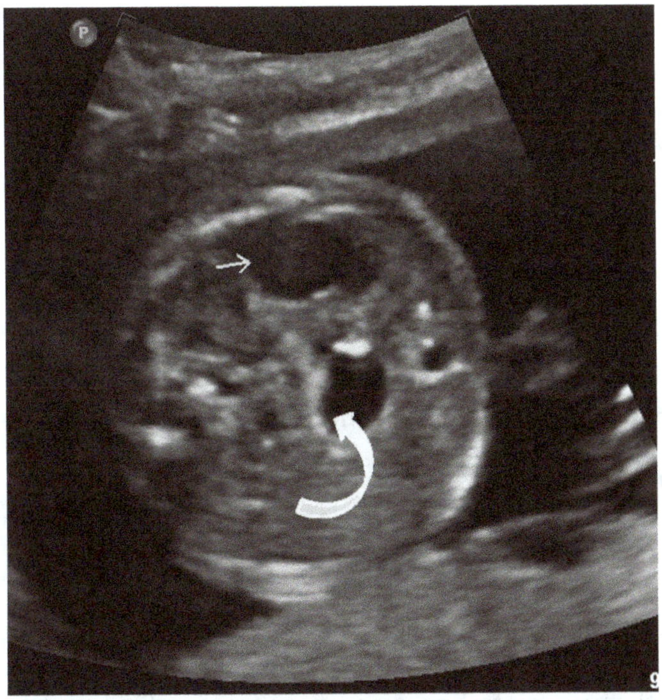

FIGURE 6.2A Duodenal atresia with stomach (straight arrow) and duodenum (curved arrow).

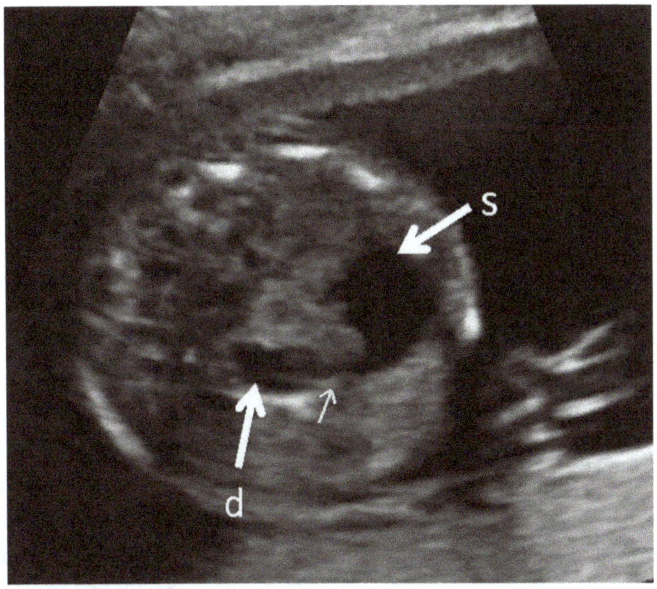


FIGURE 6.2B Duodenal atresia illustrating continuity (small straight arrow) between the stomach (s) and duodenum (d).

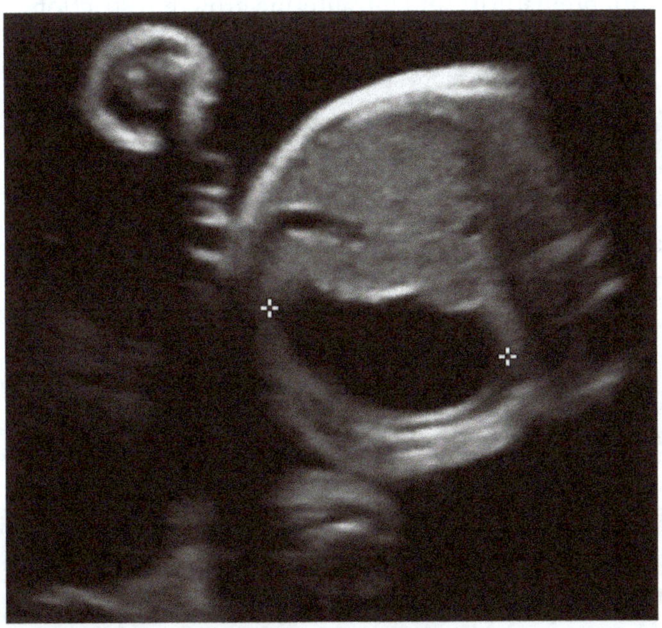

FIGURE 6.2C Duodenal atresia with an enlarged stomach (+ … +) and polyhydramnios.

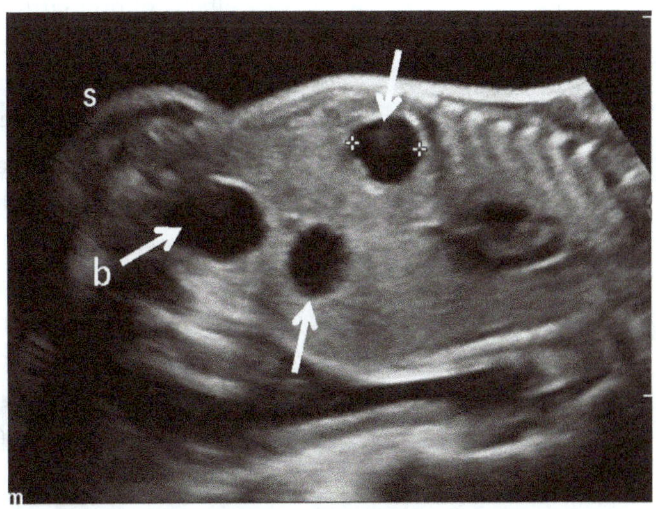


FIGURE 6.2D Duodenal atresia illustrating the double bubble (arrows) separate from the bladder (b).

# 6.3 GASTROSCHISIS

## EPIDEMIOLOGY/GENETICS

**Definition** Gastroschisis is the intrauterine evisceration of fetal intestine through a paraumbilical abdominal wall defect. No covering membrane is present.

**Epidemiology** Incidence is 1 in 2000 births (M1:F1). There is an increased rate in women under the age of 20 years and those identifying as Caucasian. Increased incidence worldwide over the last 35 years suggests an environmental effect.

**Embryology** There are multiple theories of pathogenesis, including

- Abnormal regression of the right umbilical vein
- Vascular accident
- Abnormal folding of the body wall
- Developmental disruption of the right omphalomesenteric artery

The cause is probably heterogeneous, with some cases of gastroschisis resulting from vascular accidents and some from errors in development. Thickening, edema, and matting together of the intestines occur in some cases. Originally, it was theorized that these abnormalities were due to the irritating effects of amniotic fluid, but they are more likely the result of vascular compromise of the blood vessels coming through the small paraumbilical defect. Intestinal atresias and other gastrointestinal disruptions are found in approximately 5% to 10% of cases. Malrotation is almost universal. Extraintestinal abnormalities occur in 5% to 15% of cases. Ten to 15% of affected infants have long-term developmental disabilities, most likely secondary to the effects of prematurity. Both prematurity and intrauterine growth restriction may be associated with gastroschisis. Approximately 30% of fetuses with gastroschisis are delivered prior to 37 weeks' gestation, and 30% to 50% are found to have intrauterine growth restriction.

**Inheritance Patterns** Rare familial recurrences suggest that a few families may have an autosomal dominant inheritance of isolated gastroschisis.

**Screening** Maternal serum α-fetoprotein measurement (MSAFP) will detect most gastroschisis cases. The median maternal serum α-fetoprotein level is 7.0 multiples of the median (MOM) for gastroschisis. With MSAFP and ultrasound, 90% to 97% of cases are detected prenatally.

**Teratogens** There is an association with maternal smoking and cocaine use, but it is not known if they are teratogenic or, more likely, are markers of other potential etiologies, such as poor diet.

**Prognosis** Mortality is 5% in utero, with most losses occurring before 36 weeks. There is less than a 10% neonatal death rate in the postoperative period due to complications of surgery or bowel atresia.

## SONOGRAPHY

### FREQUENT FINDINGS

- Abdominal wall defect to the right of the umbilical cord insertion
- Multiple loops of small bowel within the amniotic cavity: "cauliflower" appearance

### LESS FREQUENT

- Large bowel in the amniotic cavity
- Stomach pulled toward the abdominal defect
- Distended fetal stomach within the abdomen
- Intra-abdominal small bowel atresias
- Abnormalities of amniotic fluid volume
  - Oligohydramnios
  - Polyhydramnios

### KEY FINDINGS/PITFALLS

- The abdominal wall defect in gastroschisis is usually less than 20 mm.
- Intra-abdominal bowel dilatation in the third trimester suggests an obstruction.
- Vanishing gut involves complete necrosis of an affected loop of bowel and closure of the abdominal wall defect.
- Gastroschisis is associated with volvulus and bowel atresias.
- Bowel dilatation does not mandate early delivery.
- There is an increased risk of prematurity and intrauterine growth restriction (40%).
- Polyhydramnios may be associated with severe bowel complications.
- The fibrous peel on the intestines develops after 30 weeks' gestation.

### DIFFERENTIAL DIAGNOSIS

- Physiologic gut herniation occurs up to 12 weeks' gestation.
  - Physiologic herniation is into the base of the umbilical cord, permitting its differentiation from gastroschisis.
- Omphalocele:
  - Characteristically, this is a larger abdominal wall defect containing liver.
  - Bowel-containing omphaloceles can only be diagnosed after 12 weeks' gestation because of the physiologic herniation of bowel into the base of the umbilical cord.

## PREGNANCY MANAGEMENT

**Investigations and Consultations Required** An extended sonographic examination should be performed to exclude other anomalies and to characterize the pattern of bowel findings. The fetal size should be recorded.

Fetal echocardiography should be performed. Although the risk of chromosomal abnormalities is low, amniocentesis should be discussed with the patient. If performed, or if other fetal anomalies are present, a microarray is indicated. The family should be referred to neonatology and a pediatric surgeon for a thorough discussion of the neonatal management issues.

**Monitoring** Care should be coordinated in a tertiary center because of the potential need for early intervention. Serial ultrasonographic examinations should be performed every 4 weeks to detect thickening or dilation of the fetal bowel, and to assess fetal growth and amniotic fluid abnormalities. If abnormalities develop, ultrasound examinations may be performed more frequently. Fetal assessment, such as biophysical profiles, should be initiated if there is evidence of a lag in growth or if oligohydramnios is present.

**Pregnancy Course** The increased incidence of intrauterine growth restriction in fetuses with gastroschisis may complicate the obstetric management. Preterm labor occurs in nearly one-third of cases.

**Pregnancy Termination Issues** There are no special concerns regarding the method or location for pregnancy termination, as the diagnosis is generally clear antenatally.

**Delivery** Delivery at term is preferred, when fetal growth and amniotic fluid are reassuring. Delivery prior to 39 weeks is based on the usual obstetrical concerns for fetal growth restriction and nonreassuring antenatal testing. Vaginal delivery is appropriate with care to immediately cover the protruding bowel loops with non-latex-containing material. Delivery personnel should wear non-latex-containing gloves and carefully identify where to clamp and cut the umbilical cord. A pediatric surgeon and a tertiary neonatal intensive care unit should be available at the delivery site.

## NEONATOLOGY

**Resuscitation** Assistance with the onset of respiration is usually not required unless there is concurrent prematurity-associated respiratory distress. If assisted ventilation is required, bag-and-mask ventilation is contraindicated to avoid gaseous distension of the stomach and bowel. The major concern is the protection of the extruded bowel. Extreme care must be taken to avoid torsion of the bowel loops, which would further compromise perfusion. If there is marked distension of the bowel, perfusion can be compromised by the kinking of the mesenteric vessels as they exit through the abdominal wall defect. Prompt decompression of the stomach is important. The bowel should be covered with warmed saline-soaked gauze and supported to avoid torsion, and the trunk should be encased in a sterile plastic bag with a drawstring ("bowel bag"). The bowel bag not only reduces evaporative heat and water loss but also reduces the likelihood of surface contamination. The neonate should be positioned laterally to minimize torsion on the bowel and its mesentery, which could occur with the neonate positioned supine.

**Transport** Transfer to a tertiary center with pediatric surgery and neonatology is always indicated. Care of the bowel, as outlined, should be provided during the transport, as should gastric decompression. Reliable venous access should be established, and maintenance intravenous fluids and broad-spectrum antibiotic therapy should be instituted.

**Testing and Confirmation** Once the infant has recovered from the initial surgery and the exposed bowel is covered, additional diagnostic evaluation may be instituted if there is concern for associated anomalies.

**Nursery Management** Protection of the exposed bowel, gastric decompression, administration of broad-spectrum antibiotics, and intravenous fluid support should be maintained. In some instances, it may be necessary to provide ventilatory support in the early postoperative period, as there may be increased intra-abdominal pressure from the reduction of the extruded bowel back into the abdominal cavity. Central parenteral nutrition is required during the postoperative recovery period, as there is always a significant interval before adequate enteral intake is established.

**Surgical Management** The goal of surgical management is to reduce the eviscerated bowel into the abdominal cavity, a task complicated by the common finding of a small abdominal cavity, due to intrauterine loss of domain, and the presence of thickened bowel loops. The decision to proceed with a staged, rather than a primary, closure is dependent on the findings at the time of operative repair, specifically increased intra-abdominal pressure and its effects on ventilation and the perfusion of the intestines. A preformed, spring-loaded silo is most commonly used to protect the bowel in a staged closure, and these silos may be placed without general anesthesia, allowing placement in the neonatal intensive care unit, with gradual reduction of the intestines into the abdominal cavity over several days. A suture-less closure using the umbilical cord is a relatively new, innovative approach to the abdominal wall closure in gastroschisis. With this technique, the umbilical cord is used to plug the fascial defect with relatively rapid epithelialization of the wound. This results in a small hernia at the umbilicus that often closes with time.

## SUGGESTED READINGS

1. Badillo AT, Hedrick HL, Wilson RD, et al: Prenatal ultrasonographic gastrointestinal abnormalities in fetuses with gastroschisis do not correlate with postnatal outcomes. J Pediatr Surg 2008; 43:647-653.
2. Barisic I, Clementi M, Häusler M, et al: Evaluation of prenatal ultrasound diagnosis of fetal abdominal wall defects by 19 European registries. Ultrasound Obstet Gynecol 2001; 18:309-316.
3. Chesley PM, Ledbetter DJ, Meehan JJ, et al: Contemporary trends in the use of primary repair for gastroschisis in surgical infants. Am J Surg 2015; 209:901-906.
4. David Al, Tan A, Curry J: Gastroschisis: sonographic diagnosis, associations, management and outcome. Prenat Diagn 2008; 28:633-644.
5. Durfee SM, Benson CB, Adams SR, et al: Postnatal outcomes of fetuses with the prenatal diagnosis of gastroschisis. J Ultrasound Med 2013; 32:407-412.
6. Emami CN, Youssef F, Baird RJ, et al: A risk-stratified comparison of fascial versus flap closure techniques on the early outcomes of infants with gastroschisis. J Pediatr Surg 2015; 50:102-106.

7. Fillingham A, Ranki J: Prevalence, prenatal diagnosis and survival of gastroschisis. Prenat Diagn 2008; 28:1232-1237.
8. Langer JC, Longaker MT, Crombleholme TM, et al: Etiology of intestinal damage in gastroschisis. I: Effects of amniotic fluid exposure and bowel constriction in a fetal lamb model. J Pediatr Surg 1989; 24:992-997.
9. Mastroiacovo P, Lisi A, Castilla E, et al: Gastroschisis and associated defects: an international study. Am J Med Genet 2007; 143:660-671.
10. Overton TG, Pierce MR, Gao H, et al: Antenatal management and outcome of gastroschisis in the UK. Prenat Diagn 2012; 32:1256-1262.
11. Payne NR, Pfleghaar K, Assel B, et al: Predicting the outcome of newborns with gastroschisis. J Pediatr Surg 2009; 44:918-923.
12. Piper HG, Jaksic T: The impact of prenatal bowel dilatation on clinical outcomes in neonates with gastroschisis. J Pediatr Surg 2006; 41:897-900.
13. South AP, Stutey KM, Meinzer-Derr J: Metaanalysis of the prevalence of intrauterine fetal death in gastroschisis. Am J Obstet Gynecol 2013; 209:114.e1-13.
14. Torfs CP, Velie EM, Oechsli FW, et al: A population-based study of gastroschisis: demographic, pregnancy, and lifestyle risk factors. Teratology 1994; 50:44-53.

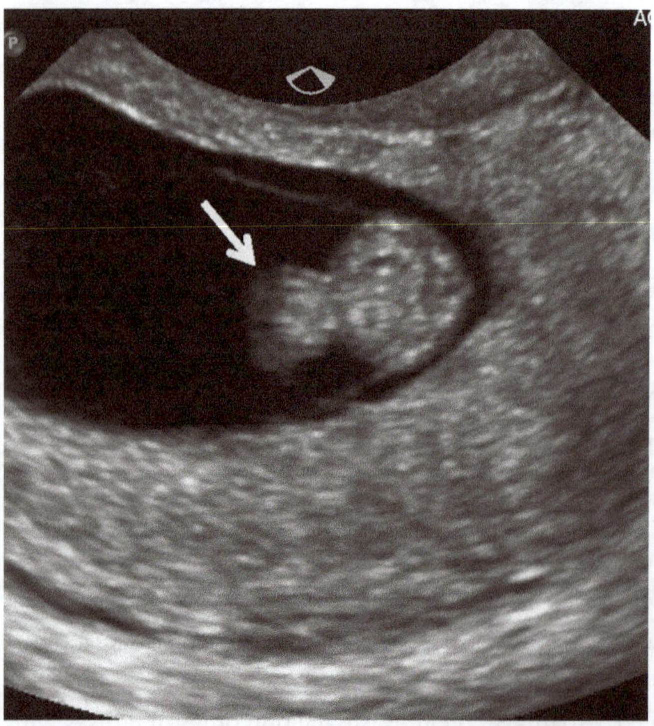

**FIGURE 6.3A** Physiologic bowel herniation at 10 weeks' gestation (arrow).

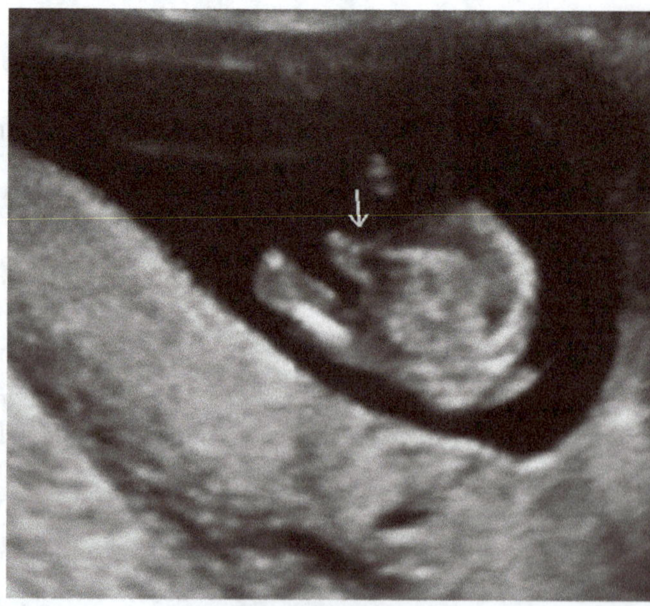

**FIGURE 6.3B** The physiologic bowel herniation seen in Figure 6.3A has resolved by 13 weeks (arrow).

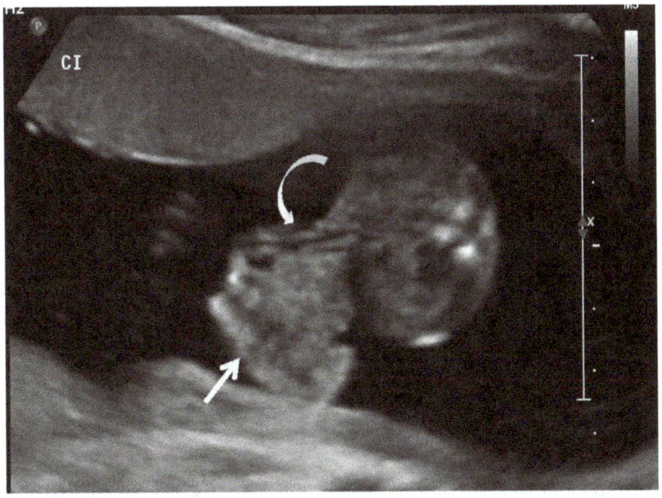

FIGURE 6.3C Gastroschisis (straight arrow) to right of umbilical insertion (curved arrow).

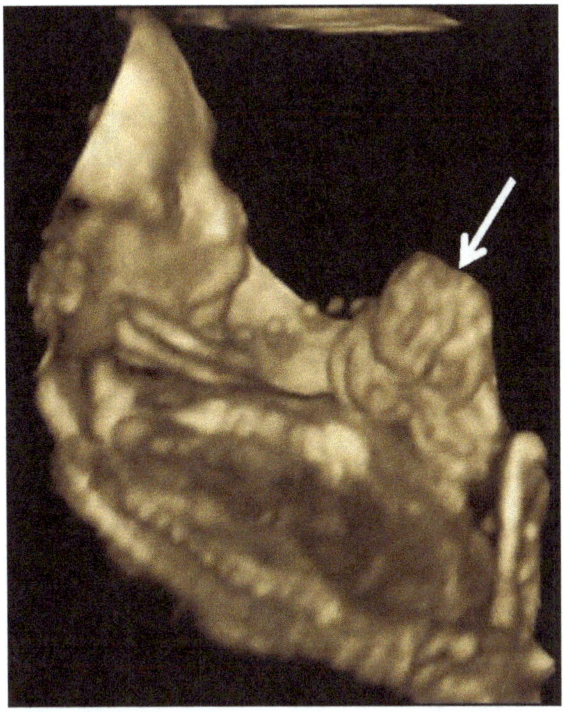

FIGURE 6.3D Three-dimensional image of gastroschisis (arrow).

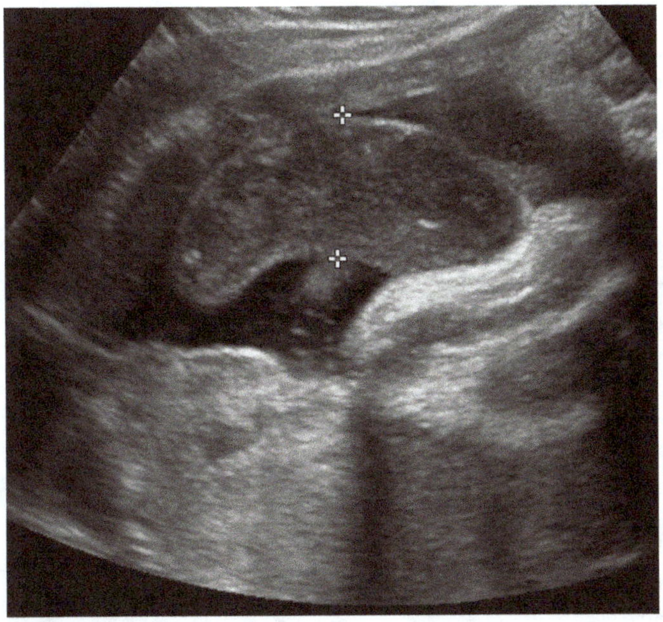

FIGURE 6.3E Gastroschisis with dilated small bowel (+ … +).

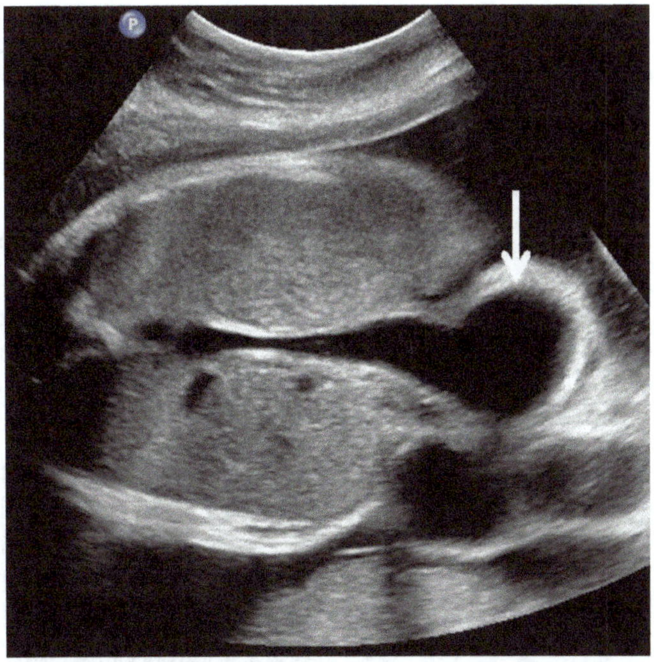

FIGURE 6.3F Stomach (arrow) protruding through the abdominal wall defect of gastroschisis.

# 6.4 HEPATIC TUMORS

## EPIDEMIOLOGY/GENETICS

**Definition** Liver tumors are the tenth most frequent pediatric tumor. Hepatic malignancy must be distinguished from benign hepatic tumors and nonneoplastic hepatomegaly. Almost 50% of primary liver tumors are benign. In older children, liver tumors more often represent metastatic disease (neuroblastoma, Wilms tumor) than primary malignancies.

**Epidemiology** Occurrence is 1.6 in 1 million births; for hepatoblastoma, incidence is M1.4:F1, and for vascular tumors it is M:1.3:F1.

**Embryology** There are three major types of hepatic tumors with the following characteristics:

- Hepatoblastomas (17%)
  - Hepatoblastomas present as an abdominal mass, with 60% detected in the first year and 90% by age 3 years.
  - They occur most frequently in the right lobe of the liver.
  - They are usually unifocal.
  - Hepatomas are locally invasive.
  - They can metastasize.
  - α-Fetoprotein is elevated.
  - The presence of embryonal or undifferentiated cell types is associated with poor prognosis.
  - Punctate calcifications may be present.
  - There is an association with the Beckwith-Weidemann syndrome, hemihypertrophy, diaphragmatic hernia, and renal abnormalities.
- Mesenchymal hamartomas (23%)
  - These are benign.
  - Etiology: They arise from an overgrowth of mature cells.
  - They can be solid, large septated, or unilocular cysts filled with mucoid material.
  - Rapid growth can lead to hydrops.
- Hemangioma (60%).
  - Types
    - Capillary and cavernous hemangioma
    - Hemangioepithelioma
    - Infantile hemangioma
  - Can be focal and multifocal lesions
  - Can be self-involuting
  - May cause consumptive coagulopathy

**Inheritance Patterns** Inheritance patterns are sporadic.

**Teratogens** None are known.

**Prognosis** Infants with vascular tumors and no evidence of heart failure or hydrops have a good prognosis. The 3-year survival rate of those with hepatoblastoma exceeds 90% in patients with initially resectable tumors, 65% in those with initially unresectable tumors treated first with chemotherapy, and only 10% to 20% in patients with metastatic disease. Survival rate for mesenchymal hamartoma is 60% or better, and for hemangioma is approximately 75%.

## SONOGRAPHY

### FREQUENT FINDINGS

- Hepatomegaly
  - Definite mass may not be detected
- Focal or multifocal lesions with complex echo pattern
  - Solid, hypoechoic
  - Cystic
  - Solid/cystic
- Multiple large dilated hepatic vessels
- Polyhydramnios

### LESS FREQUENT

- Small areas of calcification
- Nonimmune hydrops
  - Cardiomegaly
  - Pericardial effusion
  - Pleural effusion
  - Ascites
  - Anasarca
  - Placentomegaly

### KEY FINDINGS/PITFALLS

- Hepatic tumors are usually detected in the late second or third trimester.
- There is a potential for fetal intra-abdominal hemorrhage with labor.
- Multifocal, avascular liver masses may represent metastases from a neuroblastoma.
- Three-dimensional power Doppler can be used to evaluate tumor vascular anatomy.
  - Metastatic hepatic tumors have a vascular rim with a relatively avascular stroma.
  - Hepatocellular carcinomas tend to have tortuous stromal vessels.
  - Hemangiomas have a characteristic feeding vessel. High-velocity flow during systole and diastole indicates an arteriovenous shunt.
    - Smaller tumors are hypoechoic without a feeding vessel.
    - Gray-scale and Doppler characteristics cannot predict the severity of hematologic abnormalities.
- Hemangiomas may be associated with high output failure.

## PREGNANCY MANAGEMENT

**Investigations and Consultations Required** An extended ultrasound examination, including Doppler interrogation of the fetal liver for characterization of vascular flow, is required. Fetal echocardiography may be useful to detect early evidence of cardiac decompensation. Prenatal consultation with neonatology, oncology, or pediatric surgery may be useful, depending on the presumptive diagnosis.

**Fetal Intervention** None is available.

**Monitoring** Serial ultrasound examinations should be obtained to monitor growth of the mass, to detect early signs of hydrops, and to assess amniotic fluid volume. Biophysical profiles should be performed if there is evidence of fetal compromise.

**Pregnancy Course** Polyhydramnios and fetal hydrops are common complications of hepatic tumors. If hydrops develops, consideration should be given to steroid administration and early delivery.

**Pregnancy Termination Issues** Pathologic confirmation of the diagnosis is essential; an intact fetus may not be necessary to obtain appropriate tissue samples.

**Delivery** The risk of bleeding into the tumor is unknown, but accounts for much of the neonatal morbidity and mortality reported. Cesarean section should be considered and is indicated with highly vascular tumors or in cases of rapidly changing fetal status or hydrops. Delivery at a tertiary center is essential for prompt evaluation and treatment of the infant.

## NEONATOLOGY

**Resuscitation** The type, size, and systemic manifestations of a given tumor may influence the management of resuscitation. Congestive heart failure, hydrops, and consumptive coagulopathy may occur, particularly as complications of vascular hemangiomas or large, solid, infiltrative tumors. If any of these is present, the immediate postnatal management must address the pathophysiologic effects of each on the onset of respiration and circulatory transition. Abdominal enlargement is frequently present with mesenchymal hamartomas and may result in both the compression of normal intra-abdominal vasculature and significant respiratory distress, requiring immediate intubation and ventilatory support. Volume expansion, packed red cell transfusion, and correction of metabolic acidosis may be required as part of the resuscitative interventions. In the absence of any of these complications that can be anticipated from assessment of the fetus intrapartum, no special resuscitative measures are usually required.

**Transport** Transfer to a tertiary center with neonatology and surgical subspecialty capabilities is essential. Experienced neonatal personnel should conduct the transport.

**Testing and Confirmation** Vascular tumors are best delineated with a combination of MRI and ultrasound with Doppler flow studies. Solid tumors can be recognized by either computed tomography or MRI; histopathologic examination is necessary to determine cell type. α-Fetoprotein levels may be elevated in about 50% of infants with hepatoblastoma.

**Nursery Management** The most common neonatal hepatic tumor is a benign vascular hemangioma, which often involutes spontaneously during childhood. If the lesion becomes symptomatic with the presence of congestive heart failure due to hemodynamically significant shunting, thrombocytopenia, or consumptive coagulopathy, a trial of medical therapy with propranolol or corticosteroids is indicated. If the hemangioma is localized, surgical excision is recommended. Hepatic arterial ligation or embolization may be considered in the face of intractable congestive heart failure or refractory consumptive coagulopathy. While mesenchymal hamartomas typically present as an asymptomatic abdominal mass, some infants may present with hydrops, congestive heart failure, or significant abdominal distension that may compromise respiration and require ventilatory support. Surgical resection is the definitive treatment, which usually results in cure. The treatment of solid tumors varies with the histologic type. For example, treatment of hepatoblastomas requires a combination of chemotherapy and surgical resection.

**Surgical Outcomes** Even if unresectable at diagnosis, most hepatoblastomas are unifocal and chemosensitive, especially to platinum-derivative chemotherapeutic agents, minimizing the need for urgent extensive surgery in the newborn.

Although uncommon, a large, rapidly growing neonatal hemangioma can produce life-threatening complications, including cardiac failure, platelet consumption, and hypothyroidism. Congestive heart failure and abdominal compartment syndrome are associated with a significantly higher mortality rate. Initial management is usually noninvasive, consisting primarily of steroids and propranolol, and spontaneous regression occurs in most cases. Embolization, rather than surgery, is generally the next step if medical therapy fails. Relatively rarely, transplantation may be required for excision of the lesion. Standard surgical resection is rarely indicated for hepatic hemangioma.

## SUGGESTED READINGS


1. Catanzarite V, Hilfiker M, Daneshmand S, Willert J: Prenatal diagnosis of fetal hepatoblastoma. Case report and review of the literature. J Ultrasound Med 2008; 27:1095-1098.
2. Fernandez-Pineda I, Cabello-Laureano R: Differential diagnosis and management of liver tumors in infants. World J Hepatol 2014; 6:486-495.
3. Gembruch U, Baschat AA, Gloeckner-Hoffman K, et al: Prenatal diagnosis and management of fetuses with liver hemangiomata. Ultrasound Obstet Gynecol 2002; 19:454-460.
4. Huang L-C, Ho M, Chang N-C, et al: Prenatal diagnosis of fetal hepatoblastoma with a good neonatal outcome: case report and narrative review. Pediatr Hematol Oncol 2011; 28:150-154.
5. Isaacs H Jr: Fetal and neonatal hepatic tumors. J Pediatr Surg 2007; 42:1797-1803.

6. Luks FI, Yazbeck S, Brandt ML, et al: Benign liver tumors in children: a 25-year experience. J Pediatr Surg 1991; 26:1326-1330.
7. Meirwitz NB, Guzman ER, Underberg-Davis SJ, et al: Hepatic hemangioendothelioma: prenatal sonographic findings and evolution of the lesion. J Clin Ultrasound 2000; 28:258-263.
8. Mhanni AA, Chodirker BN, Evans JA, et al: Fetal hepatic haemangioendothelioma: a new association with elevated maternal serum alpha-fetoprotein. Prenat Diagn 2000; 20:432-439.
9. Samuel M, Spitz L: Infantile hepatic hemangioendothelioma: the role of surgery. J Pediatr Surg 1995; 30:1425-1429.
10. Shih J-C, Tsao P-N, Huang S-F, et al: Antenatal diagnosis of congenital hepatoblastoma in utero. Ultrasound Obstet Gynecol 2000; 16:94-97.
11. Siddiqui MA, McKenna BJ: Hepatic mesenchymal hamartoma: a short review. Arch Pathol Lab Med 2006; 130:1567-1569.
12. Weinberg AG, Finegold MJ: Primary hepatic tumors of childhood. Hum Pathol 1983; 14:512-537.

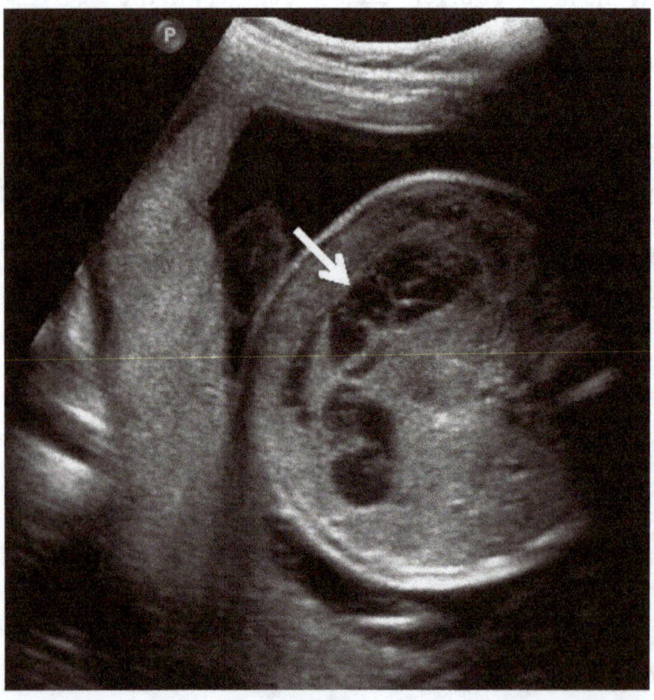


**FIGURE 6.4A** Hemangioendothelioma (arrow).

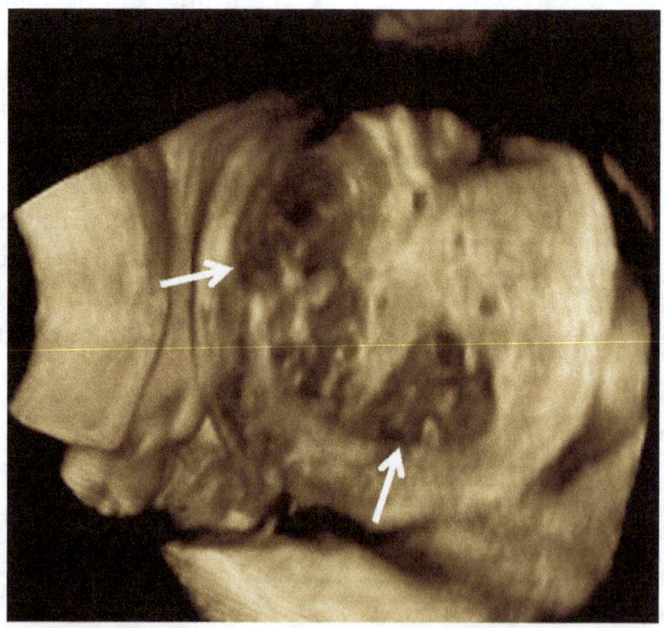

**FIGURE 6.4B** Three-dimensional image of a hemangioendothelioma (arrows).

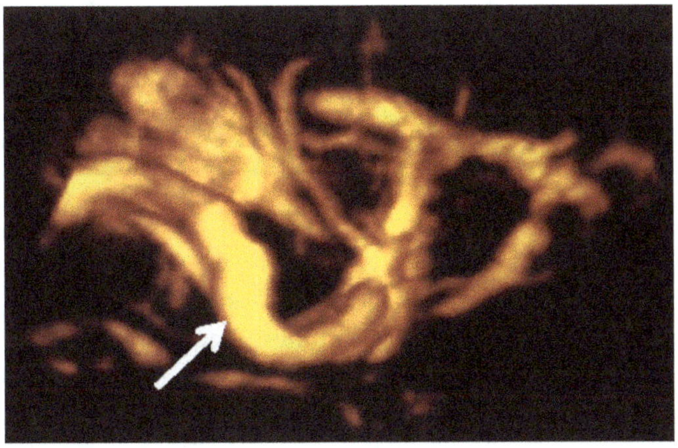

**FIGURE 6.4C** Three-dimensional power Doppler showing the feeding vessel to hemangioendothelioma (arrow).

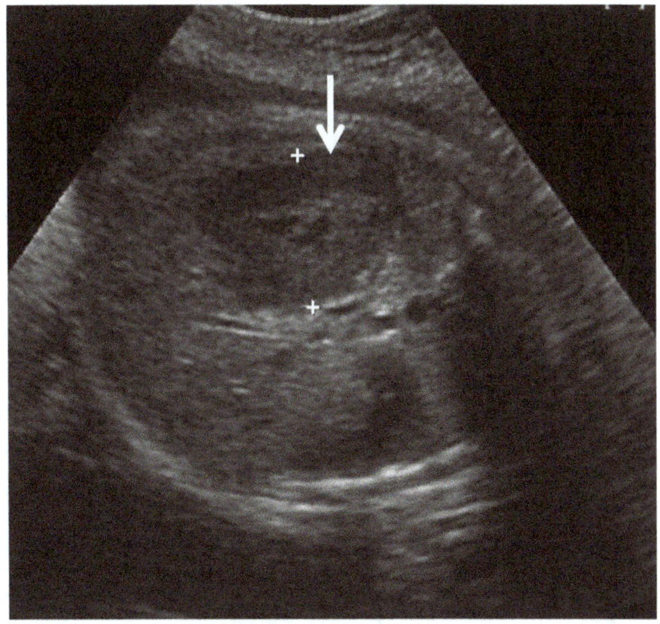

**FIGURE 6.4D** Hepatoblastoma (arrow) (+ … +).

# 6.5 HETEROTAXY

## EPIDEMIOLOGY/GENETICS

**Definition** *Heterotaxy* is defined as an abnormality where the internal thoracoabdominal organs demonstrate abnormal arrangement across the left-right axis of the body. The spleen is almost always affected, and heterotaxy syndrome is subdivided into the asplenia and polysplenia syndromes. Frequently, there is associated complex congenital heart disease.

**Epidemiology** Incidence is 1 in 10,000 births (M2:F1). Heterotaxy is diagnosed in up to 3% of infants with congenital heart disease. Because of the severity of the cardiac malformations, it accounts for 6% of cardiac defects detected in utero.

**Embryology** Heterotaxy is caused by the disruption of the right-left axis during embryonic development, resulting in the loss of the normal asymmetry of the thoracic and abdominal organs (heterotaxy). At least six gene mutations have been detected in patients with heterotaxy syndrome, including a number in ciliary development. In the nonsyndromic cases, the etiology appears to be a combination of genetic and environmental influences. In heterotaxy syndrome, there is frequently abnormal symmetry of organs that normally have some degree of asymmetry. For example, the liver is symmetrical in 76% of patients with asplenia and 67% of patients with polysplenia. Associated malformations are common (40% to 70%), including intestinal malrotation, biliary atresia, duodenal atresia, and rarely tracheoesophageal fistula. Genitourinary abnormalities are also seen, including horseshoe kidney, renal agenesis, and cryptorchidism. Vertebral abnormalities and neural tube defects have been reported in heterotaxy syndrome.

A number of genetic syndromes, as well as chromosomal abnormalities, may have laterality defects that overlap with the heterotaxy syndrome, including trisomies 13 and 18, 22q11.2 syndrome, VACTERL, and the Alagille syndrome. Laterality defects are present in a number of the ciliopathy syndromes, many of which have autosomal recessive inheritance.

**Inheritance Patterns** Most cases are sporadic, but there appears to be a strong genetic component to heterotaxy syndrome, with 10% of patients having some family history of a close relative with congenital heart disease. All three types of mendelian inheritance have been described with heterotaxy syndrome. Following the birth of a child with nonsyndromic heterotaxy, the empiric risk of recurrence of either heterotaxy syndrome or congenital heart disease in a subsequent pregnancy is approximately 5%.

**Teratogens** Maternal diabetes mellitus, cocaine, and monozygotic twinning are teratogenic.

**Prognosis** Heterotaxy includes a large spectrum of cardiac diseases, from extremely mild to extremely complex lesions. The prognosis is dependent on the severity of the cardiac abnormality. The 5-year survival rate is 30% to 74% for asplenia and 65% to 84% for polysplenia.

## SONOGRAPHY

### FREQUENT FINDINGS: LEFT ATRIAL ISOMERISM (POLYSPLENIA)

- Cardiac/visceral situs
  - Heterotaxy: 68%
  - Situs inversus: 14%
  - Normal situs: 18%
- Two vessels behind four-chamber cardiac view ("double-vessel sign")
  - Aorta
  - Interrupted inferior vena cava with azygous draining into the superior vena cava
- Midline liver
- Complex congenital heart defects
  - Atrioventricular septal defect with complete heart block is pathognomonic.

### LESS FREQUENT: LEFT ATRIAL ISOMERISM (POLYSPLENIA)

- Nonimmune hydrops
- Thickened second-trimester nuchal fold

### FREQUENT FINDINGS: RIGHT ATRIAL ISOMERISM (ASPLENIA)

- Cardiac/visceral situs
  - Heterotaxy: 60%
  - Situs inversus: 20%
  - Normal situs: 20%
- Midline liver
- Splenic artery is not identified with color Doppler.
- Transverse view is at the level of the stomach.
  - The inferior vena cava and aorta are on the same side of the spine.
- Complex congenital heart defects
  - Complete atrioventricular septal defect
  - Transposition of the great vessels
  - Double-outlet right ventricle
  - Total anomalous pulmonary venous return

### KEY FINDINGS/PITFALLS

- Right atrial isomerism
  - Loss of left-sided structures (i.e., left atrium and pulmonary veins)
    - Anomalous pulmonary venous return
    - Absent spleen
    - Gastrointestinal malformations
      - Malrotation
      - Esophageal atresia
      - Duodenal atresia
  - Single-ventricle physiology predominates
    - Complete atrioventricular canal defect
    - Pulmonary stenosis/atresia

        - Hypoplastic left ventricle
        - None or mild (ventricular septal defect) cardiac defect: 5%-10%
- Left atrial isomerism
    - Right-sided structures absent
    - Interrupted inferior vena cava
    - Absent right atrium with sinus node
        - Pulmonary veins may connect to both atria.
        - Dysrhythmias:
            - Atrial fibrillation/flutter
            - Complete heart block
    - Cardiac defects
        - Atrioseptal defects
        - Ventricular septal defects
        - Aortic coarctation
        - Sinus node dysfunction
            - Bradyarrhythmia is generally exclusive to left atrial isomerism.
- None of the findings in left or right atrial isomerism are mandatory.
- Antenatal diagnosis: 19-27 weeks
    - Cardiac malformations are the first diagnostic clue.
- In fetuses with a complex congenital heart defect, abnormal visceral situs is strongly predictive of a normal karyotype.
- Complete heart block, complex cardiac abnormalities, and fetal hydrops are poor prognostic signs.

## PREGNANCY MANAGEMENT

**Investigations and Consultations Required** At the initial diagnosis, an extended examination to search for any anomalies in other organ systems should be performed. Pediatric cardiology should be consulted for a fetal echocardiogram and to discuss with the family prognosis and neonatal management. A fetal karyotype and microarray should be done, especially if there are other organ systems involved. Prenatal consultations with other pediatric services may be warranted, depending on the findings.

**Fetal Intervention** None is available.

**Monitoring** Fetuses with heterotaxy syndrome should have regular ultrasound evaluations to assess for other abnormalities and to monitor cardiac status. Repeat fetal echocardiograms are also indicated to look for worsening of fetal cardiac status. The fetal heart rate should be assessed on a weekly basis after 28 weeks, when the probability for complete heart block is increased.

**Pregnancy Course** Maternal issues are generally not present, and the pregnancies are otherwise uncomplicated. Fetal decompensation may require early delivery.

**Pregnancy Termination Issues** A complete postmortem examination should be performed for confirmation of cardiac diagnosis, and to assess for other abnormalities.

**Delivery** In general, the fetus with heterotaxy syndrome should be delivered at a center where immediate pediatric cardiology consultation can be obtained and multiple neonatal and pediatric sub-specialists are available to care for the potentially complex problems.

## NEONATOLOGY

**Resuscitation** Infants will generally breathe spontaneously and not require resuscitation.

**Transport** Infants should be transferred to a center with pediatric cardiology and multiple pediatric surgical specialties available.

**Testing and Confirmation** Echocardiography is definitive for an accurate anatomic diagnosis. An abdominal ultrasound should be performed in suspected heterotaxy syndrome to exclude malrotation and to assess for the presence of suspected asplenia, or polysplenia, syndrome.

**Nursery Management** Management is directed toward rapid identification of the extent of organ malformation and dysfunction present while maintaining adequate cardiorespiratory support. The management of the cardiac component of the malformation complex will be dictated by the lesion(s) identified and the consequent impact on adequate cardiac function.

## SURGERY

**Preoperative Assessment** Echocardiography is generally sufficient for preoperative testing.

**Operative Indications** The indications are often similar to those discussed for individual lesions, such as complete common atrioventricular canal, double outlet, aortic stenosis, or pulmonary stenosis.

**Types of Procedures** The spectrum of heterotaxy is so variable that the reader is referred to management of each lesion in the sections where they are discussed separately.

**Surgical Results/Prognosis** The spectrum of disease and the prognosis are quite variable. Prognosis is poor in those infants with total anomalous pulmonary venous return, particularly in cases in which the return is mixed to multiple sites and in fetuses in whom there is severe systemic outflow tract obstruction. In cases in which there is severe ventricular hypoplasia, single-ventricle management is necessary, and multiple operations are required.

### SUGGESTED READINGS

1. Abuhamad AZ, Robinson JN, Bogdan D, Tannous RJ: Color Doppler of the splenic artery in the prenatal diagnosis of heterotaxic syndromes. Am J Perinatol 1999; 16:469-473.
2. Berg C, Geipel A, Kamil D, et al: The syndrome of left isomerism: sonographic findings and outcome in prenatally diagnosed cases. J Ultrasound Med 2005; 24:921-931.
3. Berg C, Geipel A, Kamil D, et al: The syndrome of right isomerism—prenatal diagnosis and outcome. Ultraschall Med 2006; 27:225-233.

4. Berg C, Geipel A, Sonreck J, et al: Prenatal diagnosis of cardiosplenic syndromes: a 10-year experience. Ultrasound Obstet Gynecol 2003; 22:451-459.
5. Brown DL, Emerson DS, Shulman LP, et al: Predicting aneuploidy in fetuses with cardiac anomalies: significance of visceral situs and non-cardiac anomalies. Ultrasound Med 1993; 12:153-161.
6. Escobar-Diaz MC, Friedman K, Salem Y, et al: Perinatal and infant outcomes of prenatal diagnosis of heterotaxy syndrome (asplenia and polysplenia). Am J Cardiol 2014:612-617.
7. Evans WN, Acherman RJ, Restrepo H: Heterotaxy in southern Nevada: prenatal detection and epidemiology. Pediatr Cardiol 2015; 36:930-934.
8. Kosaki K, Bassi MT, Kosaki R, et al: Characterization and mutation analysis of human LEFTY A and LEFTY B homologues of murine genes implicated in left-right axis development. Am J Hum Genet 1999; 64:712-721.
9. Lim JS, McCringle BW, Smallhorn JF, et al: Clinical features, management, and outcomes of children with fetal and postnatal diagnosis of isomerism syndromes. Circulation 2005; 112:2454-2461.
10. Øyen N, Poulsen G, Boyd HA, et al: Recurrence of congenital heart defects in families. Circulation 2009; 120:295-301.
11. Pepes S, Zidere V, Allen LD: Prenatal diagnosis of left atrial isomerism. Heart 2009; 95:1974-1977.
12. Zhu L, Belmont JW, Ware SM: Genetics of human heterotaxias. Eur J Hum Genet 2006; 14:17-25.

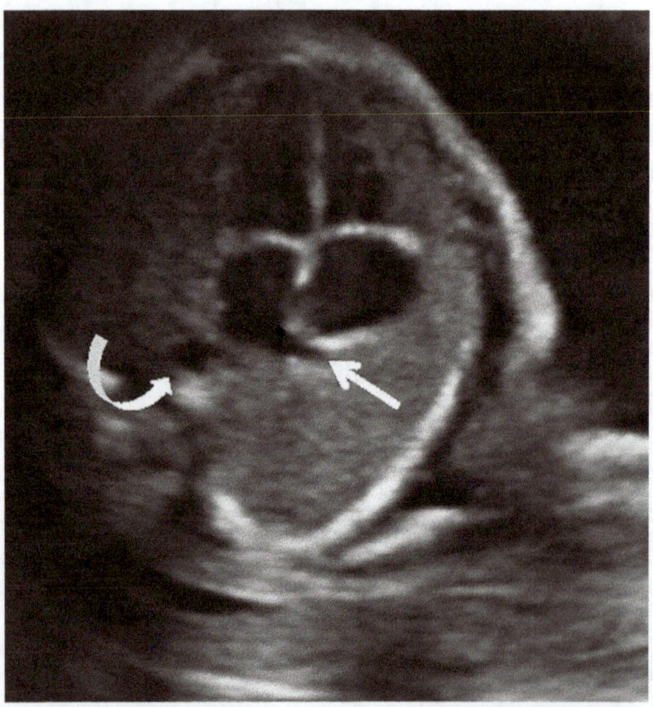

**FIGURE 6.5A** Normal four-chamber cardiac view with pulmonary veins (straight arrow). Single vessel (aorta) (curved arrow) behind the heart.

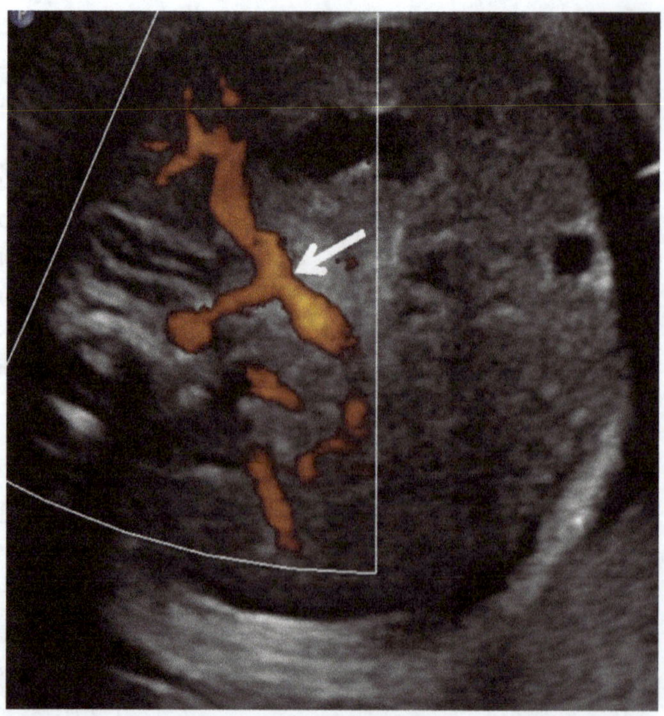

**FIGURE 6.5B** Splenic artery (arrow).

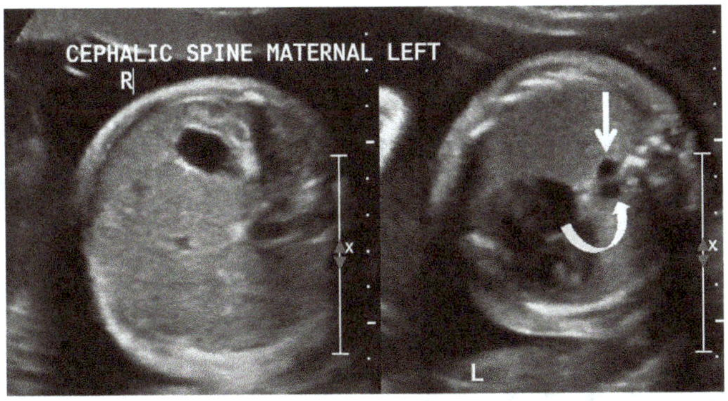


**FIGURE 6.5C** Heterotaxy (left atrial isomerism) illustrating the "two-vessel sign." The aorta (straight arrow) and azygous (curved arrow) are behind the heart.

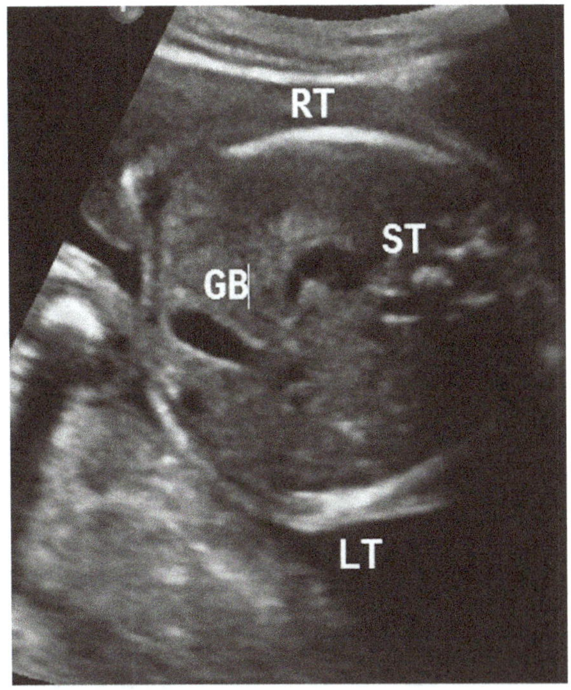


**FIGURE 6.5D** Heterotaxy with abnormally positioned right-sided stomach (ST) and gallbladder (GB) in the midline.

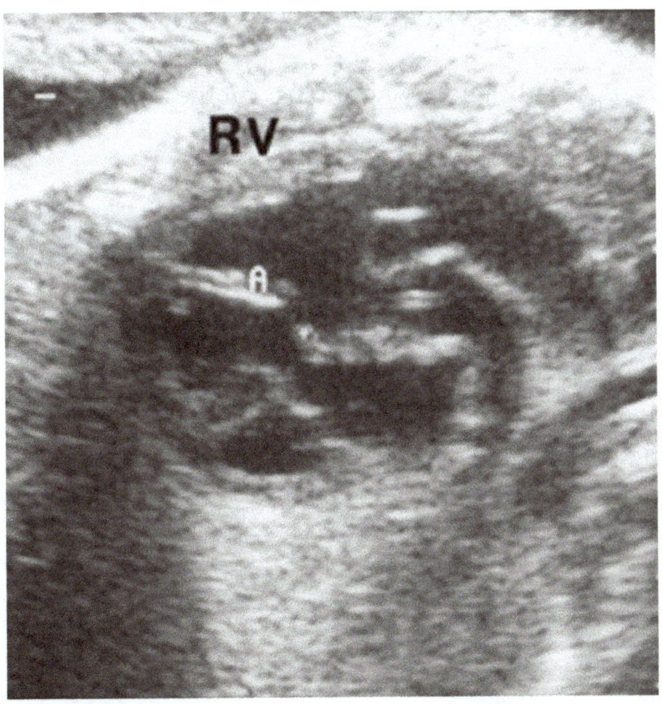


**FIGURE 6.5E** Double-outlet right ventricle (RV) with ventricular septal defect (A).

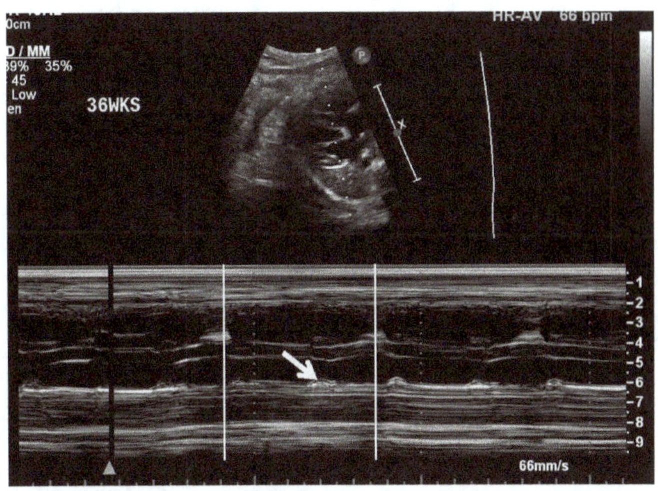


**FIGURE 6.5F** Complete heart block. The ventricular rate is between white lines, and the atrial rate is noted by the straight arrow.

# 6.6 MECONIUM ILEUS/PERITONITIS

## EPIDEMIOLOGY/GENETICS

**Definition** Meconium ileus is a congenital intestinal hypomotility/obstruction process resulting from inspissated meconium. Meconium peritonitis is a chemical peritonitis resulting from fetal bowel perforation of any cause. Continued leakage of meconium can result in pseudocyst formation.

**Epidemiology** Incidence is 1 in 3500 neonates.

**Embryology**. Inspissated meconium is thought to be caused either by bowel hypomotility or obstruction or due to an alteration in the viscosity of the meconium, as may occur in cystic fibrosis with altered electrolyte transport. Commonly associated conditions include small bowel atresias, cystic fibrosis, and volvulus. Cystic fibrosis is found in 50%, or more, of cases in northern European populations but is less likely as an etiology in other populations with a lower incidence of the disease. Altered meconium viscosity is also believed to be the etiology for the increased prevalence of second-trimester echogenic bowel in Down syndrome.

**Inheritance Patterns** Cystic fibrosis is an autosomal recessive single-gene disorder. Other conditions that have meconium ileus/peritonitis are generally sporadic.

**Teratogens** Congenital infections, especially with cytomegalovirus and parvovirus, can have echogenic bowel as one of its features, but it is not true meconium ileus.

**Prognosis** Prognosis depends on the underlying etiology for the meconium ileus/peritonitis.

## SONOGRAPHY

### FREQUENT FINDINGS: MECONIUM PERITONITIS

- Punctate echogenic foci on the periphery of the liver/spleen
- Large, intra-abdominal calcific plaques with acoustic shadowing
- Intra-abdominal walled-off cyst with an echogenic border
- Ascites

### LESS FREQUENT

- Dilated small bowel
- Hydrops
- Polyhydramnios

### KEY FINDINGS/PITFALLS

- After bowel perforation, the release of bile acids, bile salts, and lipase may cause peritoneal calcifications within approximately 4 days.
  - The calcifications that are formed are usually linear or plaque-like.

    - Pancreatic enzymes are present in only 20% of cystic fibrosis patients. Hence, there is a lower frequency of identifiable calcifications with meconium peritonitis in fetuses with cystic fibrosis.
- Dilated bowel loops filled with diffuse thick meconium suggest cystic fibrosis.
- A normal-diameter large bowel with haustra that contain homogeneous dense meconium is a normal finding associated with fetal maturity.
- The range of sonographic findings associated with meconium peritonitis is due to
  - underlying etiology;
  - time from bowel perforation to the ultrasound examination; and
  - extent of intraperitoneal leakage.
- Meconium peritonitis has been detected sonographically as early as at 15 weeks' gestation.
  - Most cases are diagnosed after 20 weeks' gestation.
  - There is no correlation between gestational age at diagnosis and outcome.
- Meconium peritonitis has been divided into
  - Simple
    - Isolated intra-abdominal calcifications.
  - Complex
    - Intra-abdominal calcifications along with additional sonographic findings (i.e., ascites, bowel dilatation, and meconium pseudocyst, hydrops, or polyhydramnios)
    - It is more likely to require postnatal surgery.
- If a small bowel perforation spontaneously seals, surgical correction in the neonatal period is frequently not required.

## PREGNANCY MANAGEMENT

**Investigations and Consultations Required** Molecular studies for cystic fibrosis should be done. The best approach is usually amniocentesis, which also can provide a karyotype and microarray. Measurement of amniotic fluid proteins, such as alkaline phosphatase, will not be helpful, as low levels would be expected in any condition that causes intestinal obstruction. If there is a question of peritonitis, amniotic fluid polymerase chain reaction for cytomegalovirus should be performed. Consultation with a pediatric surgeon is appropriate. If a diagnosis of cystic fibrosis is established, referral of the family to a center with special expertise in the management of cystic fibrosis should be made. In those circumstances in which the fetus is found to have only a single detectable mutation for cystic fibrosis, the likelihood that the fetus has cystic fibrosis is diminished, but the residual risk for cystic fibrosis ranges from 3% to 72%, depending on the ethnic background of the parents.

**Fetal Intervention** Theoretically, early delivery prior to bowel perforation might improve prognosis. At present, however, no criteria have been established to indicate when intervention would be appropriate, and having a mature infant outweighs any theoretical benefit of early delivery.

**Monitoring** Serial sonograms and regular clinical assessment are essential to detect increased amniotic fluid volume, degree of bowel dilation, amount of ascites, possible volvulus, and hydrops, as well as evidence of preterm labor. No other special fetal assessment is necessary. Prenatal care should be coordinated in a tertiary center.

**Pregnancy Course** Polyhydramnios, secondary to intestinal obstructions, may result in preterm labor.

**Pregnancy Termination Issues** There are no special concerns if a diagnosis has been established. Without a diagnosis, a complete autopsy and appropriate molecular studies on fetal tissue are essential.

**Delivery** Prenatal care and delivery should be at a tertiary center. The degree of bowel distension will rarely be significant enough to cause abdominal dystocia.

## NEONATOLOGY

**Resuscitation** No special resuscitation measures are required. If severe abdominal distension due to obstruction is present at birth, respiration may be hindered, necessitating endotracheal intubation.

**Transport** Transfer to a tertiary perinatal center with pediatric surgery is always indicated. Gastric decompression during transport is essential.

**Testing and Confirmation** The major diagnostic questions are the coexistence of an obstructive lesion or of an open perforation, allowing continuing meconium spillage. Abdominal radiography, without contrast media, is usually sufficient to answer both concerns. If meconium ileus is determined to be the cause of the obstruction leading to the perforation, then evaluation for cystic fibrosis should be initiated. Evaluation for mutations in the *CFTR* gene and iontophoresis (sweat testing) for cystic fibrosis are indicated. The sweat test is reliable after 1 week of age in term infants and is diagnostic for cystic fibrosis.

**Nursery Management** The primary issues are avoidance of aspiration by gastric decompression, maintenance of hydration and electrolyte balance, and confirmation of the diagnosis. In cases of suspected meconium ileus, a precise diagnosis and often relief of the obstruction can be obtained by use of water-soluble, high-osmolality contrast media enemas. Generally, although the recommended contrast medium has a high osmolality, it is diluted prior to use to minimize injury to the mucosa and the degree of dehydration from mobilization of fluid into the intestine.

## SURGERY

**Preoperative Assessment** Initial management includes nasogastric decompression, intravenous fluid resuscitation, and a water-soluble contrast enema radiographic study. The last technique will likely provide a diagnosis and may be therapeutic by dislodging the impacted firm meconium from the distal ileum. The hypertonic intestinal contrast material can acutely dehydrate the infant. Compensation for this fluid shift must be made with increased intravenous fluids 1.5 to 2.0 times normal maintenance levels, preferably prior to the instillation of the contrast material. It is also important to keep the neonate warm throughout the process of imaging and transport.

**Operative Indications** Failure with two separate radiographic efforts to either enter the distended impacted small bowel or evacuate the inspissated meconium is an indication for surgical exploration. The presence of peritoneal irritation or free intraperitoneal air warrants surgical management rather than an attempt at evacuation with contrast instillation.

**Types of Procedures** Surgical management includes intraoperative irrigation of the meconium-obstructed bowel via an enterotomy. Successful evacuation may be followed by primary bowel closure, depending on the extent of intraluminal irrigation and bowel manipulation required. Extensive manipulation, significant fluid shifts due to the instillation of N-acetylcysteine to liquefy the inspissated meconium, or the development of hypothermia may be indications for the creation of a stoma. Necrotic intestine, meconium peritonitis, or extensive proximal intestinal meconium blockage can necessitate the use of enteral stomas with a subsequent reanastomosis at a later time.

**Surgical Results/Prognosis** The short-term prognosis is excellent (80%), and the long-term outcome is related to the cause of the meconium ileus.

## SUGGESTED READINGS

1. Dinkes K, Crombleholme TM, Craigo SD, et al: The natural history of meconium peritonitis diagnosed in utero. J Pediatr Surg 1995; 30:979-982.
2. Dorouhar F: Meconium peritonitis: pathology, evolution, and diagnosis. Am J Clin Pathol 1982; 78:208-213.
3. Foster MA, Nyberg DA, Mahony BS, et al: Meconium peritonitis: prenatal sonographic findings and their clinical significance. Radiology 1987; 165:661-665.
4. Gorter RR, Karimi A, Sleeboom C, et al: Clinical and genetic characteristics of meconium ileus in newborns with and without cystic fibrosis. J Pediatr Gastroenterol Nutr 2010; 50:569-572.
5. Lang I, Daneman A, Cutz E, et al: Abdominal calcification in cystic fibrosis with meconium ileus: radiologic-pathologic correlation. Pediatr Radiol 1997; 27:523-527.
6. Shyu M-K, Shih J-C, Lee C-N, et al: Correlation of prenatal ultrasound and postnatal outcome in meconium peritonitis. Fetal Diagn Ther 2003; 18:255-261.
7. Zangheri G, Andreani M, Ciriello E, et al: Fetal intra-abdominal calcifications from meconium peritonitis: sonographic predictors of postnatal surgery. Prenat Diagn 2007; 27:960-963.

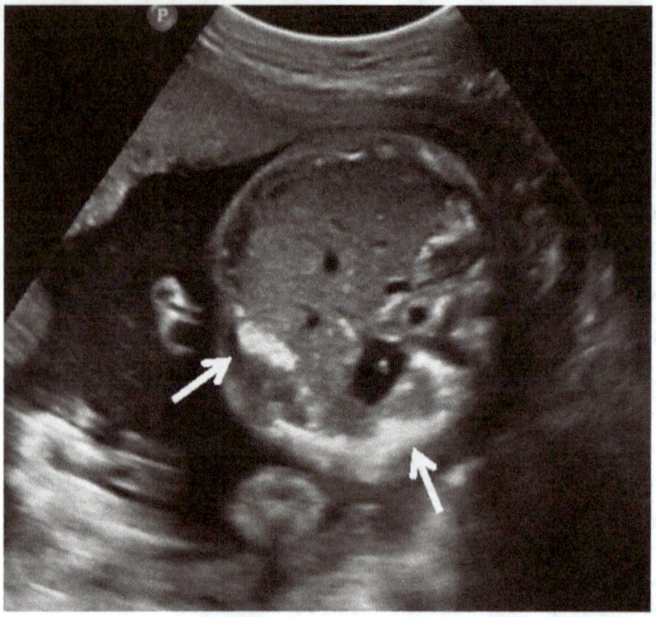

**FIGURE 6.6A** Meconium peritonitis illustrating calcified plaques (arrows).

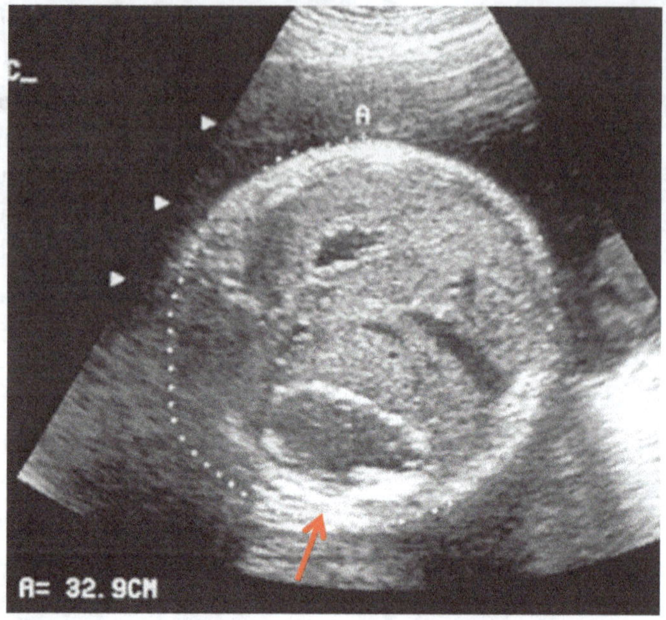


**FIGURE 6.6B** Meconium pseudocyst (arrow).

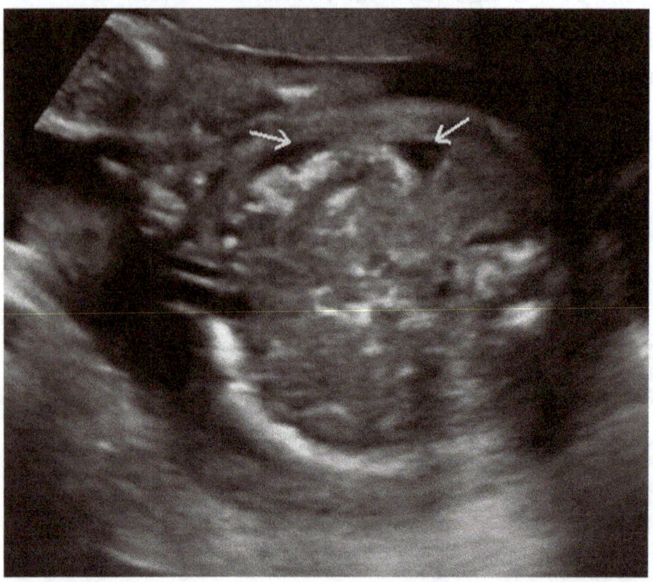

**FIGURE 6.6C** Meconium peritonitis with ascites (arrows).

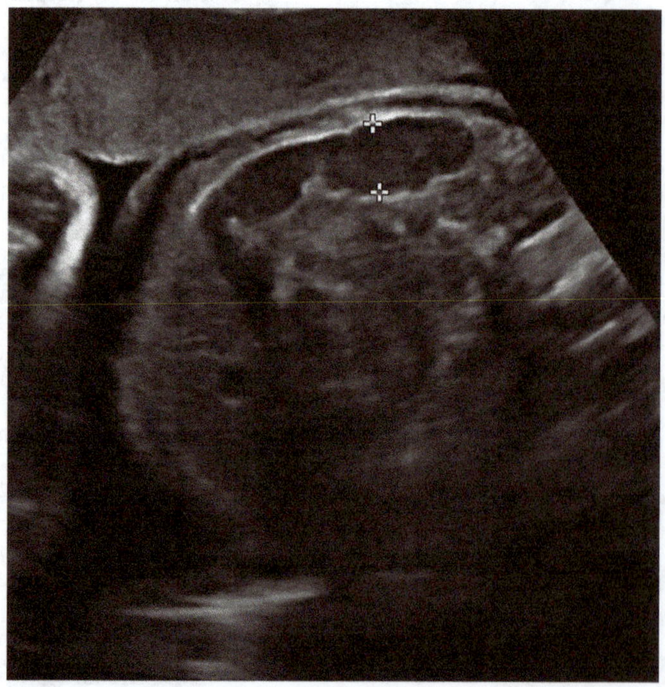

**FIGURE 6.6D** Normal large bowel diameter (+ … +).

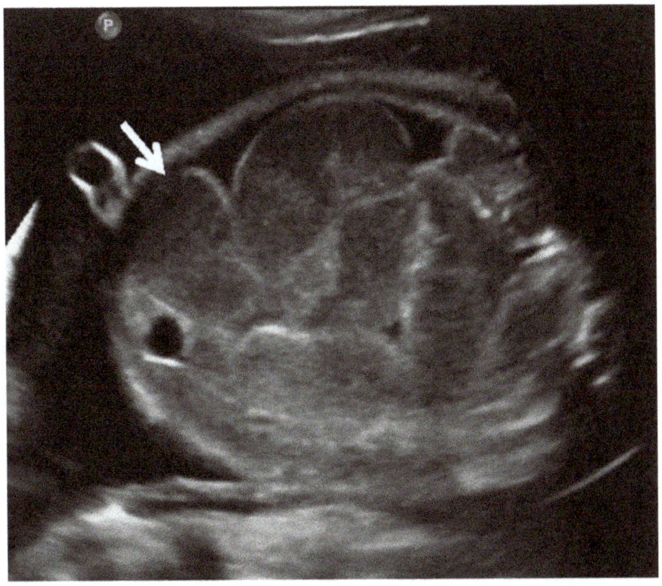

**FIGURE 6.6E** Meconium ileus with dilated bowel containing diffuse meconium (arrow). Minimal ascites is present.

# 6.7 OMPHALOCELE

## EPIDEMIOLOGY/GENETICS

**Definition** An omphalocele is a transparent sac of amnion attached to the umbilical ring that contains herniated abdominal viscera.

**Epidemiology** Omphaloceles occur in 1 in 10,000 live births (M1:F2, except in monozygotic twins, for whom there is a strong female preponderance). Incidence in the second trimester is 4 in 10,000.

**Embryology** Omphaloceles, which contain liver, are thought to result from failure of lateral body fold migration and body wall closure. A "giant" omphalocele is greater than 40 mm with liver, at least partly extruded. Omphaloceles that contain only bowel are said to result from the embryonic persistence of the body stalk. Omphaloceles have associated malformations in almost two-thirds of cases, including congenital heart defects, bladder exstrophy, imperforate anus, neural tube defects, cleft lip with or without cleft palate, and diaphragmatic hernia. In addition, approximately 25% have associated chromosomal abnormalities, especially trisomies 13 and 18. Syndromes associated with omphalocele include the Beckwith-Wiedemann syndrome (omphalocele with macrosomia, macroglossia, organomegaly, and neonatal hypoglycemia), OEIS, and a number of rare skeletal dysplasias. Beckwith-Wiedemann syndrome is found in 8% to 10% of apparently isolated cases of omphalocele.

**Inheritance Patterns** Rare autosomal dominant and X-linked recessive families have been reported with isolated omphaloceles. Some cases of the Beckwith-Wiedemann syndrome show autosomal dominant inheritance.

**Teratogens** None are known.

**Serum Screening** Measurement of maternal serum α-fetoprotein will detect approximately 70% of omphaloceles.

**Prognosis** The prognosis is generally dependent on associated malformations or the size of the defect. Of apparently isolated defects, 30% to 40% are found to have associated abnormalities or a genetic syndrome at birth. Mortality is less than 10% in isolated omphalocele but may be as high as 20% to 30% in nonisolated cases. Intrauterine growth restriction and preterm labor may complicate the pregnancy in up to a third of cases, usually those that are not isolated. Giant lesions containing both solid and hollow viscera have limited potential for successful closure.

## SONOGRAPHY

### FREQUENT FINDINGS

- Liver or bowel with a covering membrane at the cord insertion site
- Abnormal umbilical cord insertion site
- Concurrent congenital anomalies (30% to 70%)

### LESS FREQUENT

- Ascites
- Fluid within the omphalocele sac
- Polyhydramnios/oligohydramnios

### KEY FINDINGS/PITFALLS/DIFFERENTIAL DIAGNOSIS

- Liver containing omphalocele can be diagnosed at 10 weeks' gestation.
- Physiologic small bowel herniation in the first trimester must be distinguished from a bowel-containing omphalocele.
  - A bowel-containing omphalocele should not be diagnosed until at least 12 weeks' gestation.
- An increased first-trimester nuchal translucency is associated with omphalocele.
- Small isolated bowel-containing omphaloceles between 14 and 16 weeks' gestation can resolve later in pregnancy.
- An omphalocele sac may contain small bowel, liver, spleen, kidney, or bladder.
- Karyotypic abnormalities are more common with bowel-containing versus liver-containing omphaloceles.
- The absolute or relative size of an omphalocele is not associated with subsequent mortality; it appears to be better correlated with associated abnormalities.
- Three-dimensional imaging can provide additional information on possible associated congenital anomalies. In addition, the detection of a skin covering indicates an umbilical hernia in contrast to an omphalocele.
- Syndromes associated with an omphalocele have the following features:
  - Beckwith-Wiedemann syndrome is characterized by a large-for-gestational-age fetus, omphalocele, visceromegaly, macroglossia, and polyhydramnios.
  - OEIS has the following findings:
    - Failure to visualize a bladder
    - Midline abdominal wall defect
    - Lumbosacral meningomyelocele
  - Pentalogy of Cantrell has five characteristic abnormalities:
    - A defect in the lower sternum
    - Agenesis of the anterior diaphragm
    - Midline abdominal wall defect
    - Absence of diaphragmatic portion of the pericardium
    - Congenital heart defects (hallmark is ectopia cordis)

## PREGNANCY MANAGEMENT

**Investigations and Consultations Required** An extended ultrasound examination should be performed to determine if the abnormality is isolated. Further studies are indicated, including a fetal karyotype and microarray, and specific gene testing if a syndrome, such as Beckwith-Wiedemann, is suspected. The significant incidence of congenital heart disease requires fetal echocardiographic evaluation. Consultation with a neonatologist and a pediatric surgeon is helpful to plan perinatal management and to discuss the issues regarding neonatal management, such as primary versus secondary closure.

**Monitoring** No special modifications are needed. Serial ultrasonographic examinations should be done every 4 weeks to monitor growth. Fetal evaluations, such as nonstress testing, are not necessary unless there is evidence of intrauterine growth restriction.

**Pregnancy Course** There are no specific obstetric complications to be expected.

**Pregnancy Termination Issues** In cases with multiple abnormalities and in which a precise cause has not been determined, consideration should be given to using a nondestructive method of termination followed by a careful autopsy.

**Delivery** There appears to be no advantage to cesarean section, except in those cases in which there is a large lesion with the liver out of the abdomen, where rupture of the omphalocele sac during delivery is a concern. Delivery should be performed at term in a center with appropriate perinatal facilities for surgical management of the neonate.

## NEONATOLOGY

**Resuscitation** Assistance with the onset of respiration is usually not required unless there is concurrent prematurity, associated respiratory distress, or an associated anomaly that interferes with the onset of cardiorespiratory adaptation. Pulmonary hypoplasia is often present in giant omphaloceles. If assisted ventilation is required, bag-and-mask ventilation is contraindicated to avoid gaseous distension of the stomach and bowel. The major concern is to avoid trauma to, and contamination of, the omphalocele sac. Once respiration and circulation are established, the sac should be covered with warmed, saline-moistened gauze and then covered by additional wrapping to avoid evaporative heat and water loss. It is always safe to enclose the trunk and legs in a sterile plastic drawstring bag (bowel bag). Prompt decompression of the stomach is important initially, followed by intermittent gastric suction.

**Transport** Transfer to a tertiary center with pediatric surgery and neonatology is always indicated. Protection of the sac, as described, should be maintained during transport, as should gastric decompression. Reliable intravenous access should be established and infusion of a balanced electrolyte solution instituted.

**Testing and Confirmation** Because of the very high incidence of associated anomalies, appropriate diagnostic testing, including chromosomal analysis, echocardiography, and renal sonography, should be obtained expeditiously before surgical intervention.

**Nursery Management** Care of the omphalocele sac, gastric decompression, and administration of broad-spectrum antibiotics and intravenous fluids should be maintained. In some cases, it may be necessary to provide ventilatory support in the early postoperative period, as there may be increased intra-abdominal pressure from the reduction of the extruded viscera back into the abdominal cavity. Pulmonary hypoplasia may be a significant concern, especially in the setting of the larger omphalocele, and these neonates may require prolonged ventilator support, including plans for home ventilator support. Parenteral nutrition is required during the postoperative recovery period, as there is always a significant interval before adequate enteral intake can be established.

## SURGERY

**Preoperative Assessment** Preoperative and postdelivery goals include a thorough evaluation for associated anomalies, particularly of the cardiac system, including echocardiography. Preoperative broad-coverage antibiotics are administered.

**Operative Indications** Surgical repair is most commonly electively scheduled unless there has been rupture of the omphalocele sac. Surgery is generally scheduled after resuscitation and evaluation for associated anomalies. Depending on the hemodynamic and respiratory stability of the neonate, the surgeon may prefer to proceed with nonoperative management of the intact omphalocele by using frequent applications of a desiccating antiseptic solution (often iodine-based antiseptic solution, such as Betadine) and undertaking a delayed closure of the secondarily produced skin-covered hernia. This process may be associated with complications related to the difficulties in repairing the resultant large abdominal wall hernia. Because pulmonary insufficiency may be associated with a giant omphalocele, topical therapy is preferred as it may minimize further respiratory embarrassment.

**Types of Procedures** Intraoperative management consists of removal of the amniotic sac, evaluation for associated intestinal malrotation with lysis of bands obstructing the duodenum, and evaluation of the intestine for possible associated atresias. Primary fascial and abdominal wall closure can be accomplished if intra-abdominal pressure, measured by either the intragastric route using a nasogastric tube or the intravesical method using a bladder catheter, does not exceed 20 mm Hg after return of the viscera to the abdominal cavity. A temporary Silastic/Dacron extra-abdominal pouch is used if the intra-abdominal pressure is too high for primary closure. Gradual reduction of the viscera can usually be accomplished over 5 to 7 days, with subsequent surgical removal of the pouch and secondary abdominal wall closure.

Giant omphaloceles usually are associated with primary respiratory distress due to lung hypoplasia and make primary abdominal wall repair less likely. Even with the use of an initial Silastic pouch, they eventually may require mobilized lateral skin flaps with prosthetic material to achieve coverage of the exposed viscera. The alternative method is the previously described acute nonoperative therapy. Secondary closure of the remaining ventral wall defect, after either nonoperative or incomplete surgical closure of the fascia, can be achieved following further body growth and development.

**Surgical Results/Prognosis** If there are no associated anomalies, such as an intestinal atresia, resumption of postoperative intestinal function is prompt. Overall survival depends on the severity of the associated anomalies, most commonly cardiac defects and pulmonary hypoplasia, and can vary from 30% to 70%. Long-term morbidity is also related to the associated anomalies, most notably cardiac.

## SUGGESTED READINGS

1. Blazer S, Zimmer EZ, Gover A, Bronshtein M: Fetal omphalocele detected early in pregnancy: associated anomalies and outcomes. Radiology 2004; 232:191-195.
2. Bonilla-Musoles F, Machado LE, Bailão LA, et al: Abdominal wall defects. Two-versus three-dimensional ultrasonographic diagnosis. J Ultrasound Med 2001; 20:379-389.
3. Bowerman RA: Sonography of fetal midgut herniation: normal size criteria and correlation with crown-rump length. J Ultrasound Med 1993; 5:251-254.
4. Brown DL, Emerson DS, Shulman LP, Carson SA: Sonographic diagnosis of omphalocele during 10th week of gestation. Am J Roentgenol 1989; 153:825-826.
5. Corey KM, Hornik CP, Laughon MM, et al: Frequency of anomalies and hospital outcome in infants with gastroschisis and omphalocele. Early Hum Dev 2014; 90:421-424.
6. Gibbon C, Touch S, Broth RE, Berghella V: Abdominal wall defects and congenital heart disease. Ultrasound Obstet Gynecol 2003; 21:334-337.
7. Heider A, Strauss RA, Kuller JA: Omphalocele: clinical outcomes in cases with normal karyotypes. Am J Obstet Gynecol 2004; 190:135-141.
8. Hughes MD, Nyberg DA, Mack LA, Pretorius DH: Fetal omphalocele: prenatal US detection of concurrent anomalies and other predictors of outcome. Radiology 1989; 173:371-376.
9. Langer JC: Gastroschisis and omphaloceles. Sem Pediatr Surg 1996; 5:124-128.
10. Ledbetter DJ. Gastroschisis and omphalocele. Surg Clin North Am 2006; 86:249-260.
11. Nyberg DA, Fitzsimmons J, Mack LA, et al: Chromosomal abnormalities in fetuses with omphalocele. Significance of omphalocele contents. J Ultrasound Med 1989; 8:299-308.
12. Porter A, Benson CB, Hawley P, Wilkins-Haug L: Outcome of fetuses with a prenatal diagnosis of isolated omphalocele. Prenat Diagn 2009; 29:668-673.
13. Saleem I: Advances in surgery for abdominal wall defects: gastroschisis and omphalocele innovations. Clin Perinatol 2012; 39:375-386.
14. Snijders RJM, Sebire NJ, Souka A, et al: Fetal exomphalos and chromosomal defects: relationship to maternal age and gestation. Ultrasound Obstet Gynecol 1995; 6:250-255.
15. Van Eijck FC, Klein WM, Boetes C, et al: Has the liver and other visceral organs migrated to its normal position in children with giant omphalocele? A follow-up study with ultrasonography. Eur J Pediatr 2010; 169:563-567.
16. van Zalen-Sprock RM, Vugt JM, van Geijn HP: First-trimester sonography of physiological midgut herniation and early diagnosis of omphalocele. Prenat Diagn 1997; 17:511-518.

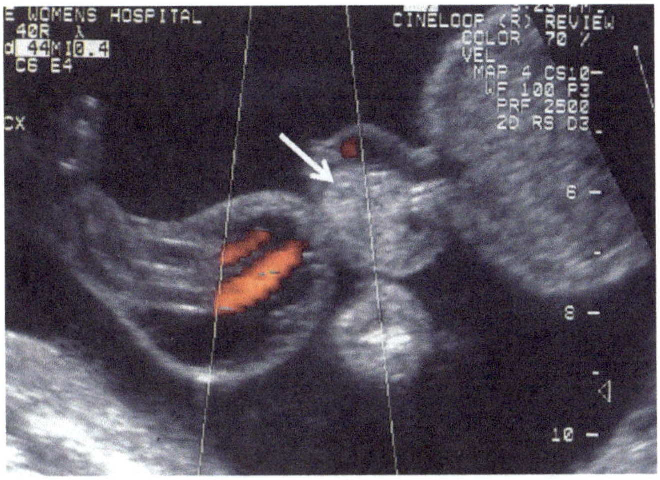


**FIGURE 6.7A** Bowel containing omphalocele (arrow) at 22 weeks.

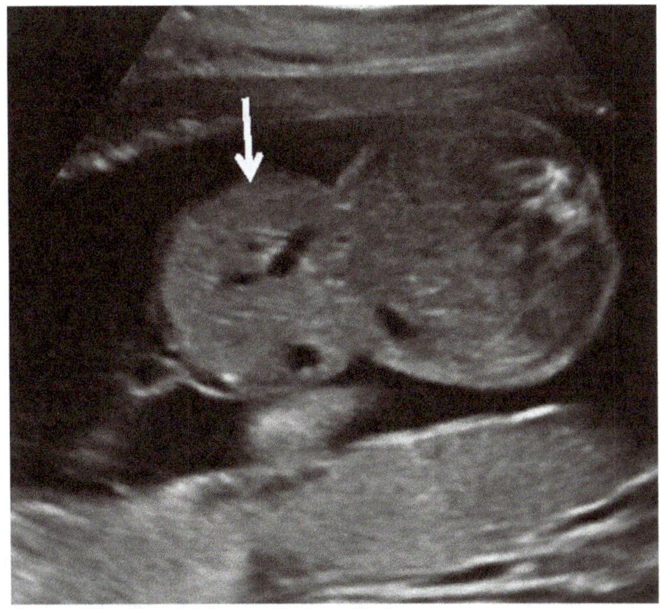

**FIGURE 6.7B** Liver containing omphalocele (arrow) at 22 weeks.

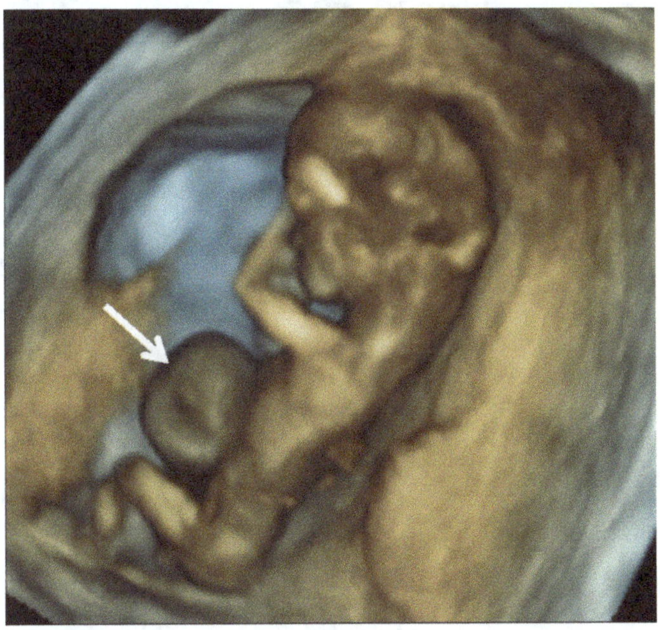

**FIGURE 6.7C** Three-dimensional image of liver containing omphalocele (arrow) at 12 weeks.

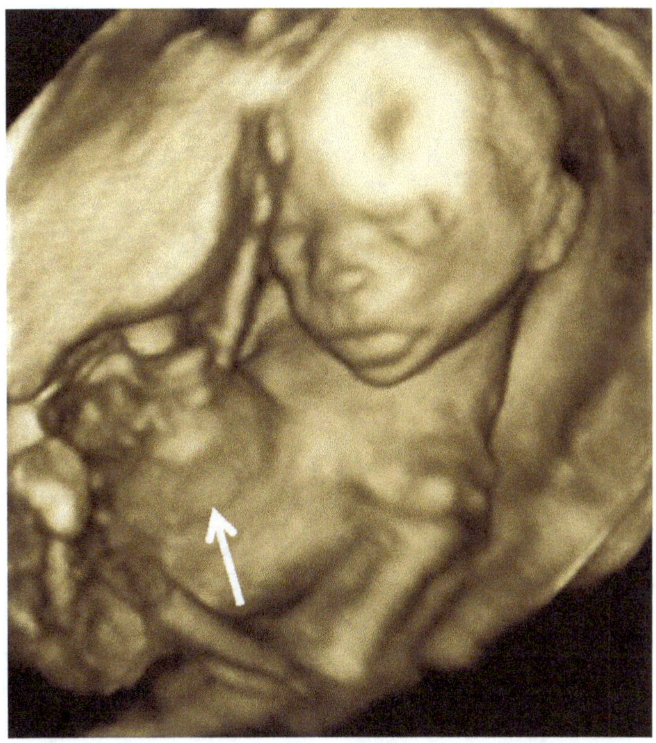

**FIGURE 6.7D** Three-dimensional image of liver containing omphalocele (arrow) at 20 weeks.

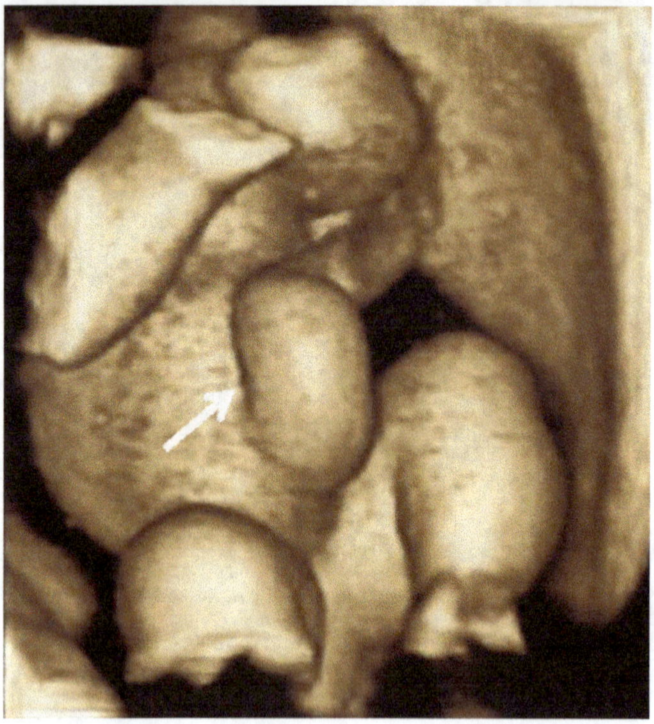

**FIGURE 6.7E** Three-dimensional image of a fetal umbilical hernia with skin covering (arrow).

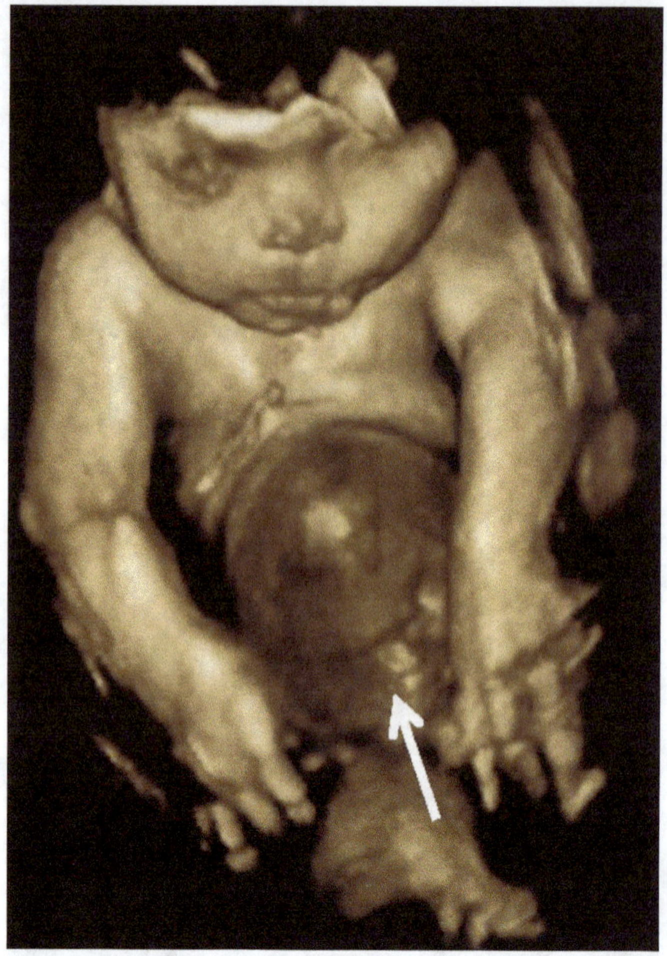

**FIGURE 6.7F** Three-dimensional image illustrating the peritoneal covering of a liver containing omphalocele (arrow).

# 6.8 SMALL BOWEL ATRESIA OR STENOSIS (INTESTINAL ATRESIA)

## EPIDEMIOLOGY/GENETICS

**Definition** Small bowel or intestinal atresia is a phrase used to describe a segmental defect of the intestine that disrupts the luminal continuity of the intestinal tube during development.

**Epidemiology** Incidence is 1 in 3000 to 1 in 5000 live births.

**Embryology** Most isolated atresias are theorized to be an in utero vascular accident due to embolic occlusion, vascular compression, or twisting of the mesenteric vessels from volvulus or intussusception. However, there is an opposing theory that the atresias are the result of a genetic mutation that disrupts a common developmental process in the embryonic gut. The location of obstruction is as follows:

- Proximal jejunum: 31%
- Distal jejunum: 20%
- Proximal ilium: 13%
- Distal ilium: 36%

Jejunoileal atresias are classified into four types:

| Type | Description |
|---|---|
| I | Mucosal |
| II | Atretic fibrous core |
| IIIa | V-shaped mesenteric defect |
| IIIb | Apple peel |
| IV | Multiple atresias |

Forty-four percent of small bowel atresias have associated findings, including small for gestational age, meconium peritonitis, meconium ileus, cystic fibrosis, omphalocele, gastroschisis, malrotation, duodenal atresia, cardiovascular defects, and chromosome abnormalities. More than 15 genetic, chromosome, and sporadic syndromes have been described with intestinal atresias.

**Inheritance Patterns** Rare autosomal recessive genetic syndromes that include multiple intestinal atresias and jejunal atresia have been described. Approximately 15% to 25% of cases of jejunal and ileal atresia have cystic fibrosis (autosomal recessive).

**Teratogens** Thalidomide and cocaine are teratogenic.

**Prognosis** Outcome is excellent if the atresia occurs as an isolated abnormality. Most of the deaths are due to the sequelae of short bowel syndrome, primarily liver failure. The prognosis is dependent on the specific associated abnormalities or syndrome diagnosis.

## SONOGRAPHY

### FREQUENT FINDINGS

- Multiple loops of dilated bowel
- Active peristalsis
- Polyhydramnios

### LESS FREQUENT

- Meconium peritonitis (6%)
- Enteric duplication cysts
- Gastroschisis
- Volvulus

### KEY FINDINGS/PITFALLS

- Sonographically, it is difficult to delineate the level of obstruction.
- The presence of intraperitoneal calcifications suggests meconium peritonitis secondary to bowel perforation.
- Polyhydramnios in association with dilated loops of small bowel is predictive of severe small bowel atresia and usually a more proximal lesion.
- This is rarely diagnosed before 24 weeks' gestation.
- Overall sonographic detection is 50.6% (95% confidence interval, 38.0% to 63.2%)
- Fetal MRI can help to determine the site of occlusion and the amount of remaining normal small bowel.

### DIFFERENTIAL DIAGNOSIS

- Volvulus: While there are multiple dilated loops of bowel, peristalsis is absent. A fluid-fluid interface may be present due to hemorrhage within the bowel.
- Meconium ileus: The dilated loops of bowel contain homogeneous debris.
- Congenital chloride and congenital sodium diarrhea are rare autosomal recessive disorders.
    - Multiple dilated loops of bowel with peristalsis and polyhydramnios are consistent with small bowel atresia.
    - On MRI, the presence of fluid in the colon as well as the small bowel suggests the presence of watery diarrhea.
    - An elevated sodium or chloride in the amniotic fluid may help to confirm this diagnosis.

## PREGNANCY MANAGEMENT

**Investigations and Consultations Required** A family history and exposure history should be sought; carrier status for cystic fibrosis should be reviewed or obtained. Chromosome studies should be performed. Fetal echocardiography should be performed to exclude associated cardiac malformations. A management plan should be devised in consultation with neonatology and pediatric surgery.

**Monitoring** Sonographic examinations should be performed every 3 to 4 weeks to detect polyhydramnios and monitor the degree of bowel dilation. Polyhydramnios is, however, rare in lesions beyond the jejunum. Careful assessment for signs of preterm labor is essential if polyhydramnios is found.

**Pregnancy Course** The risk of preterm labor is high in more proximal lesions because polyhydramnios is more common in these lesions.

**Pregnancy Termination Issues** Pregnancy termination is rarely entertained because of the third-trimester presentation of these malformations.

**Delivery** In general, management should be delivery at term in a tertiary center with appropriate support services, including neonatology and pediatric surgery availability.

## NEONATOLOGY

**Resuscitation** Infants with small bowel or intestinal atresia may present with signs of intestinal obstruction, including bilious emesis and abdominal distension. At the time of delivery, the stomach should be emptied prior to transfer of the infant from the delivery room to decompress the bowel and reduce the risk of regurgitation and aspiration. With known or suspected distal obstruction, there are usually no special resuscitation issues.

**Transport** Transfer to a tertiary center with pediatric surgery is always indicated. Orogastric decompression and maintenance of intravenous fluid infusion in transit are essential.

**Testing and Confirmation** Confirmation of the diagnosis is best established by abdominal radiographs and, when indicated, contrast studies. Air is an excellent and safe contrast medium for suspected upper tract obstruction. The typical pattern is to see multiple dilated loops and air-fluid levels proximally with no visualization of bowel distally. A contrast enema may demonstrate a microcolon and failure of the contrast to reflux into the obstructed dilated bowel segment. Additional diagnostic evaluation for associated anomalies should be obtained as indicated.

**Nursery Management** If cardiorespiratory resuscitation has been required, the first priority is to facilitate cardiorespiratory adaptation with oxygen, intravenous fluids, and ventilatory support, as needed. Intravenous access should be established, and fluid and electrolyte support should be instituted. Orogastric decompression should be maintained to minimize the risk of aspiration and respiratory complication. Parenteral nutrition is usually required in the postoperative period, as there is often a significant interval before adequate enteral intake is established.

## SURGERY

**Operative Indications** All neonates with obstructed small bowel require surgery. Generally, surgery can be safely delayed until the infant is otherwise stabilized.

**Types of Procedures** Intestinal decompression and intravenous access with maintenance fluids are begun immediately. Antibiotics are also started. Surgical repair usually consists of the excision of a portion of the dilated proximal intestine and a modified end-to-end or end-to-side primary anastomosis. If the atresia involves a large portion of bowel, it can result in potential short gut syndrome. Under these circumstances, tapering of the dilated proximal bowel with primary anastomosis is utilized. This avoids increased loss of length, facilitates early gut function, and diminishes bacterial overgrowth in the proximal intestine. The use of proximal intestinal stomas is reserved for those cases complicated by significant proximal bowel distension, with associated size mismatch between proximal and distal bowel, severe meconium peritonitis, or perforation with bacterial contamination and secondary peritonitis. In the setting of significant bowel distension, a temporary stoma with decompression may allow for decreased distension and improved size match of the anastomosis at a later surgery.

**Surgical Results/Prognosis** The long-term prognosis is primarily related to the length and functional capability of the remaining small bowel or associated defects, such as cystic fibrosis. Uncomplicated short-segment intestinal atresias have an excellent prognosis. Extensive areas of intestinal atresia can result in the short gut syndrome. Infants can be kept alive by intravenous alimentation but may undergo progressive worsening of liver function, with eventual death from portal hypertension or liver failure. Current efforts at minimizing the hepatic injury associated with parenteral nutrition and improvements in intestinal rehabilitation have resulted in better outcomes for many neonates, even with extensive loss of intestinal length.

## SUGGESTED READINGS


1. Benachi A, Sonigo P, Jouannic JM, et al: Determination of the anatomical location of an antenatal intestinal occlusion by magnetic resonance imaging. Ultrasound Obstet Gynecol 2001; 18:163-165.
2. Colombani M, Ferry M, Toga C, et al: Magnetic resonance imaging in the prenatal diagnosis of congenital diarrhea. Ultrasound Obstet Gynecol 2010; 35:560-565.
3. Dalla Vecchia LK, Grosfeld JL, West KW, et al: Intestinal atresia and stenosis. A 25-year experience with 277 cases. Arch Surg 1998; 133:490-497.
4. Hemming V, Rankin J: Small intestinal atresia in a defined population: occurrence, prenatal diagnosis and survival. Prenat Diagn 2007; 27:1205-1211.
5. Iachobelli BD, Zaccara A, Spirydakis I, et al: Prenatal counselling of small bowel atresia: watch the fluid! Prenat Diagn 2006; 26:214-217.
6. Jo YS, Jang DG, Nam SY, et al: Antenatal sonographic features of ileal atresia. J Obstet Gynaecol Res 2012; 38:215-219.
7. Nichol PF, Reeder A, Botham R: Humans, mice, and mechanisms of intestinal atresias: a window into understanding early intestinal development. J Gastrointest Surg 2011; 15:694-700.
8. Nyberg DA, Neilson IR: Abdomen and gastrointestinal tract. In: Nyberg DA, McGahan JP, Pretorius DH, et al, eds. Diagnostic Imaging of Fetal Anomalies. Philadelphia: Lippincott Williams and Wilkins; 2003: 549-572.
9. Sammour RN, Leibovitz Z, Degani S, et al: Prenatal diagnosis of small-bowel volvulus using 3-dimensional Doppler sonography. J Ultrasound Med 2008; 27:1655-1661.

10. Touloukian RJ: Intestinal atresia. Clin Perinatol 1978; 5:3-18.
11. Virgone C, D'Antonio F, Khalil A, et al: Accuracy of prenatal ultrasound in detecting jejunal and ileal atresia: systematic review and meta-analysis. Ultrasound Obstet Gynecol 2015; 45:523-529.
12. Wax JR, Hamilton T, Cantin A, et al: Congenital jejunal and ileal atresia: natural prenatal sonographic history and association with neonatal outcome. J Ultrasound Med 2006; 25:337-342.

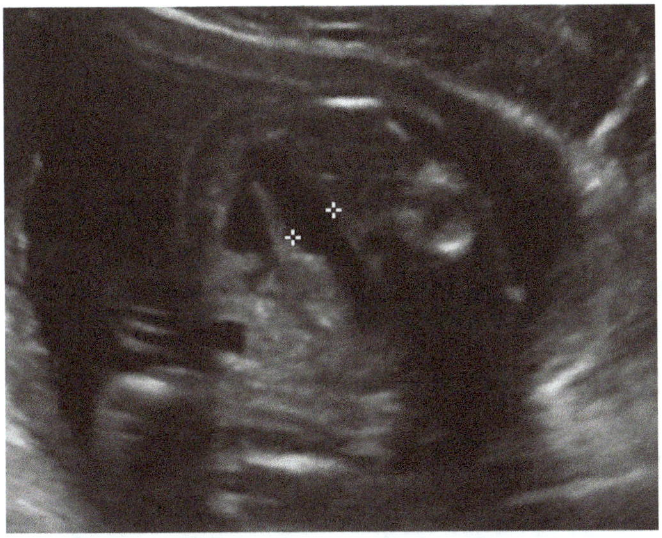

**FIGURE 6.8A** Small bowel atresia. Dilated small bowel (+ … +).

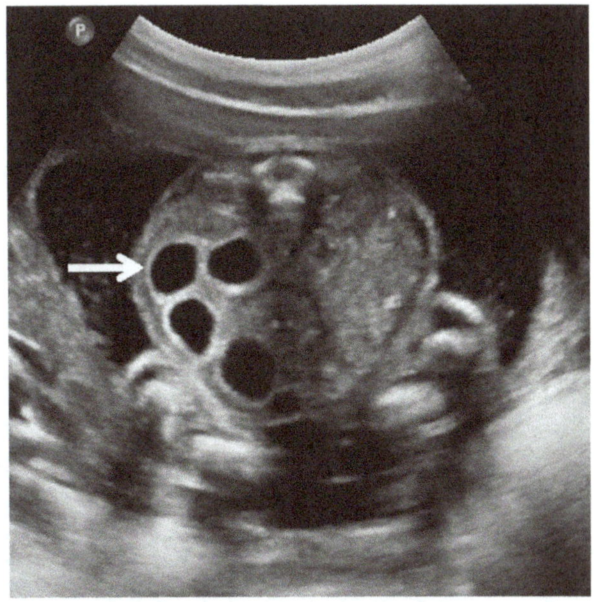

**FIGURE 6.8B** Small bowel atresia. Note the multiple loops of dilated bowel (arrow).

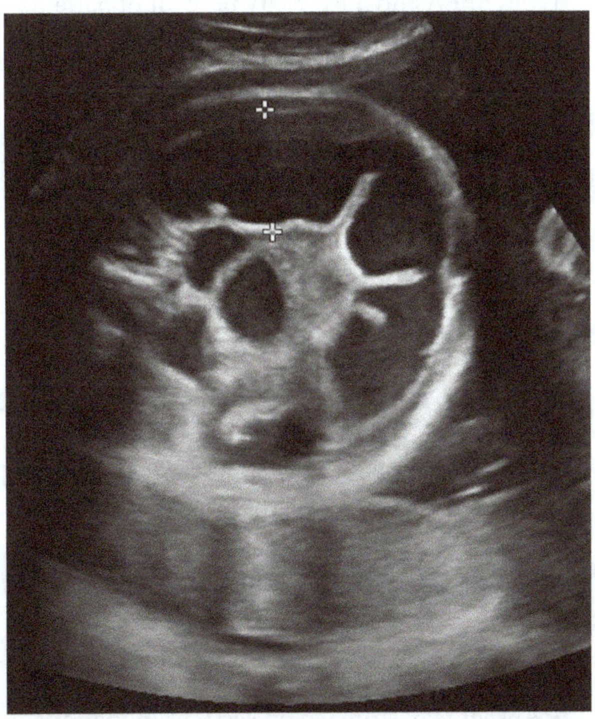

**FIGURE 6.8C** Small bowel atresia with marked bowel dilatation (+ … +).

# 6.9 TRACHEO-ESOPHAGEAL FISTULA, ESOPHAGEAL ATRESIA

## EPIDEMIOLOGY/GENETICS

**Definition** Esophageal atresia (EA) is a congenital lack of continuity of the esophagus, resulting in a blind-ending esophageal pouch. There is frequently an associated tracheo-esophageal fistula (TEF). The etiology involves a failure of the primitive foregut to divide into the esophagus posteriorly and the trachea anteriorly.

**Epidemiology** Occurrence is 1 in 2500-5000 live births (M1:F1); 90% of patients have EA with a distal TEF.

- Classification

| Type | Description | % |
|---|---|---|
| I | EA without TEF | 6-7 |
| II | EA with proximal TEF | 1-2 |
| III | EA with proximal and distal TEF | 1-5 |
| IV | EA with distal TEF | 86 |
| V | TEF without EA | 4-6 |

**Embryology** Failure of the anterior foregut to divide into the anterior trachea and posterior esophagus around the fourth week of gestation results in various types of EA and TEF. Sixty percent of patients have associated anomalies, the most common of which are cardiac (25%), genitourinary (15%), skeletal (14%), and other intestinal atresias (13%). The VACTERL association occurs in approximately 10% of cases. More than 40 genetic, chromosomal, and sporadic syndromes have been described with EA or TEF. Chromosome abnormalities account for approximately 10% of cases, with trisomy 18 the most common chromosomal abnormality.

**Inheritance Patterns** Inheritance is likely multifactorial (1% to 2% recurrence risk).

**Teratogens** Retinoic acid and alcohol are teratogenic.

**Prognosis** Survival and prognosis are determined by the cause and associated malformations. Overall survival is 85% to 90%, with more than 95% of patients with an isolated TEF surviving with a functional repair.

## SONOGRAPHY

### FREQUENT FINDINGS

- Absent fetal stomach on serial examinations
- Polyhydramnios after 24 weeks' gestation

### LESS FREQUENT

- Blind-ending esophageal pouch (10%)
  - Cervical
  - Mediastinal
- Intrauterine growth restriction

### KEY FINDINGS/PITFALLS

- Gastric secretions may give rise to a small fetal stomach with EA.
- In cases of EA with TEF, amniotic fluid may reach the stomach and stomach size may appear normal.
- The identification of an esophageal pouch requires fetal swallowing.
  - Fetal swallowing begins at 12 weeks' gestation
  - Prior to 23 weeks' gestation, the fetus does not produce enough pressure with swallowing to dilate the pouch.
  - In EA with a proximal TEF, amniotic fluid enters the trachea and the esophagus remains collapsed.
  - The duration that a pouch remains visible depends on the following:
    - Size of fistula
      - With a large fistula, the pouch will empty more quickly.
    - Fetal regurgitation
- The esophageal pouch is first detected at 23 weeks.
  - A pouch in the cervical region ("neck pouch") has a larger area of atresia and a higher probability of severe anomalies.
  - A pouch below the clavicle ("mediastinal pouch") is associated with a distal TEF; primary repair is usually possible.
- Sensitivity of ultrasound for detection of EA is 30%.
- MRI can be used to assist in the diagnosis of EA.

### DIFFERENTIAL DIAGNOSIS

- Congenital microgastria: During development, the normal stomach rotation does not occur, resulting in an absence of the greater and lesser curvatures.
- The absence of the fetal stomach and normal amniotic fluid in the third trimester should suggest that a presumptive diagnosis of EA may not be correct.

## PREGNANCY MANAGEMENT

**Investigations and Consultations Required** Most cases have an associated TEF, and the ultrasound diagnosis will be presumptive, or the condition may be suspected, but not made with certainty prenatally. If suspected, chromosome studies with microarray should be performed, as well as fetal echocardiography. Consultation with neonatology and a pediatric surgeon is appropriate.

**Fetal Intervention** No direct fetal intervention is indicated.

**Monitoring** Frequent clinical and sonographic examinations are generally necessary when considering the diagnosis and should continue once the presumptive diagnosis is made to monitor gastric size, look for an esophageal pouch, and monitor the degree of polyhydramnios.

**Pregnancy Termination Issues** Generally, this is a third-trimester diagnosis, and termination is not an option. In rare cases with an early diagnosis, the procedure for termination should provide an intact fetus for a complete autopsy.

**Delivery** Although prematurity is common, if possible, delivery should be at term in a tertiary center with appropriate support services, including neonatology and pediatric surgery availability.

## NEONATOLOGY

**Resuscitation** If the infant is born prematurely or there are associated major organ system anomalies, there may be difficulty with the onset of respiration. When the diagnosis is suspected from prenatal studies and there is delay in onset of respiration, immediate endotracheal intubation is preferable to bag-and-mask ventilation to avoid overdistension of the stomach. Excessive oral secretions may be encountered, necessitating placement of a replogle tube into the upper esophageal pouch for continuous drainage.

**Transport** Transfer to a tertiary perinatal center with a pediatric surgeon is always indicated. Depending on the size of the infant, an 8F or 10F replogle tube should be placed to continuous suction to drain the pooled secretions and avoid aspiration from the proximal pouch.

**Testing and Confirmation** Newborns present with excessive salivation, choking with feedings, and respiratory distress. Postnatal radiologic studies will define the defect. A radiopaque catheter is carefully passed into the esophagus until resistance is met. Air is injected through the catheter, and chest and abdominal radiographs are obtained. A TEF is apparent by the finding of air in the intestine on an abdominal x-ray. The lack of distal air is seen in pure EA with no distal fistula. Chromosomal analysis, if not obtained prenatally, an echocardiogram, and careful physical examination looking for any associated anomalies, such as an imperforate anus, are performed. It is critical that the echocardiogram identifies any congenital heart disease and documents the position of the aortic arch. A right-sided aortic arch makes the surgical approach more difficult, and this is key information to have preoperatively.

**Nursery Management** The priority in early care is to avoid aspiration of either oral or gastric secretions and thus to decrease the likelihood of pneumonia. Infants with a fistula between the trachea and distal esophagus are particularly prone to gastric distension and reflux of gastric contents. Continuous evacuation of esophageal secretions and avoidance of overdistension of the stomach are useful maneuvers to prevent aspiration. Intravenous access is obtained to administer intravenous fluids, as the infant will not be able to sustain enteral feedings.

If endotracheal intubation is required, an attempt should be made to locate the tip of the tube distal to the fistula insertion. This can be accomplished either by placement under endoscopic control or with careful auscultation over the stomach as a positive-pressure breath is given, advancing the tube until air is no longer heard entering the stomach. It is critical to avoid excessive bag-mask ventilation in securing the airway to minimize gastric distention and reflux up the distal fistula.

## SURGERY

**Preoperative Assessment** There are several forms of tracheoesophageal anomalies, but the most common (85%) is a combination of proximal esophageal pouch with a distal TEF. Preoperative surgical goals consist of identifying the degree of postdelivery aspiration pneumonitis and preventing further airway contamination. This includes assessment of the infant's clinical status, as well as the radiographic appearance of the lungs. The latter is a late-occurring sign and is more unreliable than clinical and metabolic (blood gas) determinations. A preoperative evaluation for all possible VACTERL anomalies is carried out with particular attention to cardiac lesions, but also including spinal and renal ultrasounds.

**Operative Indications** It is rare in the setting of EA/TEF without associated duodenal atresia to need to perform an urgent gastrostomy to relieve gastric distention and potential aspiration due to reflux. Most commonly, the neonate can be prepared for either thoracoscopy or thoracotomy for division of the TEF and a primary anastomosis of the EA. Operative planning is more difficult in the setting of a right-sided aortic arch, as the approach is generally through the right chest, and the right-sided arch makes identification and dissection on the proximal pouch difficult. It is critical to carefully evaluate the upper pouch for any evidence of a proximal fistula, as this may be difficult to identify preoperatively. In the setting of pure EA without fistula, most often a thoracotomy or thoracoscopy is deferred, and a gastrostomy is placed to allow growth, with the anticipation that by waiting 6-12 weeks a primary anastomosis can be completed.

**Types of Procedures** Classically, a right thoracotomy via a retropleural approach is used to facilitate better control of postoperative drainage in instances of an esophageal leak (5% to 20%). The TEF is divided and the tracheal opening closed carefully to prevent airway stenosis. Care must be exercised so that a tracheal fistula involving the upper pouch is not missed intraoperatively. A retropleural chest tube to act as a passive drain is left in position for any potential esophageal leakage.

**Surgical Results/Prognosis** The early complications include respiratory infection, esophageal anastomotic leak, and recurrent TEF, as well as potential complications associated with the VACTERL anomalies. Late complications consist of esophageal strictures, gastroesophageal reflux, dysphagia, and various manifestations of reactive airway disease, such as recurrent bronchitis or asthmatic symptoms. The symptoms of gastroesophageal reflux can be difficult to treat.

### SUGGESTED READINGS

1. Centini G, Rosignoli L, Kenanidis A, Petraglia F: Prenatal diagnosis of esophageal atresia with the pouch sign. Ultrasound Obstet Gynecol 2003; 21:494-497.
2. de Jong EM, de Haan MAM, Gischler SJ, et al: Pre- and postnatal diagnosis and outcome of fetuses and neonates with esophageal atresia and tracheoesophageal fistula. Prenat Diagn 2010; 30:274-279.

3. Depaepe A, Dolk H, Lechat MF, and a EUROCAT Working Group: The epidemiology of tracheo-oesophageal fistula and oesophageal atresia in Europe. Arch Dis Child 1993; 68:743-748.
4. Engum SA, Grosfeld JL, West KW, et al: Analysis of morbidity and mortality in 227 cases of esophageal atresia and/or tracheoesophageal fistula over two decades. Arch Surg 1995; 130:502-508.
5. Estroff JA, Parad RB, Share JC, Benacerraf BR: Second trimester prenatal findings in duodenal and esophageal atresia without tracheoesophageal fistula. J Ultrasound Med 1994; 13:375-379.
6. Goyal A, Jones MO, Couriel JM, Losty PD: Oesophageal atresia and trachea-oesophageal fistula. Arch Dis Child Fetal Neonatal Ed 2006; 91:F381–F384.
7. Hill LM: Congenital microgastria: absence of the fetal stomach and normal third trimester amniotic fluid volume. J Ultrasound Med 1994; 13:894-896.
8. Kalache DK, Wauer R, Mau H, et al: Prognostic significance of the pouch sign in fetuses with prenatally diagnosed esophageal atresia. Am J Obstet Gynecol 2000; 162:978-981.
9. Koivusalo AI, Pakarinen MP, Rintala RF: Modern outcomes of oesophageal atresia: single centre experience over the last twenty years. J Pediatr Surg 2013; 48:297-303.
10. Konkin DE, O'Hali WA, Webber EM, Blair GK: Outcomes in esophageal atresia and tracheoesophagel fistula. J Pediatr Surg 2003; 38:1726-1729.
11. Langer JC, Hussain H, Khan A, et al: Prenatal diagnosis of esophageal atresia using sonography and magnetic resonance imaging. J Pediatr Surg 2001; 36:804-807.
12. Shulman A, Mazkerath R, Zalel Y, et al: Prenatal identification of esophageal atresia: the role of ultrasonography for evaluation of functional anatomy. Prenat Diagn 2002; 22:669-674.
13. Spitz L: Esophageal atresia. Lessons I have learned in a 40-year experience. J Pediatr Surg 2006; 41:1635-1640.
14. Stringer MD, McKenna KM, Goldstein RB, et al: Prenatal diagnosis of esophageal atresia. J Pediatr Surg 1995; 30:1258-1263.
15. Tsukerman GL, Krapiva GA, Kirillova IA: First-trimester diagnosis of duodenal stenosis associated with esophageal atresia. Prenat Diagn 1993; 13:371-376.

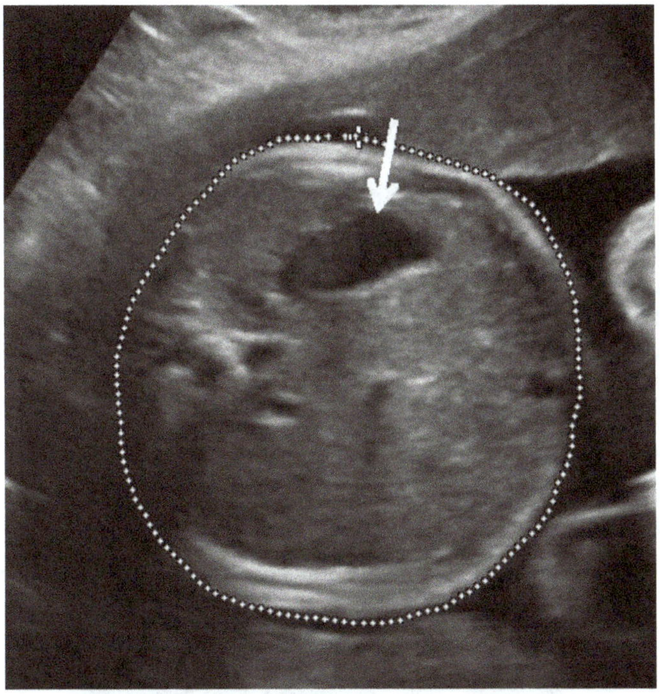

FIGURE 6.9A Normal stomach (arrow).

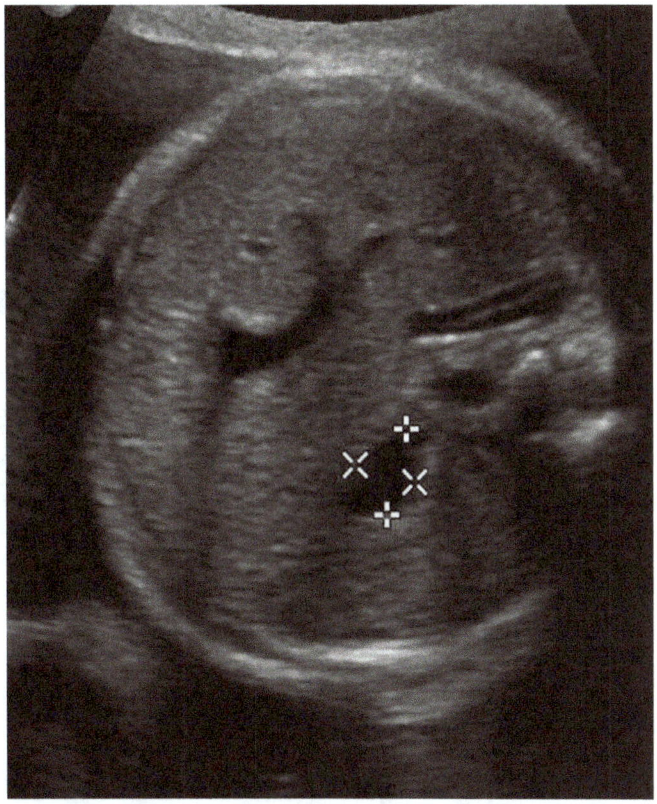

FIGURE 6.9B Small stomach (x … x; + … +) due to esophageal atresia with a tracheoesophageal fistula.

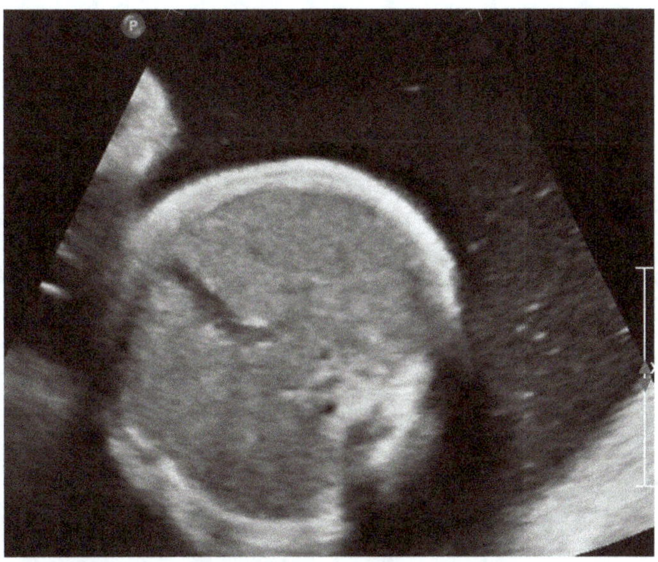

FIGURE 6.9C Absent fetal stomach and polyhydramnios.

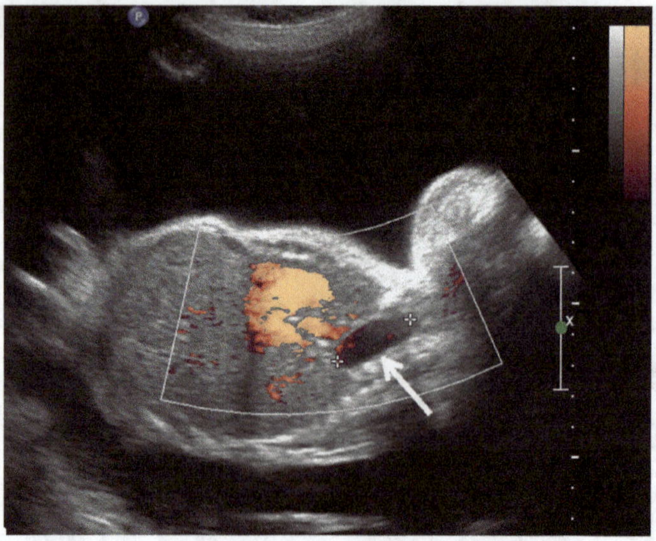

**FIGURE 6.9D** Mediastinal pouch (arrow). Note the polyhydramnios.

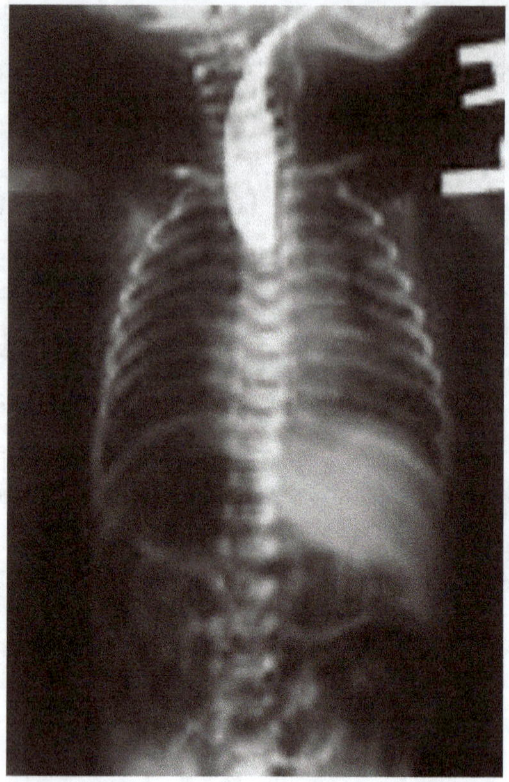

**FIGURE 6.9E** Neonatal image of esophageal atresia.

# CHAPTER 7

# NECK AND FACE

# 7.1 CLEFT LIP AND PALATE

## EPIDEMIOLOGY/GENETICS

**Definition** A facial cleft involving the upper lip or palate, usually occurring to the left or right of midline, the cleft lip or cleft palate may occur as an isolated malformation or as part of a multiple-malformation syndrome. Midline facial clefts may be associated with underlying brain malformations, especially holoprosencephaly.

**Epidemiology** Occurrence is 1 in 1000 births (M2:F1) for cleft lip or cleft palate and 0.65 in 1000 births for isolated cleft palate (M2:F3). There is marked ethnic and racial variation in incidence (Caucasian 1 to African American 0.6). Some studies suggested that maternal preconceptional folic acid supplementation decreases the incidence of nonsyndromic clefts. Medial facial clefts account for less than 1% of all facial clefts.

**Embryology** The primary palate (anterior to incisive foramina) and secondary palate (posterior to the incisive foramina) are embryologically distinct. The upper lip and primary palate have usually fused by the seventh week of gestation. Formation of the secondary palate occurs by fusion of the palatal shelf by the 12th week. Cleft lip and cleft palate are due to a failure of union of the frontonasal process of the face with the lateral maxillary prominences at about 7 weeks' gestation. Approximately 60% of cases are isolated. Almost 300 multiple-malformation syndromes have been described with cleft lip or cleft palate. Chromosomal abnormalities may be found in 3.9% of isolated cleft lip and palate and in up to 63% when associated anomalies are present. A variety of chromosomal abnormalities have been implicated, including the 22q11 deletion. The most common associated anomalies are those involving the lumbar and cervical spine (33%) and heart (24%).

Midline facial clefts are the result of a deficient frontonasal development process that is normally induced by the underlying brain. Midline facial clefts with underlying brain abnormalities are seen in trisomy 13, as well as other chromosomal abnormalities and genetic syndromes.

**Inheritance Patterns** Most isolated cleft lips or cleft palates show multifactorial inheritance, but up to 20% are a component of dominant, recessive, and X-linked syndromes (including van der Woude syndrome). Determining the pattern of inheritance depends on an accurate diagnosis.

**Teratogens** Alcohol, smoking, maternal phenylketonuria, hyperthermia, hydantoin, trimethadione, aminopterin, carbamazepine, valproate, retinoic acid, and methotrexate are teratogenic.

**Prognosis** The prognosis for a good cosmetic and functional repair with isolated cleft lip or cleft palate is excellent. Otherwise, the prognosis is dependent on any associated malformations or a syndrome diagnosis. Midline clefts, if they are associated with underlying brain malformations, usually carry a poor prognosis.

## SONOGRAPHY

### FREQUENT FINDINGS

- Unilateral cleft lip with or without cleft palate
  - A space is identified in the soft tissue of the lip and may be seen just on the inferior surface of the lip (incomplete cleft) versus into the nostril (complete cleft).
  - The alae of the nose are often inferiorly displaced with a complete cleft.
  - The hard palate (alveolar ridge) can often be imaged just posterior to the lip, and a defect in this region appears as a space between the tooth buds.
- Bilateral cleft lip with or without palatal defect
  - Bilateral cleft lip is almost universally found in the setting of a bilateral cleft palate as well.
  - There are soft tissue clefts seen on each half of the upper lip.
  - The bilateral clefting in the palate causes the central alveolar ridge segment to lose its bony attachment to the remainder of the maxilla, resulting in an anterior displacement of the lip and palate. This can be seen sonographically as a premaxillary protuberance that is characteristic of bilateral cleft lip and palate.
- Isolated cleft palate or cleft soft (secondary) palate
  - The presence of isolated cleft palate (not associated with cleft lip) or cleft soft (secondary) palate is difficult to identify prenatally.
  - This diagnosis is most commonly established in the neonatal period.
- Median cleft lip and palate
  - There is an absence of the central maxilla and upper lip with a deformed nose that may be absent or replaced by a proboscis.
  - The facial profile is often flat.
  - This type of cleft lip and palate is almost always associated with other facial abnormalities, such as hypotelorism or cyclopia, and brain abnormalities, particularly holoprosencephaly.
- Atypical facial clefts
  - Typically, these are the result of amniotic bands.
  - The appearance of the lip and face is quite variable, although often defects seen in this setting are severe.
  - Close evaluation for additional fetal deformations related to amniotic bands is warranted.

### KEY FINDINGS/PITFALLS

- Three-dimensional (3-D) sonography has been demonstrated to more accurately diagnose facial clefting anomalies. The 3-D surface view can more clearly demonstrate a more life-like appearance of the defect, which is key in confirming the diagnosis and counseling the family.
- The presence of cleft lip and palate can be identified as early as the late first trimester, particularly when transvaginal imaging is performed.
- Bilateral cleft lip and palate may be mistaken for a facial mass, such as a teratoma or proboscis.

- It may be difficult to accurately image the lip and palate in a fetus that is in a prone position facing the maternal back or when image quality is poor secondary to large maternal body habitus.
- With 3-D sonography, movement artifacts, or overlapping fetal parts, may mimic a facial cleft.

### DIFFERENTIAL DIAGNOSIS

- Epignathus (facial teratoma)
  - The mass is asymmetrical and enters the mouth.
  - There is no associated soft tissue cleft.

## PREGNANCY MANAGEMENT

**Investigations and Consultations Required** Chromosome studies, with microarray, should be done in all cases, including apparently isolated cleft lip/palate. Because of the strong association with cardiac abnormalities, fetal echocardiography is an important component of the evaluation. The parents should be examined by a pediatric dysmorphologist for possible genetic disorders that are inherited in an autosomal dominant fashion. Coordinated prenatal care with a fetal anomaly center, genetics, neonatology, and pediatric plastic surgery is recommended.

**Monitoring** Because of the significant risk of other abnormalities that may not be detected on the initial sonographic evaluation, serial ultrasound is recommended. A follow-up ultrasound examination at the beginning of the third trimester, with 3-D assessment, may provide a more accurate surface image of the fetal face, which can be helpful for counseling.

**Pregnancy Course** No specific obstetric complications should be expected in the fetus with cleft lip/palate. Mild polyhydramnios may occur occasionally.

**Pregnancy Termination Issues** An intact fetus is necessary for pathologic assessment to confirm the ultrasound findings and to assess for additional anomalies that can provide a precise syndrome diagnosis.

**Delivery** Delivery should occur at a center experienced in taking care of neonates with facial clefting. A medical geneticist should also be available to assess for additional dysmorphic features or genetic syndromes.

## NEONATOLOGY

**Resuscitation** Fetal distress is not expected with isolated facial clefting. However, infants found to have additional anomalies often need additional support, including respiratory assistance. The decision to intervene is based on the prognosis for the specific syndrome or anomaly complex.

**Transport** Referral to a tertiary center following birth is not indicated for isolated facial clefts unless a satisfactory feeding technique cannot be established. With multiple anomalies, referral for more extensive diagnostic evaluation is appropriate.

**Testing and Confirmation** Assessment of the type, and extent, of the cleft is recommended following delivery. Because clefts in the soft palate cannot typically be identified antenatally, a careful assessment of the lip and hard and soft palate is recommended. Because of the increased prevalence of associated anomalies, which may not have been detected antenatally, a thorough neonatal evaluation for additional anomalies is warranted.

**Nursery Management** Establishing a successful oral feeding technique and facilitating parental adaptation are the initial objectives in management. There are multiple special devices available for use, and use of a customized prosthetic device for large palatal defects may help some infants. Referral to a center with a multidisciplinary orofacial team for long-term management, including surgical repair and rehabilitation, is essential.

## SURGERY

**Surgical Reconstructive Procedures** All patients with orofacial clefts will require surgical interventions, which may continue until they reach skeletal maturity. Surgical procedures, and timing, are based on the child's diagnosis and the presence of any comorbid conditions.

**Primary Lip/Nose Reconstruction** Incomplete cleft lips and less-severe complete cleft lips are repaired generally between 3 and 6 months of age. The primary repair includes approximation of the lip elements, including muscle and skin, as well as the nasal cartilages and tissues. For more severe, or wide complete, clefts of the lip and alveolus, treatment may involve staged interventions.

**Primary Palate Repair** Children with cleft palate generally undergo primary palatoplasty, or palate repair, between 9 and 18 months of age. Palatoplasty is necessary for a child to develop normal speech and velopharyngeal competence.

**Maxillary Alveolar Cleft Reconstruction** Children who are born with complete cleft lip with alveolar involvement will undergo reconstruction of their alveolar defect between 6 and 10 years of age.

**Surgical Results/Prognosis** Surgery usually restores facial aesthetics and functional speech. The rate of complications from cleft palate closure, requiring late palatal lengthening or fistula closure, ranges from 8% to 20%. The more extensive the deformities are, the greater the number of procedures that will be required to achieve the desired results. Surgical procedures may extend into the end of the craniofacial growth period in the teenaged years.

### SUGGESTED READINGS

1. Babcook CJ, McGahan JP: Axial ultrasonographic imaging of the fetal maxilla for accurate characterization of facial clefts. J Ultrasound Med 1997; 16:619-625.
2. Bardach J, Morris HL: Multidisciplinary Management of Cleft Lip and Palate. Philadelphia: Saunders; 1990.
3. Benacerraf BR, Mulliken JB: Fetal cleft lip and palate: sonographic diagnosis and postnatal outcome. Plast Reconstr Surg 1993; 92:1045-1051.

4. Berge SJ, Plath H, Vondel PT: Fetal cleft lip and palate: sonographic diagnosis, chromosomal abnormalities, associated anomalies, and postnatal outcome in 70 fetuses. Ultrasound Obstet Gynecol 2001; 18:422-431.
5. Bronshtein M, Mashiah N, Blumenfeld I, et al: Pseudoprognathism: an auxiliary ultrasonographic sign for transvaginal ultrasonographic diagnosis of cleft lip and palate in the early second trimester. Am J Obstet Gynecol 1991; 165:1314-1316.
6. Chervenak FA, Tortora M, Mayden K, et al: Antenatal diagnosis of median cleft face syndrome: sonographic demonstration of cleft lip and hypertelorism. Am J Obstet Gynecol 1984; 149:94-97.
7. Cockell A, Lees M: Prenatal diagnosis and management of orofacial clefts. Prenat Diagn 2000; 20:149-151.
8. Dufresne C, Jelks G: Classification of craniofacial anomalies. In Smith B, ed. Ophthalmic Plastic and Reconstructive Surgery. Philadelphia: Mosby-Year Book; 1987: 1185.
9. Dufresne C, So I: Facial clefting malformations. In Dufresne C, Carson B, Zinreich SJ, eds. Complex Craniofacial Problems. New York: Churchill Livingstone; 1992: 195.
10. Maarse W, Rozendaal AM, Pajkrt E, et al: A systematic review of associated structural and chromosomal defects in oral clefts: when is prenatal genetic analysis indicated? J Med Genet 2012; 49:490-498.
11. Michel B, Debauche C, Hutchings G, et al: Pregnancy and neonatal outcome following an antenatal diagnosis of cleft lip and palate. J Perinat Med 2012; 41:1-8.
12. Mossey P, Little J, Munger R, et al: Cleft lip and palate. Lancet 2009; 374:1773-1785.
13. Nyberg DA, Hegge FN, Kramer D, et al: Premaxillary protrusion: a sonographic clue to bilateral cleft lip and palate. J Ultrasound Med 1993; 12:331-335.
14. Stoll C, Alembic Y, Dobb B, et al: Associated malformations in cases with oral clefts. Cleft Palate Craniofac J 2000; 37:41-47.
15. Watkins SE, Meyer RE, Strauss RP, Aylsworth AS: Classification, epidemiology, and genetics of orofacial clefts. Clin Plast Surg. 2014; 41:149-163.

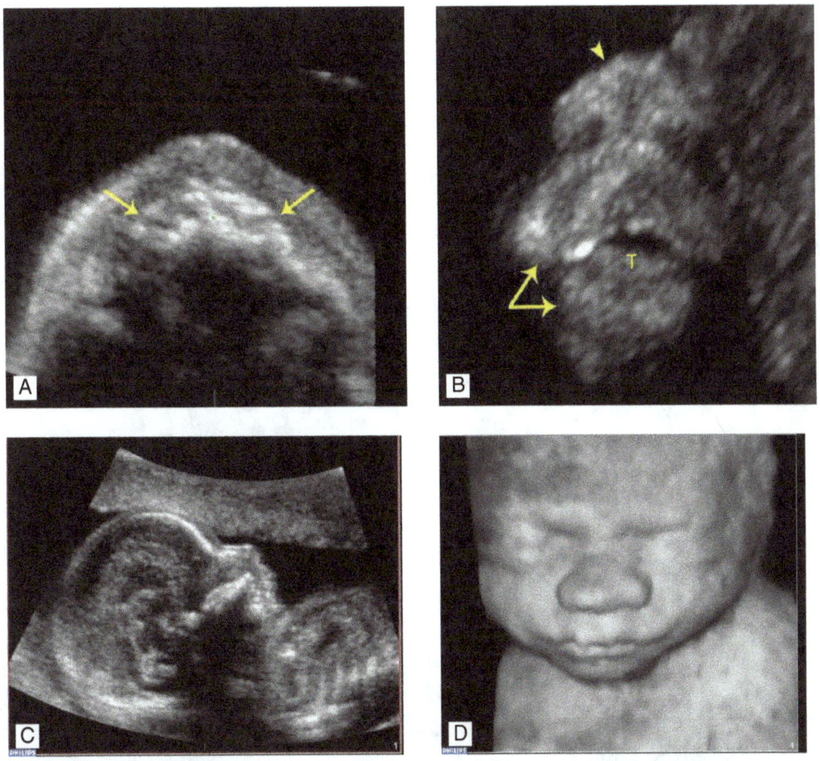


**FIGURE 7.1A-D** Sonographic images of normal face: (A) axial view of intact hard palate with tooth buds (arrow); (B) coronal view demonstrating tip of nose (triangle), nostrils, upper lip (arrow), tongue, and lower lip (arrow); (C) sagittal view demonstrating normal fetal profile; (D) 3-D surface rendering of superficial facial features.

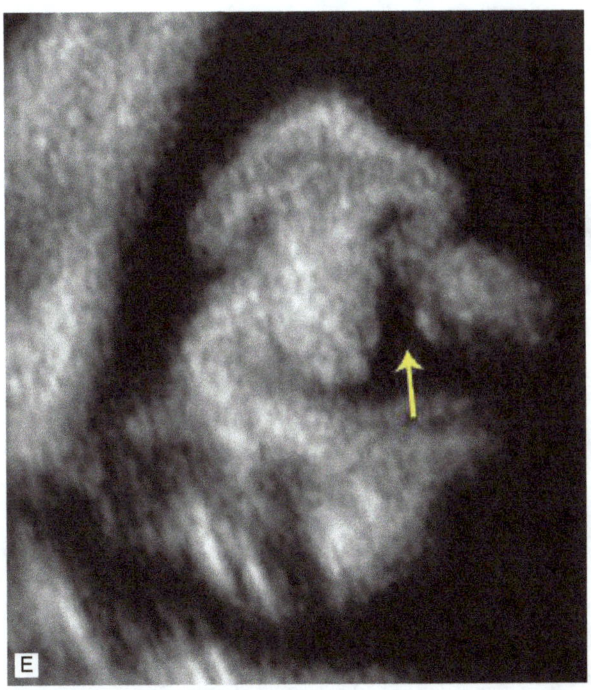


**FIGURE 7.1E** Ultrasound showing a hypoechoic space (arrow) disrupting the normal lip contour, indicating cleft lip.

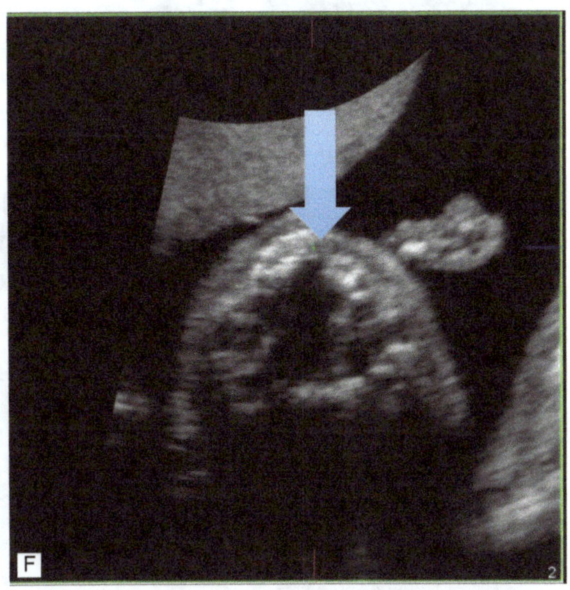


**FIGURE 7.1F** Ultrasound demonstrating disruption of the alveolar ridge (hard palate), (arrow) indicating a unilateral cleft palate.

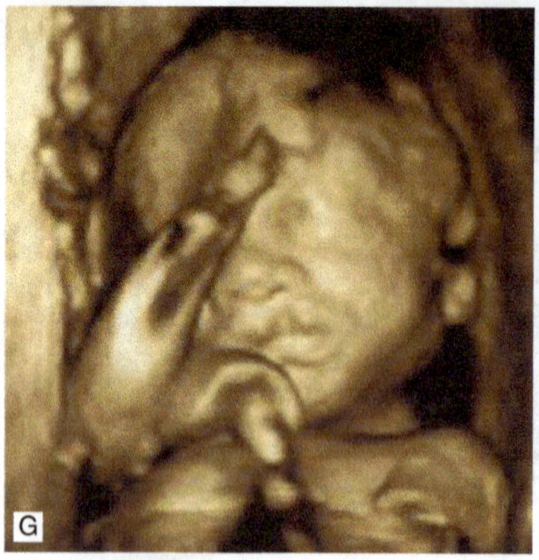


**FIGURE 7.1G** Three-dimensional surface-rendered image demonstrating unilateral incomplete cleft lip.

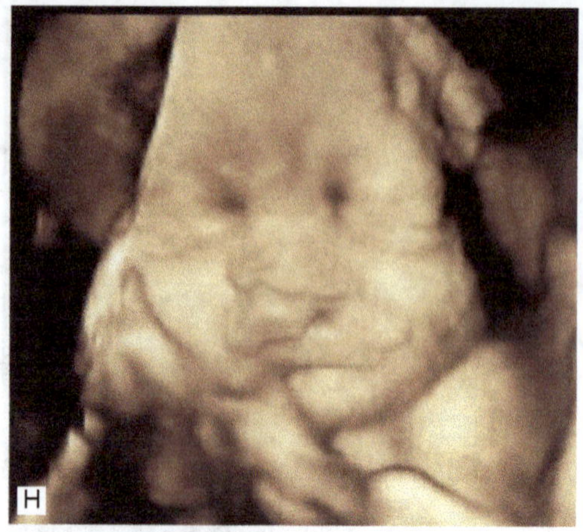


**FIGURE 7.1H** Three-dimensional surface-rendered images of third-trimester fetus with unilateral cleft lip. Note deformation of ipsilateral nostril.

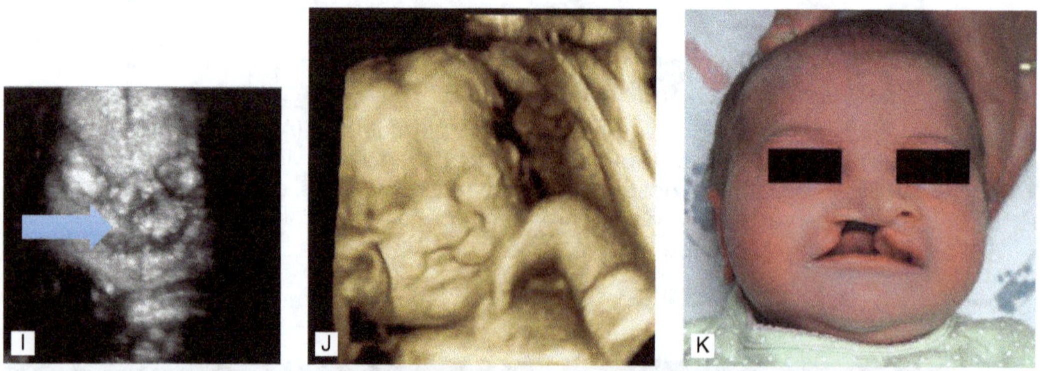


**FIGURE 7.1I-K** Ultrasound and postnatal correlation: (I) skeletal setting demonstrating wide cleft palate (arrow); (J) 3-D surface rendering demonstrating wide cleft lip; (K) postnatal correlation.

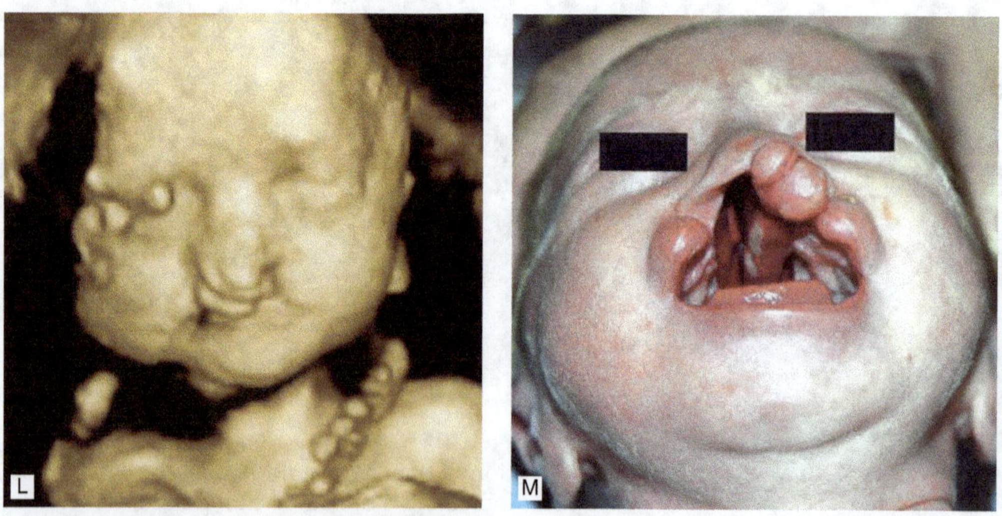


**FIGURE 7.1L-M** Bilateral cleft lip and palate (L). Third-trimester surface-rendered image with neonatal correlation (M).

# 7.2 CYSTIC HYGROMA

## EPIDEMIOLOGY/GENETICS

**Definition** Nuchal cystic hygromas (CHs) are characterized by single or multiple congenital cysts of the lymphatic system, most commonly found within the soft tissues of the posterior and lateral neck.

**Epidemiology** Incidence is 1 in 285 first-trimester fetuses.

**Embryology** Nuchal cystic hygromas are the clinical consequence of a delay in development, or absence, of the communications that normally develop between the jugular lymph sacs and the internal jugular veins at approximately 5-6 weeks' gestation. Failure of communication between the lymphatic and venous systems leads to enlarged lymphatic sacs and channels. They are most commonly seen in the subcutaneous region of the posterior fetal neck but may also extend to the lateral neck. As the pressure within the lymphatic system increases, lymphatic fluid can be visualized within the subcutaneous tissue, the pleural space, and the pericardial space and within the abdominal cavity (nonimmune fetal hydrops), which is frequently lethal. Late manifestations of the cystic hygroma, if the fetus survives, include redundancy of posterior nuchal skin, neck webbing, and elevation and anterior rotation of the ears. Occasionally, the cystic hygroma is only unilateral. These cases are generally not associated with chromosomal abnormalities or other genetic conditions.

**Inheritance Patterns** Multiple-malformation syndromes with cystic hygromas include multiple-pterygium syndrome (autosomal recessive, X linked); Noonan syndrome (autosomal dominant); Roberts syndrome (autosomal recessive); as well as others. Chromosomal abnormalities associated with cystic hygroma include Turner syndrome; trisomies 13, 18, and 21; Klinefelter syndrome, and other aneuploidies.

**Teratogens** No teratogens are reported.

**Prognosis** Almost all fetuses with cystic hygroma and hydrops die antenatally. Survivors with lymphatic recanalization may present with a webbed neck or redundant nuchal skin. Even for chromosomally normal fetuses that survive, the prevalence of congenital anomalies, some of which may not be identifiable antenatally, is significantly increased.

## SONOGRAPHY

### FREQUENT FINDINGS

- Cystic hygromas present as septated fluid collections in the subcutaneous tissue of the posterior fetal neck.
  - They may extend laterally to the sides of the neck and inferiorly down the fetal back.
  - In the second trimester, they are often large and can exceed the size of the fetal calvarium.

- Skin thickening
  - Secondary to subcutaneous lymphedema
  - Often develops in the second trimester but can also be seen in the late first trimester
  - Presents as diffuse anasarca, which can be present throughout the fetal skin
- Hydrops
  - With large hygromas, fetal nonimmune hydrops often develops.
  - The presence of nonimmune hydrops in a fetus with a cystic hygroma is a particularly ominous sign, and fetal death often occurs within several weeks.

### LESS FREQUENT

- Oligohydramnios in cases of hydrops is less frequent.

### KEY FINDINGS/PITFALLS

- Often, cystic hygromas are first identifiable in the middle of the first trimester (after 10 weeks' gestation).
- Because small cystic hygromas can spontaneously disappear, patients who had cystic hygromas early on may later appear normal and yet have syndromes, such as Turner or Down syndrome, at birth.
- The resolution of a cystic hygroma does not eliminate the risk for genetic syndromes or aneuploidy.

### DIFFERENTIAL DIAGNOSIS

- Thickened nuchal translucency (NT) may have a similar appearance.
  - A simple NT is confined to the occipital region and does not contain septations.
  - As the size of the fluid collection behind the neck increases, the distinction between a thickened NT and a cystic hygroma is lost.
  - The association with an abnormal karyotype, or other structural abnormalities, is the same for an NT above the 99th centile (3.5 mm) and a cystic hygroma.
- Encephalocele or meningocele
  - The mass is seen focally at the posterior occiput or midline upper spine.
  - Both cases almost always also demonstrate abnormal intracranial findings.
- Unfused amniotic membrane
  - Before 13 weeks, an unfused amniotic membrane may lie adjacent to the fetus and be confused with a cystic hygroma.
- Lymphangioma
  - Lymphangioma may have a similar multiseptated appearance.
  - However, a lymphangioma is typically unilateral and develops later in pregnancy.

## PREGNANCY MANAGEMENT

**Investigations and Consultations Required** Approximately 50% of fetuses with a cystic hygroma will be found to have a chromosomal abnormality. The most common chromosomal abnormalities identified are trisomy 21, 45X, and trisomy 18. Noonan syndrome may account for up to 15% of cases. A gene panel for genes associated with Noonan syndrome should be done if chromosome analysis and microarray studies are negative. For those fetuses found to be euploid, up to 30% will have additional anomalies, most commonly affecting the cardiac, skeletal, and genitourinary systems. A detailed anatomic survey in midgestation, as well as a fetal echocardiogram, is recommended. Only approximately 15% of fetuses found to have a cystic hygroma will be born alive, with no long-term sequelae.

**Fetal Intervention** In utero drainage procedures have no role in management. Spontaneous resolution may occur, although is difficult to predict. Progression to fetal hydrops suggests impending fetal death in most cases.

**Monitoring** Serial sonography every 3-4 weeks may be helpful to assess for the development of nonimmune hydrops, evaluate for the appearance of additional anomalies, and assess for fetal death.

**Pregnancy Course** Cystic hygroma with hydrops is almost always a lethal combination, with death within a short time period. Cystic hygromas without hydrops may regress; however, the fetus is still at risk for undiagnosed genetic syndromes or other anomalies.

**Pregnancy Termination Issues** Unless a precise diagnosis has been established prenatally, the method of termination should be nondestructive, and examinations by both a fetal pathologist and a dysmorphologist should be performed.

**Delivery** Except in the case of markedly excessive size, the presence of a cystic hygroma should not necessitate a cesarean section. Delivery should occur in a tertiary center with capabilities for managing any complications that may arise.

## NEONATOLOGY

**Resuscitation** Airway compromise at birth occurs infrequently because the cystic hygroma is typically posteriorly located and should not affect the anterior neck.

**Transport** Once the neonate is stabilized, transfer to a tertiary care center with pediatric subspecialties, including genetics, neonatology, and surgery, is recommended.

**Testing and Confirmation** Cystic hygroma is usually obvious on physical examination in the newborn unless the hygroma is small. A webbed neck and excessive nuchal skin, suggesting a resolved antenatal cystic hygroma, may also be noted on the newborn examination. Diagnostic evaluation should be directed toward excluding other coexisting abnormalities, as indicated by prenatal findings and physical examination. Computerized tomographic (CT) scanning or magnetic resonance imaging (MRI) of the neck and upper thorax is used to delineate the extent and anatomic location of the neck mass.

## SURGERY

The treatment for cystic hygromas in the neonate is typically surgical excision. However, sclerotherapy and medical therapy with anti-inflammatory agents have been used. Because of the abnormal lymphatic connections, even if the hygroma can be resected, the recurrence rate is high, and children may require multiple procedures.

## SUGGESTED READINGS


1. Adams MT, Saltzman B, Perkins J: Head and neck lymphatic malformation treatment: a systematic review. Otolaryngol Head Neck Surg 2012; 147:627-639.
2. Azar GB, Snijders RJM, Gosden C, Nicolaides KH: Fetal nuchal cystic hygromata: associated malformations and chromosomal defects. Fetal Diagn Ther 1991; 6:46-57.
3. Bronshtein M, Bar-Hava I, Blumenfeld I, et al: The difference between septated and nonseptated nuchal cystic hygroma in the early second trimester. Obstet Gynecol 1993; 81:683-687.
4. Byrne J: The significance of cystic hygroma in fetuses. Hum Pathol 1984; 15:61-67.
5. Chervenak FA, Isaacson G, Blakemore KJ, et al: Fetal cystic hygroma: cause and natural history. N Engl J Med 1983; 309:822-825.
6. Croonen EA, Nillesen WM, Stuurman KE, et al: Prenatal diagnostic testing of the Noonan syndrome genes in fetuses with abnormal ultrasound findings. Eur J Hum Genet 2013; 21:936-942.
7. Gallagher PG, Mahoney MJ, Gosche JR: Cystic hygroma in the fetus and newborn. Semin Perinatal 1999; 23:341-356.
8. Johnson MP, Johnson A, Holzgreve W, et al: First-trimester simple hygroma: cause and outcome. Am J Obstet Gynecol 1993; 168:156-161.
9. Langer JC, Fitzgerald PG, Desa D, et al: Cervical cystic hygroma in the fetus: clinical spectrum and outcome. J Pediatr Surg 1990; 25:58-61.
10. Malone FD, Ball RH, Nyberg DA, et al: First trimester septated cystic hygroma: prevalence, natural history, and pediatric outcome. Obstet Gynecol 2005; 106:288-294.
11. Ninh TN, Ninh TX: Cystic hygroma in children: a report of 126 cases. J Pediatr Surg 1974; 9:191-195.
12. Scholl J, Durfee SM, Russell MA, et al: First trimester cystic hygroma: relationship of nuchal translucency thickness and utcomes. Obstet Gynecol 2012; 120:551-558.
13. Van Zalen-Sprock MM, Van Vugt JMG, Van der Harten HJ, Van Geijn HP: Cephalocele and cystic hygroma: diagnosis and differentiation in the first trimester of pregnancy with transvaginal sonography: report of two cases. Ultrasound Obstet Gynecol 1992; 2:289-292.
14. Zimmer EZ, Drugan A, Ofir C, et al: Ultrasound imaging of fetal neck anomalies: implications for the risk of aneuploidy and structural anomalies. Prenat Diagn 1997; 17:1055-1058.

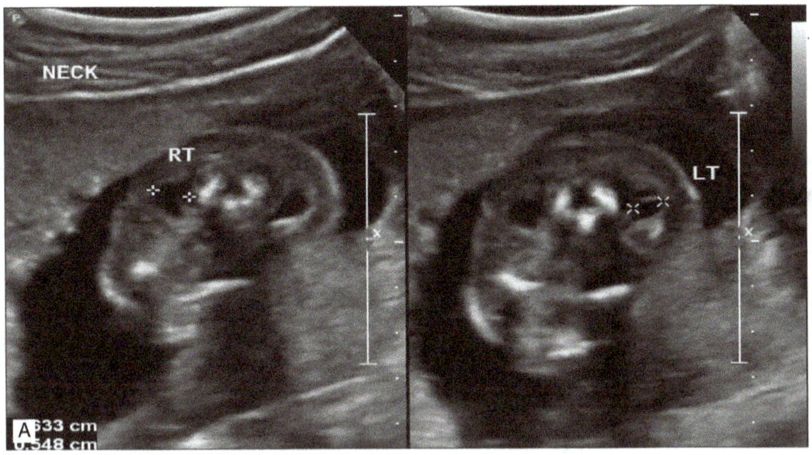


FIGURE 7.2A Distended jugular lymphatics: right (RT) and left (LT).

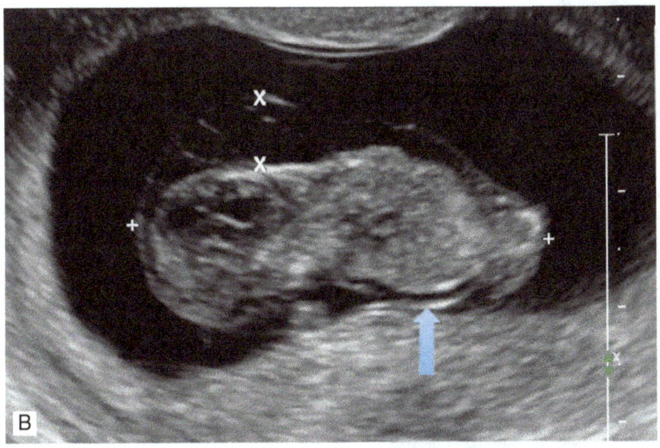


FIGURE 7.2B First-trimester fetus with cystic hygroma (x … x). There is also subcutaneous edema (arrow). Chorionic villus sampling revealed trisomy 18.

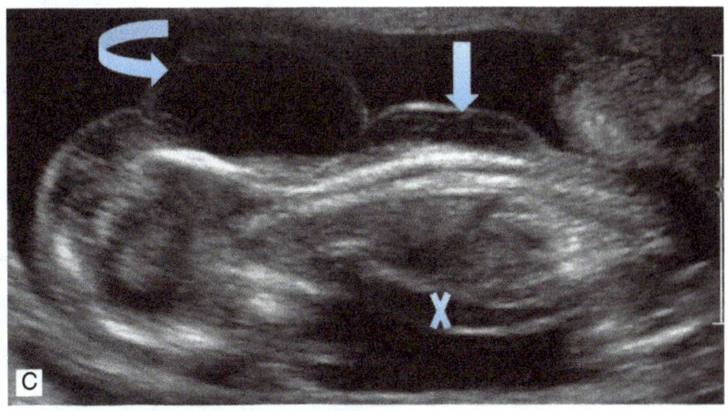


FIGURE 7.2C Sagittal view of fetus demonstrating large cystic hygroma (curved arrow). There is diffuse subcutaneous edema (straight arrow) and ascites (X), consistent with nonimmune hydrops.

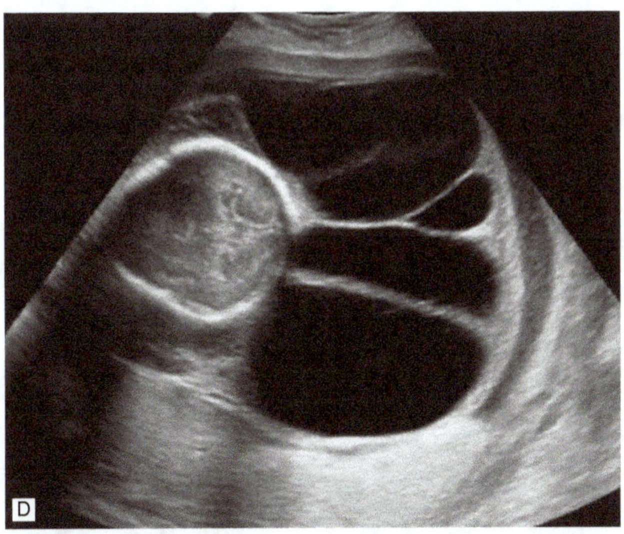


FIGURE 7.2D Axial view of the head of an 18-week fetus demonstrating extremely large, multiseptated cystic hygroma.

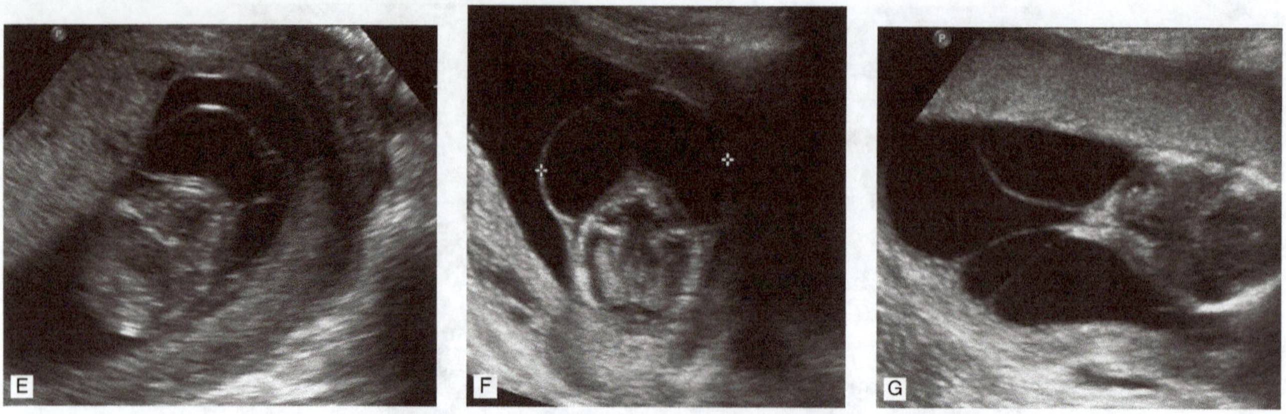

FIGURE 7.2E-G Axial views of the fetal head at 12 weeks', 16 weeks', and 20 weeks' gestation in the same fetus. Note progression of the hygroma over time. Fetal demise was diagnosed at the 20-week study.

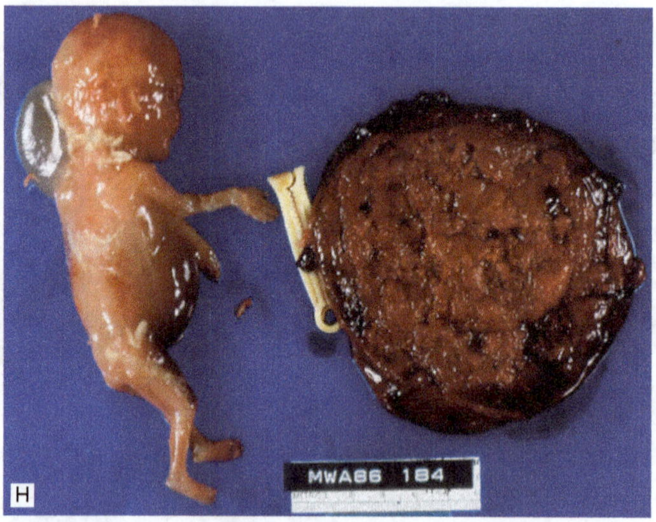


FIGURE 7.2H Fetus with cystic hygroma.

# 7.3 FACIAL ASYMMETRY, GOLDENHAR SYNDROME (OCULO-AURICULO-VERTEBRAL SPECTRUM)

## EPIDEMIOLOGY/GENETICS

**Definition** Goldenhar syndrome features significant facial asymmetry involving the maxilla and mandible, often with associated ipsilateral ocular and auricular abnormalities.

**Epidemiology** Birth frequency is estimated to be 1 in 3000 to 1 in 5000, with a male-to-female ratio of at least 3:2 and a 3:2 predilection for right-sided involvement.

**Embryology** The malformation involves the embryologic structures of the first and second pharyngeal arches. Goldenhar syndrome features a wide range of manifestations, including facial asymmetry; ipsilateral abnormalities of the external ear (anotia, microtia, preauricular abnormalities); ocular defects (epibulbar lipodermoid, lid coloboma); cardiac abnormalities (30%); renal malformations (30%); and vertebral anomalies, often with torticollis (50%). Approximately 30% of children have some bilateral involvement. The etiology is unknown but likely represents a combination of genetic and environmental effects.

**Inheritance Patterns** Goldenhar syndrome is generally sporadic, with an estimated 2% to 3% recurrence risk.

**Teratogens** Maternal diabetes, multiple gestations, and vasoactive medications, especially in association with smoking, are teratogenic.

**Differential Diagnosis** Treacher-Collins syndrome, craniosynostosis syndromes, acrofacial dysostoses, and chromosome 4p- syndrome may have facial asymmetry with auricular abnormalities. There have been several cases of apparent hemifacial microsomia that have had 22q1.2 deletions detected.

**Prognosis** Minor degrees of facial asymmetry may improve over time. More severe forms of facial asymmetry require major reconstructive surgery. Intelligence in most patients with Goldenhar syndrome is normal unless the central nervous system is involved. In the presence of microphthalmia, the syndrome is more likely to include intellectual disability. There is an increased frequency of conductive hearing loss on the affected side.

## SONOGRAPHY

### FREQUENT FINDINGS

- Craniofacial microsomia
  - Hemifacial maldevelopment
    - Small, malformed ear
    - Preauricular skin tag
    - Anopthalmia
    - Hypertelorism

  - Micrognathia
  - Ipsilateral cleft lip/palate
  - Unilateral hypoplasia of the mandible
  - Midface hypoplasia

### LESS FREQUENT

- Ventriculomegaly
- Cerebellar hemisphere hypoplasia
- Congenital cardiac defects
  - Ventricular septal defect
  - Tetralogy of Fallot
  - Atrial septal defect
- Esophageal atresia
- Pyelocaliectasis
- Renal agenesis
- Hemivertebrae
- Scoliosis
- Spina bifida
- Polydactyly
- Hypoplasia of the thumb
- Polyhydramnios
- Oligohydramnios

### KEY FINDINGS/PITFALLS

- The association of polyhydramnios with Goldenhar syndrome is due to difficulties in swallowing and is usually not diagnosed until after 24 weeks' gestation.
- In utero diagnosis has been made as early as 15 weeks' gestation.
- Three-dimensional multiplanar and rendered images are effective in evaluating the facial abnormalities associated with Goldenhar syndrome.

## PREGNANCY MANAGEMENT

**Investigations and Consultations Required** Precise prenatal diagnosis is unlikely; therefore, chromosomal studies, including microarray, and fetal echocardiography should be performed to exclude other genetic conditions. Consultation with a medical geneticist to discuss differential diagnosis and possible testing options is recommended.

**Fetal Intervention** None is indicated or necessary.

**Monitoring** Normal obstetric management is appropriate in most cases. Should there be significant fetal micrognathia, monthly sonographic assessment of amniotic fluid volume may be beneficial to detect polyhydramnios. An early third-trimester scan to assess fetal growth should be performed in all cases.

**Pregnancy Course** Usually, pregnancy course is uncomplicated. Occasionally, there will be prenatal growth deficiency.

**Pregnancy Termination Issues** If termination is chosen, an intact fetus is essential to establish this diagnosis.

**Delivery** Site of delivery will depend on the presence of cardiac malformations, the degree of micrognathia, and the presence of other associated malformations. If the micrognathia is severe enough, evaluation for an EXIT (ex utero intrapartum treatment) procedure may be indicated. In most cases, delivery at a tertiary center is the most prudent option.

## NEONATOLOGY

**Resuscitation** Several components of the spectrum of anomalies may necessitate special consideration for resuscitation. Mandibular hypoplasia is the most common of the group, although difficulties with maintaining an adequate airway have not been reported in neonates. Much less frequent are cardiac anomalies and anomalies of the foregut derivatives, such as tracheoesophageal fistula and developmental bronchopulmonary defects. If this diagnosis is made prenatally, then delivery room management of the onset of respiration should follow the directions for the individual anomalies.

**Transfer** Transport to a tertiary center with neonatology; genetics; ophthalmology; cardiology; ear, nose, and throat; craniofacial; and surgical subspecialty capabilities is indicated in the neonatal period to confirm the diagnosis, identify all the component abnormalities, and initiate a multidisciplinary long-term care plan.

**Testing and Confirmation** The specific diagnostic imaging to be performed will be dictated by the associated abnormalities suspected from the clinical course and physical examination. The initial evaluation in all infants should include imaging of the cervical spine, echocardiogram, renal ultrasound, ophthalmologic evaluation, and hearing screen.

**Nursery Management** The specifics of management will be dictated by the spectrum of anomalies present in an individual infant. Priority should be given to establishing a long-term plan for craniofacial reconstructive surgery and sensorineural habilitation.

## SURGERY

**Preoperative Assessment** The goal of treatment in patients with mandibular deformities, as seen in Goldenhar syndrome, is improvement of function and optimization of aesthetic facial appearance and symmetry when craniofacial growth is completed. Treatment includes correction of the secondary deformities of the maxilla and orbit and improvement of the deficiencies of the facial soft tissues. Treatment varies according to the age of the patient, the degree of malformation, and the anticipated distortion of future growth potential. Surgical management is based on analysis of facial skeletal radiographs in the frontal, sagittal, and transverse planes. Three-dimensional CT scanning provides the best evaluation of the frontal plane. A lateral cephalogram offers a demonstration of the sagittal plane. The submental vertex radiograph helps to evaluate the transverse plane.

**Operative Indications** The main objectives of surgical management are (1) improvement of symmetry of the mandible; (2) provision for downgrowth of the maxilla by lengthening of the anteromedial displacement; (3) restoration of functional dental occlusion by proper positioning of the mandibular symphyseal midlines; and (4) expansion of the facial skeleton at an early age to fill out the soft tissue on the affected side of the face.

**Types of Procedures** In the surgical phase of treatment, the mandible is reconstructed by either elongation or extension of the mandible. Elongation is performed on patients who have a functioning temporomandibular joint.

**Surgical Results/Prognosis** The key to success in this type of craniofacial surgery is the realization that the osteotomies and grafts are part of a complex treatment plan with interventions required at specific stages of craniofacial growth. Decisions regarding timing of surgery are based on the character of the anatomic deformities.

## SUGGESTED READINGS

1. Beleza-Meireles A, Clayton-Smith J, Saraiva JM, Tassabehiji M: Oculo-auriculo-vertebral spectrum: a review of the literature and genetic update. J Med Genet 2014; 51:635-645.
2. Castori M, Brancati F, Rinaldi R, et al: Antenatal presentation of the oculo-auricular-vertebral spectrum (OAVS). Am J Med Genet 2006; 140A:1573-1579.
3. DeCatte L, Laubach M, Legein J, Goossens A: Early prenatal diagnosis of oculoauriculovertebral dysplasia or the Goldenhar syndrome. Ultrasound Obstet Gynecol 1996; 8:422-424.
4. Digilio MC, McDonald-McGinn DM, Heike C, et al: Three patients with oculo-auriculo-vertebral spectrum and microdeletion 22q11.2. Am J Med Genet 2009; 149A:2860-2864.
5. Hartsfield JK: Review of the etiologic heterogenecity of the oculo-aureculo-vertebral spectrum (hemifacial microsomia). Orthod Craniofacial Res 2007; 10:121-128.
6. Martinelli P, Maruotti GM, Agangi A, et al: Prenatal diagnosis of hemifacial microsomia and ipsilateral cerebellar hypoplasia in a fetus with oculoauriculo-vertebral spectrum. Ultrasound Obstet Gynecol 2004; 124:199-201.
7. Volpe P, Gentile M: Three-dimensional diagnosis of Goldenhar syndrome. Ultrasound Obstet Gynecol 2004; 24:798-800.
8. Werler MM, Starr JR, Cloonan YK, Speltz ML: Hemifacial microsomia: from gestation to childhood. J Craniofac Surg 2009; 20:664-669.

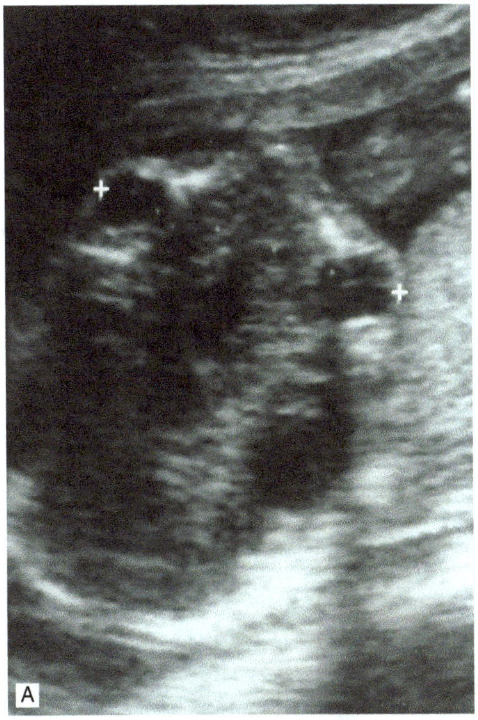

**FIGURE 7.3A** Hypertelorism (+ … +).

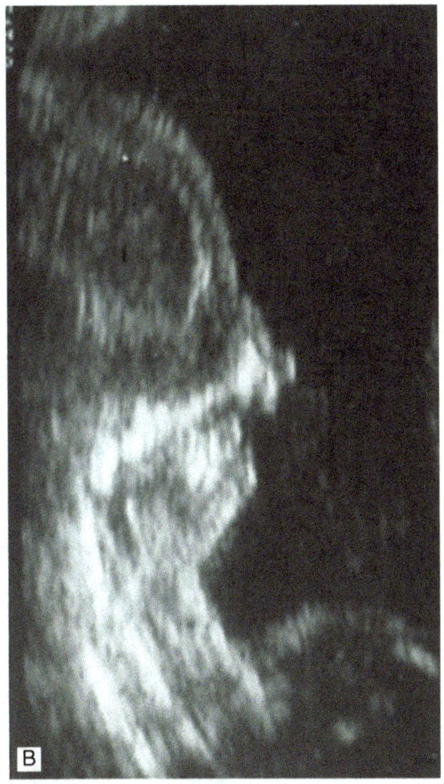

**FIGURE 7.3B** Micrognathia with midface hypoplasia.

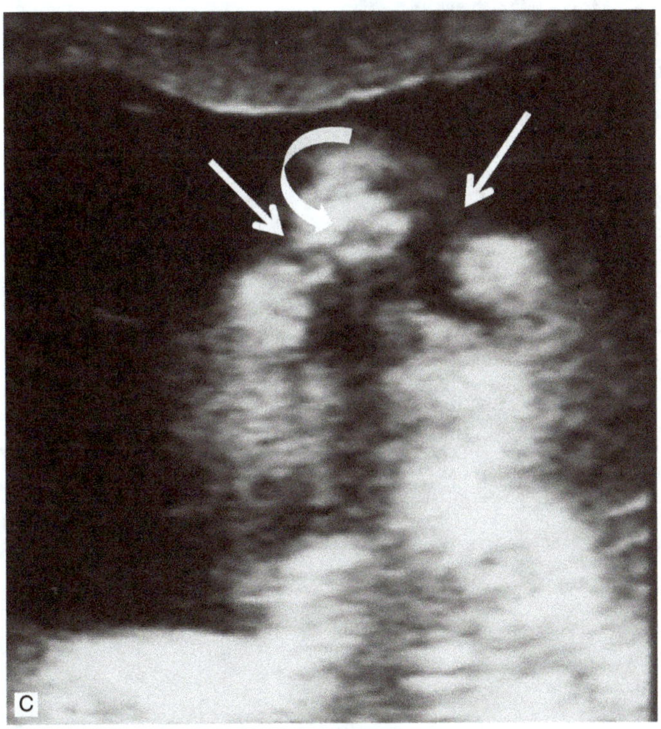

**FIGURE 7.3C** Bilateral cleft lip (straight arrows) with premaxillary protrusion (curved arrow).

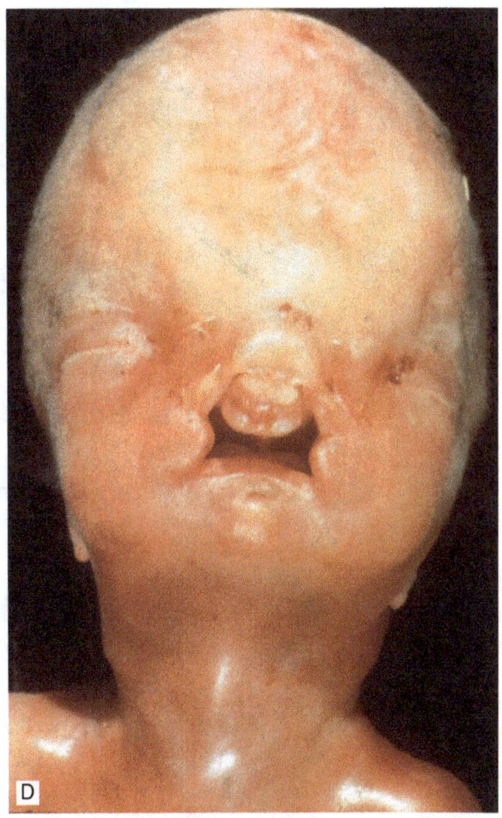

**FIGURE 7.3D** Fetus with bilateral cleft lip/palate, premaxillary protrusion, micrognathia, and midface hypoplasia.

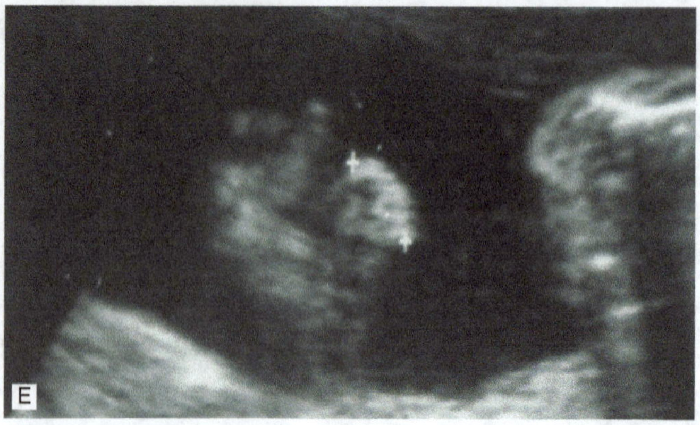

**FIGURE 7.3E** Microtia. Note the small, anomalous ear (+ … +).

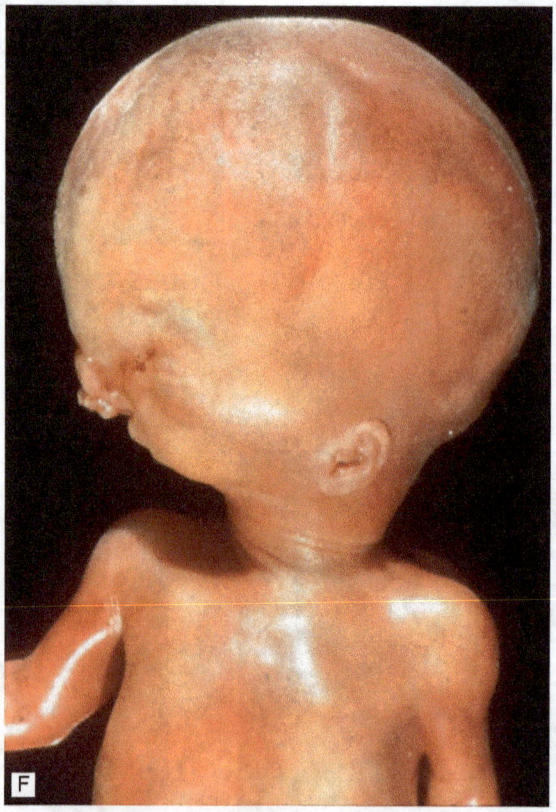

**FIGURE 7.3F** Fetus with low-set, small ear, micrognathia, and midface hypoplasia.

# 7.4 PIERRE ROBIN SEQUENCE

## EPIDEMIOLOGY/GENETICS

**Definition** The Pierre Robin sequence (PRS) consists of the triad of micrognathia (a small, symmetrically receded mandible), glossoptosis (posteriorly displaced tongue), and cleft palate. The presence of airway obstruction is also considered by many to be required for diagnosis. It may be identified as an isolated finding or as part of a syndrome.

**Epidemiology** One in 8500 to 1 in 14,000 births (M1:F1) are affected.

**Embryology** It is hypothesized that severe micrognathia is the initiating event. The severely small mandible displaces the tongue posteriorly and superiorly, which prevents closure of the palatine shelves during embryogenesis at 9-10 weeks' gestation. Approximately 50% to 60% of fetuses with PRS will be found to have associated genetic syndromes, chromosomal abnormalities, or other structural anomalies. Abnormalities in the cardiovascular system, central nervous system, and musculoskeletal system are most frequently cited.

**Inheritance Patterns** Inheritance is dependent on the cause; it is autosomal dominant for the Stickler syndrome.

**Teratogens** Retinoic acid and alcohol are teratogenic.

**Prognosis** Prognosis depends on the cause and syndrome association. Patients with isolated, nonsyndromic cases often have a good outcome with normal cognitive function and very low risk of death. Patients with genetic syndromes, concomitant anomalies, or chromosome abnormalities have a higher risk of death in the neonatal period. The respiratory and feeding difficulties are more severe in these cases than when isolated.

## SONOGRAPHY

### FREQUENT FINDINGS

- Micrognathia is characterized by a small mandible and receding chin.
- Retrognathia is characterized by a receding, though normal size, mandible.
- Fetuses with PRS may demonstrate both micrognathia and retrognathia.
- Mild or severe polyhydramnios is common (70%), presumably due to poor swallowing ability.

### KEY FINDINGS/PITFALLS

- Micro-/retrognathia is most commonly identified initially by subjective assessment of the fetal profile.
- Objective measures have been utilized to characterize this more specifically.
  - The mandible and maxilla width can be measured, and nomograms for mandibular width/maxillary width are available to help diagnose micrognathia.
  - This is a difficult measurement to obtain, however.
- The inferior facial angle may be used to assess retrognathia.

- With this technique, an angle is drawn from a line perpendicular to the forehead and a line from the tip of the mentum and most protruding lip.
- A normal facial angle is 65°. An abnormal facial angle, defined as those less than 50°, can identify retrognathia accurately.
- Most fetuses with PRS will have an abnormal inferior facial angle.

- Neither the cleft in the posterior palate nor the glossoptosis usually can be identified sonographically.
- Three-dimensional sonography has been useful in identifying micro-/retrognathia.
  - The surface-rendered image can provide a lifelike view of the fetus for the parents and craniofacial team to review.
  - Using 3-D reconstruction of the orthogonal planes, true orthogonal planes can be identified so that the exact midline profile view can be ensured.
- Three-dimensional ultrasound has been used to diagnose isolated clefts of the soft palate rarely, but.
  - The examination may be limited by fetal position and shadowing from adjoining structures, resulting in an overall sensitivity of only 30%.
- If the profile is not imaged in a true midline position, the mandible may appear small or recessed.
- A small percentage of normal fetuses may have an abnormal inferior facial angle, most commonly attributable to a large upper lip.
- Suspicion for micro-/retrognathia may be raised as early as the late first trimester. However, most diagnoses are made in the second trimester.

### DIFFERENTIAL DIAGNOSIS

- Stickler syndrome: This is found in approximately 15% to 20% of fetuses with PRS.
- Velocardiofacial syndrome: A 22q11 deletion is found in approximately 5% of fetuses with PRS.
- Chromosome abnormalities: Trisomies 13 and 18 and microdeletions are found in approximately 2%.
- Treacher-Collins syndrome: The features include severe micrognathia, malar hypoplasia, and malformation of the external ears. Cleft palate may be present.
- Goldenhar syndrome: The facial structures are asymmetrical.
- Pena-Shokeir syndrome
- Multiple pterygium syndrome
- Nager acrodysostosis

## PREGNANCY MANAGEMENT

**Investigations and Consultations Required** Chromosomal studies with microarray should be offered. Fetal echocardiography and an extended fetal anatomic survey are recommended. Consultation with neonatology and an expert in craniofacial abnormalities is recommended.

**Fetal Intervention** No fetal intervention is indicated.

**Monitoring** In some severe cases, polyhydramnios may develop. Monthly sonographic evaluations should be performed to detect changes in amniotic fluid volume and to assess for other anomalies that may have been missed on earlier examinations.

**Pregnancy Course** No significant changes are expected unless polyhydramnios develops. Polyhydramnios may be associated with preterm labor. Severe polyhydramnios may be a sign of more severe airway obstruction, and plans should be made so that specialists in neonatal intubation are present in the delivery room.

**Pregnancy Termination Issues** Should a couple choose pregnancy termination, labor induction and delivery of an intact fetus are essential to establish a precise diagnosis.

**Delivery** Delivery should occur in a tertiary center because severe respiratory complications and difficult intubation may result from the more severe cases of mandibular hypoplasia.

## NEONATOLOGY

**Resuscitation** Airway obstruction from mandibular hypoplasia and glossoptosis is the primary concern and may be life threatening in severe cases. Initial support involves prone positioning so that the mandible and tongue fall forward, allowing for the airway to open. The majority of infants with nonsyndromic PRS can establish spontaneous respirations in the prone position. If this is not successful, an oral airway, nasal continuous positive pressure ventilation, or nasopharyngeal or endotracheal intubation may be required. When the diagnosis is known prior to delivery, arrangements should be made for a physician skilled in neonatal airway management to be present at delivery. Emergency tracheostomy is rarely required.

**Transport** Immediate transport by an experienced neonatal transport team to a tertiary center with pediatric otolaryngology expertise may be indicated.

**Testing and Confirmation** The diagnostic triad of mandibular hypoplasia, glossoptosis, and a large, usually U-shaped, palatal defect forms the basis of the diagnosis. Careful physical examination will confirm the presence, or absence, of other abnormalities. The triad of findings occurs in isolation in approximately one-third of cases, as a component of Stickler syndrome in another 15% to 20%, and as part of other multiple-malformation syndromes in the remaining. The concomitant occurrence of airway obstruction and feeding difficulties is more frequent and more severe in infants with associated anomalies or other genetic syndromes. The presence of other malformations or organ malfunction will dictate the other diagnostic studies needed to complete the assessment.

**Nursery Management** The major objectives of care are to establish a definitive diagnosis, a stable airway, and an adequate feeding modality as expeditiously as possible. Concurrent abnormalities in other systems should raise the concern for a syndromic diagnosis. Flexible endoscopy or fiber-optic nasal laryngoscopy/bronchoscopy is recommended to determine the most appropriate management approach if airway obstruction is a significant issue. Oral feeding is often a difficult problem because of the combination of airway issues, palatal defect, and abnormal tongue position. Frequently, prone positioning with the head forward will ameliorate the airway obstruction and allow for oral feeding. In the more severe cases, nasogastric feeding, use of specialized feeding systems, or gastrostomy tube placement may be required.

## SURGERY

**Preoperative Assessment** The primary goal of treatment in patients with PRS is stabilization of the airway. Aesthetic facial reconstruction is an adjunctive goal. Treatment includes correction of the secondary deformities of the maxilla and orbit and improvement of the deficiencies of the facial soft tissues. Treatment varies according to the age of the patient, the degree of malformation, and the anticipated distortion of future growth potential. Surgical management is based on analysis of facial skeletal radiographs and often a 3-D CT scan.

**Types of Procedures** Several surgical options are available for neonates with PRS. Tongue-lip adhesion glossoplexy, in which the ventral surface of the tongue is anchored to the lower lip and the lateral surface of the tongue anchored to the mandible, functions to pull the tongue forward to prevent airway obstruction. Mandibular distraction is another alternative. In this procedure, the mandible is gradually lengthened with a mechanical apparatus. This brings the tongue base forward, thus relieving the airway obstruction. In rare cases, tracheostomy may be required as the definitive procedure.

**Surgical Results/Prognosis** For most infants, tongue-lip adhesion or mandibular distraction will resolve the airway obstruction until the child can grow. Repair of the soft tissue facial features constitutes a secondary surgery, after the facial skeleton has been restored. This leads to an overall favorable prognosis, but one that requires multiple surgeries over an extended period of time.

### SUGGESTED READINGS


1. Costa M, Tu MM, Murage KP, et al: Robin sequence: mortality, causes of death, and clinical outcomes. Plast Reconstr Surg 2014; 134:738-745.
2. Evans K, Sie KC, Hopper RA, et al: Robin sequence: from diagnosis to development of an effective management plan. Pediatrics 2011; 127:936-948.
3. Izumi K, Konczal LL, Mitchell AL, Jones MC: Underlying genetic diagnosis of Pierre Robin sequence: retrospective chart review at two children's hospitals and a systematic literature review. J Pediatr 2012; 160:645-650.
4. Marques IL, Barbieri MA, Bettol H: Etiopathogenesis of isolated Robin sequence. Cleft Palate Craniofac J 1998; 35:517-525.
5. Myers CM III, Reed MJ, Cotton RT, et al: Airway management in Pierre Robin sequence. Otolaryngol Head Neck Surg 1998; 118:630-635.
6. Otto C, Platt LD: The fetal mandible measurement: an objective determination of fetal jaw size. Ultrasound Obstet Gynecol 1991; 1:12-17.

7. Paladini D, Morra T, Teodoro A, et al: Objective diagnosis of micrognathia in the fetus: the jaw index. Obstet Gynecol 1999; 93:382-386.
8. Perkins JA, Sie KCY, Milczuk H, Richardson MA: Airway management in children with craniofacial anomalies. Cleft Palate Craniofac J 1997; 34:135-140.
9. Rotten D, Levaillant JM, Martinez H, et al: The fetal mandible: a 2-D and 3-D sonographic approach to the diagnosis of retrognathia and micrognathia. Ultrasound Obstet Gynecol 2002; 19:122-130.
10. Scott A, Tibesar R, Sidman J: Pierre Robin sequence: evaluation, management, indications for surgery, and pitfalls. Otolaryngol Clin N Am 2012; 45: 695-710.
11. Tan TY, Kilpatrick N, Farlie PG: Developmental and genetic perspectives on Pierre Robin Sequence. Am J Med Genet C Semin Med Genet 2013; 163C:295-305.
12. Tomaske SM, Zalzal GH, Saal HM: Airway obstruction in the Pierre Robin sequence. Laryngoscope 1995; 105:111-114.

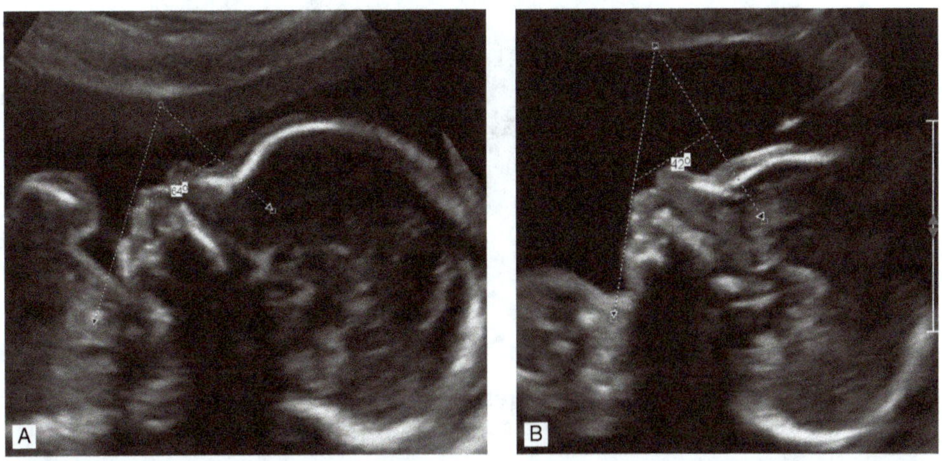


**FIGURE 7.4A-B** Normal (A) and abnormal (B) inferior facial angles. The fetus on the right had Pierre Robin sequence.

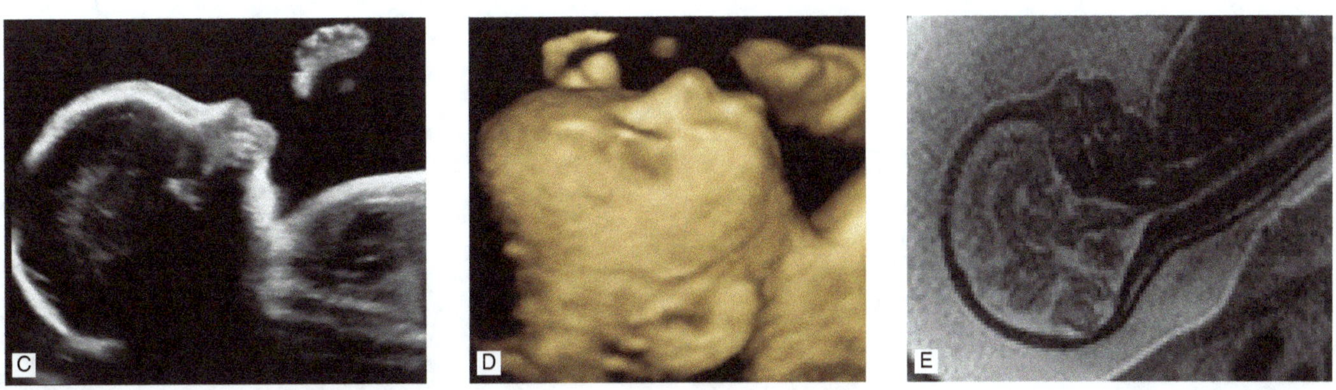


**FIGURE 7.4C-E** Conventional 2-D ultrasound, 3-D ultrasound, and fetal MRI (left to right) at 24 weeks' gestation of fetus with severe Pierre Robin sequence. Fetus was also noted to have additional abnormalities (note abnormal-appearing ear on 3-D study).

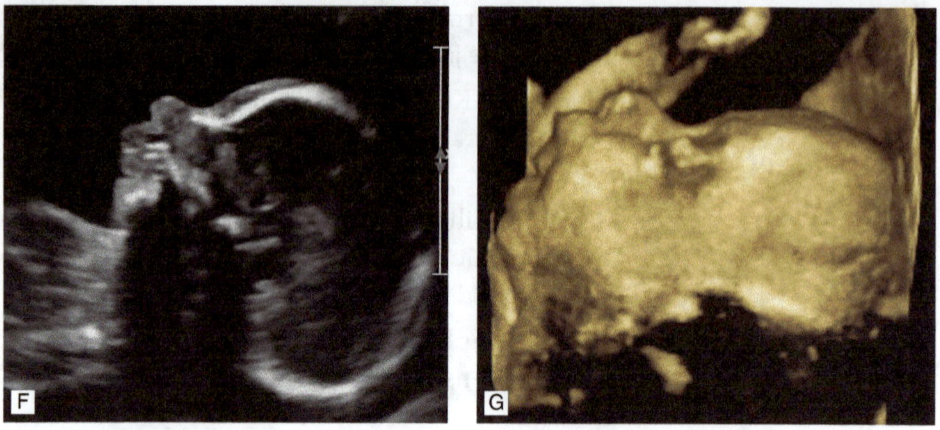


**FIGURE 7.4F-G** The 2-D (F) and 3-D (G) profile views of the same fetus with isolated Pierre Robin sequence. Note the significant micrognathia.

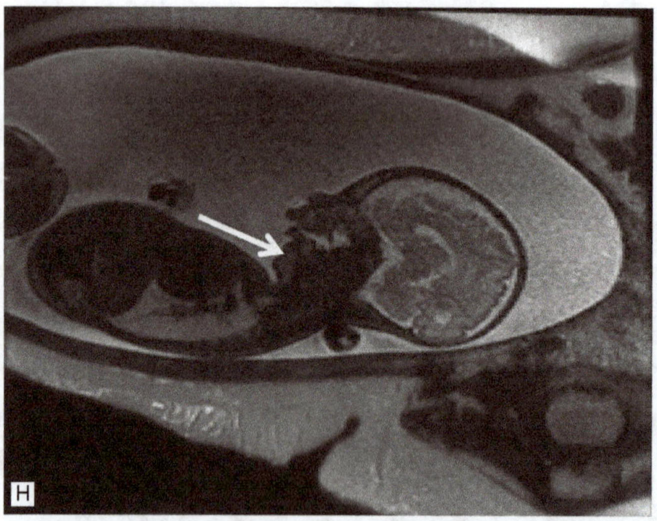


**FIGURE 7.4H** Magnetic resonance image of fetus with micrognathia (arrow) and severe polyhydramnios.

# 7.5 THYROID ENLARGEMENT/GOITER

## EPIDEMIOLOGY/GENETICS

**Definition** A goiter is an enlarged thyroid gland.

**Epidemiology** Occurrence is 1 in 40,000 deliveries.

**Embryology** Goiters can be associated with hypothyroidism (most common), hyperthyroidism, or a euthyroid state. Goiters associated with hypothyroidism are due to iodine deficiency, iodine intoxication, maternal antithyroid medications, or inborn errors in thyroid hormone synthesis. Goiters associated with hyperthyroidism are the result of transplacental passage of maternal thyroid-stimulating antibodies, whether or not the mother has active Graves' disease. One in 70 women with Graves' disease will have a fetus with a goiter.

**Inheritance Patterns** Generally, inheritance is sporadic. The Pendred syndrome, however, is an autosomal recessive disorder with sensorineural deafness and goiter caused by an inborn error in thyroid hormone synthesis.

**Teratogens** Propylthiouracil, iodine preparations, and lithium are teratogenic.

**Prognosis** The prognosis depends on the cause of the goiter. Polyhydramnios may induce prematurity.

## SONOGRAPHY

### FREQUENT FINDINGS

- The enlarged fetal thyroid gland will appear as a large, bilobed, symmetric, homogeneously echogenic anterior neck mass, maintaining the contour of the thyroid.
  - Normative tables of fetal thyroid size (circumference and width) across gestational ages are available.
- On 3-D sonography, the thyroid appears as a thick collar across the front of the neck.
- Color Doppler often demonstrates significantly increased vascular flow to the enlarged thyroid.

### LESS FREQUENT

- In cases of severe enlargement, the fetal head may be extended posteriorly, resulting in a "stargazer" posture of the fetus.
- In some cases, there may be altered ossification of the skeletal system (craniosynostosis) or tachycardia.
- Polyhydramnios may occur if the esophagus is compressed.
- Intrauterine growth restriction may occur.

### KEY FINDINGS/PITFALLS

- Small goiters are difficult to identify sonographically.
- Due to fetal position, it may be difficult to evaluate the anterior neck late in the third trimester.
- Fetal goiter has been reported as early as 14 weeks' gestation.

### DIFFERENTIAL DIAGNOSIS

- Cervical teratoma
  - Masses tend to be larger, containing both solid and cystic components.
  - Asymmetric.
  - Often extend into the lower jaw or upper mediastinum.
  - Often demonstrate rapid growth.
- Cystic hygroma
  - Primarily cystic with septations
  - Located in the posterior neck/occipital region; may extend laterally
- Lymphangioma
  - Primarily cystic, though may have solid elements
  - Typically located in the lateral neck
  - Most often unilateral

## PREGNANCY MANAGEMENT

**Investigations and Consultations Required** A maternal history and complete ultrasound evaluation of the fetus may give clues as to the etiology of the goiter, and whether it is associated with fetal hyper- or hypothyroidism. Because measurement of thyroid hormone in fetal blood is more reliable than amniotic fluid thyroid concentrations, cordocentesis is used to determine thyroid status prior to considering fetal therapy. Fetal MRI may help establish the diagnosis, and evaluate possible airway compromise at delivery. The goiter will appear homogeneous and hyperintense in T1-weighted images, but the trachea and esophagus are more easily seen on T-2 weighted images.

**Fetal intervention** Fetal intervention is beneficial in decreasing the size of the goiter in both hyperthyroid and hypothyroid fetuses. Levothyroxine injected into the amniotic fluid every 1-2 weeks has been shown to improve fetal thyroid status, and decrease the size of the fetal goiter.

**Monitoring** Serial sonography every 3-4 weeks may be helpful to assess fetal thyroid size, as well as amniotic fluid volume and fetal growth. If fetal therapy has been instituted, closer follow up is warranted.

**Pregnancy Termination Issues** In the absence of a precise diagnosis, termination should be performed by a nondestructive approach.

**Delivery** Because of the increased possibility for respiratory complications, delivery should be in a tertiary center. Cesarean section may be required as a result of the excessive extension of the fetal head. If airway compromise is suspected, cesarean section with an EXIT procedure may, rarely, be required.

## NEONATOLOGY

**Resuscitation** In the delivery room, the establishment of an adequate airway is the major concern. Rarely does this require emergency tracheostomy, but if the mass is very large, endotracheal intubation can be difficult. Once an airway is secured, other specific resuscitative measures usually are not required.

**Transport** Referral to a tertiary perinatal center is always indicated for diagnostic evaluation and treatment. If airway compromise is present, emergency transfer by an experienced neonatal transport team is important.

**Testing and Confirmation** Thyroid enlargement will be visible on clinical examination. Radionuclide scanning, thyroid function studies, and cervical sonography are useful to define both the anatomy and the functional status of the gland.

**Nursery Management** Once adequate ventilation is ensured, the focus of care is the diagnosis of the functional abnormality in thyroid production causing the goiter. Prompt relief of a congenital hypothyroid state or control of neonatal thyrotoxicosis is necessary to suppress the stimulus for hyperplasia and cause resolution of the goiter.

## SUGGESTED READINGS

1. Achiron R, Rotstein Z, Lipitz S, et al: The development of the foetal thyroid: in utero ultrasonographic measurements. Clin Endocrinol 1998; 48:259-264.
2. Agrawal P, Ogilvy-Stuart A, Lees C: Intrauterine diagnosis and management of congenital goitrous hypothyroidism. Ultrasound Obstet Gynecol 2002; 19:501-505.
3. Asteria C, Rajanayagam O, Collingwood TN, et al: Prenatal diagnosis of thyroid hormone resistance. J Clin Endocrinol Metab 1999; 84:405-410.
4. Belfar HL, Foley TP Jr, Hill LM, Kislak S: Sonographic findings in maternal hyperthyroidism. J Ultrasound Med 1991; 10:281-284.
5. Blumenfeld Y, David A, Milan K, et al: Conservatively managed fetal goiter: an alternative to in utero therapy. Fetal Diagn Ther 2013: 34;184-187.
6. Bromley B, Frigoletto FD Jr, Cramer D: The fetal thyroid: normal and abnormal sonographic measurements. J Ultrasound Med 1992; 11:25-28.
7. Corbacioglu Esmer A, Gul A, Dagdeviren H, et al: Intrauterine diagnosis and treatment of fetal goitrous hypothyroidism. J Obstet Gynaecol Res 2013; 39:720-723.
8. Hanono A, Shah B, David R, et al: Antenatal treatment of fetal goiter: a therapeutic challenge. J Matern Fetal Neonatal Med 2009; 22:76-80.
9. Hubbard AM, Crombleholme TM, Adzick NS: Prenatal MRI evaluation of giant neck masses in preparation for the fetal exit procedure. Am J Perinatol 1998; 15:253-257.
10. Ranzini A, Ananth C, Smulian J, et al: Ultrasonography of the fetal thyroid: nomograms based on biparietal diameter and gestational age. J Ultrasound Med 2001; 20:613-617.
11. Volumenie JL, Polak M, Guibourdenche J, et al: Management of fetal thyroid goiters: a report of 11 cases in a single perinatal unit. Prenat Diagn 2000; 20:799-806.

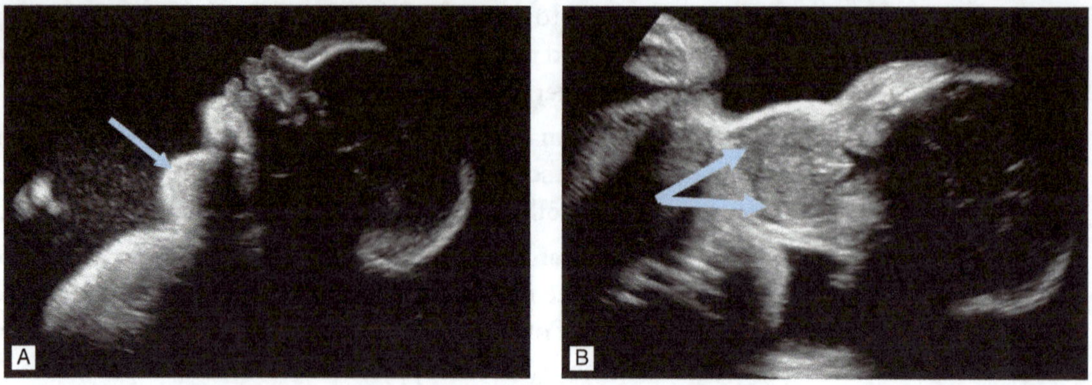

**FIGURE 7.5A-B** Sagittal (A) and coronal (B) view of a large fetal goiter noted by the arrows. Note the homogeneous, solid, goiter neck mass and an extended fetal head in the sagittal view (A) and the bilobed mass in the coronal view (B).

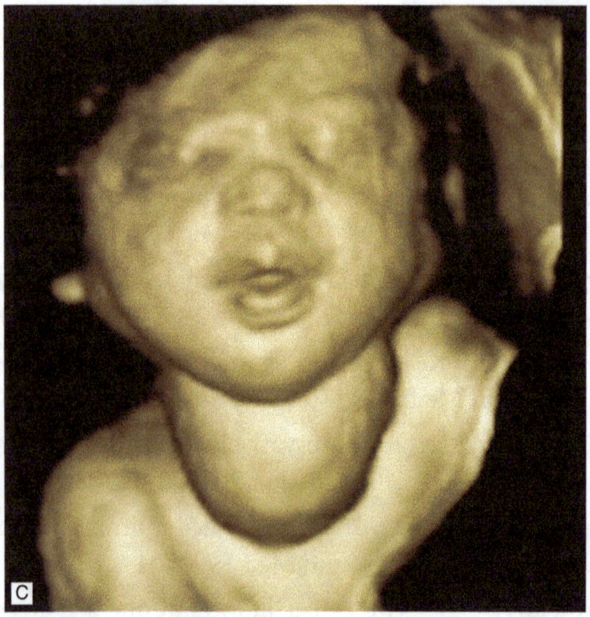

**FIGURE 7.5C** Three-dimensional view of 28-week fetus with large goiter. Note the collar-like appearance of the goiter across the anterior neck.

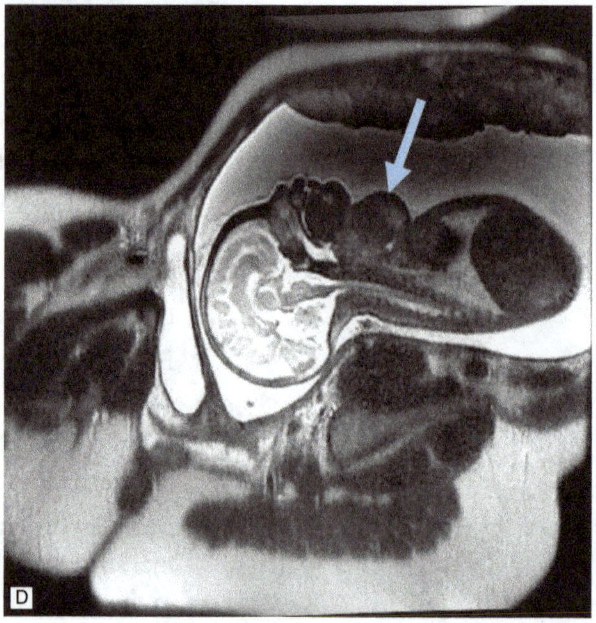

**FIGURE 7.5D** T2-weighted fetal MRI demonstrating fetal goiter (arrow). A portion of the esophagus and airway can also be seen in this image.

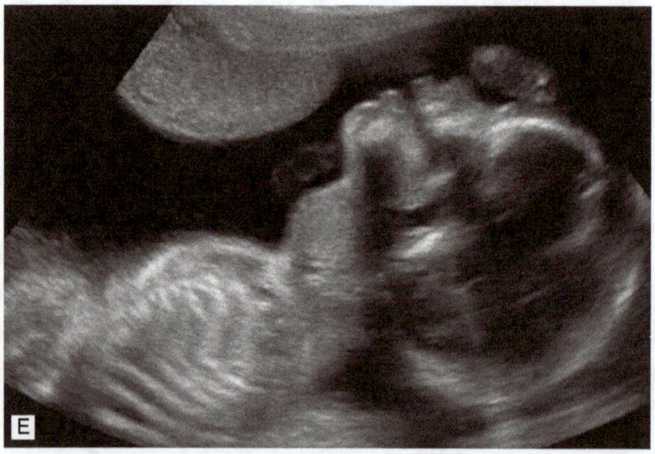

**FIGURE 7.5E** Fetus in "stargazer" position with extended fetal head due to goiter.

# CHAPTER 8

# SKELETAL ABNORMALITIES

# 8.0 INTRODUCTION

## DIAGNOSTIC APPROACH TO SUSPECTED SKELETAL DYSPLASIAS

The overall incidence of a lethal skeletal dysplasia is 1/10,000. A detailed fetal anatomic survey is required to satisfactorily evaluate a fetus for a suspected skeletal dysplasia. However, specific key measurements, ratios, and anatomic landmarks will aid the sonographer/sonologist in determining not only if a skeletal dysplasia is present, but also if it is lethal.

- Because of the rarity of lethal skeletal dysplasias, a femur length less than 2 SD (standard deviations) of the mean is not necessarily diagnostic. However, when the femur length is 5 mm below 2 SD, the diagnosis of a skeletal dysplasia can be confirmed.
- When a skeletal dysplasia is suspected, all of the long bones should be measured bilaterally to exclude a focal skeletal abnormality.
- The appearance of the long bones (i.e., bowing, fractures, or degree of mineralization) may provide important clues in classifying the type of skeletal dysplasia.
- Pre- or postaxial polydactyly and clubbed feet are associated with specific skeletal dysplasias.
- The femur length/abdominal circumference ratio is normally between 0.20 and 0.24. A ratio of less than 0.16 in a population at risk is consistent with a severe skeletal dysplasia.
- In a normal fetus, the femur and foot are of comparable length. A femur length/foot ratio of less than 0.87 discriminates between intrauterine growth restriction and a severe skeletal dysplasia.
- A thoracic circumference at the level of the four-chamber view below fifth centile or a thoracic/abdominal circumference ratio less than 0.83 is consistent with severe skeletal dysplasia. A narrow chest and protruding abdomen subjectively suggest a diagnosis of severe skeletal dysplasia.
- The presence of severe femur length shortening, in isolation, is insufficient to diagnose a severe skeletal dysplasia. Utilizing the previous criteria, the sonographic detection of lethal skeletal dysplasias is greater than 90%. However, the ability to accurately diagnosis the type of severe skeletal dysplasia is only 50%. A thorough postdelivery evaluation of the fetus is therefore required to confirm a diagnosis and to provide appropriate counseling to the family.

## SUGGESTED READINGS


1. Brons JTJ, van der Harten JJ, van Geijn HP, et al: Ratios between growth parameters for the prenatal ultrasonographic diagnosis of skeletal dysplasias. Eur J Obstet Gynecol Reprod Biol 1990; 34:37-46.
2. Hadlock FP, Harris RB, Shah Y, Park SK: The femur length/head circumference relation in obstetric sonography. J Ultrasound Med 1984; 3:439-442.
3. Hersh JH, Angle B, Pietrantoni M, et al: Predictive value of fetal ultrasonography in the diagnosis of a lethal skeletal dysplasia. Southern Med J 1998; 91:1137-1142.

4. Krakow D, Lachman LS, Rimoin DL: Guidelines for the prenatal diagnosis of fetal skeletal dysplasia. Genet Med 2009; 11:127-133.
5. Kurtz AB, Needleman L, Wapner RJ, et al: Usefulness of a short femur in the in-utero detection of skeletal dysplasias. Radiology 1990; 177:197-200.
6. Orioli I, Castilla EE, Barbosa-Neto JG: The birth prevalence rates for the skeletal dysplasias. J Med Genet 1986; 23:328-332.
7. Parilla BV, Leeth EA, Kambich MP, et al: Antenatal detection of skeletal dysplasias. J Ultrasound Med 2003; 22:255-258.
8. Ramus RM, Martin LB, Twickler DM: Ultrasonographic prediction of fetal outcome in suspected skeletal dysplasias with use of the femur length-to-abdominal circumference ratio. Am J Obstet Gynecol 1998; 179:1348-1352.

# 8.1 ACHONDROGENESIS

## EPIDEMIOLOGY/GENETICS

**Definition** Achondrogenesis is a group of lethal skeletal dysplasias characterized by severe limb and trunk shortening, with a disproportionately large head.

**Epidemiology** Achondrogenesis is rare.

**Embryology** There are two main subtypes. In type I, there is gross shortening of the limbs (micromelia) with flaring of the ribs, or fractures, and lack of ossification of the calvarium and spine. Micrognathia may be present. Hydrops may occur. Type I is subdivided into type IA, which has multiple rib fractures, and type IB, in which rib fractures do not occur. In type II (Langer-Saldino), there is no flaring of the ribs or rib fractures, and there is a relatively normal skull ossification, but otherwise the features are similar (i.e., severe micromelia, trunk shortening, edema of the soft tissues, and a disproportionately large head). Ossification of the lumbar vertebrae is minimal (type I) or absent (type II), and the sacral, pubic, and ischial bones show little ossification. Characteristic craniofacial features include micrognathia, flat face, and frontal bossing. Type II is occasionally associated with other abnormalities, including cleft palate, postaxial polydactyly of the feet, cystic hygroma, and cardiac defects. Type IA is caused by mutations in the thyroid hormone receptor interactor gene. Mutations in the diastrophic dysplasia sulfate transporter (*DTDST*) gene cause achondrogenesis type IB. Both type IA and type IB are inherited in an autosomal recessive fashion. Molecular defects in type II collagen have been found in cases of type II achondrogenesis with dominant inheritance. Consultation with a geneticist or genetic counselor is recommended when this group of disorders is suspected.

**Inheritance Patterns** Type I is inherited as an autosomal recessive disorder. Type II achondrogenesis is a new dominant mutation. Recurrence in some families has been reported, likely due to germ cell mosaicism.

**Teratogens** None are known.

**Prognosis** Achondrogenesis is lethal antenatally or in the newborn period.

## SONOGRAPHY

### FREQUENT FINDINGS

- Decreased/absent fetal movement
- Extremities
  - Micromelia
  - Brachydactyly
  - Clubfeet
  - Club hands
  - Long bones poorly calcified
    - Both sides of the long bones are visualized (no acoustic shadowing).
    - Because of significant demineralization, some bones may not be identifiable sonographically.

- Head
  - Short neck
  - Midface hypoplasia
  - Normal-to-absent calcification of the skull
  - Cystic hygroma
- Chest
  - Small, bell-shaped ribs that do not extend beyond the cardiac atrium
  - Rib fractures
  - Pulmonary hypoplasia
- Protuberant abdomen
- Spine: normal-to-poor calcification

### LESS FREQUENT

- First-trimester increased nuchal translucency
- Microcephaly
- Cleft palate
- Ventricular septal defect or other cardiac defects
- Pyelocaliectasis
- Hydrops

### KEY FEATURES/PITFALLS

- Three-dimensional (3-D) imaging accurately portrays facial features, brachydactyly, and the relative disproportion of limb segments.
- Rib fractures may help to differentiate type IA.

## PREGNANCY MANAGEMENT

**Investigations and Consultations Required** There are two goals of further investigations: determining whether the skeletal dysplasia is lethal and, if possible, determining which skeletal dysplasia the case represents. If the precise skeletal dysplasia is uncertain, other investigations are warranted, including a fetal echocardiogram. Congenital heart disease is a feature of a number of skeletal dysplasias and may be seen in type II achondrogenesis. Once a diagnosis of a lethal condition is established, and if the pregnancy is beyond the legal limits for termination, the family should meet with a neonatologist to discuss neonatal management.

**Monitoring** Further ultrasound examinations looking for relative growth and mineralization of the spine, ribs, and long bones may help to establish the diagnosis. Once a diagnosis of a lethal condition has been established, routine supportive maternal care should be provided. No attempts to treat preterm labor or to monitor fetal status are appropriate.

**Pregnancy Course** Polyhydramnios is a common complicating factor and may result in preterm labor. In addition, nonimmune hydrops may develop. If the polyhydramnios is significant and symptomatic, delivery should be undertaken. No tocolysis should be administered for preterm labor.

**Pregnancy Termination Issues** An intact fetus must be delivered, and the postmortem examination, including radiologic, morphologic, biochemical, and molecular studies, must be performed by individuals with extensive experience in skeletal dysplasias. Determining a precise diagnosis is essential to counseling the family regarding recurrence risk and for offering the appropriate prenatal diagnosis in subsequent pregnancies.

**Delivery** Vaginal delivery without electronic monitoring is appropriate. Some forms of achondrogenesis have relative macrocephaly, which may make vaginal delivery difficult. Delivery should occur in a center with expertise in the diagnostic evaluation of skeletal dysplasias or one with an interest and expertise in fetal pathology.

## NEONATOLOGY

**Neonatal Resuscitation** When the diagnosis is known prior to delivery, a prenatal decision for nonintervention, made after discussion with the family, is appropriate. If the diagnosis is uncertain, it is appropriate to support respiration to allow time for diagnostic evaluation and parental adaptation to occur.

**Neonatal Transport** Referral to a tertiary perinatal center is appropriate for confirmation of a diagnosis. Mechanical ventilatory support is often required during the transport.

**Testing and Confirmation** Postnatal radiographs can help determine the specific type of achondrogenesis.

**Nursery Management** Confirmation of the diagnosis, comfort care for the infant, and counseling and support of the family are the primary goals. Provision of mechanical life support in the interim is appropriate. Live-born infants that do not receive life support usually do not survive beyond the immediate newborn period.

### SUGGESTED READINGS


1. Borochowitz Z, Lachman R, Adomian GE, et al: Achondrogenesis type I: delineation of further heterogeneity and identification of two distinct subgroups. J Pediatr 1988; 112:23-31.
2. Borochowitz Z, Ornoy A, Lachman R, Rimoin DL: Achondrogenesis II—hypochondrogenesis: variability versus heterogeneity. Am J Med Genet 1986; 24:273-288.
3. Graham D, Tracey J, Winn K, et al: Early second trimester sonographic diagnosis of achondrogenesis. J Clin Ultrasound 1983; 11:336-338.
4. Krakow D, Williams J III, Poehl M, et al: Use of three-dimensional ultrasound imaging in the diagnosis of prenatal-onset skeletal dysplasias. Ultrasound Obstet Gynecol 2003; 21:467-472.
5. Mahony BS, Filly RA, Cooperberg PL: Antenatal sonographic diagnosis of achondrogenesis. J Ultrasound Med 1984; 3:333-335.

6. Nagendran S, Richards AJ, McNinch A, et al: Somatic mosaicism and phenotypic expression of the COL2A1 mutations. Am J Med Genet 2012; 158A:1204-1207.

7. Tretter AE, Sanders RC, Meyers CM, et al: Antenatal diagnosis of lethal skeletal dysplasias. Am J Med Genet 1998; 75:518-522.

8. Wataganara T, Sutanthavibool A, Limwongse C: Real-time three-dimensional sonographic features of an early third trimester fetus with achondrogenesis. J Med Assoc Thai 2006; 89:1762-1765.

9. Whitley CB, Gorlin RJ: Achondrogenesis: nosology with evidence of genetic heterogeneity. Radiology 1983; 148:693-698.

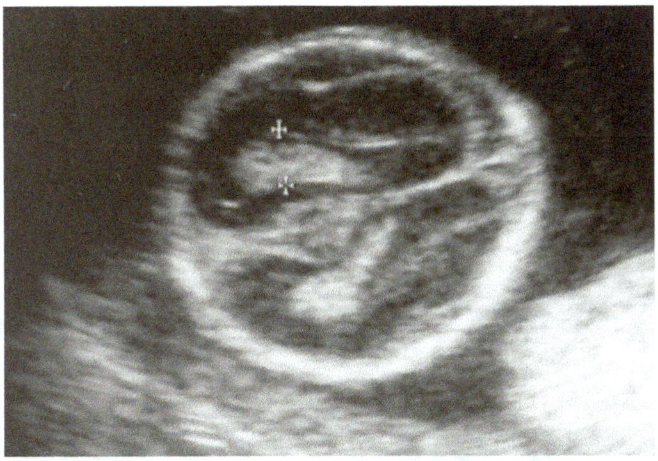

FIGURE 8.1A Achondrogenesis. Calvarial hypomineralization with excellent visualization of anterior lateral ventricle (+ … +) and no acoustic shadowing from skull.

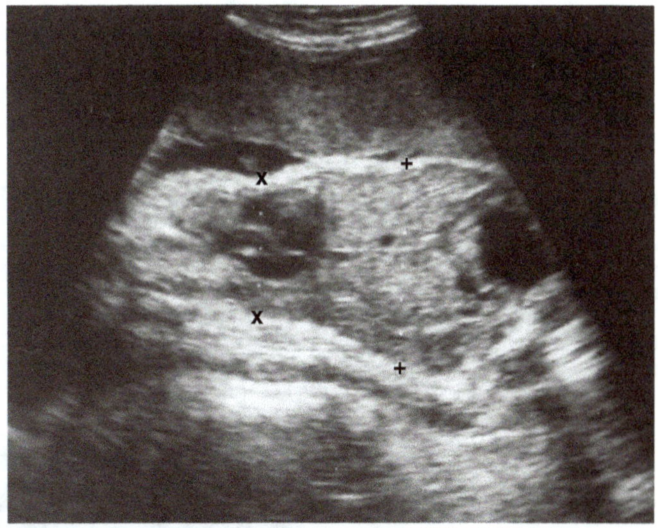

FIGURE 8.1B Achondrogenesis with small chest (x … x) and protuberant abdomen (+ … +).

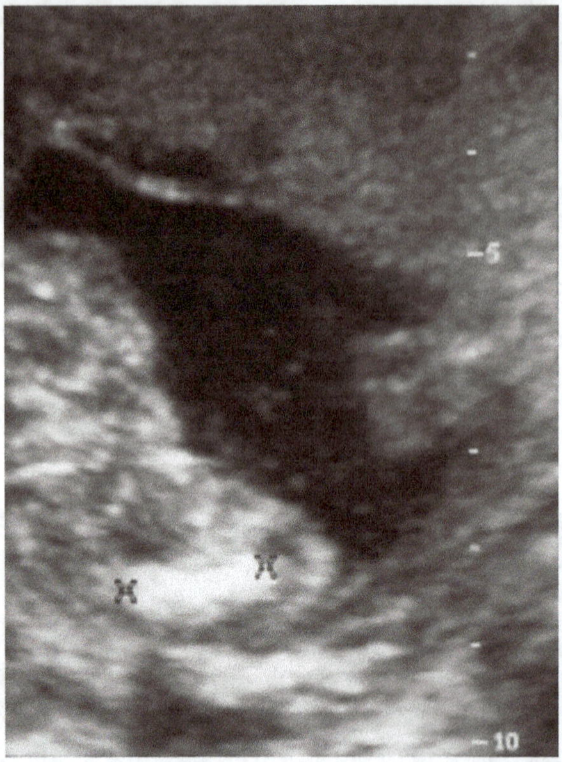


**FIGURE 8.1C** Short femur (x … x) in achondrogenesis.

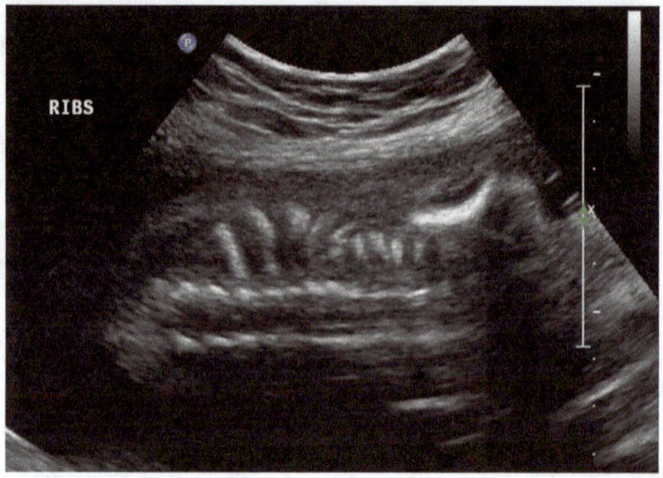


**FIGURE 8.1D** Severe rib shortening in achondrogenesis.

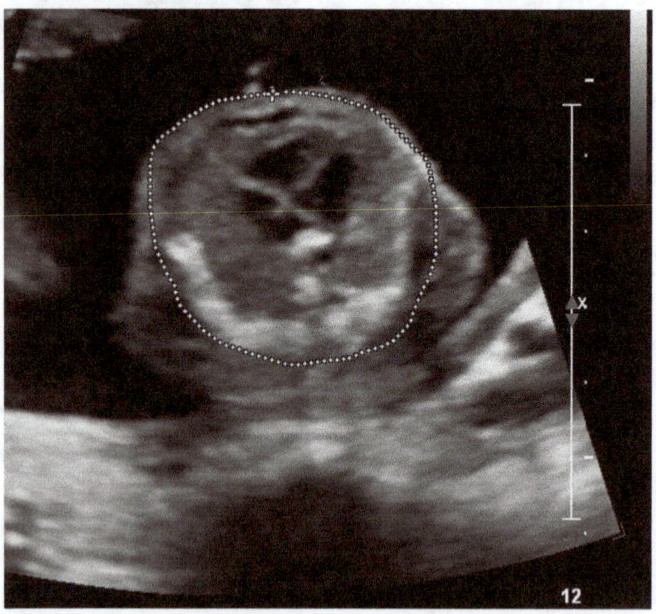


**FIGURE 8.1E** Short rib and narrow chest in achondrogenesis.

# 8.2 ACHONDROPLASIA

## EPIDEMIOLOGY/GENETICS

**Definition** Achondroplasia is the most common skeletal dysplasia and is characterized by rhizomelic limb shortening with macrocephaly.

**Epidemiology** Occurrence is 1 in 15,000 live births (M1:F1).

**Embryology** The phenotype is due to decreased endochondral ossification and is characterized by rhizomelic micromelia, macrocephaly with frontal bossing, and midface hypoplasia. The macrocephaly is due to anatomic megalencephaly secondary to an increase in the number of brain cells. Achondroplasia is due to mutations in the fibroblast growth factor receptor 3 (*FGFR3*) gene that maps to the distal end of chromosome 4p. Almost all cases demonstrate the same single base-pair substitution.

**Inheritance Patterns** Inheritance is autosomal dominant, with nearly 90% of cases representing new gene mutations. Recurrence risk in subsequent pregnancies is approximately 5% because of germ cell mosaicism.

**Teratogens** None are known.

**Prognosis** Intelligence and life span are usually normal. Affected individuals are at risk for neurologic complications, including spinal cord compression at the foramen magnum and the thoracolumbar region. Other complications include obstructive sleep apnea and obesity. The average life expectancy is decreased by 15 years. Homozygosity for achondroplasia, which occurs when both parents are affected, is lethal, with either stillbirth or early neonatal death from pulmonary hypoplasia.

## SONOGRAPHY

### FREQUENT FINDINGS

- Head
  - Relative macrocephaly
  - Frontal bossing
  - Depressed nasal bridge
  - Midface hypoplasia
- Chest
  - Small, but within the normal range
- Extremities
  - Mild-to-moderate rhizomelic shortening
  - Femur length initially within the normal range
  - Late second and early third trimester: femur length between –2 and –3 SD
  - Bowing of femur
- Hands/feet
  - Brachydactyly (short fingers)
  - Trident hand

        - Separation of second and third digit
        - Inability to approximate third and fourth fingers
    - Equal-length fingers

### LESS FREQUENT

- Spine
    - Lordosis
- Central nervous system
    - Ventriculomegaly

### KEY FEATURES/PITFALLS

- Ultrasound does not provide a firm diagnosis until the third trimester.
- When achondroplasia is suspected, a femur length/abdominal circumference (FL/AC) ratio of less than 0.16 in the third trimester is not a reliable indicator of severe skeletal dysplasia.

### DIFFERENTIAL DIAGNOSIS

- Severe intrauterine growth restriction: The limbs will not be as short, and there may be markedly decreased fluid.
- Thanatophoric dwarfism: Similar appearance, but it develops earlier and is much more severe (see Section 8.14).
    - The pattern of long-bone growth will readily distinguish these two diagnoses.
        - With thanatophoric dysplasia, long-bone shortening begins in the first trimester, in contrast to the late second or early third trimester with achondroplasia.

## PREGNANCY MANAGEMENT

**Investigations and Consultations Required** Achondroplasia may present with mild shortening of the long bones in fetal life, and there is significant overlap with normal. Unless the fetus is at risk (one of the parents has achondroplasia), this would represent a new mutation, and the diagnosis may be in doubt. As such, an evaluation for other causes of shortened long bones, particularly early-onset intrauterine growth restriction, should be undertaken. An amniocentesis for DNA testing, looking for the most common mutations causing this disorder, may be useful. Fetal echocardiography and chromosomal studies should be performed to exclude other conditions with mild shortening of the long bones. Consultation with a pediatric geneticist should be done to assist the family with an understanding of the disorder and the implications for further care.

**Monitoring** Serial ultrasound examinations looking for growth of the long bones may be necessary to make the diagnosis, but once it is made, no further exams are needed unless obstetrical complications arise. No change in standard obstetric practice is necessary.

**Pregnancy Course** Mild polyhydramnios may develop, but preterm labor or other obstetric complications are unusual.

**Pregnancy Termination Issues** Generally, this diagnosis is not made until the third trimester. It may be made sooner in families at risk, but for those individuals, termination of pregnancy is generally not desired. If the termination is contemplated and a DNA diagnosis to confirm is available, any method of termination is available. If the diagnosis is in doubt, an intact fetus and an autopsy, as well as x-ray studies, would be necessary.

**Delivery** Delivery should occur in a tertiary center with full capabilities for neonatal resuscitation in the event of an incorrect diagnosis. Because of the narrow foramen magnum and upper cervical spine, spinal cord compression is a significant risk with neck manipulation. Respiratory distress in the neonatal period is not uncommon, also necessitating a tertiary center for delivery.

## NEONATOLOGY

**Resuscitation** In the absence of known homozygosity, there are no contraindications to full resuscitative efforts following delivery if there is delay in spontaneous onset of respiration.

**Transport** The primary indication for referral in the immediate neonatal period is for confirmation of the diagnosis and evaluation by pediatric subspecialists, including genetics, orthopedics, and neurology.

**Testing and Confirmation** Postnatal skeletal radiographs are pathognomonic and can confirm the clinical phenotype.

**Nursery Management** Hydrocephalus may develop, although not usually in the neonatal period.

### SUGGESTED READINGS

1. Andersen PE Jr, Hauge M: Congenital generalized bone dysplasias: a clinical, radiological, and epidemiological survey. J Med Genet 1989; 26:37-44.
2. Bellus GA, Hefferon TW, Ortiz de Luna RI, et al: Achondroplasia is defined by recurrent G380R mutations of FGFR3. Am J Hum Genet 1995; 56:368-373.
3. Chitty LS, Griffin DR, Meaney C, et al: New aids for the non-invasive prenatal diagnosis of achondroplasia: dysmorphic features, charts of fetal size and molecular confirmation using cell-free fetal DNA in maternal plasma. Ultrasound Obstet Gynecol 2011; 37:283-289.
4. Cohen MM Jr: Achondroplasia, hypochondroplasia and thanatophoric dysplasia: Clinically related skeletal dysplasias that are also related at the molecular level. Int J Oral Maxillofax Surg 1998; 27:451-455.
5. Horton WA, Hall JG, Hecht JT: Achondroplasia. Lancet 2007; 370:162-172.

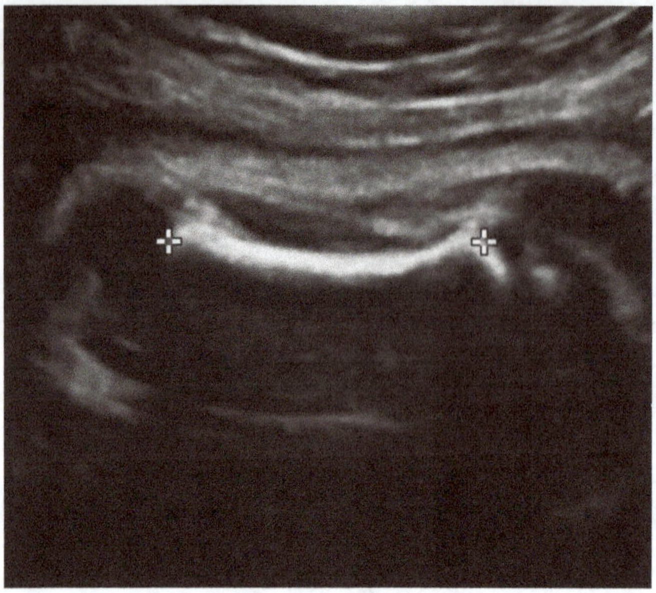

FIGURE 8.2A Achondroplasia with femur length of 41mm (23 weeks 2 days) at 25 weeks' gestation (fourth centile).

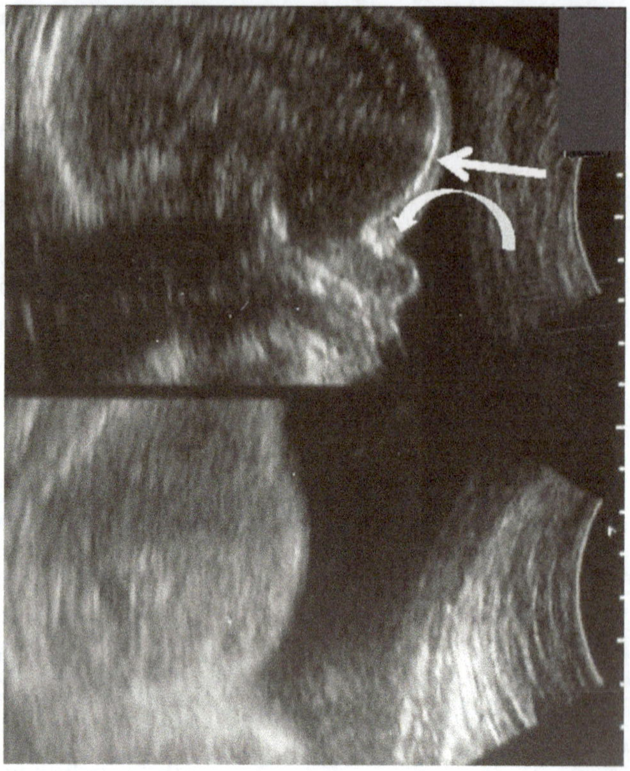

FIGURE 8.2B Achondroplasia illustrating frontal bossing (straight arrow) and depressed nasal bridge (curved arrow).

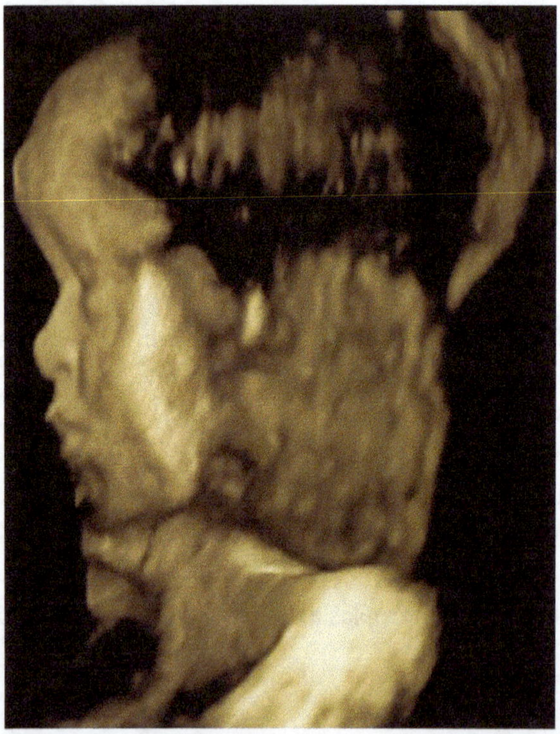

FIGURE 8.2C Achondroplasia with frontal bossing (3-D).

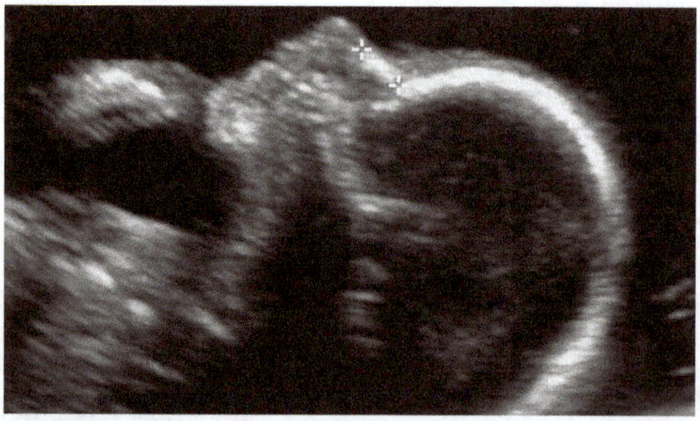

FIGURE 8.2D Normal fetal profile.

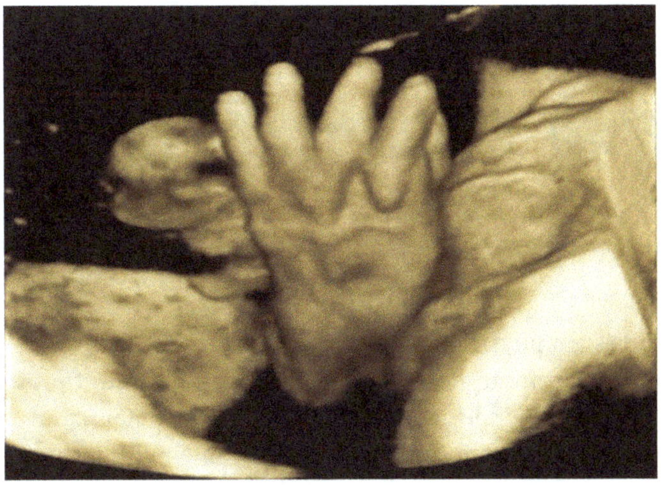

FIGURE 8.2E Trident hand.

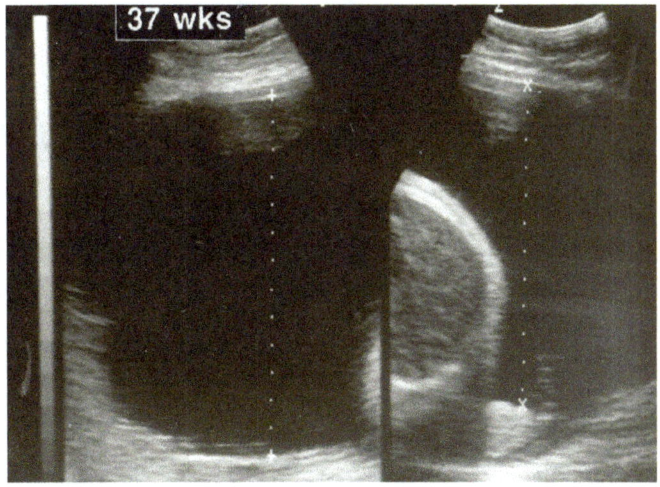


FIGURE 8.2F Achondroplasia illustrating marked polyhydramnios.

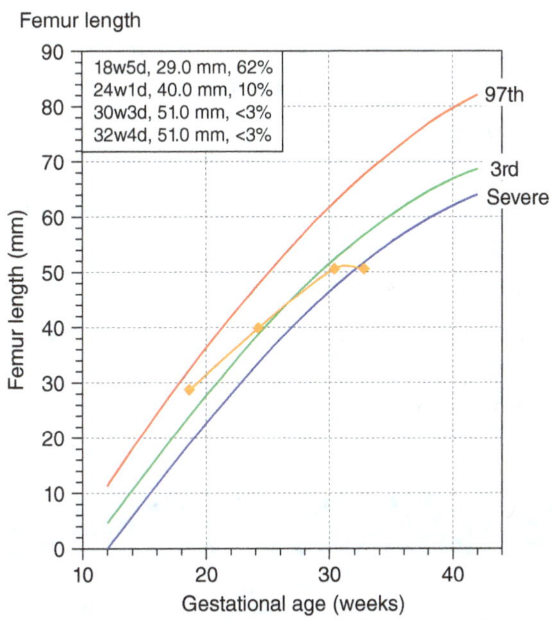


FIGURE 8.2G Graph illustrating lag in femur length growth with achondroplasia.

# 8.3 ARTHROGRYPOSIS

## EPIDEMIOLOGY/GENETICS

**Definition** Arthrogryposis is a term for a group of disorders characterized by congenital, usually nonprogressive, joint contractures at multiple sites.

**Epidemiology** Occurrence is 1 to 3 in 10,000 births (M1:F1).

**Embryology** Arthrogryposis is a physical finding that results from a heterogeneous group of disorders. The arthrogryposes can be divided into three groups: (1) limb involvement only; (2) generalized neuromuscular involvement; and (3) central nervous system, as well as neuromuscular, involvement. There are more than 300 genetic, chromosomal, and sporadic multiple-malformation syndromes that have congenital contractures as a feature. Possible etiologies include a vascular event, neurologic or myopathic process, connective tissue abnormalities, chromosomal abnormalities, intrauterine compression, or a teratogenic exposure. Only one-half of children with arthrogryposis receive a specific diagnosis. Trisomy 18 is the most common chromosomal diagnosis. Myotonic dystrophy is an autosomal dominant disorder with a severe arthrogrypotic congenital form. It occurs only in offspring of mothers with myotonic dystrophy.

**Inheritance Patterns** Autosomal dominant, recessive, and X-linked syndromes have been described.

**Teratogens** Maternal hyperthermia and congenital infections are teratogenic.

**Prognosis** The prognosis is dependent on an accurate diagnosis and may range from perinatal lethal disorders to those with only mild-to-moderate orthopedic limitations.

## SONOGRAPHY

### FREQUENT FINDINGS

- Extremities
  - Limited joint mobility
  - May involve one or more joints
  - Clubfeet
  - Clenched hands
  - Ulnar deviation
  - Extension at the elbow
  - Flexed wrists
  - Hypoplastic muscles
- Head/Neck
  - Fixed hyperextension
  - Micrognathia
- Umbilical cord
  - Short, due to decreased movement

- Polyhydramnios
- Intrauterine growth restriction
- First-trimester thickened nuchal translucency

### LESS FREQUENT

- Cleft palate
- Ventriculomegaly
- Microcephaly
- Agenesis of the corpus callosum
- Holoprosencephaly
- Pulmonary hypoplasia
- Pleural effusions
- Hydrops
- Tracheoesophageal fistula
- Scoliosis
- Oligohydramnios

### KEY FINDINGS/PITFALLS

- The hallmark is bilateral clubbed feet and decreased fetal movement.
- Diagnosis usually is made in the second trimester.
- Four-dimensional (4-D) ultrasound permits the diagnosis of motor failure, even in the latter part of the first trimester.
- In some cases, there are only mild orthopedic limitations.

### DIFFERENTIAL DIAGNOSIS

- Pena-Shokeir syndrome: a perinatal lethal form of multiple contractures
  - There is nuchal thickening or generalized edema in all cases of Pena-Shokeir syndrome.
  - The stomach is small to absent due to decreased swallowing.
  - While pulmonary hypoplasia is always present with Pena-Shokeir syndrome, it does not occur in mild forms of arthrogryposis.

## PREGNANCY MANAGEMENT

**Investigations and Consultations Required** The extent and direction of further evaluation will depend in part on associated ultrasound findings, which suggest whether the arthrogryposis is isolated or part of a syndrome. Fetal karyotype, microarray analysis, and studies to rule out congenital infections should be done, especially if additional malformations are detected. Fetal echocardiography may also be helpful in establishing a diagnosis. Consultations with a medical geneticist should be done to determine if specific molecular testing should be done.

**Monitoring** Standard obstetric care is appropriate unless there are features consistent with the lethal forms of the disorder. Serial ultrasound examinations to assess the possible progression of limb abnormalities may be helpful for prognostic purposes. The presence or absence of polyhydramnios and nonimmune hydrops can also be evaluated during these follow-up ultrasound examinations.

**Pregnancy Course** No changes are expected. The finding of severe polyhydramnios is highly suggestive of the lethal forms of the condition, and amnioreduction, except for maternal indications, should not be considered. If a lethal form of arthrogryposis is suspected, consultation with a neonatologist to discuss neonatal management is appropriate.

**Pregnancy Termination Issues** Arthrogryposis may be part of a heterogeneous group of disorders; a complete autopsy on an intact fetus should be performed. Accurate recurrence risk counseling requires a precise diagnosis.

**Delivery** Breech presentation is common in fetuses with arthrogryposis. The mode of delivery should be based on obstetric indications. Delivery at a tertiary center is appropriate as an exact diagnosis may not be established prenatally, and a team prepared to handle complex neonatal issues should be available.

## NEONATOLOGY

**Resuscitation** The decision not to offer resuscitation is easiest when there is a definite diagnosis of a concomitant lethal condition. In all other circumstances, resuscitation should be initiated and support continued, if needed, while a diagnostic evaluation is completed.

**Transport** Referral to a tertiary perinatal center for diagnostic evaluation is appropriate. With an otherwise-asymptomatic infant, referral for outpatient evaluation and treatment planning is also acceptable.

**Testing and Confirmation** Because the long-term prognosis is heavily influenced by associated or coexisting disorders, complete diagnostic evaluation and etiologic determination are the top priorities. Muscle biopsy and nerve conduction studies are important in determining the potential for habilitation.

**Nursery Management** Treatment is directed toward achieving stable, functional weight-bearing and manual dexterity. Initially, positioning, physical therapy, and bracing are used, followed by surgery in later infancy and childhood.

### SUGGESTED READINGS


1. Bui TH, Lindholm H, Demir N, Thomassen P: Prenatal diagnosis of distal arthrogryposis type I by ultrasonography. Prenat Diagn 1992; 12:1047-1053.
2. Fahy MJ, Hall JG: A retrospective study of pregnancy complications among 828 cases of arthrogryposis. Genet Couns 1990; 1:3-11.
3. Filges I, Hall JG: We are failing to identify disorders of fetal movement—why? Prenat Diagn 2012; 32:919-920.
4. Filges I, Hall JG: Failure to identify antenatal multiple congenital contractures and fetal kinesia—proposal of guidelines to improve diagnosis. Prenat Diagn 2013; 33:61-74.

5. Geifman-Holtzman O, Fay K: Prenatal diagnosis of congenital myotonic dystrophy and counseling of the pregnant mother: case report and literature review. Am J Med Genet 1998; 78:250-253.
6. Gorczyca DP, McGahan JP, Lindfors KK, et al: Arthrogryposis multiplex congenita: prenatal ultrasonographic diagnosis. J Clin Ultrasound 1989; 17:40-44.
7. Hoellen F, Schröer A, Lelling K, et al: Arthrogryposis multiplex congenital and Pena-Shokeir phenotype: challenge of prenatal diagnosis—report of 21 cases, antenatal findings and review. Fetal Diagn Ther 2011; 30:289-298.
8. Hyett J, Noble P, Sebire NJ, et al: Lethal congenital arthrogryposis presents with increased nuchal translucency at 10-14 weeks of gestation. Ultrasound Obstet Gynecol 1997; 9:310-313.
9. Kwjak A, Vacek N, Hafner T, et al: Prenatal diagnosis: what does four-dimensional ultrasound add? J Perinat Med 2002; 30:57-62.
10. Rink BD: Arthrogryposis: a review and approach to prenatal diagnosis. Obstet Gynecol Surv 2011; 66:369-377.
11. Scott H, Hunger A, Bedard B: Non-lethal arthrogryposis multiplex congenital presenting with cystic hygroma at 13 weeks gestational age. Prenat Diagn 1999; 19:966-971.
12. Silberstein EP, Kakulas BA: Arthrogryposis multiplex congenita in Western Australia. J Paediatr Child Health 1998; 34:518-523.

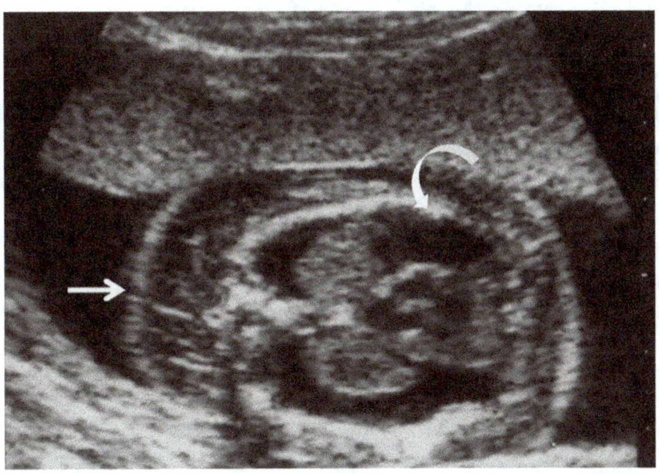

**FIGURE 8.3A** Arthrogryposis with hydrops-anasarca (straight arrow) and effusion (curved arrow).

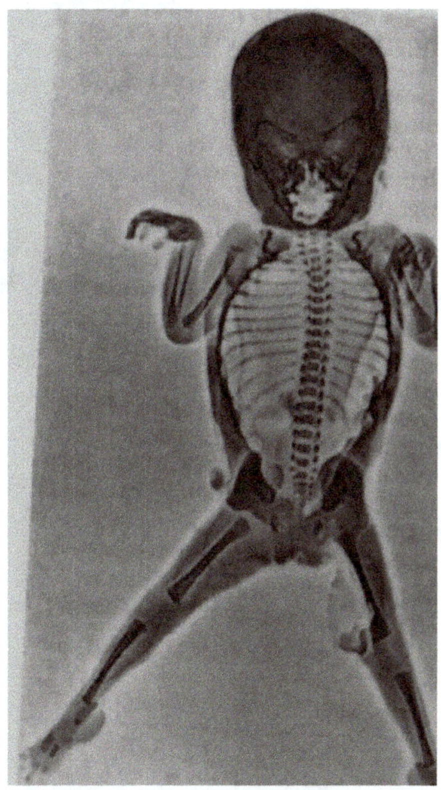

**FIGURE 8.3B** X-ray of fetus with arthrogryposis.

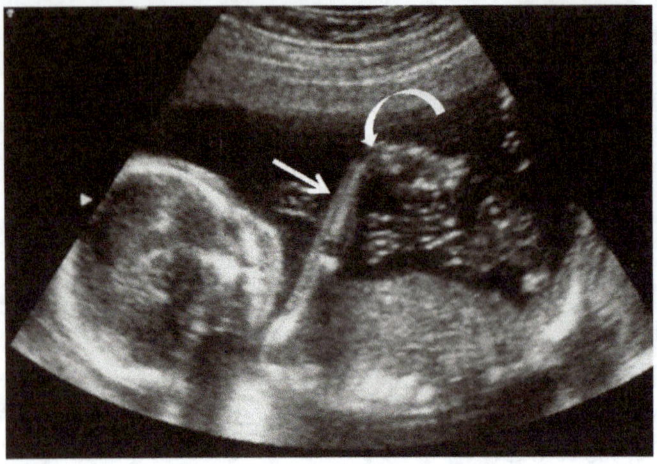

**FIGURE 8.3C** Arthrogryposis with extension at elbow, muscular atrophy (straight arrow), and ulnar deviation (curved arrow).

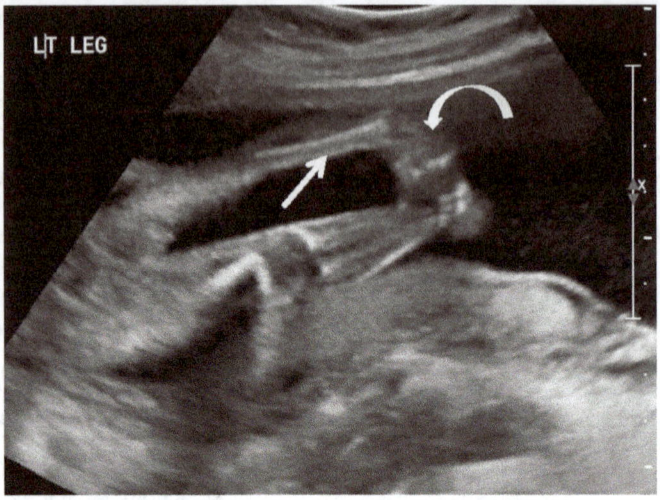


**FIGURE 8.3D** Arthrogryposis illustrating extended legs, clubfoot (curved arrow), and muscular atrophy (straight arrow).

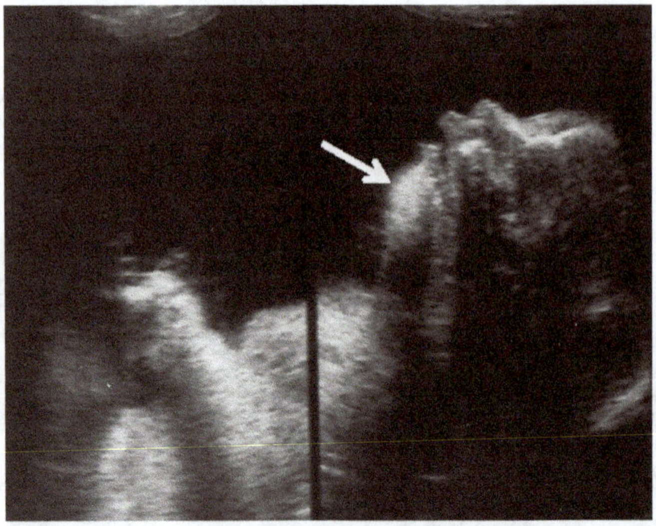

**FIGURE 8.3E** Arthrogryposis with micrognathia (arrow) and polyhydramnios.

# 8.4 CAMPOMELIC DYSPLASIA

## EPIDEMIOLOGY/GENETICS

**Definition** Campomelic dysplasia is a skeletal dysplasia usually characterized by bowing deformities of the femur and tibia.

**Epidemiology** Incidence: rare. Phenotypic sex ratio, M1:F3; karyotypic sex ratio, M1:F1.

**Embryology** Infants with campomelic dysplasia have a flat facial profile, cleft palate, and tracheal abnormalities. Other abnormalities that have been associated are cardiac and renal anomalies. There is a less-common form of the disorder, known as acampomelic campomelic dysplasia, that has milder skeletal abnormalities and lacks long-bone curvature. An apparent preponderance of females is due to 46,XY males with sex reversal. The gene associated with the disorder is located on chromosome 17 and is designated *SOX*-9 (*SRY*-related *HMG*-box 9) gene. Mutations in the gene are responsible for both forms of campomelic dysplasia.

**Inheritance Patterns** Inheritance is autosomal dominant, with all cases representing new mutations. Campomelic dysplasia is due to mutations in the *SOX9* gene on chromosome 17q. Recurrence in families has been reported on the basis of both somatic mutations and germ cell mutations in the parents. Consultation with a geneticist or genetic counselor concerning antenatal testing should be done in suspected cases.

**Teratogens** None are known.

**Prognosis** Usually, this is lethal in the neonatal period. Survival duration is related to the degree of respiratory compromise at birth. Infants with less-severe manifestations may occasionally survive into early infancy and beyond, but with significant respiratory and feeding difficulties. All have severe intellectual disability.

## SONOGRAPHY

### FREQUENT FINDINGS

- Extremities
  - Moderate to markedly shortened femur and tibia
  - Anteriorly bowed femur and/or tibia
    - Skin dimpling over the convex surface of the bone at the point of maximum deformity
  - Abnormal ratio of upper to lower limb
    - Upper limbs normal to shortened 25% versus 50% to 70% shortening of the lower limbs
  - Upper long bones occasionally bowed
  - Normal bone echogenicity
  - Hypoplastic/absent fibula
  - Hypoplastic scapula
  - Clubfeet

- Thorax
  - Bell shaped
  - Mild narrowing
  - Eleven pairs of ribs
- Face
  - Protuberant forehead
  - Micrognathia
  - Flattened nasal bridge
  - Low-set ears
- Genitourinary
  - Ambiguous genitalia
- Polyhydramnios

### LESS FREQUENT

- Upper long bones bowed
- Hypotelorism
- Cleft palate
- Cloverleaf skull
- Ventriculomegaly
- Pyelocaliectasis
- Ventricular septal defect
- Aortic stenosis
- Kyphoscoliosis

### KEY FINDINGS/PITFALLS

- Three-dimensional imaging provides additional information that assists in the diagnosis of campomelic dysplasia. For example, 3-D skeletal mode can be used to evaluate the fetus for the 11 pairs of ribs associated with campomelic dysplasia.

## PREGNANCY MANAGEMENT

**Investigations and Consultations Required** There are two goals of further investigations: determining whether the skeletal dysplasia is lethal and, if possible, determining which skeletal dysplasia the case represents. Campomelic dysplasia is particularly difficult, as some cases have been survivors, but most are lethal. If the precise skeletal dysplasia is uncertain, other investigations are warranted, including a fetal echocardiogram. Congenital heart disease is a rare feature of campomelic dysplasia. As gender may be phenotypically reversed, a karyotype is a useful adjunct to determining the diagnosis of campomelic dysplasia. Molecular testing on amniocytes can be done if there is a high suspicion of campomelic dysplasia. Once a diagnosis is established, and if the pregnancy is beyond the legal limits for termination, the family should meet with a neonatologist to discuss neonatal management. Consultation with a pediatric dysmorphologist may be beneficial to the family to discuss the natural history of those infants who survive.

**Monitoring** If the diagnosis is uncertain, follow-up ultrasound examinations may be helpful to look for features of the bones, such as the degree of bowing and the number of ribs, which may help to determine the diagnosis. Once the diagnosis is made, ultrasound examinations may be helpful to monitor facial features, such as a small chin, which may affect airway management at birth. Chest size is also a predictor of lethality and may be useful to monitor.

**Pregnancy Course** Mild polyhydramnios may develop, but preterm labor or other obstetric complications are unusual.

**Pregnancy Termination Issues** An intact fetus must be delivered, and the postmortem examination, including radiologic, morphologic, biochemical, and molecular studies, must be performed by individuals with extensive experience in skeletal dysplasias. Tissue for DNA testing should be obtained.

**Delivery** The site for delivery should be one where all personnel are comfortable with a nonaggressive approach to labor, delivery, and neonatal care, if elected by the family. Respiratory complications are common, and intubation may be complicated because of micrognathia. Delivery should occur in a tertiary center.

## NEONATOLOGY

**Resuscitation** When the diagnosis is known prior to delivery, a prenatal decision for nonintervention, made after discussion with the family, is appropriate. If the diagnosis is uncertain, resuscitation and ventilatory support are instituted to allow time for diagnostic evaluation and parental adaptation.

**Transport** Referral to a tertiary perinatal center is appropriate for confirmation of a diagnosis. Mechanical ventilatory support is often required during the transport.

**Testing and Confirmation** Skeletal radiographs postnatally will establish the diagnosis.

**Nursery Management** Confirmation of the diagnosis and counseling and support of the family are the primary goals. Provision of mechanical life support initially is appropriate, with concurrence of the family. Redirection of care with comfort measures only may be offered if severe respiratory insufficiency persists.

### SUGGESTED READINGS

1. Cordone M, Lituania M, Zampatti C, et al: In utero ultrasonographic features of camptomelic dysplasia. Prenat Diagn 1989; 9:745-750.
2. Dreyer SD, Zhou G, Lee B: The long and short of it: developmental genetics of the skeletal dysplasias. Clin Genet 1998; 54:454-473.
3. Gentilin B, Forzano F, Bedeschi MF, et al: Phenotype of five cases of prenatally diagnosed campomelic dysplasia harboring novel mutations of the *SOX9* gene. Ultrasound Obstet Gynecol 2010; 36:315-323.
4. Gillerot Y, Vanheck CA, Foulon M, et al: Camptomelic syndrome: manifestations in a 20 week fetus and case history of a 5-year-old child. Am J Med Genet 1989; 34:589-592.

5. Houston CS, Opitz JM, Spranger JW, et al: The camptomelic syndrome: review, report of 17 cases, and follow-up on the currently 17-year-old boy first reported by Maroteaux et al in 1971. Am J Med Genet 1983; 15:3-28.
6. Mansour S, Offiah AC, McDowell S, et al: The phenotype of survivors of campomelic dysplasia. J Med Genet 2002; 39:597-602.
7. McDowall S, Argentaro A, Ranganathan S, et al: Functional and structural studies of wild type *SOX9* and mutations causing camptomelic dysplasia. J Biol Chem 1999; 274:24023-24030.
8. Seow K-M, Huang L-W, Lin Y-H, et al: Prenatal three-dimensional ultrasound diagnosis of a camptomelic dysplasia. Arch Gynecol Obstet 2004; 269:142-144.
9. Tongsong T, Wanapirak C, Pongsatha S: Prenatal diagnosis of camptomelic dysplasia. Ultrasound Obstet Gynecol 2000; 15:428-430.
10. Tretter AE, Sanders RC, Meyers CG, et al: Antenatal diagnosis of lethal skeletal dysplasias. Am J Med Genet 1998; 75:518-522.
11. Winter R, Rosenkranz W, Hofmann H, et al: Prenatal diagnosis of camptomelic dysplasia by ultrasonography. Prenat Diagn 1985; 5:1-8.

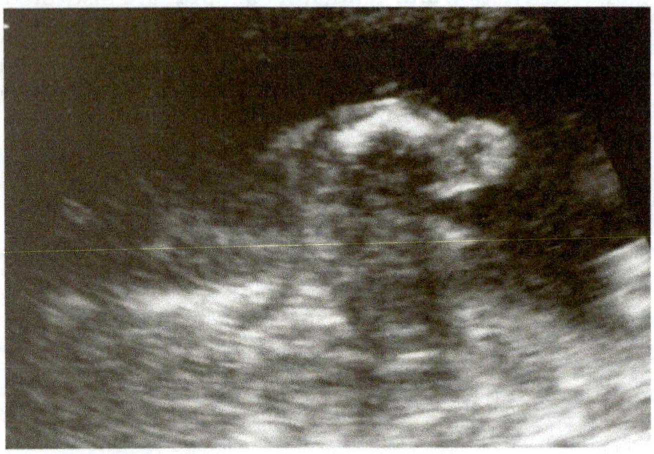

**FIGURE 8.4A** Campomelic dysplasia with shortened bowed femur length.

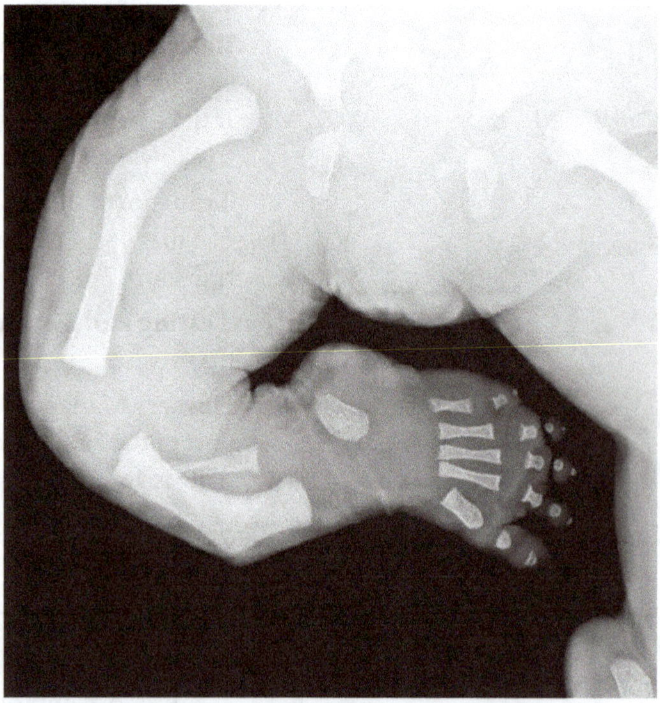

**FIGURE 8.4B** X-ray of fetus with campomelic dysplasia. Note the bowed femur and tibia.

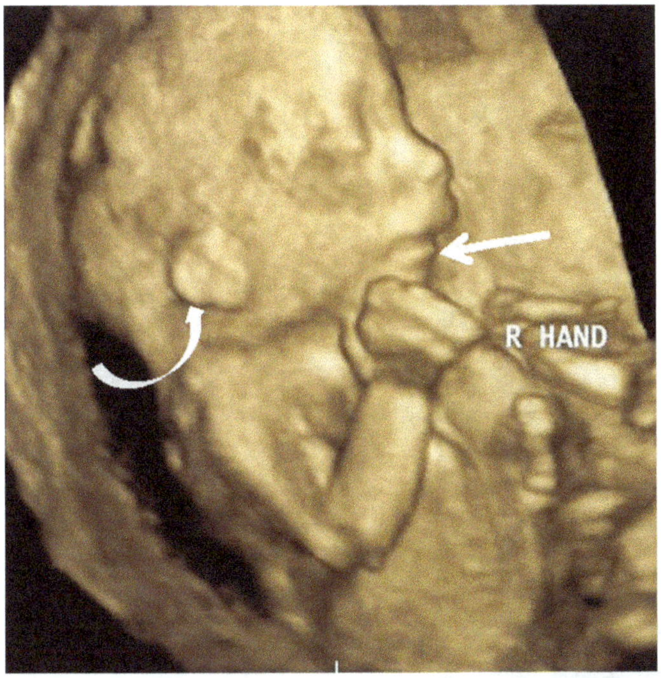


FIGURE 8.4C Three-dimensional ultrasound of a fetus with campomelic dysplasia illustrating micrognathia (straight arrow) and low-set ear (curved arrow).

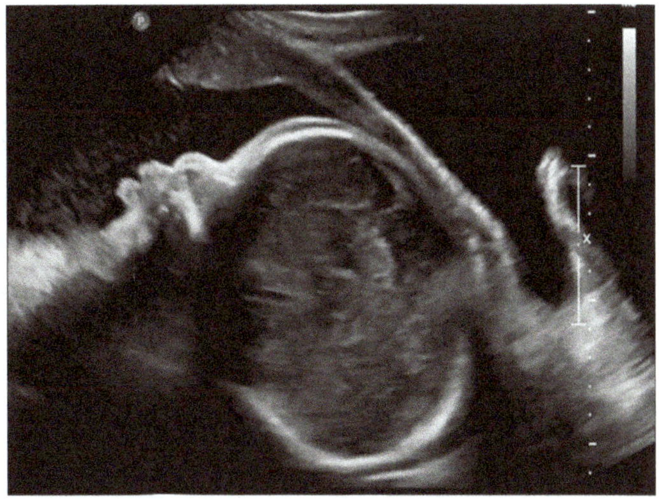

FIGURE 8.4D Campomelic dysplasia with protuberant forehead.

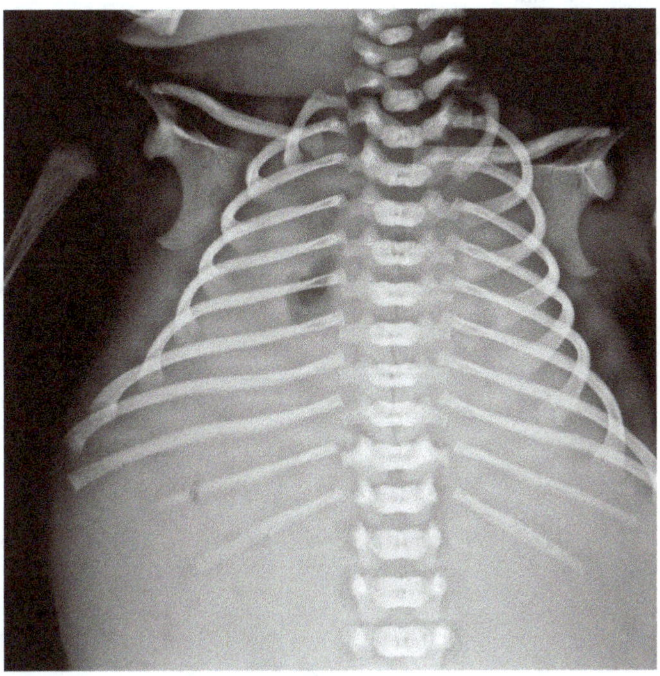

FIGURE 8.4E Campomelic dysplasia with bell-shaped chest and 11 pairs of ribs.

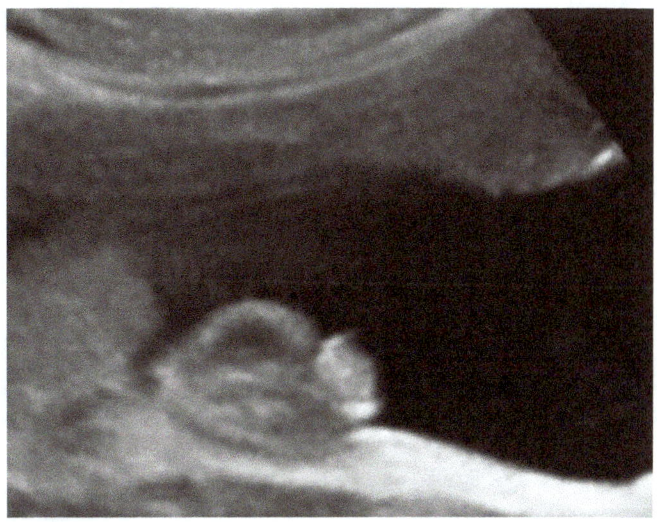

FIGURE 8.4F Campomelic dysplasia illustrating ambiguous genitalia.

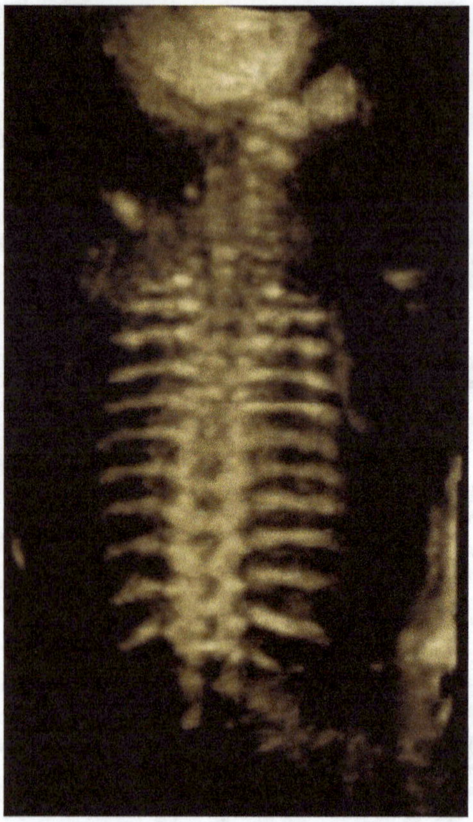

**FIGURE 8.4G** Three-dimensional skeletal mode of fetal ribs in campomelic dysplasia.

# 8.5 CLUB- AND ROCKER-BOTTOM FEET

## EPIDEMIOLOGY/GENETICS

**Definition** Clubfoot is characterized by abnormal bone formation in the foot. There are four variations of clubfoot, including talipes varus, talipes valgus, talipes equinus, and talipes calcaneus. In talipes varus, the most common form of clubfoot, the foot generally turns inward. In talipes valgus, the foot rotates outward. In talipes equinus, the foot points downward. In talipes calcaneus, the foot points upward, with the heel pointing down.

A rocker-bottom foot is the phenotypic description of a foot characterized by dorsiflexion of the forefoot, equinus of the heel, and a convex sole.

**Epidemiology** Clubfoot occurs with a frequency of 1 to 3 in 1000 live births (M2:F1), making it the most common musculoskeletal abnormality. The frequency of rocker-bottom feet is unknown, but it is much less common.

**Embryology** Clubfoot can occur as an isolated abnormality or as part of more than 200 chromosomal, genetic, or sporadic multiple-malformation syndromes. The incidence of associated abnormalities has been reported to be between 24% and 50%. It is frequently secondary to lower extremity paralysis from a neural tube defect. There are also extrinsic causes of clubfoot, such as oligohydramnios, uterine cavity abnormality (leiomyomas), and amniotic bands. Rocker-bottom feet have been described in association with more than 30 chromosomal, genetic, or sporadic multiple-malformation syndromes, especially trisomy 18. Other more common causes of rocker-bottom feet are arthrogryposis syndromes and the multiple pterygium syndrome.

**Inheritance Patterns** Inheritance is dependent on the cause of the foot abnormalities.

**Teratogens** None are reported.

**Prognosis** Prognosis is dependent on the cause of the foot abnormalities. The outcome of an isolated clubfoot is excellent.

## SONOGRAPHY

### FINDINGS: CLUBFEET

- Tibia and fibula visualized with the lateral aspect of the foot.
- The foot is flexed or extended and fixed in position.
  - Recheck the foot on a second scan to ensure it is not positioned to give the appearance of a clubfoot.
- When a clubfoot is detected, the fetus should be evaluated for other congenital anomalies/syndromes. In many cases of suspected isolated clubfoot, associated anomalies may be undetected prenatally.

### FINDINGS: ROCKER-BOTTOM FEET

- These are characterized by prominent calcaneus (heel) and a convex, rounded bottom of the foot.
- Well-defined criteria are not established.
  - "Subjective" impression
- Essentially, they are always in association with other abnormalities.

## PREGNANCY MANAGEMENT

**Investigations and Consultations Required** Because these defects are frequently part of a syndrome, attention should be directed toward other ultrasound findings. A fetal echocardiogram should be performed, as cardiac defects are associated with a number of the possible etiologic conditions. Fetal karyotype and microarray should be done, especially if other malformations are detected. Prenatal consultations should be obtained based on associated anomalies detected, the presumptive diagnosis, and the need for neonatal medical or surgical therapy. For most cases of isolated clubfoot, orthopedic services alone are sufficient, but a prenatal consultation is useful in preparing the parents for postnatal therapy.

**Fetal Intervention** None is indicated.

**Monitoring** Ultrasonographic examinations should be performed periodically throughout the pregnancy to reassess the findings and to assess movement, limb development, and the presence of other abnormalities that may have been missed on earlier examinations. Follow-up of apparently isolated clubfoot, or clubfeet, is particularly helpful to confirm this diagnosis, as it may be overdiagnosed due to fetal position.

**Pregnancy Termination Issues** Unless a clear diagnosis has been established prenatally, the method of termination should provide an intact fetus for a complete morphologic and radiologic examination.

**Delivery** If a multiple-malformation syndrome is suspected, delivery and neonatal management at a tertiary center are required. In cases of isolated clubfoot/clubfeet, delivery can be at a community hospital.

## NEONATOLOGY

**Resuscitation** Infants with clubfeet as an isolated anomaly generally breathe spontaneously and do not require resuscitation.

**Transport** Infants with an isolated clubfoot/clubfeet or rocker-bottom feet do not require transfer to a tertiary center in the immediate newborn period.

**Testing and confirmation** The diagnosis of neonatal clubfoot is made on clinical examination, with uncorrectable hindfoot equinus and rigid forefoot adductus. The entire foot is internally rotated relative to the tibia. Radiographs of clubfeet in the neonatal period are less helpful because the bones are largely nonossified. The physical findings in rocker-bottom feet are more subtle. The arch of the foot is "flat." In a true vertical talus, the foot is rigid, not flexible.

Radiographic confirmation of the vertical talus is required to confirm the diagnosis. In a true vertical talus, stress plantar flexion lateral views of the foot show that the first metatarsal never lies in line with the long axis of the talus. Other causes of flat foot should be considered in the preoperative assessment, including tarsal coalition, flexible flat foot, and benign calcaneovalgus flat foot (from intrauterine molding).

**Nursery Management** Referral, as an outpatient, to a tertiary center with pediatric orthopedics is indicated in isolated cases of clubfeet or rocker-bottom feet. Intervention is not required prior to discharge from the nursery.

## SURGERY

**Preoperative Assessment** See the previous Testing and Confirmation section.

**Operative Indications** Nearly every foot with vertical talus will require surgery to obtain a plantigrade, shoe-able foot. Treatment for clubfoot always begins with serial casting. Idiopathic cases may require only tenotomy of the Achilles tendon, but syndromic cases often require extensive posteromedial surgical release.

**Types of Procedures** The initial treatment for clubfoot or vertical talus is serial casting. This helps to stretch the contracted soft tissues in preparation for surgery. The optimal age for surgery is 6 to 12 months. For both disorders, surgery consists of tendon lengthenings combined with ligament releases. This allows the bones to be repositioned into normal alignment. Usually, small, temporary steel pins are inserted to hold the alignment for the first 6 weeks after surgery. Casts are worn for 6 to 12 weeks after surgery. In more severe cases, follow-up bracing is used to prevent recurrence, particularly in neurogenic and severe cases associated with syndromes. For idiopathic clubfoot, the Ponseti method is commonly performed. This method uses serial casting, percutaneous Achilles tenotomy, and prolonged splinting with a foot abduction orthosis.

**Surgical Results/Prognosis** For most idiopathic cases, the results of surgery are a nearly normal foot. Recurrence after surgery is not unusual, especially in neurogenic cases.

### SUGGESTED READINGS

1. Bronshtein M, Zimmer EZ: Transvaginal ultrasound diagnosis of fetal club feet at 13 weeks, menstrual age. J Clin Ultrasound 1989; 17:518-520.
2. Carroll SCM, Lockyer H, Andrews H: Outcome of fetal talipes following in utero sonographic diagnosis. Ultrasound Obstet Gynecol 2001; 18:437-441.
3. Dobbs MB, Gurnett CA: Update on clubfoot: etiology and treatment. Clin Orthop Relat Res 2009; 467:1146-1153.
4. Hartge DR, Gaertner S, Weichart J: Prenatal detection and postnatal outcome of congenital talipes equinovarus in 106 fetuses. Arch Gynecol Obstet 2012; 286:831-842.
5. Malone F, Marion T, Bianchi DW, et al: Isolated clubfoot diagnosed prenatally: is karyotyping indicated? Obstet Gynecol 2000; 95:437-440.

6. Offerdal K, Jebons N, Blaas HGK, Eik-Nes SH: Prenatal ultrasound detection of talipes equinovarus in a non-selected population of 49,314 deliveries in Norway. Ultrasound Obstet Gynecol 2007; 30:838-844.
7. Paley D, Herzenberg JE: Applications of external fixation to foot and ankle reconstruction. In: Myerson MS, ed. Foot and Ankle Disorders. Philadelphia: Saunders; 1999: 1135-1188.
8. Ponseti IV: Clubfoot management. J Pediatr Orthop 2000; 20(6):699-700.
9. Rijhsinghani A, Yankowitz J, Kanis AB, et al: Antenatal sonographic diagnosis of club foot with particular attention to the implications and outcomes of isolated club foot. Ultrasound Obstet Gynecol 1998; 11:103-106.
10. Tillett RL, Fisk NM, Murphy D, Hunt DM: Clinical outcome of congenital talipes equinovarus diagnosed antenatally by ultrasound. J Bone Joint Surg Br 2000; 82:976-980.
11. Woodrow N, Tran T, Umstad M, et al: Mid-trimester ultrasound diagnosis of isolated talipes equinovarus: accuracy and outcome for infants. Aust NZ J Obstet Gynaecol 1998; 38:301-305.

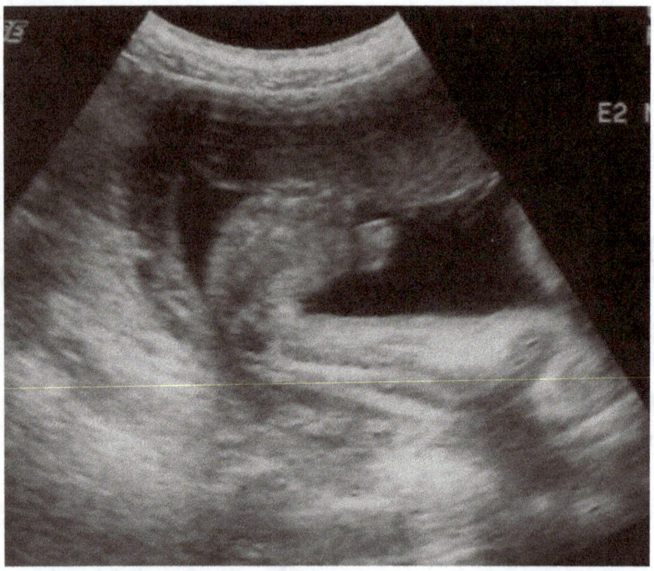


**FIGURE 8.5A** Clubfoot.

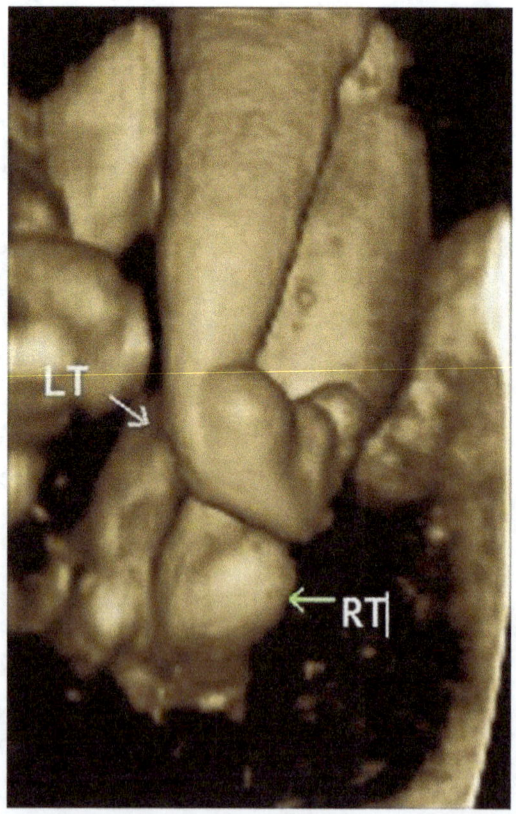


**FIGURE 8.5B** Three-dimensional views of left (LT) and right (RT) clubfeet.

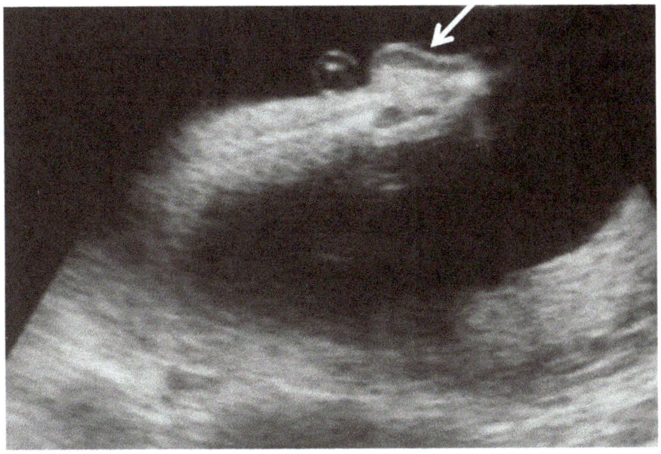

**FIGURE 8.5C** Rocker-bottom foot (arrow) in fetus with arthrogryposis.

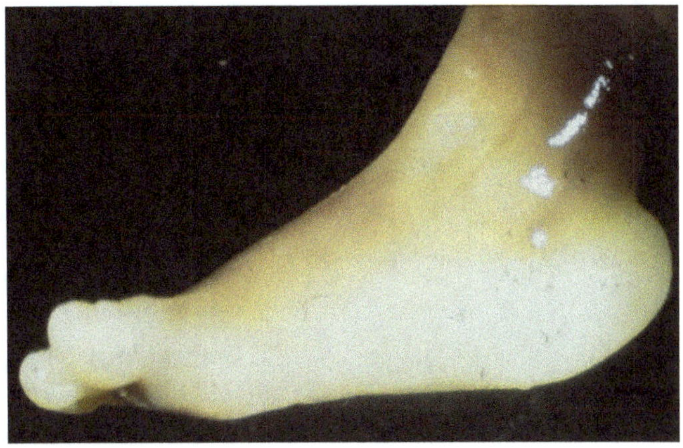

**FIGURE 8.5D** Fetus with rocker-bottom foot.

# 8.6 DIASTROPHIC DYSPLASIA

## EPIDEMIOLOGY/GENETICS

**Definition** Diastrophic dysplasia is a short-limbed skeletal dysplasia characterized by clubfeet, ear swelling, and progressive joint and spine deformity.

**Epidemiology** Diastrophic dysplasia is very rare (M1:F1).

**Embryology** Diastrophic dysplasia is characterized by clubfeet, an abducted "hitchhiker" thumb, hypertrophied auricular cartilage, and cleft palate. The great toes also are abducted. Micrognathia and laryngeotracheal stenosis are occasionally present. The gene for diastrophic dysplasia has been cloned and is called the diastrophic dysplasia sulfate transporter (*DTDST*) gene and is located on chromosome 5q31-34. Consultation with a geneticist should be sought to determine the status of antenatal DNA mutation analysis.

**Inheritance Patterns** Inheritance is autosomal recessive.

**Teratogens** None are known.

**Prognosis** Respiratory obstruction due to either laryngeal stenosis or the Pierre Robin sequence (micrognathia and glossoptosis with or without a cleft palate) can result in a mortality rate of up to 25% in early infancy. For survivors, most will have a normal life span and intellectual development. Adult height is generally less than 4 feet, with severe orthopedic abnormalities and neurologic complications from spine abnormalities.

## SONOGRAPHY

### FREQUENT FINDINGS

- Micromelia
- Short hands/fingers
- Hitchhiker thumb
- Ulnar deviation of the hands
- Extension limitation at the elbows and knees
- Cleft palate (50%)
- Clubfeet
- Kyphoscoliosis
- "Buddha" position of lower limbs
- Thickened nuchal translucency in the first trimester

### LESS FREQUENT

- Micrognathia
- Congenital heart defects
- Polyhydramnios

### KEY FINDINGS/PITFALLS

- Biometry and specific morphologic criteria permit detection at the end of the first trimester.
- Fetuses with a severe skeletal dysplasia have a femur length greater than 5 mm below 2 SD.
  - With diastrophic dysplasia, femur length is 40% to 80% of the mean for gestational age.
- Three-dimensional ultrasound can be utilized to help confirm the diagnosis.

## PREGNANCY MANAGEMENT

**Investigations and Consultations Required** The gene for diastrophic dysplasia has been identified, and prenatal diagnosis is available for at-risk families. Fetal echocardiography should be performed; the presence of a congenital heart defect suggests a type of skeletal dysplasia other than diastrophic dysplasia. A neonatology consultation should be obtained to assist in planning perinatal management.

**Monitoring** Preterm labor secondary to polyhydramnios may occur. Therefore, obstetric care should be coordinated by a perinatologist. Despite the severity of the disorder, it is not usually lethal, and severe prematurity will only further complicate management.

**Pregnancy Course** Polyhydramnios is an occasional complication of this skeletal dysplasia and may result in preterm labor. As is the case for all skeletal dysplasias, the lethal forms should be excluded before an obstetric management plan is established.

**Pregnancy Termination Issues** An intact fetus must be delivered and the postmortem examination, including radiologic, morphologic, biochemical, and molecular studies, must be performed by individuals with extensive experience in skeletal dysplasias. Tissue should be obtained for DNA analysis.

**Delivery** Respiratory complications are common, and intubation may be complicated because of micrognathia. Delivery should occur in a tertiary center with the capabilities to manage these complications.

## NEONATOLOGY

**Resuscitation** Initiation of resuscitation in live-born infants is appropriate when the prognosis is in doubt.

**Testing and Confirmation** Confirmation of the diagnosis and determining the prognosis are the first priorities. Careful physical examination, skeletal radiographs, echocardiography, and genetic testing are useful in the evaluation.

**Nursery Management** Respiratory insufficiency, secondary to laryngeal obstruction, appears to be the mode of death in the lethal variant. Response to ventilatory support and a mechanical airway is unknown. The long-term treatment plan for survivors is directed toward orthopedic correction of the clubfeet and kyphoscoliosis, should the latter develop.

## SUGGESTED READINGS


1. Canto MJ, Buixeda M, Palau J, Ojeda F: Early ultrasonographic diagnosis of diastrophic dysplasia at 12 weeks of gestation in a fetus without previous family history. Prenat Diagn 2007; 27:976-978.
2. Chitty LS, Altmann DG: Chart of fetal size: limb bones. Br J Obstet Gynaecol 2002; 109:919-929.
3. Gembruch U, Niesen M, Kehrberg H, Hansmann M: Diastrophic dysplasia: a specific prenatal diagnosis by ultrasound. Prenat Diagn 1988; 8:539-545.
4. Goncalves L, Jeanty P: Fetal biometry of skeletal dysplasia: a multicenter study. J Ultrasound Med 1994; 13:977-985.
5. Gustavson K-H, Holmgren G, Jagell S, Jorulf H: Lethal and non-lethal diastrophic dysplasia. A study of 14 Swedish cases. Clin Genetics 1985; 28:321-334.
6. Kurtz AB, Needleman L, Wapner RJ, et al: Usefulness of a short femur in the in utero detection of skeletal dysplasias. Radiology 1990; 177:197-200.
7. Ngo C, Viot G, Aubry MC, et al: First- trimester ultrasound diagnosis of skeletal dysplasia associated with increased nuchal translucency thickness. Ultrasound Obstet Gynecol 2007; 30:221-226.
8. Sepulveda W, Sepulveda-Swatson E, Sanchez J: Diastrophic dysplasia: prenatal three-dimensional ultrasound findings. Ultrasound Obstet Gynecol 2004; 23:312-314.
9. Severi FM, Bocchi C, Sanseverino F, Petraglia F: Prenatal ultrasonographic diagnosis of diastrophic dysplasia at 13 weeks of gestation. J Matern-Neonat Med 2003; 13:282-284.
10. Tongsong T, Wenapirak C, Sirichotiyakul S, Chanpropaph P: Prenatal sonographic diagnosis of diastrophic dwarfism. J Clin Ultasound 2002; 30:103-105.
11. Wax JR, Carpenter M, Smith W, et al: Second-trimester sonographic diagnosis of diastrophic dysplasia. J Ultrasound Med 2003; 22:805-808.

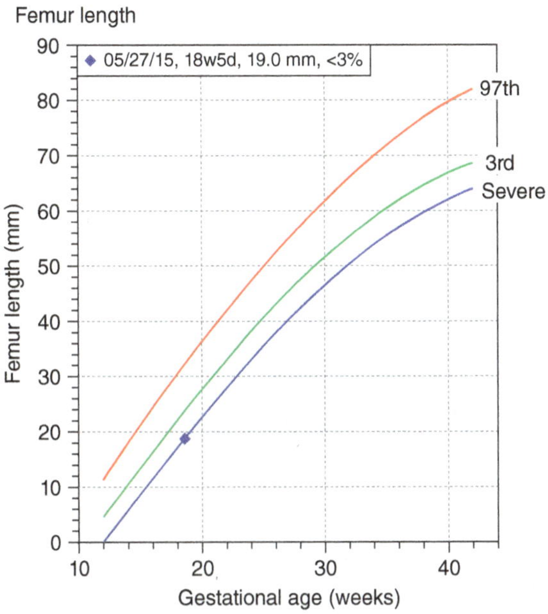


**FIGURE 8.6A** Graph of femur length in a fetus with diastrophic dysplasia.

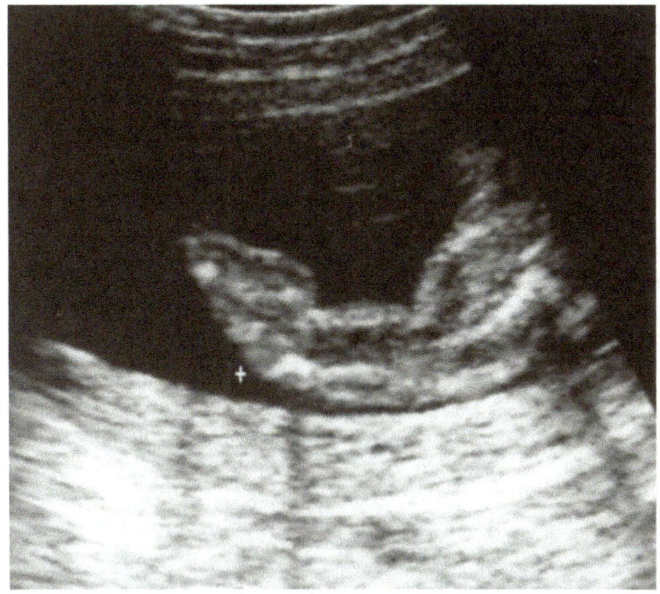

**FIGURE 8.6B** Micromelia of lower extremity.

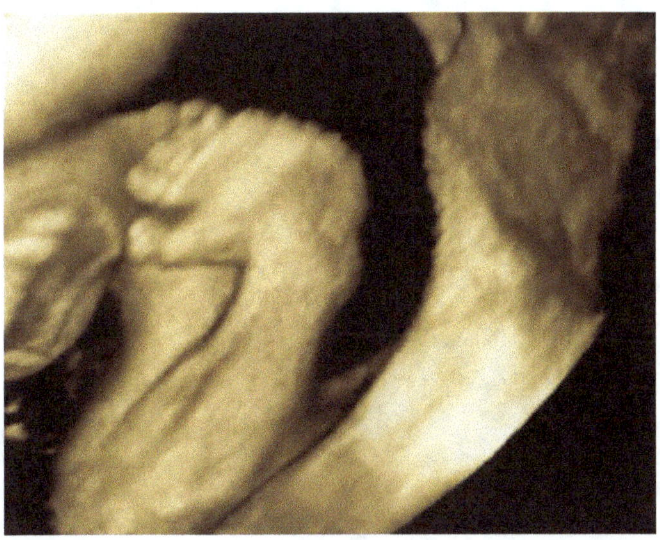

**FIGURE 8.6C** Three-dimensional ultrasound illustrating clubfoot.

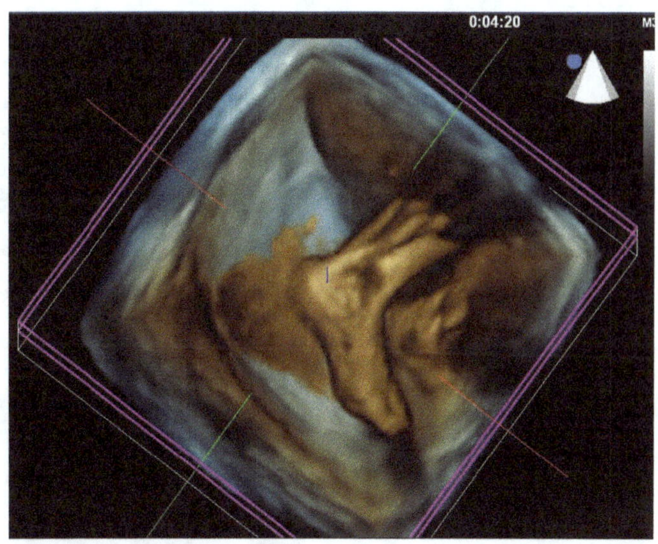


**FIGURE 8.6D** Three-dimensional ultrasound illustrating the normal foot orientation.

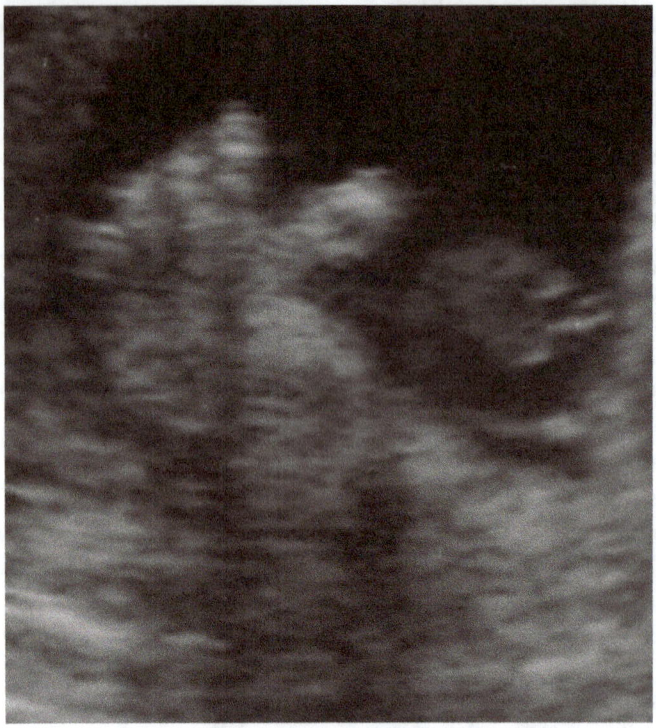

**FIGURE 8.6E** "Hitchhiker" big toe in diastrophic dysplasia.

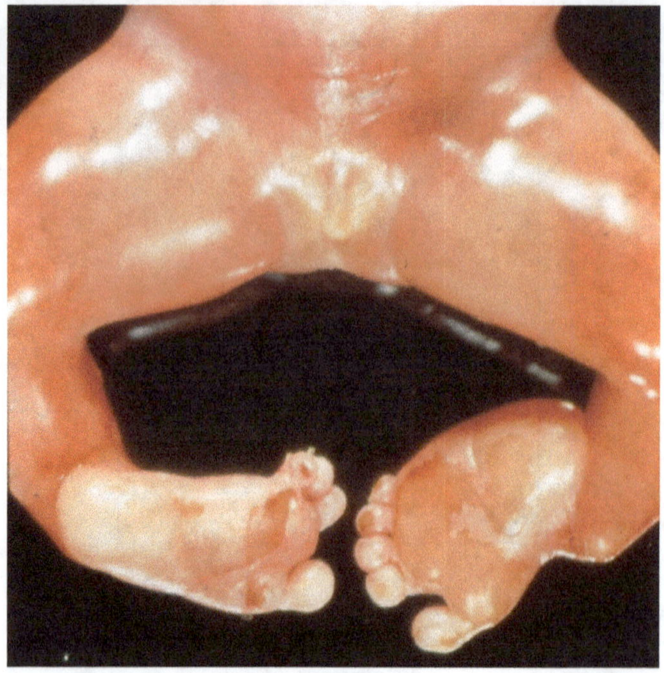

**FIGURE 8.6F** Buddha position of lower extremities in a second-trimester pathologic specimen with diastrophic dysplasia.

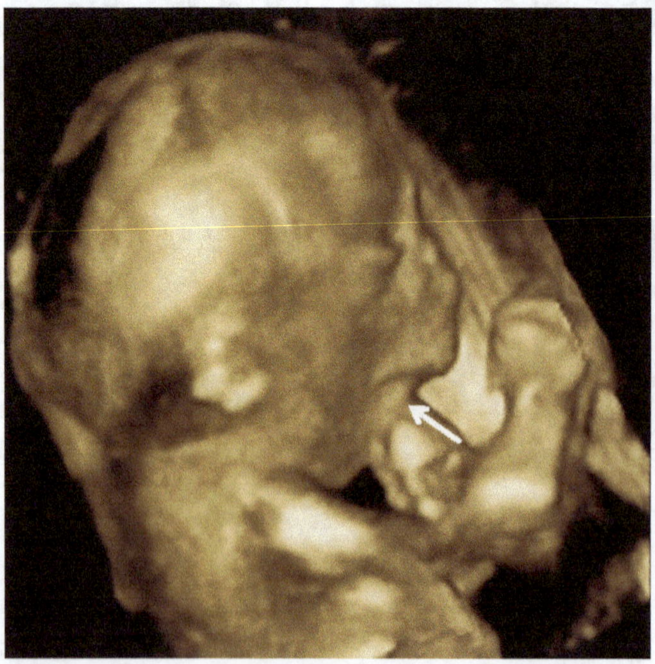

**FIGURE 8.6G** Three-dimensional ultrasound of micrognathia in a fetus with diastrophic dysplasia.

# 8.7 FOCAL FEMORAL HYPOPLASIA

## EPIDEMIOLOGY/GENETICS

**Definition** Focal femoral hypoplasia (FFH) is characterized by shortening or deformity of the femur.

**Epidemiology** Occurrence is 1 to 2 per 100,00 live births (M1: F1).

**Embryology** Focal femoral hypoplasia is a physical finding that may be seen in more than 25 genetic and sporadic multiple-malformation syndromes, including a number of skeletal dysplasias. Congenital hypoplasia of the femur is a part of four malformation syndromes that account for most cases: (a) proximal focal femoral deficiency, (b) femur/fibula/ulnar hypoplasia, (c) femoral hypoplasia/unusual facial syndrome, and (d) limb/pelvis-hypoplasia/aplasia syndrome. There are often associated abnormalities of the ipsilateral tibia and fibula.

**Inheritance Patterns** Inheritance is dependent on diagnosis, but includes dominant and recessive genetic syndromes. Most cases are sporadic.

**Teratogens** Maternal diabetes, thalidomide, and congenital viral infections are teratogenic.

**Prognosis** Prognosis is dependent on the cause and can range from lethal skeletal dysplasias (rare) to disorders with only mild orthopedic abnormalities.

## SONOGRAPHY

### FREQUENT FINDINGS

- Unilateral or bilateral femoral shortening
- Bowing of femur

### LESS FREQUENT

- Absence or partial absence of other long bones
- Bowing of the tibia may occur if the fibula is absent
- Acetubulum affected in the severe form
- Restrictive range of motion
- Lateral rotation of thigh

### KEY FINDINGS/PITFALLS

- A normal fetus with only one femur less than the fifth centile is diagnostic of focal femoral deficiency.
- The ratio of the short limb to the normal limb remains constant throughout gestation.
- Limb length at term or at skeletal maturity can be determined by multiplying the current femur length by a predetermined gestational age multiplier.

- Three-dimensional imaging illustrates discrepancy in limb length; skeletal mode evaluates the acetabulum.
- Four-dimensional imaging evaluates range of motion.

### DIFFERENTIAL DIAGNOSIS

- Femur-fibula-ulna complex consists of bilateral femoral hypoplasia and partial or complete absence of the fibula and ulna. There may be partial or complete absence of the arm.
- The femoral hypoplasia/unusual facies syndrome consists of cleft palate, micrognathia, short or absent femurs, and vertebral and genitourinary malformations such as ambiguous genitalia.

## PREGNANCY MANAGEMENT

**Investigations and Consultations Required** As this diagnosis may be a diagnosis of exclusion, other syndromes or clinical scenarios with a shortened femur should be sought. Fetal echocardiography should be performed, as the presence of a congenital heart defect would prompt a reassessment of the diagnosis of FFH. Karyotyping or microarray should be considered if other anomalies are detected. An orthopedic surgeon should meet with the family to discuss the prognosis for the child and initiate planning for postnatal management.

**Monitoring** Serial ultrasound examinations are useful to confirm that the findings are limited to the femur and not part of generalized limb shortening as would be found in either intrauterine growth restriction or a skeletal dysplasia syndrome. The absence of other abnormalities can also be reassessed. Because the severity of the shortening can be predicted by the rate of growth of the femur, serial ultrasonographic studies may be worthwhile for surgical preparation.

**Pregnancy Course** No specific obstetric complications are associated with FFH.

**Pregnancy Termination Issues** An intact fetus should be delivered so that the diagnosis can be confirmed. There would be no increased risk for recurrence if FFH is the only finding.

**Delivery** There should be no perinatal complications associated with FFH that would require special management in a tertiary center unless there are associated malformations requiring evaluation and management.

## NEONATOLOGY

**Resuscitation** No specific resuscitation measures are required.

**Transport** Referral in the immediate neonatal period is not necessary unless there are associated malformations requiring evaluation and management.

**Testing and Confirmation** The diagnostic evaluation should include careful physical examination, skeletal radiographs, and pediatric orthopedic consultation. These may be obtained through an outpatient referral.

## SURGERY

**Preoperative Assessment** The predicted leg length discrepancy is estimated by measuring the length of the long and short legs following birth and expressing the difference as a percentage of the longer. The percentage of shortening tends to remain constant, whereas the absolute discrepancy increases with age. Radiographs define both length and angular deformities. Next, determine the stability of the hip and knee and look for contractures.

**Operative Indications** All children with this diagnosis will require some form of surgery. Problems to be addressed may include the following: femoral shortening, tibial shortening, unstable knee, varus hip, acetabular insufficiency, and external rotation deformity. Usually, the necessary corrective surgeries are staged over a series of years. The most important decision to make is whether to lengthen or to amputate. Traditional thinking recommends amputation and prosthetic rehabilitation. The indications for leg lengthening are evolving, but the tendency is to recommend lengthening for predicted discrepancies of up to 20 cm and even more. For mild cases, epiphysiodesis (growth arrest) of the normal side can easily equalize length.

**Types of Procedures** The management controversy for this diagnosis has been reconstruction with lengthening and deformity correction versus Symes amputation with above-knee prosthetic fitting. A modification of amputation has been described in which the joint is removed and the foot and ankle rotated 180 degrees, thus becoming a "knee" and allowing below-knee prosthetic fitting. Recently, it has been demonstrated that femoral lengthening can be performed as early as 2-4 years of age.

**Surgical Results/Prognosis** The main risk of lengthening is the loss of knee motion. When a hip and knee are present, the results of lengthening are potentially excellent. It is possible, in most children, to equalize the leg length, maintain the function of the knee and hip, and restore the patient to a normal gait pattern. Amputation surgery is reliable and reduces the need for additional surgical procedures. Long-term outcome studies are needed to determine the relative indications for amputation versus lengthening.

### SUGGESTED READINGS

1. Camer G, Dodero D, Parodi M, et al: Anatenatal ultrasongraphic diagnosis of a proximal femoral focal deficiency. J Clin Ultrasound 1993; 21:475-479.
2. Filly AL, Robnett-Filly B, Filly RA: Syndromes with focal femoral deficiency. Strengths and weaknesses of prenatal sonography. J Ultrasound Med 2004; 23:1511-1516.

3. Florio I, Wisser J, Huch R, Huch A: Prenatal ultrasound diagnosis of a femur-fibula-ulna complex during the first half of pregnancy. Fetal Diagn Ther 1999; 14:310-312.
4. Goncalves LF, De Luca GR, Vitorello DA, et al: Prenatal diagnosis of bilateral proximal femoral hypoplasia. Ultrasound Obstet Gynecol 1996; 8:127-139.
5. Mailath-Pokorny M, Timor-Tritsch IE, Monteagudo A, et al: Prenatal diagnosis of unilateral proximal femoral focal deficiency at 19 weeks' gestation: case report and review of the literature. Ultrasound Obstet Gynecol 2011; 38:594-597.
6. Otera Y, Morokuma S, Yumoto Y, et al: Prenatal three-dimensional images of proximal focal femoral deficiency produced by helical computed tomography. Fetal Diagn Ther 2009; 25:349-353.
7. Paley J, Gelman A, Paley D, Herzenberg J: The prenatal multiplier method for prediction of limb length discrepancy. Prenat Diagn 2005; 25:435-438.
8. Radler C, Myers AK, Hunter RJ, et al: Prenatal diagnosis of congenital femoral deficiency and fibular hemimelia. Prenat Diagn 2014; 34:940-945.
9. Sabharwal S, Paley D, Bhave A, Herzenberg JE: Growth patterns after lengthening of congenitally short lower limbs in young children. J Pediatr Orthop 2000; 20:137-145.


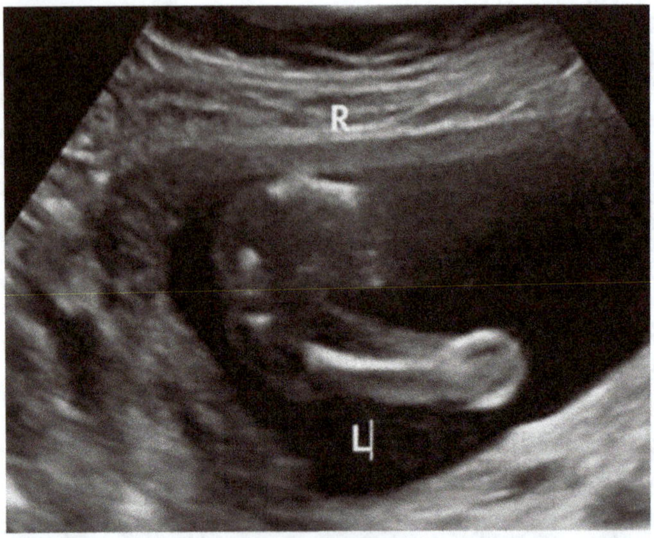


**FIGURE 8.7A** Shortened right femur (R) and normal left femur (L) in focal femoral hypoplasia.

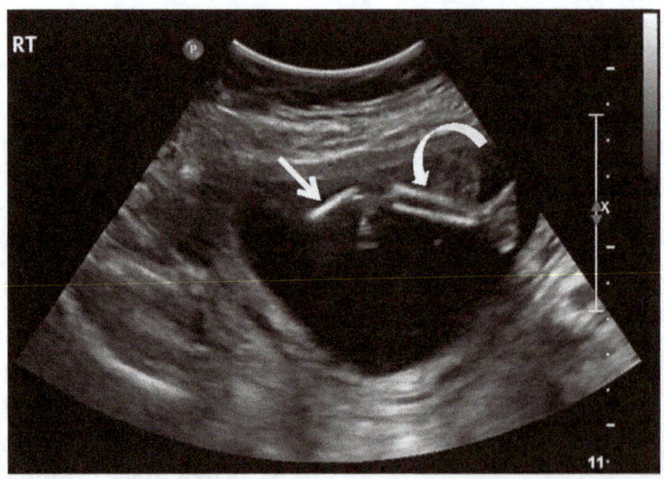


**FIGURE 8.7B** Short femur (straight arrow) with normal tibia/fibula (curved arrow).

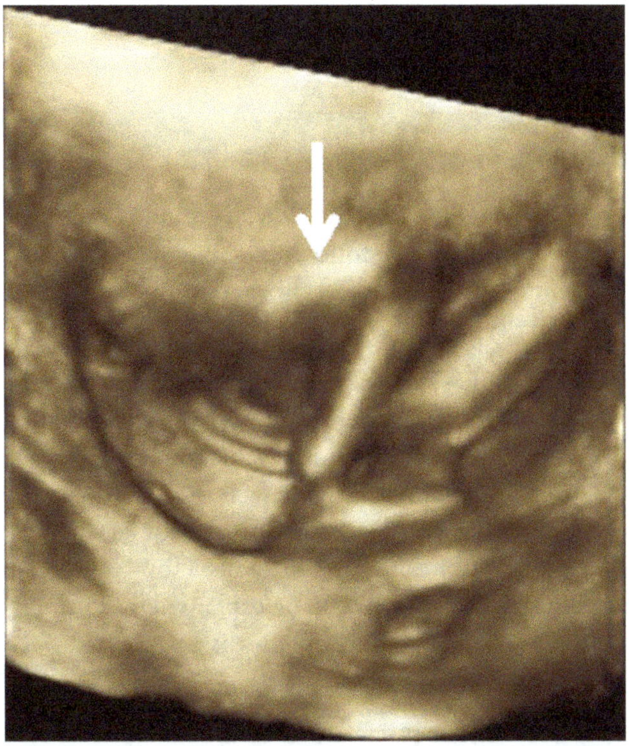

**FIGURE 8.7C** Three-dimensional ultrasound of short femur (arrow).

# 8.8 LIMB–BODY WALL COMPLEX

## EPIDEMIOLOGY/GENETICS

**Definition** Limb–body wall complex is generally defined as consisting of two of the three following abnormalities: (1) exencephaly/encephalocele with facial clefts; (2) thoraco- or abdominoschisis; and (3) limb defects (any type).

**Epidemiology** Birth prevalence is 0.235 to 3.3 per 10,000.

**Embryology** There are two phenotypes, likely reflecting two different etiologies: (1) The limb–body wall complex likely is due to early vascular disruption; it includes craniofacial defects. (2) The body stalk complex results from defective folding of the embryonic disk; it has no craniofacial defects, but there are placental abdominal adhesions. However, recently it has been suggested that all the malformations can be explained by a primary defect, or deficiency, of the ectoderm of the embryonic disk.

**Inheritance Patterns** Inheritance is sporadic.

**Teratogens** None are known.

**Prognosis** This condition is lethal in those cases with the full manifestation of the limb—body wall complex. Milder forms of what may be termed amniotic band syndrome, with gastroschisis and absent limb, for example, may be part of the limb—body wall complex but have a better prognosis.

## SONOGRAPHY

### FINDINGS

**Characteristic Triad**

- Limb anomalies
  - Abnormal position
  - Absent limb
  - Limb hypoplasia
  - Oligodactyly
- Abdominal wall defect
  - The abdominal wall defect is characteristically lateral rather than centrally located.
  - Liver, small bowel, kidneys, or bladder are exteriorized.
    - Extruded organs attached to the placenta or uterine wall
    - Absent diaphragm
    - Bowel atresia
- Craniofacial defects
  - Cranioplacental attachment
  - Anencephaly
  - Encephalocele

**Frequent Findings**

- Myelomeningocele
- Kyphoscoliosis
- Pulmonary hypoplasia
- Short, straight umbilical cord
- Single umbilical artery
- First-trimester thickened nuchal translucency

**Less Frequent**

- Primitive cardiac ventricle
- Ectopic cordis
- Common atrium
- Atrial septal defect
- Ventricular septal defect
- Unilateral/bilateral renal agenesis
- Cloaca

### DIFFERENTIAL DIAGNOSIS

- Cloacal exstrophy: A large omphalocele, distorted spine, clubfeet, and meningomyelocele are features of cloacal exstrophy. Partial or complete absence of an extremity is not present with cloacal exstrophy. An absent bladder is a feature of cloacal exstrophy that does not occur with limb–body wall complex.
- Amniotic Band Sequence: This may be one manifestation of the limb–body wall complex and not a separate entity.

## PREGNANCY MANAGEMENT

**Investigations and Consultations Required** No specific antenatal evaluations or consultations are necessary. The pattern and severity of the malformations are inconsistent with common chromosome abnormalities, but chromosomal studies should be considered to exclude chromosome rearrangements if the diagnosis is in doubt.

**Monitoring** Routine prenatal care aimed at maternal comfort and support is appropriate. Follow-up ultrasound examinations are only indicated if the diagnosis is in doubt after the initial examination.

**Pregnancy Course** This condition is always lethal at birth or shortly thereafter. No specific obstetric complications should be expected.

**Pregnancy Termination Issues** To establish a precise diagnosis, a termination technique should be used that allows an intact fetus to be delivered.

**Delivery** There are no special conditions regarding delivery. A diagnosis of limb–body wall complex should be an indication for vaginal delivery only, without fetal monitoring. Despite the short umbilical cord and a high incidence of malpresentation, vaginal delivery is generally possible and is preferred.

## NEONATOLOGY

**Resuscitation** Resuscitation is not indicated because this anomaly is lethal.

**Transport** Transport is not indicated unless the fetus survives delivery and the diagnosis is uncertain.

**Testing and Confirmation** Careful physical examination and sonography are usually all that are required to determine the extent of organ involvement.

**Nursery Management** Supportive care is appropriate until the diagnosis is confirmed and time has been allowed for parental adaptation to the lethal prognosis.

## SUGGESTED READINGS

1. Aquirre-Pascual E, Epelman M, Johnson AM, et al: Prenatal MRI evaluation of limb–body wall complex. Pediatr Radiol 2014; 44:1412-1420.
2. Colpaert C, Bogers J, Hertveldt K, et al: Limb–body wall complex: four new cases illustrating the importance of examining placenta and umbilical cord. Pathol Res Pract 2000; 196:783-790.
3. Hunter AG, Seaver LH, Stevenson RE: Limb–body wall defect. Is there a defensible hypothesis and can it explain all the associated anomalies? Am J Med Genet A. 2011; 155A: 2045-2059.
4. Martinez-Frias ML, Bermejo E, Rodriguez-Pinilla E: Body stalk defects, body wall defects, amniotic bands with and without body wall defects and gastroschisis. Comp Epidemiol Am J Med Genet 2000; 92:13-18.
5. Moerman P, Fryns J-P, Vanderberghe K, Lauweryns JM: Constrictive amniotic bands, amniotic adhesions, and limb–body wall complex: discrete disruption sequences with pathogenetic overlap. Am J Med Genet 1992; 42:470-479.
6. Russo R, D'Armiento M, Angrisani P, Vecchione R: Limb–body wall complex: a critical review and a nosological proposal. Am J Med Genet 1993; 47:893-900.

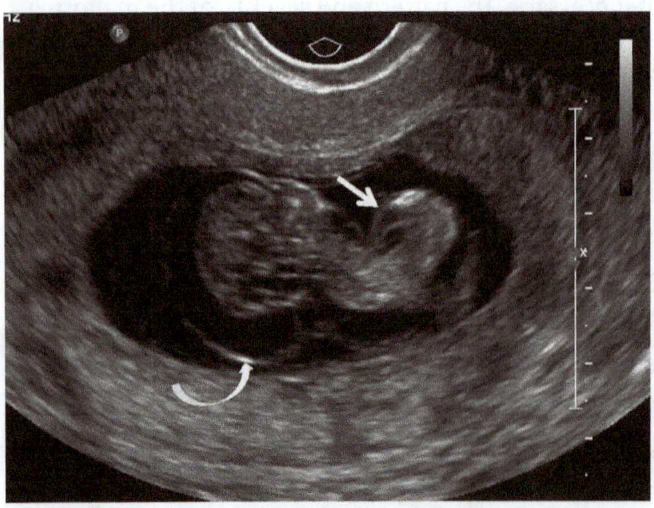

**FIGURE 8.8A** Limb–body wall complex with ectopia cordis (straight arrow) and cystic hygroma (curved arrow).

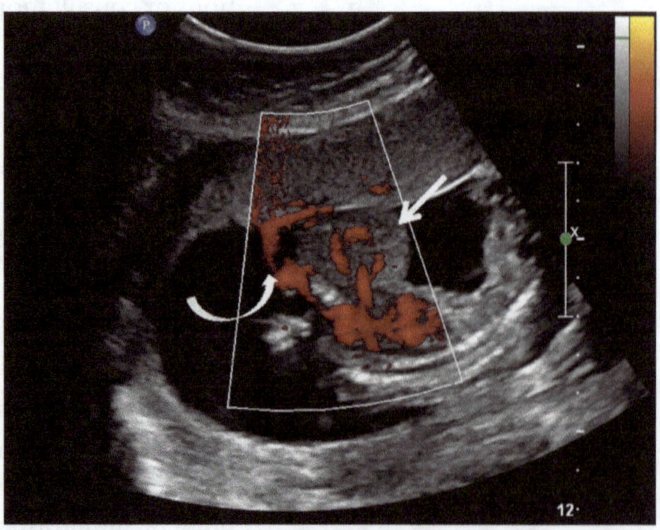

**FIGURE 8.8B** Limb–body wall complex with an abdominal wall defect attached to the placenta (straight arrow) and short umbilical cord (curved arrow).

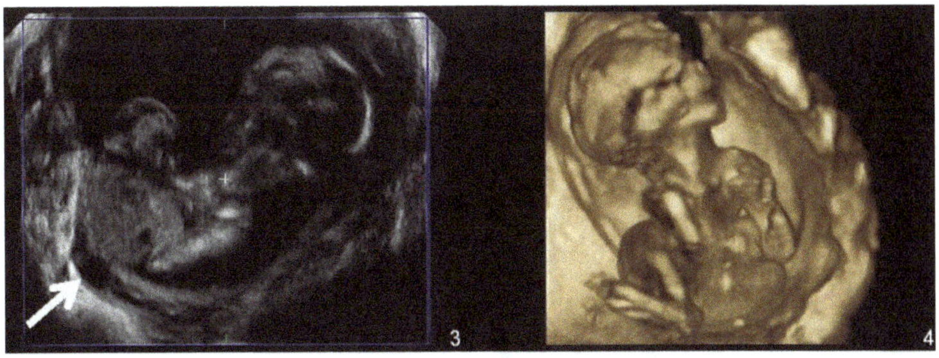


**FIGURE 8.8C** Two- (left) and three-dimensional (right) images of limb–body wall complex attached to uterine wall (arrow).

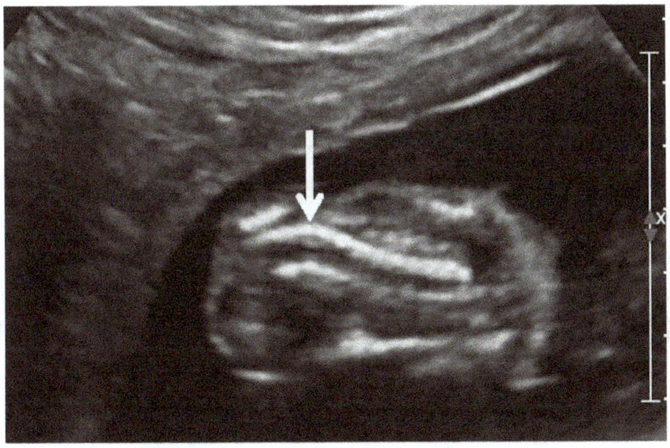

**FIGURE 8.8D** Limb–body wall complex illustrating kyphoscoliosis (arrow).

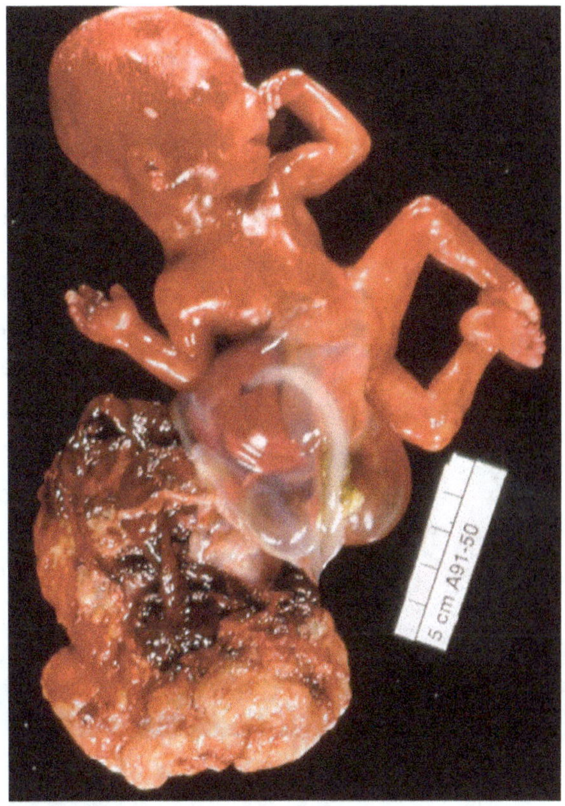


**FIGURE 8.8E** Fetus with an abdominal wall defect attached to the placenta.

# 8.9 MULTIPLE PTERYGIUM SYNDROMES

## EPIDEMIOLOGY/GENETICS

**Definition** The multiple pterygium syndromes are a heterogeneous group of disorders characterized by pterygia, or webbing, across the neck and other joints.

**Epidemiology** Incidence is rare (M1:F1).

**Embryology** Pterygia, or webs that occur across joint spaces, are thought to be the result of limited in utero movement. More than 25 multiple-malformation syndromes have been described with pterygia and have been divided into lethal and nonlethal forms. The lethal forms generally have growth restriction, cystic hygroma, or fetal hydrops.

**Inheritance Patterns** Most nonlethal cases are sporadic, but there is an autosomal dominant form (Escobar syndrome). Lethal cases usually show autosomal recessive inheritance. X-linked recessive families also have been reported. Mutations in the *CHRNG* gene have been identified in approximately 10% of lethal cases and in about 25% of those with Escobar syndrome. Other families have been found to have mutations in the *MYH3* gene. Because of the rapid progress in mapping genes and in the subsequent development of genetic testing, consultation with a medical geneticist or genetic counselor to determine the availability of clinical genetic testing for this disorder (or disorders) is advised.

**Teratogens** None are known.

**Prognosis** Lethal cases usually die in utero from hydrops and in the immediate neonatal period, secondary to pulmonary hypoplasia. Life span and intellectual development in nonlethal cases are generally normal. Ambulation and function are dependent on the severity of the pterygia and the success of the orthopedic correction.

## SONOGRAPHY

### FINDINGS

**Classic Triad**

- Decreased/absent movement
- Cystic hygroma
- Hydrops

**Frequent Findings**

- Polyhydramnios
- Midface hypoplasia
- Micrognathia
- Low-set ears
- Bilateral clubbed hands/clubbed feet

- Flexion deformities across joints
- Pterygium (skin webbing) across joints
- Lack of muscle movement
- Scoliosis
- Short umbilical cord

**Less Frequent**

- Cleft palate
- Cataracts
- Cardiac defects
- Diaphragmatic hernia
- Pulmonary hypoplasia
- Intrauterine growth restriction

**Key Findings/Pitfalls**

- Three-dimensional imaging permits a better spatial recognition of the multiple malformations.

## PREGNANCY MANAGEMENT

**Investigations and Consultations Required** Chromosomal studies should be done, as trisomy 18 may present with a similar clinical picture. Fetal echocardiography should be performed, as cardiac hypoplasia is a frequent feature.

**Monitoring** Standard obstetric care without fetal assessment is appropriate. No attempt to abate preterm labor should be made.

**Pregnancy Course** Polyhydramnios is a common complication and may be severe, resulting in preterm labor or maternal respiratory compromise. Maternal complications are an indication for delivery.

**Pregnancy Termination Issues** Delivery of an intact fetus and neuropathological evaluation are essential to establish a precise diagnosis.

**Delivery** The site of delivery should be one where the staff is comfortable with a noninterventional approach to labor management and newborn resuscitation. Fetal monitoring during labor is not appropriate.

## NEONATOLOGY

**Resuscitation** If a lethal variant is suspected from prenatal diagnosis, a decision for nonintervention at delivery is appropriate with concurrence of the family. There may be difficulty in establishing a reliable airway if jaw mobility is affected.

**Transport** Referral to a tertiary perinatal center in the immediate neonatal period is appropriate for diagnostic evaluation and confirmation of the prognosis. Mechanical respiratory support during transport may be needed for infants with the lethal variant.

**Testing and Confirmation** The diagnostic evaluation should include careful physical examination, genetic consultation, and skeletal radiographs.

**Nursery Management** Mechanical life support, to allow time for diagnostic evaluation and parental adaptation, is appropriate. Death in the lethal variant results from respiratory failure secondary to pulmonary hypoplasia. Therefore, long-term mechanical ventilation is unlikely to be beneficial. The long-term treatment goal for an infant without respiratory failure is to establish joint mobility with physical therapy and soft tissue release surgery.

## SUGGESTED READINGS

1. Anthony J, Mascarenhas L, O'Brien J, et al: Lethal multiple pterygium syndrome—the importance of fetal posture in mid-trimester diagnosis by ultrasound: discussion and case report. Ultrasound Obstet Gynecol 1993; 3:212-216.
2. Barros FS, Júnion EA, Rolo LC, Narduzza LMM: Prenatal diagnosis of lethal multiple pterygium syndrome using two- and three-dimensional ultrasonography. J Clin Imaging Sci 2012; 2:65. doi:10.4103/2156-7514.103055. Epub 2012 Oct 31.
3. Chen M, Chan GSW, Lee DP, Tang MHY: Sonographic features of lethal multiple pterygium syndrome at 14 weeks. Prenat Diagn 2005; 25:475-478.
4. Chong JX, Burrage LC, Beck AE, et al: Autosomal-dominant multiple pterygium syndrome is caused by mutations in MYH3. Am J Hum Genet 2015; 96:841-849.
5. de Die-Smulders CEM, Vonsee HJ, Zandvoort JA, Fryns JP: The lethal multiple pterygium syndrome: Prenatal ultrasonographic and post-mortem findings: a case report. Eur J Obstet Gynecol Reprod Biol 1990; 35:283-289.
6. Froster UG, Stallmach T, Wisser J, et al: Lethal multiple pterygrium syndrome: suggestion for a consistent pathological workup and review of reported cases. Am J Med Genet 1997; 68:82-85.
7. Hertzberg BS, Ktiewer MA, Paulyson-Nunez K: Lethal multiple pterygium syndrome: antenatal ultrasonographic diagnosis. J Ultrasound Med 2000; 19:657-662.
8. Moerman P, Fryns JP, Cornelis A, et al: Pathogenesis of the lethal multiple pterygium syndrome. Am J Med Genet 1990; 35:415-421.
9. Sciarrone A, Verdiglione P, Botta G, et al: Prenatal diagnosis of lethal multiple pteryium syndrome in mid-pregnancy. Ultrasound Obstet Gynecol 1998; 12:218-219.
10. Vogt J, Morgan NJ, Rehal P, et al: CHRNG genotype-phenotype correlations in multiple pterygium syndrome. J Med Genet 2012; 49:21-26.

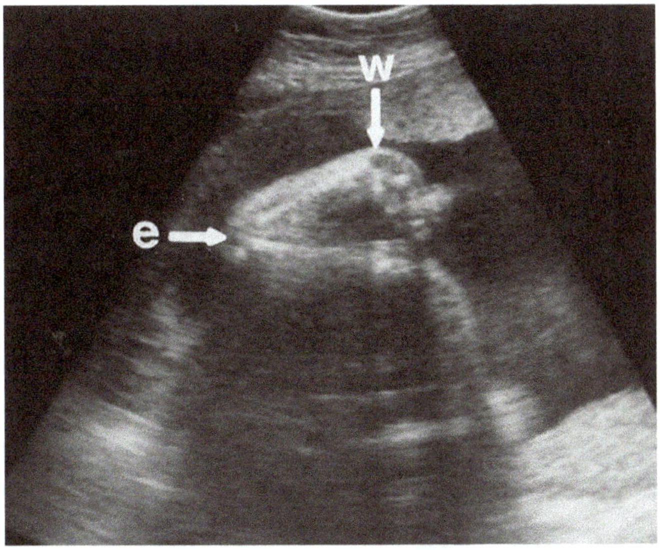


FIGURE 8.9A Multiple pterygium syndrome with flexion deformity at elbow (e) and clubbed hand and wrist (w).

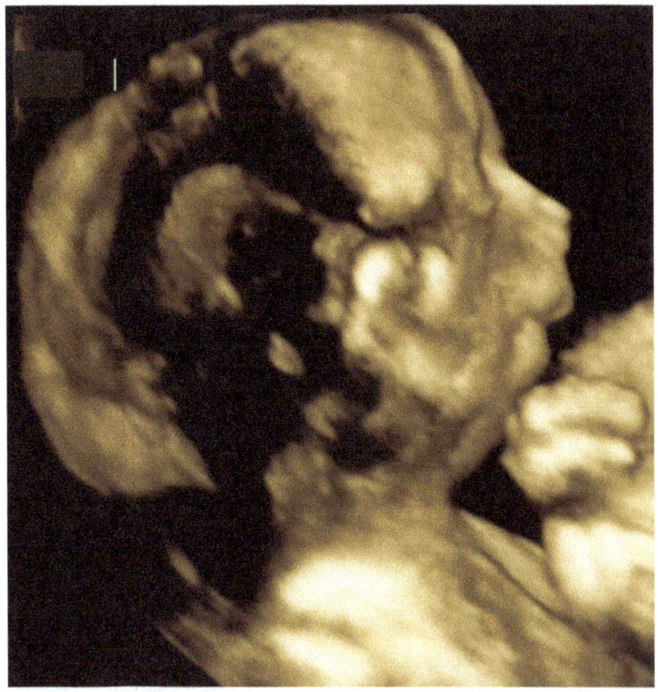

FIGURE 8.9B Micrognathia in fetus with multiple pterygium syndrome.

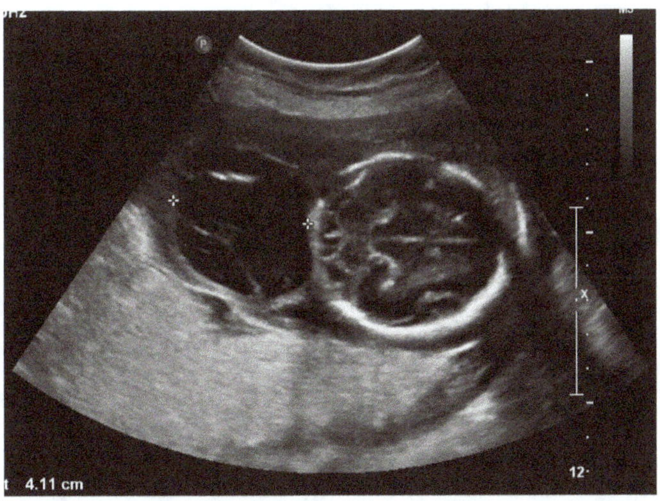


FIGURE 8.9C Cystic hydroma (+ … +) associated with multiple pterygium syndrome.

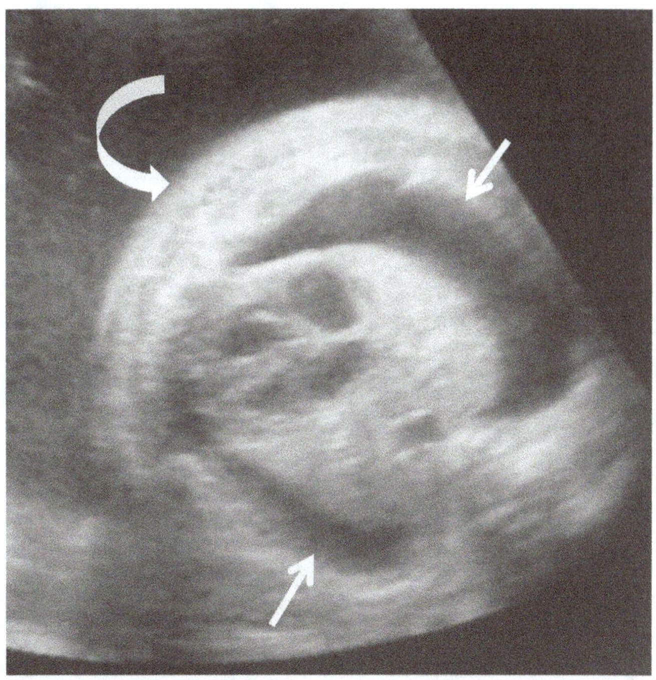

FIGURE 8.9D Multiple pterygium syndrome. Bilateral pleural effusions (straight arrow), anasarca (curved arrow), and polyhydramnios.

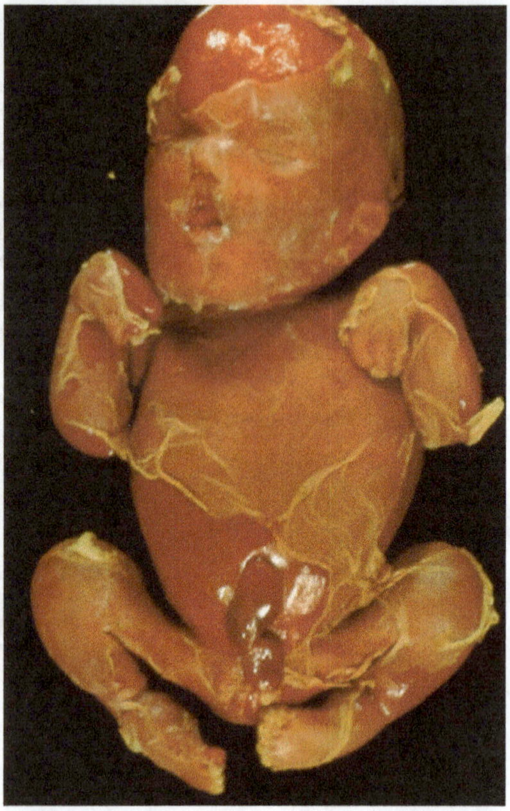

**FIGURE 8.9E** Autopsy of a fetus with multiple pterygium syndrome. Flexion deformity at the elbows, club hands, clubfeet, midface hypoplasia, and low-set ears.

# 8.10 OSTEOGENESIS IMPERFECTA

## EPIDEMIOLOGY/GENETICS

**Definition** Osteogenesis imperfecta is a heterogeneous group of brittle bone diseases characterized by an excessive tendency to antenatal or postnatal fractures. There are currently 13 types that are recognized, but types I, II, and III are the most common.

**Epidemiology** An Australian study found an incidence of 1.6 to 3.5 in 100,000 live births (M1:F1).

**Embryology** Of osteogenesis imperfecta cases, 90% are due to mutations in *COL1A1*/*COL1A2* genes. The phenotype is highly variable, depending on the specific mutation. The Sillence classification is used to divide these disorders into phenotypic groups. Type I is the classic form of osteogenesis imperfecta, with moderate fractures, blue sclera, variable degrees of hearing loss, and dentinogenesis imperfecta; type II is a severe neonatal lethal form with multiple antenatal fractures; type III is a progressively deforming disorder with severe disability by early adulthood.

**Inheritance Patterns** Most families demonstrate autosomal dominant inheritance. In the lethal forms, the mutations are new dominant mutations, but the presence of germ-line mosaicism results in recurrence risks for the family that range from approximately 2% to 5%. Much higher risks have been reported if there are two previously affected children. These families almost always represent autosomal recessive conditions that have been associated with mutations in genes other than *COL1A1*/*COL1A2*, but look phenotypically like osteogenesis imperfecta type III.

**Teratogens** None are known.

**Screening** If the precise abnormality in a particular family is known, biochemical analysis of type I collagen or another biochemical or DNA marker may be studied in future pregnancies. If the DNA mutation is known, the testing can be done by chorionic villus sampling (CVS) or amniocentesis. If the previous child had only collagen biochemical testing and a DNA mutation is not known, the subsequent prenatal diagnosis can only be done on CVS material (villi have collagen that can be assayed; amniotic fluid cells do not). Collagen and mutational analysis always should be done on any fetus or infant with a presumptive diagnosis of osteogenesis imperfecta to allow for future prenatal diagnosis.

**Prognosis** Prognosis is highly variable, depending on clinical type. Infants with type II disease are born with multiple fractures, and most often die in the neonatal period from respiratory compromise. Type III usually presents with multiple fractures at birth, with progressive bone deformities through childhood and adolescence. In type I, fractures may not occur until later in life.

## SONOGRAPHY

### FINDINGS

- Type I
  - Mild limb shortening to normal bone length
  - One or two fractures
  - Long-bone bowing rather than fractures
  - Demineralization not apparent until after 24 weeks' gestation
- Type II
  - There is severe micromelia (– 3 SD in second trimester).
  - The long bones are "transparent," with the back wall of the long bones visible without acoustic shadowing.
  - Hypomineralization is apparent in the second trimester.
  - There are more fractures in the lower extremities than in the upper extremities.
  - There are multiple rib fractures.
  - A small bell-shaped thorax is present.
  - Hypomineralization of the calvarium
    - Visualization of near-field fetal brain
    - Pressure deformity of the skull with transducer
  - First-trimester thickened nuchal translucency exists.
- Type III
  - Macrocephaly
  - Moderate-to-severe limb shortening
  - Multiple fractures in the third trimester
  - Hypomineralization
  - Lower extremities affected more than the upper extremities

### KEY FINDINGS/PITFALLS

- Three-dimensional ultrasound can be used to evaluate the face and extremities of fetuses with suspected osteogenesis imperfecta.
- Type I is rarely diagnosed prenatally unless there is a strong suspicion because of an affected parent.

## PREGNANCY MANAGEMENT

**Investigations and Consultations Required** In a family known to be at risk, with a known mutation, prenatal genetic analysis is indicated by either CVS or amniocentesis. This approach does not apply for de novo cases. Many of the skeletal dysplasias, but not osteogenesis imperfecta, are associated with congenital heart disease. Therefore, a fetal echocardiogram should be obtained if the diagnosis is in doubt. If a lethal dwarfism is expected, a neonatologist should be consulted to plan perinatal management.

**Monitoring** Follow-up ultrasound examinations are useful in nonlethal cases to monitor the extent of prenatal fractures. These examinations are also useful if the diagnosis is in doubt. No obstetric intervention should be performed for the fetus with osteogenesis imperfecta type II or with type III if the findings are consistent with a lethal condition. Other types should not be lethal; they are associated with a less-severe deformity, and standard obstetric management should be employed.

**Pregnancy Course** Polyhydramnios may occur but, if present, is usually mild. It can be more significant in osteogenesis imperfecta type II.

**Pregnancy Termination Issues** An intact fetus must be delivered for a complete postmortem evaluation, including radiologic, morphologic, biochemical, and molecular studies. There is a special need to determine the exact molecular or biochemical defect so that early diagnosis will be possible in future pregnancies.

**Delivery** For the nonlethal forms of osteogenesis imperfecta, cesarean delivery theoretically might be of benefit to decrease the risk of fractures and intracranial hemorrhage. However, experience with de novo cases finds no increase in morbidity with vaginal delivery. Operative vaginal delivery would be contraindicated. Delivery should occur in a tertiary center.

## NEONATOLOGY

**Resuscitation** Given that the prenatal differentiation between the various types may be difficult, it is appropriate to initiate resuscitative efforts. However, if the prenatal diagnosis of osteogenesis imperfecta type II is definite, a prenatal decision for nonintervention, after discussion with the parents, is appropriate.

**Transport** Referral to a tertiary perinatal center for confirmation of the diagnosis is always indicated for a live-born infant with osteogenesis imperfecta. Mechanical ventilatory support may be required during transport. Caution in handling is required to reduce the risk of inadvertent fractures.

**Testing and Confirmation** Careful physical examination and skeletal radiographs are helpful in determining classification. Multiple prenatal fractures and blue sclerae at birth strongly suggest osteogenesis imperfecta type II, the ultimately lethal form.

**Nursery Management** Consultation with pediatric genetics and orthopedics is indicated. Long-term ventilatory support is possible, but controversial, in rare infants with osteogenesis imperfecta type II and less-severe pulmonary hypoplasia. Survival beyond early childhood has not been reported.

### SUGGESTED READINGS

1. Bulas DI, Stern JH, Rosenbaum KN, et al: Variable prenatal appearance of osteogenesis imperfecta. J Ultrasound Med 1994; 13:419-427.
2. Krakow D, Rimoin DL: The skeletal dysplasias. Genet Med 2010; 12:327-341.
3. McEwing RL, Alton K, Johnson J, et al: First-trimester diagnosis of osteogenesis imperfecta type II by three-dimensional sonography. J Ultrasound Med 2003; 22:311-314.

4. Palmer TM, Rouse GA, Song A, DeLange M: Transparent bone and concave ribs: additional sonographic features of lethal osteogenesis imperfecta. J Diagn Med Sonogr 1998; 14:246-250.
5. Pepin M, Atkinson M, Starman BJ, Byers PH: Strategies and outcomes of prenatal diagnosis for osteogenesis imperfecta: a review of biochemical and molecular studies completed in 129 pregnancies. Prenat Diagn 1997; 17:559-570.
6. Tongsong T, Pongthsa S: Early prenatal diagnosis of congenital hypophosphatasia. Ultrasound Obstet Gynecol 2000; 15:252-255.
7. Tretter AE, Sanders RC, Meyers CM, et al: Antenatal diagnosis of lethal skeletal dysplasias. Am J Med Genet 1998; 75:518-522.
8. Van Dijk FS, Sillence DO: Osteogenesis imperfecta: clinical diagnosis, nomenclature, and severity assessment. Am J Med Genet 2014; 164A:1470-1481.
9. Warmon ML, Cormier-Daire V, Hall C, et al: Nosology and classification of genetic skeletal disorders: 2010 revision. Am J Genet A. 2010; 155:943-968.
10. Willing MC, Pruchno CJ, Byers PH: Molecular heterogeneity in osteogenesis imperfecta. Am J Med Genet 1993; 45:223-227.

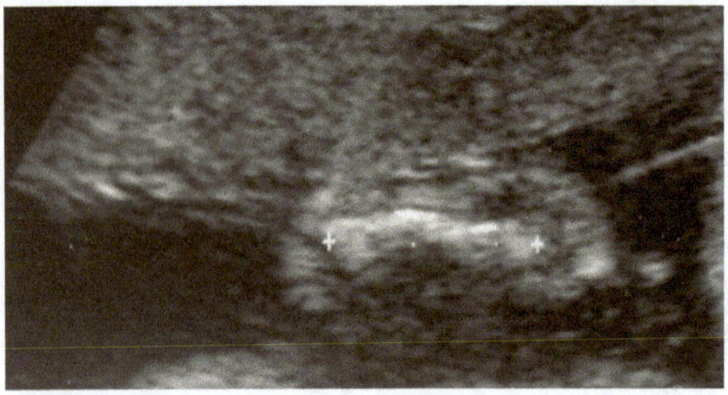

**FIGURE 8.10A** Osteogenesis imperfecta with short, irregularly shaped humerus due to fractures (+ … +).

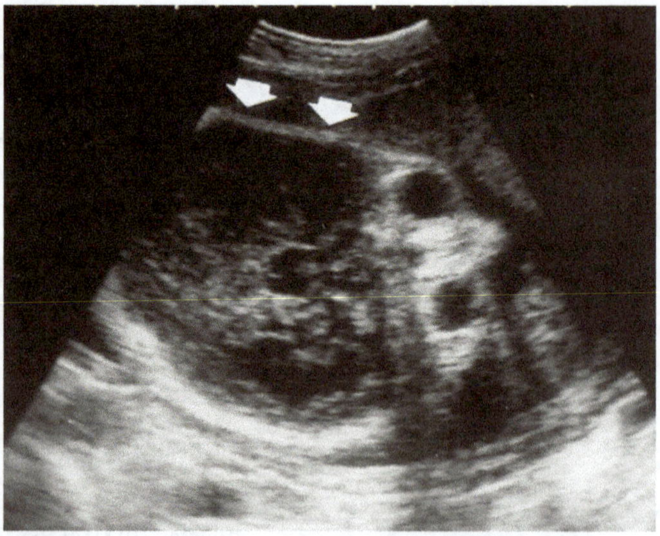

**FIGURE 8.10B** Osteogenesis imperfecta illustrating the pressure deformity of the skull from the ultrasound transducer (arrows).

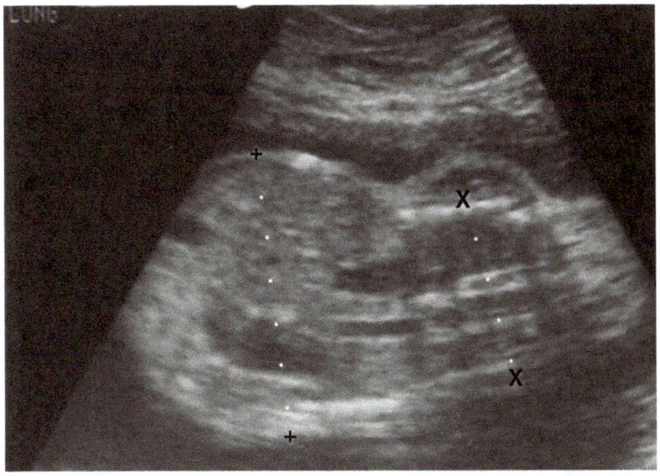

FIGURE 8.10C Osteogenesis imperfecta with a small, bell-shaped thorax (x … x) and protruding abdomen (+ … +).

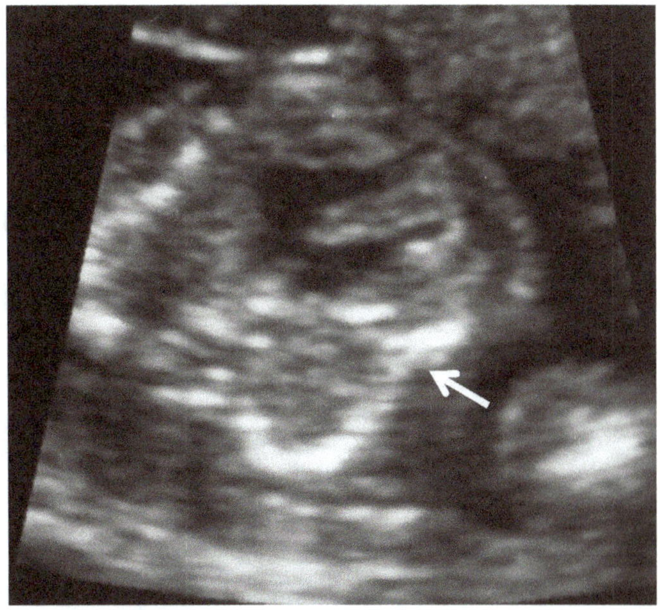

FIGURE 8.10D Transverse view of narrow chest with rib fractures (arrow).

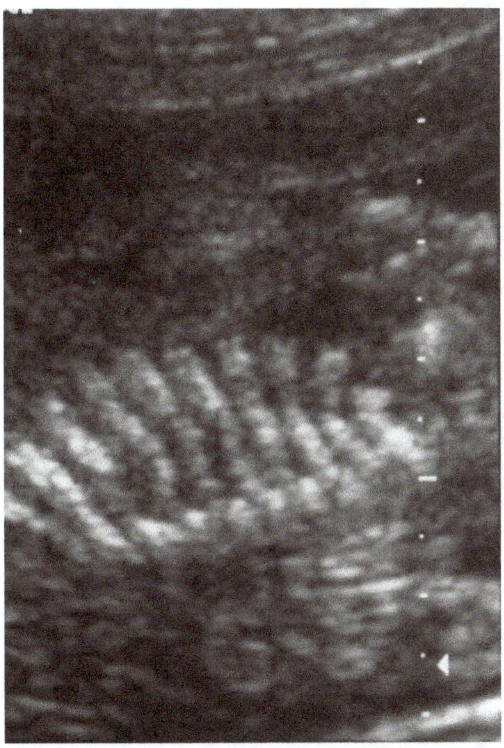

FIGURE 8.10E Osteogenesis imperfecta type II illustrating multiple rib fractures.

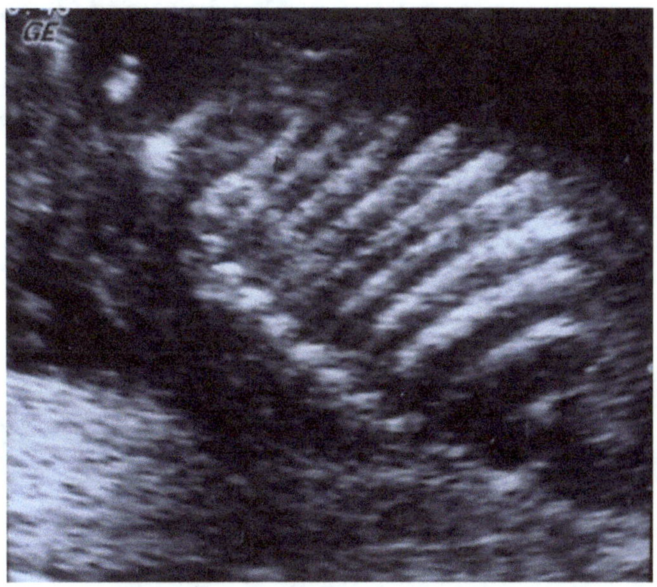

FIGURE 8.10F Normal rib appearance.

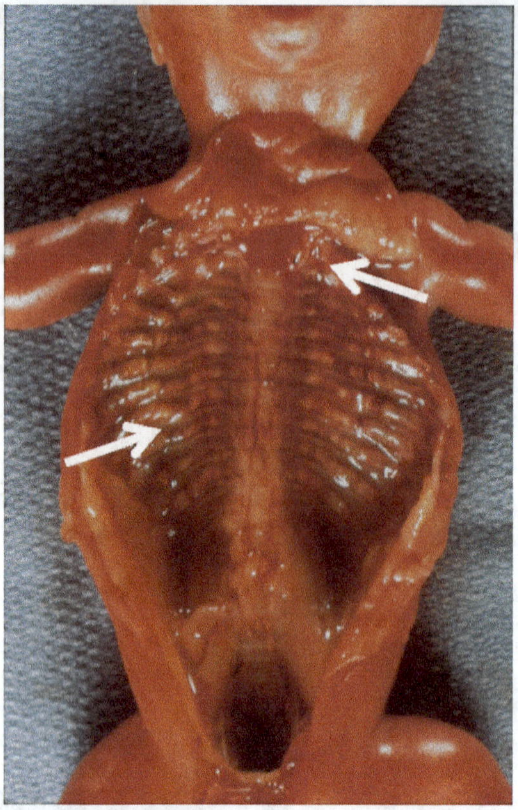

**FIGURE 8.10G** Fetus with osteogenesis imperfecta that has narrow chest and multiple rib fractures (arrows).

# 8.11 POLYDACTYLY

## EPIDEMIOLOGY/GENETICS

**Definition** Polydactyly is a phenotypic abnormality of the limbs characterized by excessive partitioning of the digital rays of the hands and feet. This is clinically manifest as extra digits, broad digits, or bifid digits.

**Epidemiology** Postaxial (ulnar or fibular side of the limb) polydactyly occurs in 1 in 3000 live births of white infants but is 10 times more common in blacks than whites (M1.5:F1). Preaxial (radial or tibial side of limb) polydactyly is much less common, with a frequency in whites of 0.15 in 1000.

**Embryology** More than 100 multiple-malformation syndromes have been described with polydactyly, including many short-limbed skeletal dysplasias and chromosome abnormalities, including trisomies 13, 18, and 21. The combination of low maternal serum estriol, postaxial polydactyly, and congenital heart disease should raise the suspicion for the Smith-Lemli-Opitz syndrome. Antenatal testing for this autosomal recessive defect in cholesterol metabolism is available. The prevalence of associated anomalies is 11.8% in postaxial polydactyly and 20% with preaxial polydactyly.

**Inheritance Patterns** Isolated postaxial polydactyly is most often inherited as an autosomal dominant trait. Isolated preaxial polydactyly is most often unilateral and not familial.

**Teratogens** Alcohol, valproate, and maternal diabetes are teratogenic.

**Prognosis** Prognosis is excellent for isolated polydactylies; otherwise, it is dependent on the associated abnormalities and syndrome diagnosis.

## SONOGRAPHY

### FINDINGS

- Hands or feet have one or more extra digits.
  - Extra digits may consist of soft tissue or contain bone.
  - An extra digit may be normal size or small, abnormally located and angled toward or away from the palm.
  - The extra digit may be located proximal to the rest of the digits on the radial or tibial side (preaxial) or on the ulna or fibular side (postaxial).

### KEY FINDINGS/PITFALLS

- Three-dimensional ultrasound can be utilized to improve visualization of the hands and feet.
- First-trimester transvaginal sonography may detect polydactyly.
- Preaxial polydactyly is less frequent and has a higher association with syndromes.
- Central polydactyly is rare and usually associated with syndactyly.

### DIFFERENTIAL DIAGNOSIS

- Meckel-Gruber syndrome: Look for renal abnormalities and encephalocele.
- Ellis van Creveld syndrome: Short extremities, narrow chest with short ribs, and cardiac defects are characteristics.
- Skeletal dysplasias: Short-rib polydactyly, chondroectodermal dysplasia, and asphyxiating thoracic dystrophy are associated dysplasias.
- Smith-Lemli-Opitz syndrome. See previous discussion.
- Trisomy 13: Look for stigmata; polydactyly commonly present.

## PREGNANCY MANAGEMENT

**Investigations and Consultations Required** Although some cases are autosomal dominant and parents may provide a history supporting this, many cases of polydactyly are part of a syndrome, and steps to determine this are warranted. Chromosomal analysis to exclude trisomy 13 may be necessary. Fetal echocardiography should be performed to detect congenital heart disease. Additional consultations will depend on the associated abnormalities found.

**Monitoring** Unless the condition can clearly be established as lethal, obstetric management should not be modified. No further ultrasound monitoring is necessary.

**Pregnancy Course** Obstetric complications will vary, depending on the associated abnormalities. Obstetric complications are not expected on the basis of polydactyly alone.

**Pregnancy Termination Issues** Except for cases with trisomy 13, all other situations require a nondestructive termination procedure and a complete postmortem evaluation by a fetal pathologist and a dysmorphologist.

**Delivery** Isolated polydactyly does not require any change in delivery mode. If concern for an undiagnosed syndrome is present, delivery should occur at a center with specialists available to evaluate a neonate with multiple malformations.

## NEONATOLOGY

**Resuscitation** There are no specific measures required.

**Transport** Transfer of the newborn is not indicated in cases of isolated polydactyly.

**Testing and Confirmation** Most infants with polydactyly, even if it appears to be isolated, should be evaluated by a pediatric geneticist.

**Nursery Management** There are no special care requirements for the newborn. Referral to pediatric plastic surgery or hand surgery for outpatient evaluation is indicated.

## SUGGESTED READINGS

1. Bromley B, Shipp TD, Benacerraf B: Isolated polydactyly: prenatal diagnosis and perinatal outcome. Prenat Diagn 2000; 20:905-908.
2. Castilla EE, Lugarinho R, da Graca Dutra M, Salgado LJ: Associated anomalies in individuals with polydactyly. Am J Med Genet 1998; 80:459-465.
3. Filges I, Kang A, Hench J, et al: Fetal polydactyly. A study of 24 cases ascertained by prenatal sonography. J Ultrasound Med 2011; 30:1021-1029.
4. Guschmann M, Horn D, Gasiorek-Wiends A, et al: Ellis-van Creveld syndrome: examination at 15 weeks' gestation. Prenat Diagn 1999; 19:879-883.
5. Kratz LE, Kelley RI: Prenatal diagnosis of the RSH/Smith-Lemli-Opitz syndrome. Am J Med Genet 1999; 82:376-381.
6. Paladini D, Graco E, Sglavo G, et al: Congenital anomalies of upper extremities: prenatal diagnosis, significance, and outcome. Am J Obstet Gynecol 2010; 202:596 e1-10.
7. Zimmer EZ, Bronshtein M: Fetal polydactyly diagnosis during early pregnancy: clinical applications. Obstet Gynecol 2000; 183:755-758.

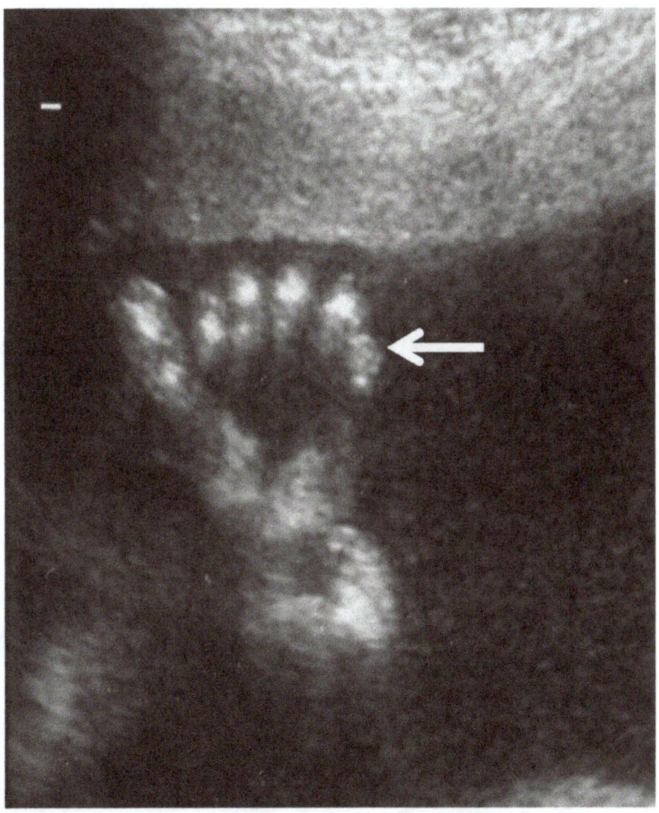

FIGURE 8.11A Postaxial polydactyly (arrow).

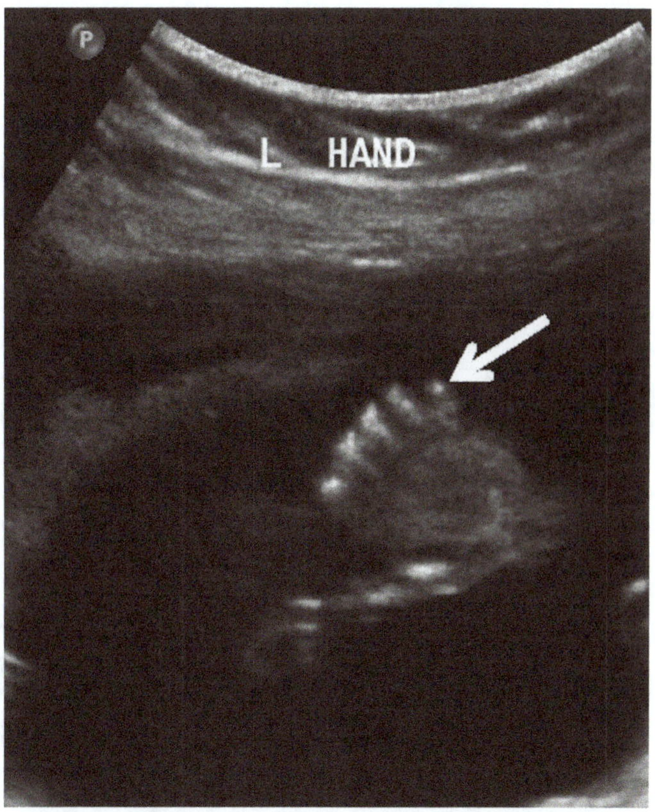


FIGURE 8.11B Postaxial polydactyly (arrow).

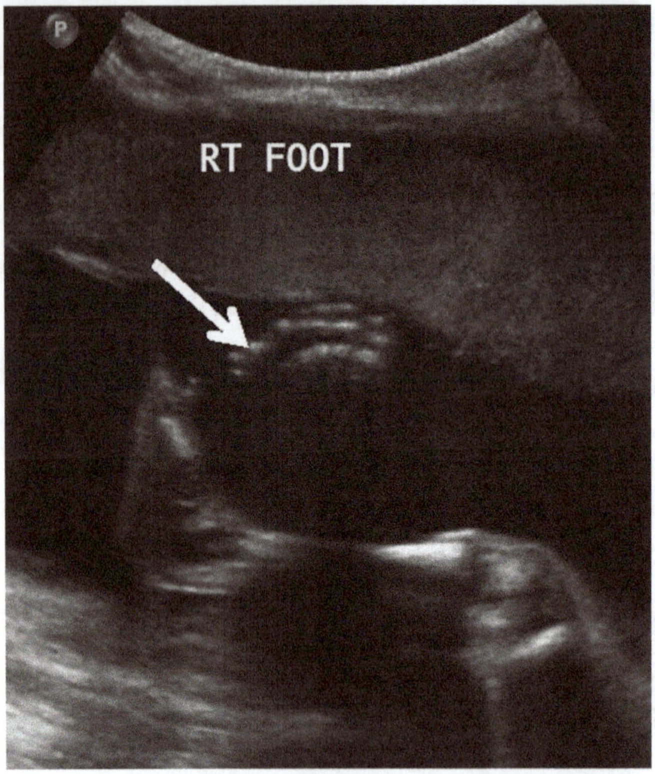


FIGURE 8.11C Postaxial polydactyly (arrow) of right foot.

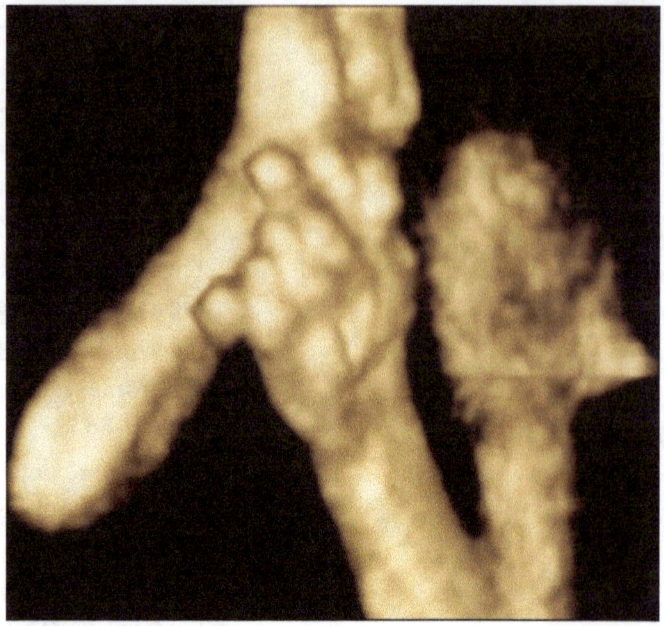

FIGURE 8.11D Three-dimensional ultrasound of postaxial polydactyly.

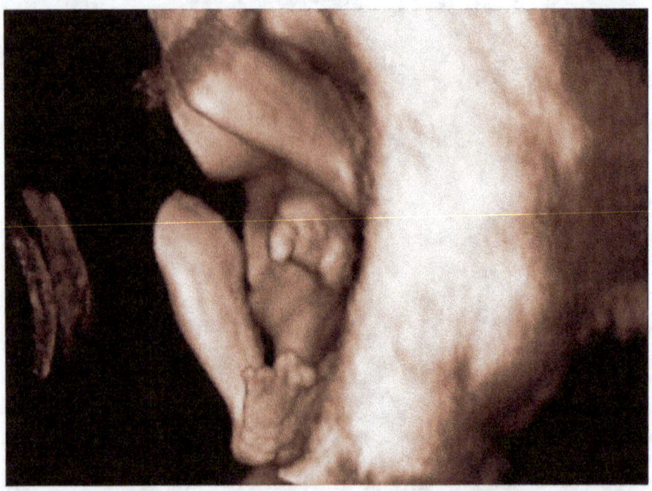

FIGURE 8.11E Three-dimensional scan of foot polydactyly.

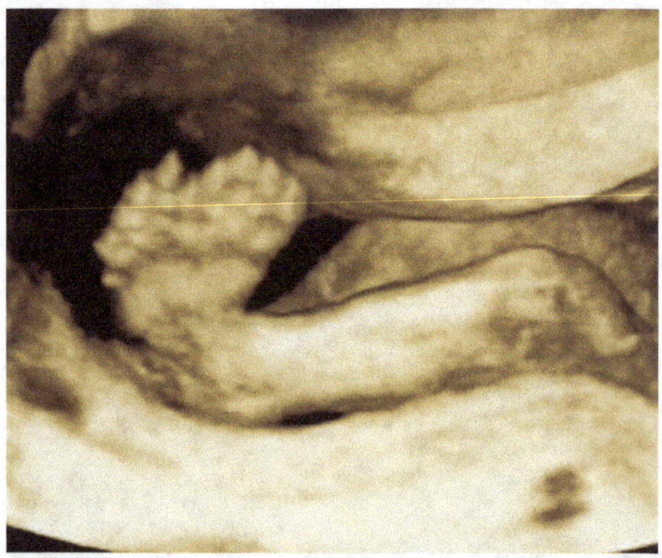

FIGURE 8.11F Three-dimensional ultrasound illustrating 10 toes on one foot.

# 8.12 RADIAL RAY ANOMALIES

## EPIDEMIOLOGY/GENETICS

**Definition** Radial aplasia/hypoplasia is a physical and radiographic abnormality characterized by partial or complete absence of the radius or radial ray structures (thumb and radial carpal bones). The etiology is heterogeneous, with most defects being unilateral and sporadic.

**Epidemiology** Occurrence is 0.3 to 0.8 per 10,000 births.

**Embryology** The distal upper limbs are composed of two major developmental fields: a radial (preaxial) field and an ulnar (postaxial) field. Most major limb defects result from abnormalities in one of these fields, causing pre- or postaxial limb defects. Defects occurring at the junction of these fields result in split hand (ectrodactyly) malformations.

**Inheritance Patterns** Most radial defects are unilateral and sporadic, with bilateral defects much more likely to be part of a multiple-malformation syndrome. Syndromes with radial aplasia/hypoplasia (see Appendix 1) include hematologic syndromes such as Fanconi anemia, Aase syndrome, and thrombocytopenia–absent radius (TAR) syndrome. Sporadic associations include the VACTERL (vertebral defects, anal atresia, cardiac defects, tracheoesophageal fistula, renal anomalies, limb abnormalities) association and the Goldenhar syndrome. Chromosome syndromes include trisomies 13 and 18 and triploidy, as well as several microduplication/microdeletion syndromes. Miscellaneous syndromes that have polydactyly are acrofacial dysostoses, Baller-Gerold syndrome, Cornelia de Lange syndrome, Townes-Brock syndrome, and Holt-Oram syndrome. Because of the rapid progress in mapping of genes and subsequent development of genetic testing, consultation with a medical geneticist or genetic counselor to determine the availability of clinical genetic testing for this disorder (or disorders) is advised.

**Teratogens** Thalidomide, cocaine, valproate, and vitamin A are teratogenic.

**Prognosis** Prognosis is dependent on associated abnormalities and syndromic diagnosis. Good function is possible in most cases with aggressive orthopedic treatment.

## SONOGRAPHY

### FREQUENT FINDINGS

- Partial-to-complete absence of the radius with or without deficiency of the thumb
  - The hand is in marked radial (medial) deviation.
  - As the radial defect worsens from slightly short to absent, the curve of the ulna (i.e., the remaining support of the wrist) increases.
    - An awkward angle results in limited finger motion.

### KEY FINDINGS/PITFALLS

- Unilateral or bilateral forearm defects with other anomalies increase the likelihood of aneuploidy.
- Almost all cases are part of a specific syndrome.

## PREGNANCY MANAGEMENT

**Investigations and Consultations Required** Because this defect is most often part of a syndrome, attention should be directed toward other ultrasound findings that may help to identify a specific syndrome. A fetal echocardiogram should be done, as cardiac defects are associated with a number of the possible etiologic conditions. A careful history is essential to assess for the presence of limb or cardiac abnormalities in the parents or previous children. The history also should include information regarding consanguinity because many of the disorders are autosomal recessive. Any potential teratogen exposure, specifically valproic acid, should be ascertained. A consultation with a medical geneticist should be done to determine possible genetic testing options. Fetal karyotype and microarray should be performed, especially if other malformations are detected. Cordocentesis should be performed to assess fetal hematologic status, which may identify TAR syndrome, Fanconi anemia, or Aase syndrome. Other consultations should be based on the presumptive diagnosis and the need for neonatal medical or surgical therapy.

**Fetal Intervention** None is indicated.

**Monitoring** Ultrasound examinations should be performed periodically throughout the pregnancy to assess limb development and to look for the presence of other abnormalities.

**Pregnancy Termination Issues** Unless a precise diagnosis has been established prenatally, the method of termination should provide an intact fetus for a complete morphologic and radiologic examination.

**Delivery** The complex nature of these multiple-malformation conditions requires that delivery and neonatal management occur in a tertiary center. In cases of TAR syndrome and Fanconi anemia with platelet counts less than 50,000/mm$^3$, consideration must be given to elective cesarean section or platelet transfusion just prior to elective induction of labor.

## NEONATOLOGY

**Resuscitation** In general, any special issues for resuscitation are determined by the associated or underlying cause of the skeletal defect.

**Transport** Referral to a tertiary perinatal center following birth is indicated for definitive diagnosis, particularly if cardiac or chromosomal abnormalities are suspected.

**Testing and Confirmation** In general, careful physical examination, blood cell morphology, extremity radiographs, an echocardiogram, and chromosomal analysis (particularly if there are other dysmorphic features) complete the basic evaluation.

**Nursery Management** The primary issue is a definitive etiologic diagnosis. Long-term prognosis is determined by the associated or underlying cause. Palliative procedures are possible to create a prehensile grasp.

## SUGGESTED READINGS


1. Auerbach AD, Sagi M, Adler B: Fanconi anemia: prenatal diagnosis in 30 fetuses at risk. Pediatrics 1985; 76:794-800.
2. Brons JTJ, Van Der Harten JH, Van Geijn HP, et al: Prenatal ultrasonographic diagnosis of radial-ray reduction malformations. Prenat Diagn 1990; 10:279-288.
3. Cox H, Viljoen D, Versfeld G, Beighton P: Radial ray defects and associated anomalies. Clin Genet 1989; 35:322-330.
4. Koshimies E, Lindfors N, Gissler M, et al: Congenital upper limb deficiencies and associated malformations in Finland: a population study. J Hand Surg Ann 2011; 36:1058-1065.
5. Kozin SH: Upper-extremity congenital anomalies. J Bone Joint Surg Ann 2003; 85-A(8):1564-1576.
6. Meizner I, Bar-Ziv J, Barki Y, Abeliovich D: Prenatal ultrasonic diagnosis of radial-ray aplasia and renal anomalies (acro-renal syndrome). Prenat Diagn 1986; 6:223-225.
7. Tongsong T, Chanprapaph P: Prenatal sonographic diagnosis of Holt-Oram syndrome. J Clin Ultrasound 2000; 28:98-100.
8. Tongsong T, Sirichotiyakul S, Chanprapaph P: Prenatal diagnosis of thrombocytopenia-absent-radius (TAR) syndrome. Ultrasound Obstet Gynecol 2000; 15:256-258.
9. Wood VE: Congenital thumb deformities. Clin Orthop 1985; 195:7-25.
10. Ylagan LR, Budorick NE: Radial ray aplasia in utero: a prenatal finding associated with valproic acid exposure. J Ultrasound Med 1994; 13:408-411.


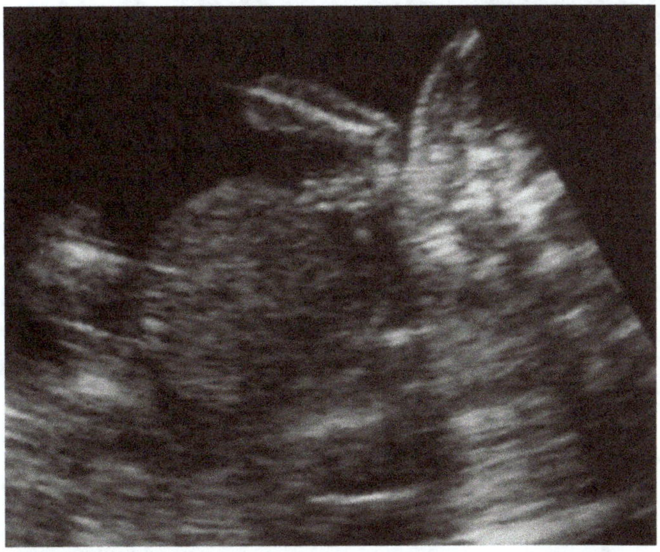

**FIGURE 8.12A** Radial ray anomaly with absent radius and hand in medial rotation.

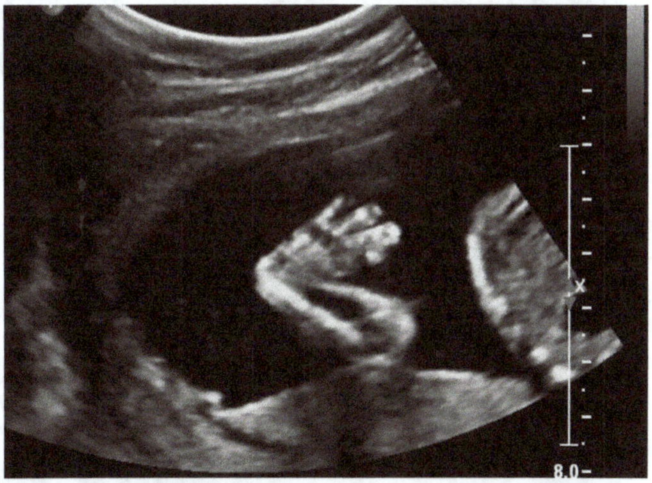


**FIGURE 8.12B** Radial ray anomaly with absent radius and thumb.

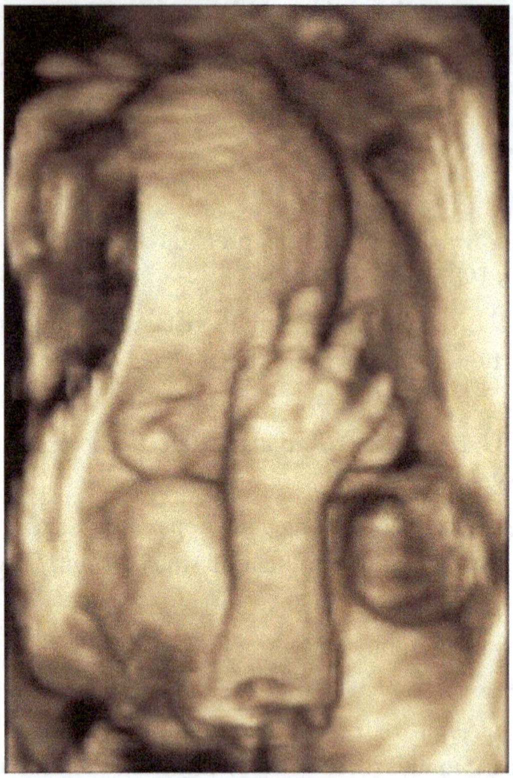

**FIGURE 8.12C** Three-dimensional image of normal hand/wrist orientation.

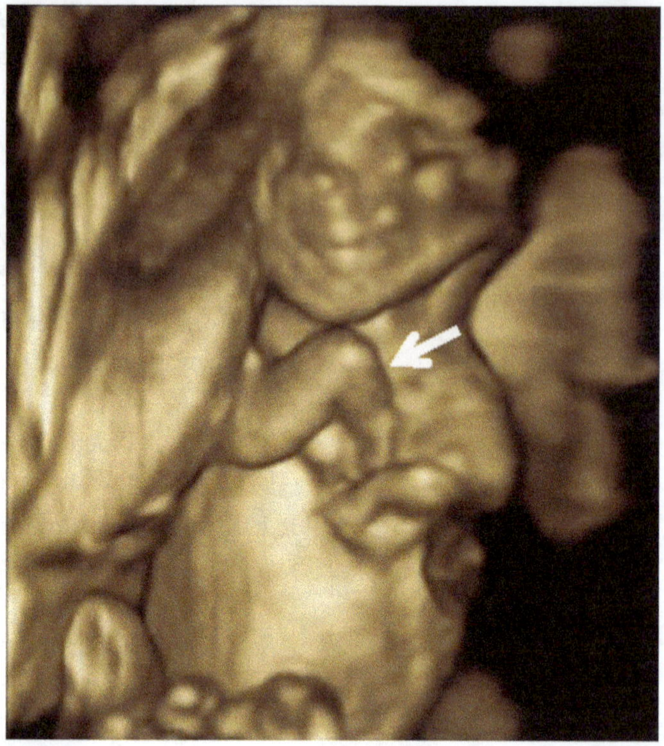

**FIGURE 8.12D** Three-dimensional image of radial ray anomaly with absent radius (arrow).

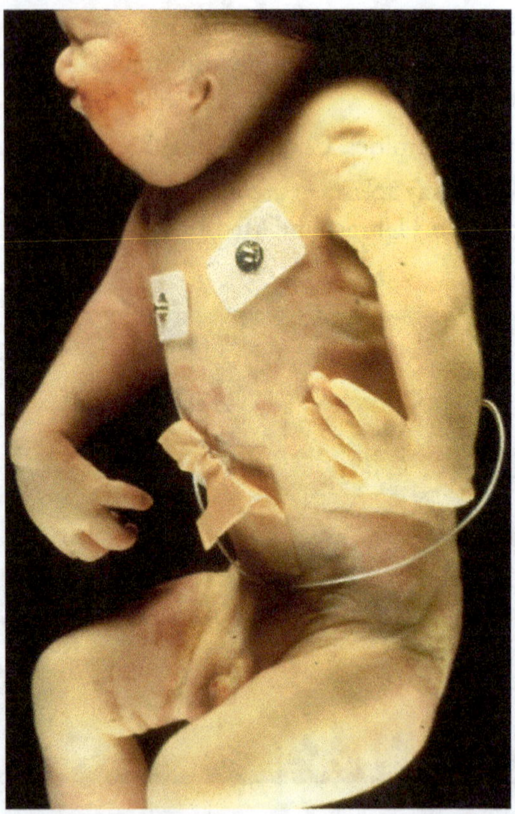

**FIGURE 8.12E** Fetus with absent radius and thumb.

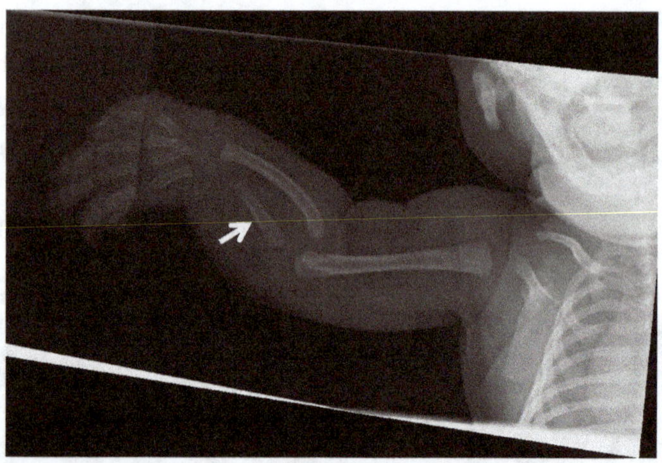

**FIGURE 8.12F** X-ray of hypoplastic radius (arrow), curvature of the ulna, and radial deviation at the wrist.

# 8.13 SHORT-RIB POLYDACTYLY SYNDROMES

## EPIDEMIOLOGY/GENETICS

**Definition** Short-rib polydactyly syndrome (SRPS) refers to a group of skeletal dysplasias characterized by short, horizontal ribs and either pre- or postaxial polydactyly in most cases. The four types of SRPS are

- Type I: Saldino-Noonan
- Type II: Majewski
- Type III: Verma-Naumoff
- Type IV: Beemer-Langer

**Epidemiology** The estimate frequency of the so-called ciliary chondrodysplasias is approximately 1 in 200,000. For SRPSs, the exact incidence is not known, but they are rare.

**Embryology** These disorders are among the birth defects known as ciliopathies. Primary cilia are key to the transduction of signal in the hedgehog pathway that is of critical importance in skeletal development. Other disorders in this group include Jeune thoracic dystrophy and Ellis-van Creveld syndrome. Multiple genes in the hedgehog signaling pathway have been found to be associated with the SRPSs. Consultation with a medical geneticist should be obtained to discuss potential genetic testing.

**Inheritance Pattern** All are inherited in an autosomal recessive fashion.

**Teratogens** None are known.

**Prognosis** Death from respiratory insufficiency, secondary to pulmonary hypoplasia, occurs in the first few days of life.

## SONOGRAPHY

### FREQUENT FINDINGS

- Frontal bossing
- Pre- and post-axial polydactyly
- Short horizontal ribs
- Severe tibial shortening
- Thickened first-trimester nuchal translucency

### LESS FREQUENT

- Ventriculomegaly
- Median cleft lip/palate
- Low-set ears
- Ambiguous genitalia/sex reversal
- Hydrops
- Transposition of the great vessels

- Endocardial cushion defect
- Ventricular septal defect
- Esophageal atresia
- Enlarged echogenic kidneys

### KEY FINDINGS/PITFALLS

- Three-dimensional imaging can be utilized to better assess the face and extremities.
- Transvaginal sonography can be utilized to diagnose SRPS in the first trimester.
- Amniotic fluid: Polyhydramnios or oligohydramnios may be present, depending on the type of SRPS and the associated abnormalities.

## PREGNANCY MANAGEMENT

**Investigations and Consultations Required** There are two goals of further investigations: determining whether the skeletal dysplasia is lethal and, if possible, determining which skeletal dysplasia the case represents. If the precise skeletal dysplasia is uncertain, other investigations are warranted, including a fetal echocardiogram. Congenital heart disease is a feature of a number of skeletal dysplasias and may be present in SRPS. Once a diagnosis of a lethal condition is established, and if the pregnancy is beyond the legal limits for termination, the family should meet with a neonatologist to discuss neonatal management.

**Monitoring** Further ultrasound examinations looking for relative growth of the ribs and long bones and confirmation of polydactyly, if it was difficult to image, may help to establish the diagnosis. Once a diagnosis of a lethal condition has been established, routine supportive maternal care should be provided. No attempts to treat preterm labor or to monitor fetal status are appropriate.

**Pregnancy Course** Polyhydramnios, oligohydramnios, or nonimmune hydrops may develop. No treatment or further investigation for these complications should be undertaken.

**Pregnancy Termination Issues** An intact fetus must be delivered, and the postmortem examination, including radiologic, morphologic, biochemical, and molecular studies, must be performed by individuals with extensive experience in skeletal dysplasias. As SRPSs are recessively inherited, this will be of particular importance to the family.

**Delivery** Vaginal delivery without electronic monitoring is appropriate. Delivery should occur in a center with expertise in the diagnostic evaluation of skeletal dysplasias or one with an interest and expertise in fetal pathology.

## NEONATOLOGY

**Resuscitation** Given a uniformly lethal prognosis, resuscitation is not indicated.

**Transport** Transport should not be a consideration given the prognosis.

**Testing and Confirmation** Careful physical examination, complemented by a detailed postmortem examination, will confirm the spectrum of abnormalities.

**Nursery Management** In the rare circumstance of fetal survival beyond delivery, comfort measures only are indicated. Support for parental grieving and genetic counseling for future pregnancies are essential.

## SUGGESTED READINGS

1. Elçioglu NH, Hall CM: Diagnostic dilemmas in the short rib-polydactyly syndrome group. Am J Med Genet 2002; 111:392-400.
2. Eleftheriades M, Iazzo C, Manolakos E, et al: Recurrent short rib polydactyly syndrome. J Obstet Gynaecol 2013; 33:14-16.
3. Hill LM, Leary J: Transvaginal sonographic diagnosis of short-rib polydactyly dysplasia at 13 weeks' gestation. Prenat Diagn 1998; 18:1198-1201.
4. Krakow D, Rimoin DL: The skeletal dysplasias. Genet Med 2010; 12:327-341.
5. Meng HW, Pao LK, Shio JL: Prenatal diagnosis of recurrence of short rib polydactyly syndrome. Am J Med Genet 1995; 55:279-284.
6. Rösing B, Kempe A, Berg C, et al: Orofaciodigital syndrome type IV (Mohr-Majewski): early prenatal diagnosis in siblings. Ultrasound Obstet Gyhnecol 2008; 31:457-460.
7. Schmidts M: Clinical genetics and pathobiology of ciliary chondrodysplasias. J Pediatr Genet 2014: 3:46-94.
8. Sillence D, Kozlowski K, Bar-Ziv J, et al: Perinatally lethal short rib polydactyly syndrome. 1. Variability in known syndromes. Pediatr Radiol 1987; 17:474-480.
9. Suer PS, Kumar CP, Gurushi S: Case report: short rib polydactyly syndrome—type 2 (Majewski syndrome). Indian J Radiol Imaging 2010; 20:134-142.

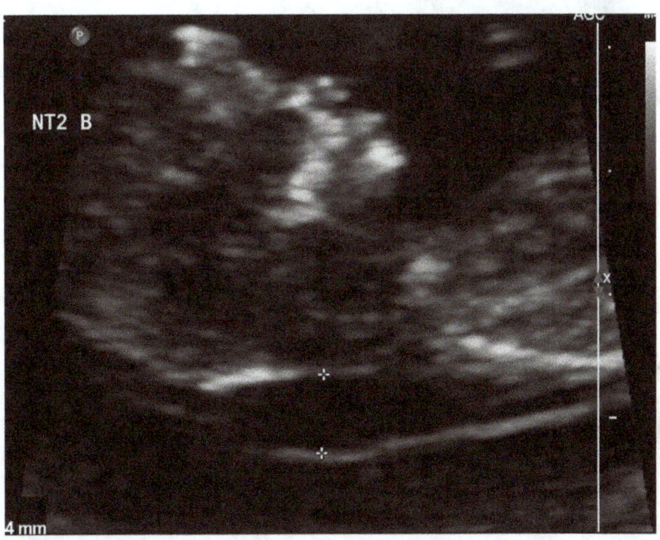


**FIGURE 8.13A** Thickened nuchal translucency (+ … +) in fetus with short-rib polydactyly syndrome.

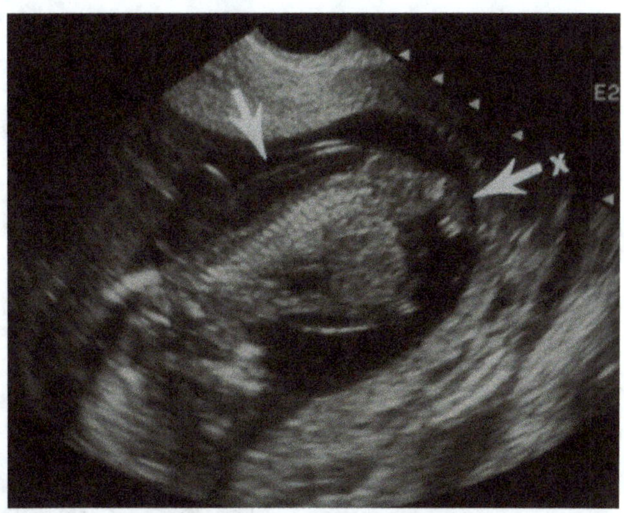


**FIGURE 8.13B** A 13-week ultrasound image of thickened nuchal/anasarca (arrow); markedly shortened lower extremity (X).

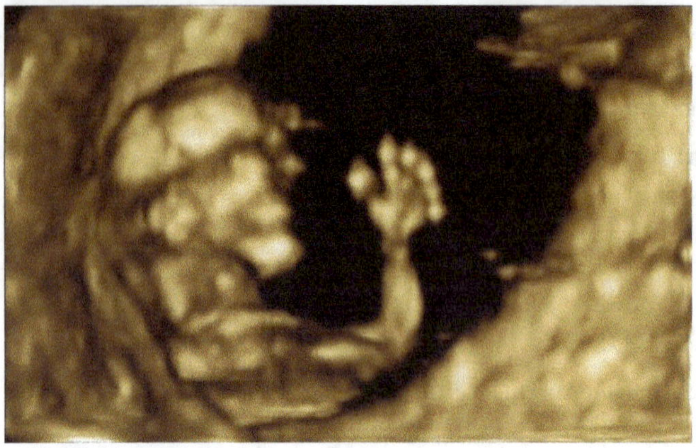

**FIGURE 8.13C** Three-dimensional image of polydactyly.

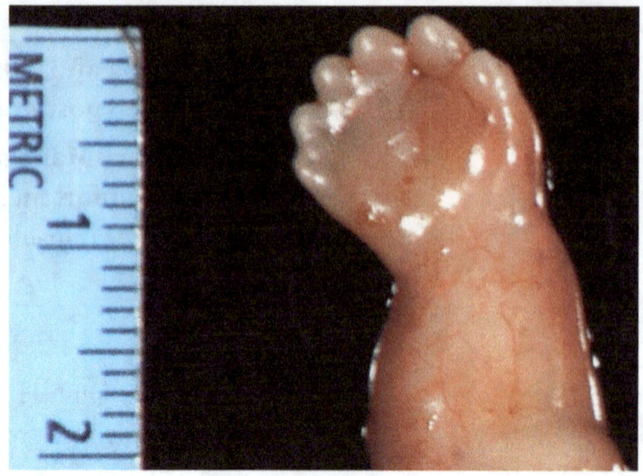


**FIGURE 8.13D** Hand of fetus with short-rib polydactyly syndrome.

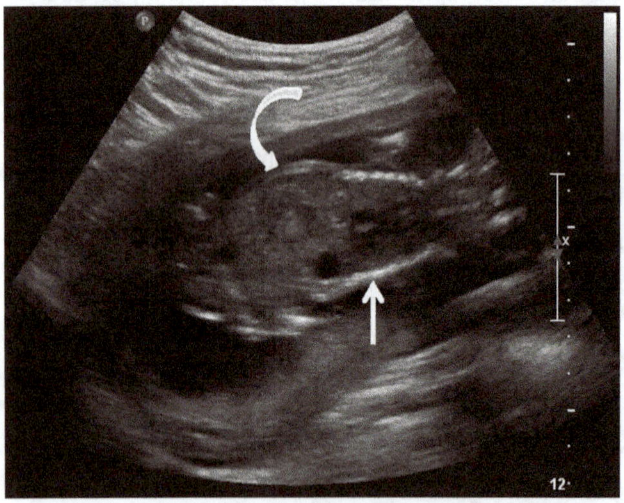

**FIGURE 8.13E** Narrow chest (straight arrow) and protuberant abdomen (curved arrow).

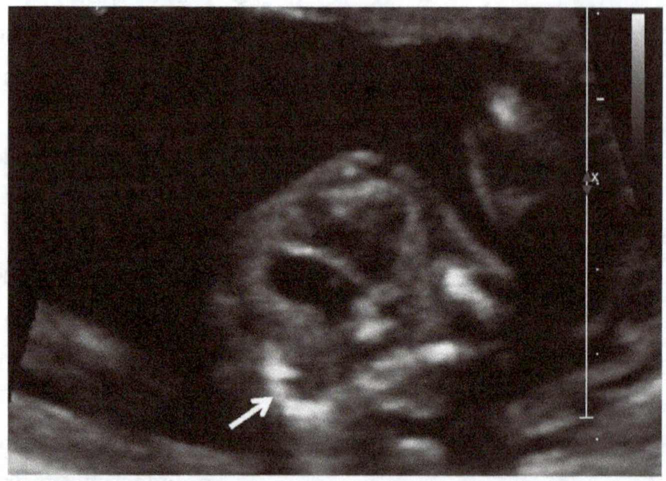

**FIGURE 8.13F** Short ribs (arrow) with a normal heart filling the chest cavity.

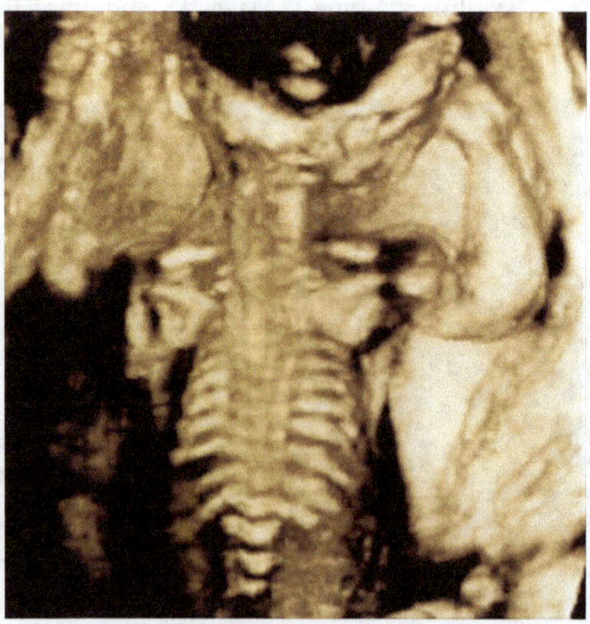

**FIGURE 8.13G** Three-dimensional examination of a fetus with short-rib polydactyly (19 weeks).

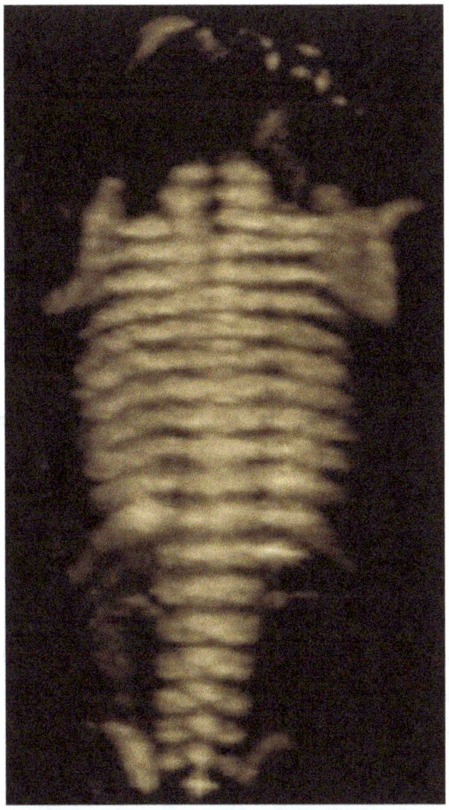

FIGURE 8.13H Three-dimensional study of normal ribs and spine (19 weeks).

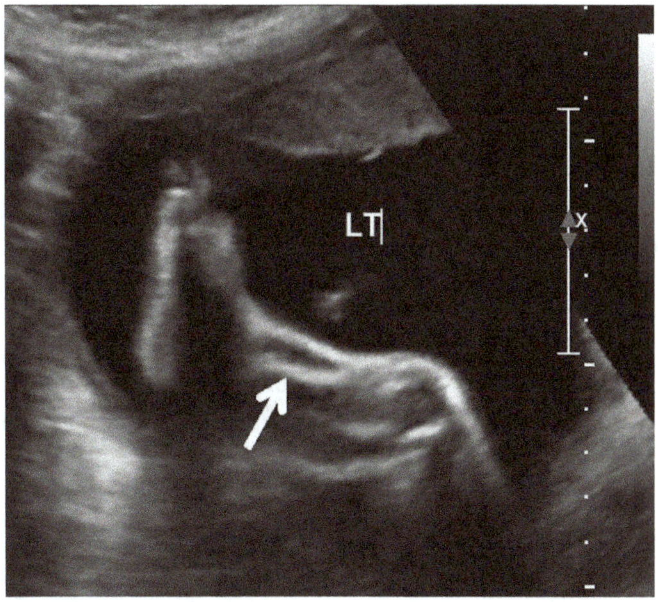


FIGURE 8.13I Disproportionately shortened tibia (arrow).

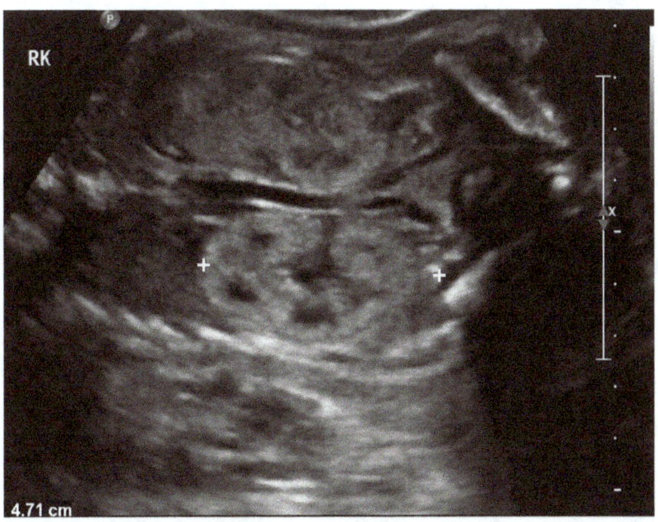


FIGURE 8.13J Enlarged echogenic kidney (+ … +).

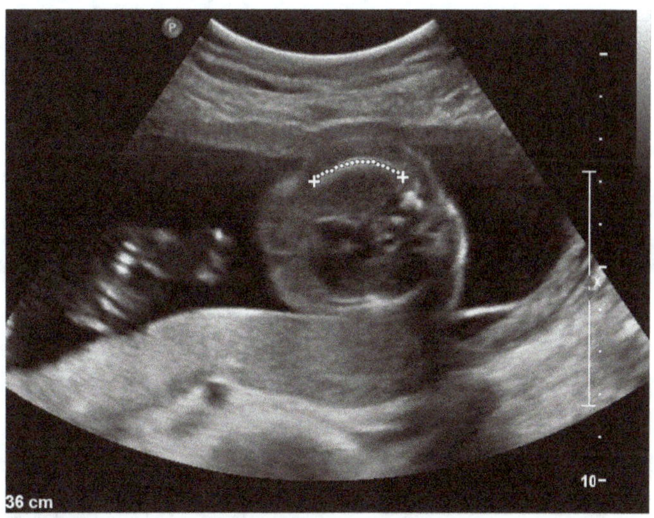


FIGURE 8.13K Short rib (+ … +) in a fetus with short-rib polydactyly syndrome.

# 8.14 THANATOPHORIC DYSPLASIA

## EPIDEMIOLOGY/GENETICS

**Definition** Thanatophoric dysplasia is the most common lethal short-limbed skeletal dysplasia and is characterized by micromelia, narrow thorax, and a relatively large head.

**Epidemiology** Occurrence is 1 in 40,000 live births.

**Embryology** Thanatophoric dysplasia is divided into two types. Type I (85%) has characteristic radiographic findings, including telephone receiver–shaped (bowed) femurs and short ribs. Type II has short long bones, but they are straighter and longer than for type I. A cloverleaf skull is seen almost exclusively in type II.

**Inheritance Patterns** All cases are sporadic and represent new dominant mutations in the *FGFR*-3 gene on chromosome 4p. Antenatal diagnosis using DNA mutation analysis is widely available. Because of germ cell mosaicism, recurrence risk in subsequent pregnancies is approximately 5%.

**Prognosis** Thanatophoric dysplasia is invariably fatal, usually shortly after birth.

## SONOGRAPHY

### FREQUENT FINDINGS

- Severe (<4 SD) micromelia
- Abnormal sulcation of temporal and occipital lobes (pathognomonic)
- Relatively large calvarium (95th centile)
- Frontal bossing
- Depressed nasal bridge
- Chest circumference less than fifth centile
- Protuberant abdomen
- Extremities
  - Reduced movement
  - Positioned at right angles to the body
  - Redundant skin
- Hands
  - Trident shape
  - Short, stubby fingers that are widely separated
- Spine
  - Flattened vertebral bodies (platyspondyly)

### LESS FREQUENT

- Proptosis
- Ventriculomegaly
- Partial agenesis of the corpus callosum

### KEY FINDINGS/PITFALLS

- Three-dimensional imaging provides an improved overall assessment of the stigmata associated with thanatophoric dysplasia.
- Severe polyhydramnios is present in the late second or third trimester.
- It has been detected as early as 13 weeks' gestation.

## PREGNANCY MANAGEMENT

**Investigations and Consultations Required** Fetal echocardiography, to detect congenital heart defects, may assist in establishing a precise diagnosis. A neonatologist should be consulted to plan perinatal management.

**Monitoring** Follow-up ultrasound examinations may be required if the diagnosis is in doubt, but are otherwise unnecessary. No obstetric intervention should be undertaken for fetal indications.

**Pregnancy Course** Nearly 75% of cases of thanatophoric dwarfism will be complicated by severe polyhydramnios. Any ensuing preterm labor should not be treated, and significant maternal discomfort or respiratory distress is an indication for delivery.

**Pregnancy Termination Issues** If a molecular diagnosis is made, no confirmatory postmortem studies are necessary. Otherwise, an intact fetus must be delivered for confirmation of the prenatal diagnosis. A complete postmortem evaluation of the fetus, including radiologic, morphologic, biochemical, and molecular studies, should be performed by individuals with extensive experience in skeletal dysplasias to confirm the diagnosis and provide information for subsequent pregnancies.

**Delivery** Cesarean section is contraindicated, except in cases of dystocia or for other maternal indications.

## NEONATOLOGY

**Resuscitation** When the diagnosis is known prior to delivery, a prenatal decision for nonintervention, made after discussion with the family, is appropriate. If the diagnosis is uncertain, resuscitation and ventilatory support should be provided to allow time for diagnostic evaluation and parental adaptation.

**Transport** Referral to a tertiary perinatal center is appropriate for confirmation of a diagnosis. Mechanical ventilatory support is often required during the transport.

**Testing and Confirmation** Postnatal skeletal radiographs and careful physical examination will establish the diagnosis.

**Nursery Management** Confirmation of the diagnosis, comfort care for the infant, and counseling and support of the family are the primary goals. Provision of mechanical life support in the interim is appropriate.

## SUGGESTED READINGS

1. Chen C, Schu-Revn C, Shih J: Prenatal diagnosis and genetic analysis of type 1 and type 2 thanatophoric dysplasia. Prenat Diagn 2001; 21:89-95.
2. Chitty LS, Khalil A, Barrett AN, et al: Safe, accurate prenatal diagnosis of thanatophoric dyplasia using ultrasound and free fetal DNA. Prenat Diagn 2013; 33:416-423.
3. Fink AM, Hingston T, Sampson A, et al: Malformation of the fetal brain in thanatophoric dysplasia: US and MRI findings. Pediatr Radiol 2010; 40(Suppl 1):S134-S137.
4. Parilla BV, Leeth EA, Kambich MP, et al: Antenatal detection of skeletal dysplasias. J Ultrasound Med 2003; 22:255-258.
5. Schild RL, Hunt GH, Moore J, et al: Antenatal sonographic diagnosis of thanatophoric dysplasia: a report of three cases and a review of the literature with special emphasis on differential diagnosis. Ultrasound Obstet Gynecol 1996; 8:62-67.
6. Tsai P-Y, Chang C-H, Yu C-H, et al: Thanatophoric dysplasia: role of 3-dimensional sonography. J Clin Ultrasound 2009; 37:31-34.
7. Wang DC, Shannon P, Toi A, et al: Temporal lobe dysplasia: a characteristic sonographic finding in thanatophoric dysplasia. Ultrasound Obstet Gynecol 2014; 94:588-594.

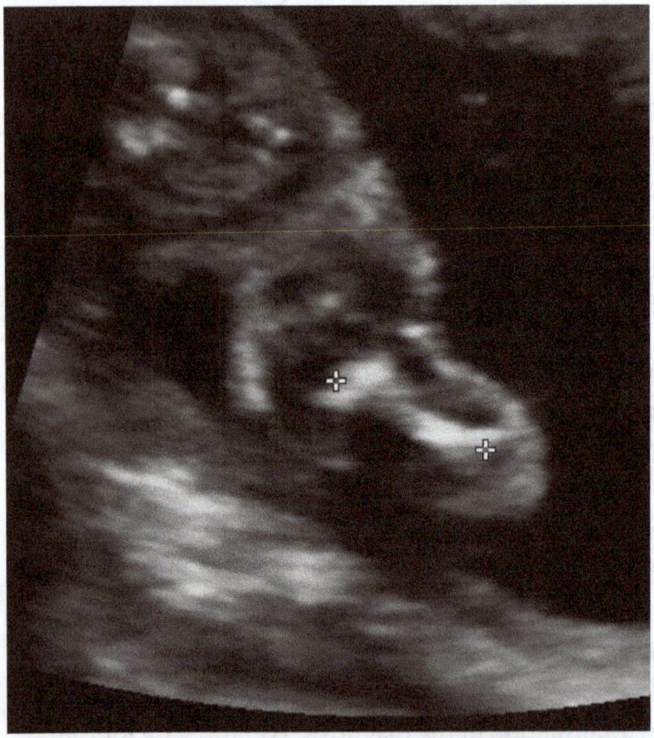

**FIGURE 8.14A** Thanatophoric dysplasia illustrating a short femur (+ … +).

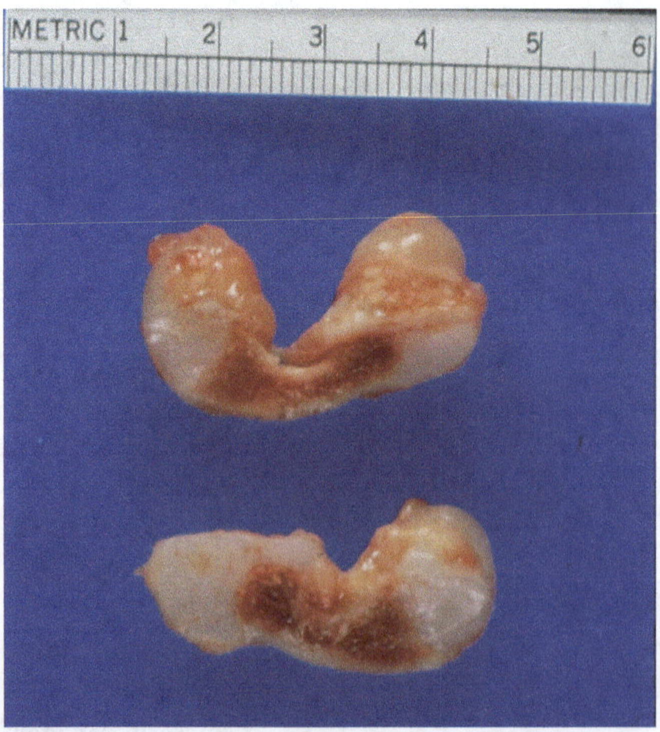


**FIGURE 8.14B** Femurs from fetus with thanatophoric dysplasia illustrating the telephone receiver appearance.

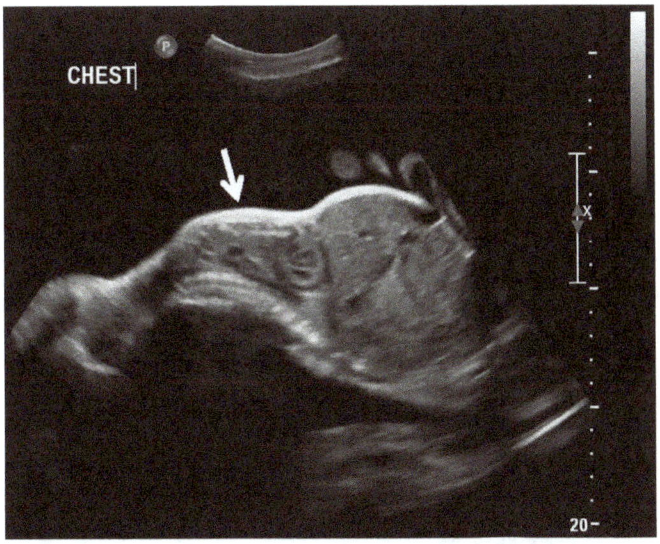


**FIGURE 8.14C** Thanatophoric dysplasia with narrow chest (arrow), pulmonary hypoplasia, and polyhydramnios.

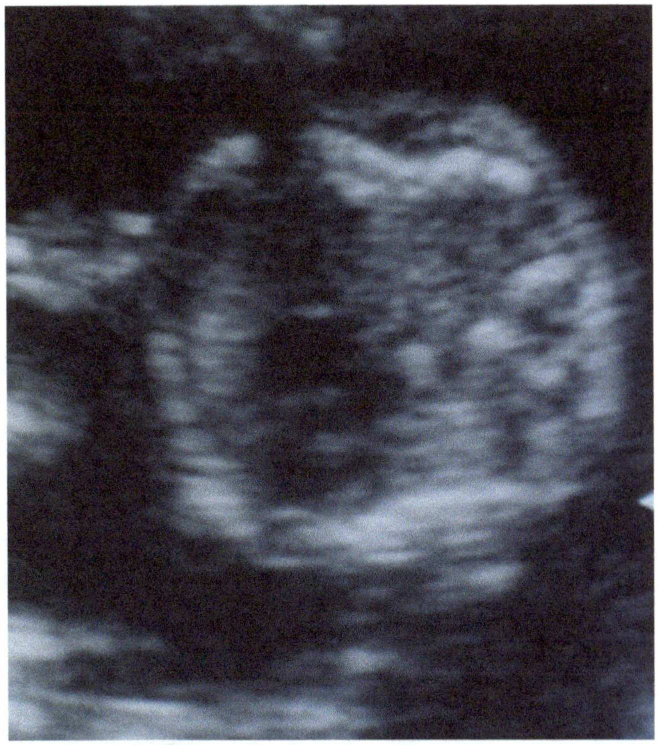

**FIGURE 8.14D** Thanatophoric dysplasia showing narrow, bell-shaped chest.

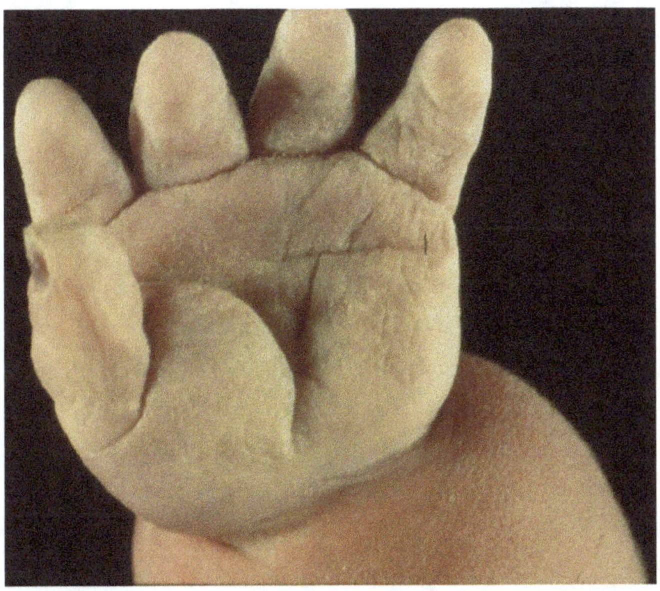

**FIGURE 8.14E** Fetus with thanatophoric dysplasia and trident hand with short, stubby fingers that are widely separated.

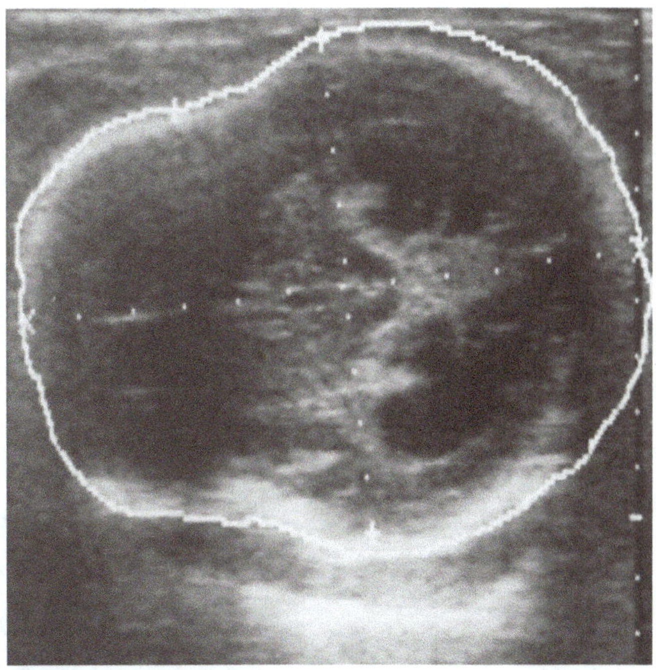

**FIGURE 8.14F** Cloverleaf skull in thanatophoric dysplasia.

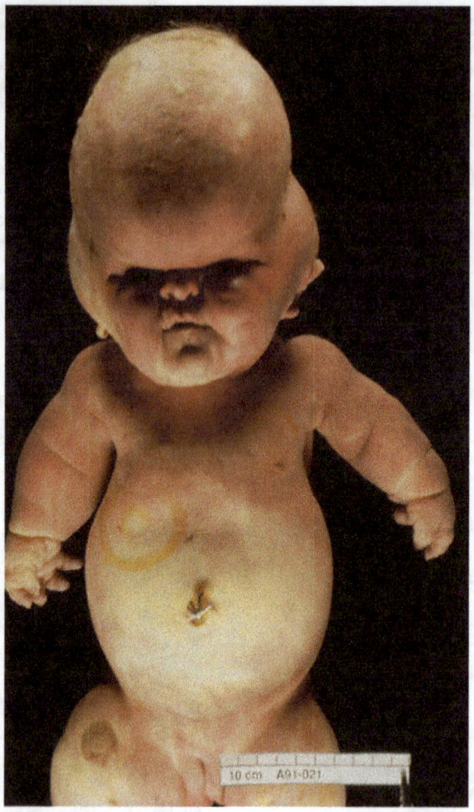


**FIGURE 8.14G** Fetus with thanatophoric dysplasia and classic feature of cloverleaf skull, narrow chest, and micromelia.

# CHAPTER 9

# INFECTIONS

# 9.1 CYTOMEGALIC INCLUSION DISEASE

## EPIDEMIOLOGY/GENETICS

**Definition** Cytomegalovirus (CMV) is a large, enveloped DNA herpesvirus. Adult infection is frequently asymptomatic, but fetal infection may cause severe damage to multiple organ systems. CMV is transmitted in adults by bodily secretions. Fetal exposure occurs transplacentally.

**Epidemiology** CMV is the most common cause of in utero infection; approximately 0.5% to 1% of pregnant women are infected. Maternal CMV infection usually presents with few, if any, side effects. When first infected, some people may have symptoms similar to mononucleosis (i.e., fatigue, weakness, fever, lymphadenopathy). Most people in the United States are infected during childhood or as adults if they work around children. Pregnant women who have not been infected with CMV in the past and become infected during pregnancy (i.e., a primary infection) are at particularly increased risk of fetal CMV infection. Of note, recurrent or reactivation CMV infection in women can also cause fetal CMV infection, although the likelihood and severity of fetal infection is lower and less severe than with primary maternal CMV infection. For pregnant women, the two most common exposures to CMV are through sexual contact and through contact with the urine of young children with CMV infection. Most CMV infections encountered in pregnant women are asymptomatic, even during the acute stage. Less than 5% of pregnant women with primary infection are reported to be symptomatic, and an even smaller percentage suffer from a mononucleosis syndrome

**Prognosis** The severity of disease and its manifestations are determined by the timing of infection and the affinity of nervous tissue to different CMV strains. A normal second-trimester scan does not exclude an abnormal ultrasound examination later in gestation.

## SONOGRAPHY

### FREQUENT FINDINGS

- Hepatic calcifications
- Splenic calcifications
- Hydrops
  - Pleural effusions
  - Ascites
  - Anasarca
  - Scalp edema
  - Placentomegaly
- Cardiomegaly
- Ventriculomegaly

### LESS FREQUENT

- Central nervous system
  - Microcephaly
  - Periventricular echogenic halo, indicating white matter necrosis
  - Linear calcifications in the basal ganglia
  - Punctate cerebellar calcifications
  - Intraventricular hemorrhage
  - Porencephaly
  - Lissencephaly
  - Subependymal cysts
  - Microphthalmia
- Echogenic small bowel
- Hepatomegaly
- Splenomegaly
- Punctate calcifications
  - Pericardial
  - Placental
- Echogenic nephropathy

## PREGNANCY MANAGEMENT

**Investigations and Consultations Required** Maternal blood serologic testing is helpful in delineating the acuity of CMV infection. Serologic testing for CMV may be considered for women who develop influenza-like illness or a viral hepatitis-like illness during pregnancy or following detection of sonographic findings suggestive of CMV infection. Maternal blood ought to be tested for CMV immunoglobulin (Ig) M, IgG, and IgG avidity. To ascertain if fetal infection has occurred, amniocentesis can be performed, with testing of amniotic fluid for CMV-specific polymerase chain reaction (PCR). Amniocentesis should be timed for at least 7 weeks after the presumed time of maternal infection and at 21 weeks or more of gestation. This interval is important because it takes 5 to 7 weeks following fetal infection, and subsequent replication of the virus in the kidney, for a detectable quantity of the virus to be secreted to the amniotic fluid.

If CMV is suspected, diagnosed because of fetal ultrasound findings, or the fetus is symptomatic, a more aggressive approach is warranted. An extended ultrasound should be performed. Consultations with maternal fetal medicine, neonatology, or infectious disease are useful for counseling parents about prognosis and outlining an approach to pregnancy management and neonatal issues.

**Maternal Treatment** Currently, there are no licensed treatments for pregnant women who become infected with CMV during pregnancy. Treatments that are effective against CMV infection in the nonpregnant population have serious side effects, are not approved for use in pregnant women, and have not been shown to prevent CMV infection in the fetus. Likewise, treatment with hyperimmune globulin does not significantly modify the course of primary CMV infection during pregnancy.

**Fetal Intervention** Symptomatic fetuses will not have the course of their infection altered by currently available treatments in utero. Intrauterine transfusion is a successful treatment for the rare case of fetal anemia secondary to CMV infection, although in these cases prognosis is poor with or without transfusion.

**Monitoring** In the setting of confirmed fetal CMV infection, interval ultrasound examinations should be performed to measure growth and exclude the development of sequelae of infection in the fetus, particularly in the central nervous system. In addition, the fetus can be monitored for the development of hydrops. These findings confer a worsening prognosis and warrant reconsultation with the parents and pediatric subspecialists and transfer to a tertiary center for delivery.

**Pregnancy Course** Most women with CMV are asymptomatic. Among those with influenza-like or hepatitis-like illness, supportive care ought to be given. Pregnancy course otherwise is unaltered.

**Pregnancy Termination Issues** If pregnancy termination is undertaken, fetal and placental tissues should be tested for CMV by PCR and have histopathologic examination.

**Delivery** The mode of delivery should be based on obstetric indications and will vary depending on the condition of the fetus. Delivery should be at a tertiary center for symptomatic fetuses.

## NEONATOLOGY

**Resuscitation** In the absence of respiratory distress, significant hydrops, or severe anemia, resuscitative efforts are usually not required. Premature infants born with congenital CMV are more likely to present with pneumonitis and may require respiratory support

**Transport** In symptomatic infants, transfer to a tertiary center with neonatology and pediatric infectious disease subspecialists is indicated. Infants with hydrops or CMV pneumonitis may require ventilatory assistance in transit.

**Testing and Confirmation** Laboratory diagnosis of congenital CMV infection is accomplished by isolation or molecular detection of CMV from urine or saliva samples collected within the first 3 weeks of life. Both viral culture and PCR tests have high sensitivity and specificity for detection of CMV in infected neonates.

**Nursery Management** Although infants born prematurely or with severe disease at birth have an increased risk of morbidity and mortality, most infants with congenital CMV infection are asymptomatic. Approximately 10% of infected neonates have symptoms at birth. Clinical findings may include petechiae, jaundice, hepatosplenomegaly, small for gestational age, and microcephaly. In symptomatic infants with congenital CMV, common laboratory findings include thrombocytopenia, hemolytic anemia, elevated transaminases, and conjugated hyperbilirubinemia. Abdominal ultrasound may demonstrate intrahepatic calcifications. Findings on cranial imaging (magnetic resonance imaging [MRI], head ultrasound, or computed tomographic [CT] scan) include periventricular intracranial calcifications, ventriculomegaly, lenticulostriate vasculopathy, migrational abnormalities, or periventricular leukomalacia. Chorioretinitis is the most common ophthalmologic abnormality in symptomatic infants. Abnormalities on cranial imaging or the presence of chorioretinitis correlates with poor neurodevelopmental outcome.

Congenital CMV is the leading cause of sensorineural hearing loss in infants. Sensorineural hearing loss occurs in 33% to 50% of symptomatic infants. Infants with symptomatic congenital CMV require routine serial hearing screens, as the sensorineural hearing loss may be progressive.

Antiviral treatment with ganciclovir and valganciclovir is recommended for symptomatic infants with virologically proven CMV infection and at least one end-organ symptom. Antiviral treatment in symptomatic infants has been shown to improve both long-term audiologic and neurodevelopmental outcomes.

## SUGGESTED READINGS

1. Benoist G, Salomon LJ, Mohlo M, et al: Cytomegalovirus in related fetal brain lesions: comparison between targeted ultrasound examination and magnetic resonance imaging. Ultrasound Obstet Gynecol 2008; 32:900-905.
2. Benoist G, Salomon LJ, Jacquemard F, et al: The prognostic values of ultrasound abnormalities and biologic parameters in blood of fetuses infected with cytomegalovirus. Br J Obstet Gynaecol 2008; 115:823-829.
3. Benoist G, Ville Y: Features of the congenital CMV infection in the unborn and newborn infant. Fetal Matern Med Rev 2007; 18:181-199.
4. Casteels A, Naessens A, Gordts F, et al: Neonatal screening for congenital cytomegalovirus infections. J Perinat Med 1999; 27:116-121.
5. Drose JA, Dennis MA, Thickman D: Infection in utero: US findings in 19 cases. Radiology 1991; 178:369-374.
6. Fakhry J, Khoury A: Fetal intracranial calcifications: the importance of periventricular hyperechoic foci without shadowing. J Ultrasound Med 1991; 10:51-54.
7. Goderis J, De Leenheer E, Smets K, et al. Hearing loss and congenital CMV infection: a systematic review. Pediatrics 2014; 134:972-982.
8. Guerra B, Lazzarotto T, Quarta S, et al: Prenatal diagnosis of symptomatic congenital cytomegalovirus infection. Am J Obstet Gynecol 2000; 183:476-482.
9. Hohlfeld P, Vial Y, Maillard-Brignon C, et al: Cytomegalovirus fetal infection: prenatal diagnosis. Obstet Gynecol 1991; 78:615-618.
10. Kimberlin DW, Jester PM, Sánchez PJ, et al. Valganciclovir for symptomatic congenital cytomegalovirus disease. N Engl J Med 2015; 372:933-943.
11. Kumar ML, Nankervis GA, Jacobs IB, et al: Congenital and postnatally acquired cytomegalovirus infections: long-term follow-up. J Pediatr 1984; 104:675-679.
12. Lazzarotto T, Varani S, Guerra B, et al: Prenatal indicators of congenital cytomegalovirus infection. J Pediatr 2000; 137:90-95.
13. Liesnard C, Donner C, Brancart F, et al: Prenatal diagnosis of congenital cytomegalovirus infection: prospective study of 237 pregnancies at risk. Obstet Gynecol 2000; 95:881-888.

14. Malinger G, Lev D, Zahalka N, et al: Fetal cytomegalovirus infections of the brain: the spectrum of sonographic findings. Am J Neuroradiol 2003; 24:28-32.

15. Revello MG, Lazzarotto T, Guerra B, et al. CHIP Study Group. A randomized trial of hyperimmune globulin to prevent congenital cytomegalovirus. N Engl J Med. 2014; 370:1316-1326.

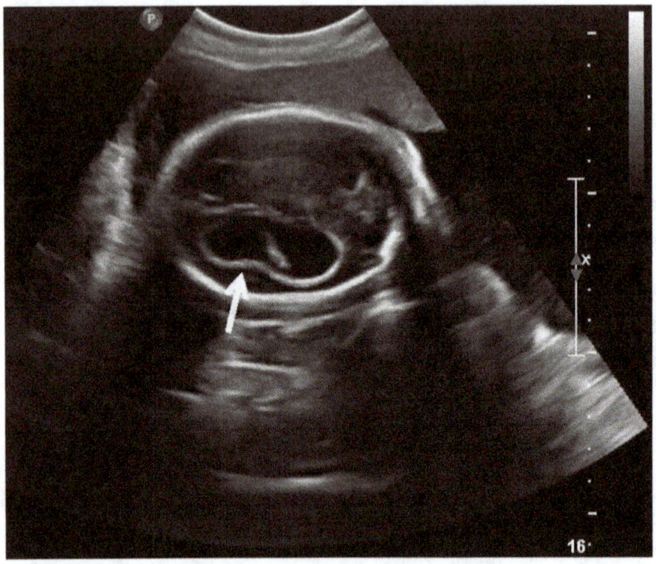


**FIGURE 9.1A** Cytomegalovirus. Periventricular "halo" (arrow) associated with white matter necrosis.

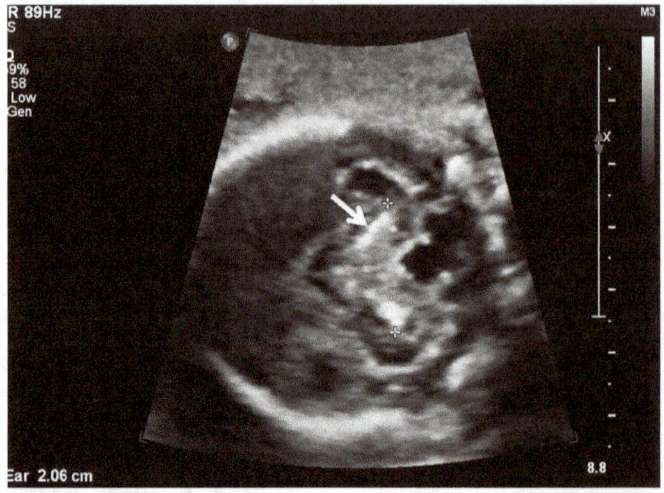


**FIGURE 9.1B** Cytomegalovirus. Cerebellar calcifications (arrow).

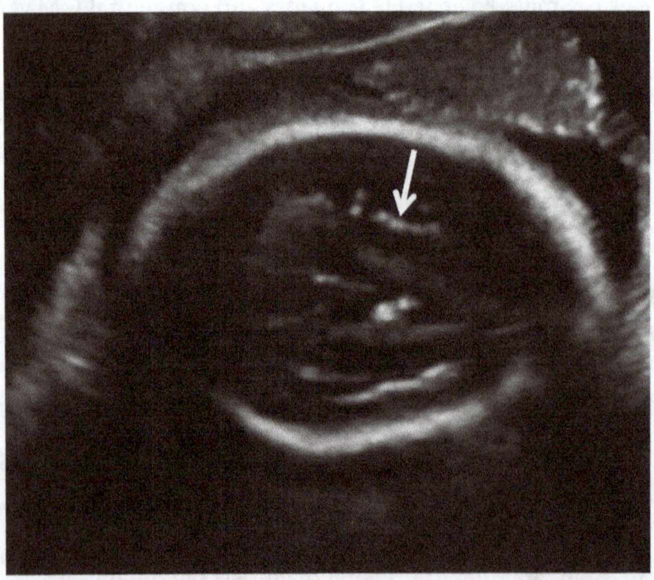

**FIGURE 9.1C** Cytomegalovirus. Periventricular calcifications (arrow).

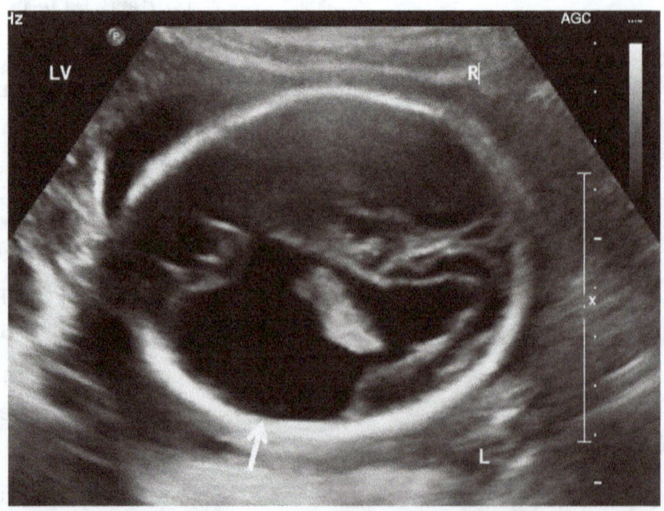


**FIGURE 9.1D** Cytomegalovirus. Porencephalic cyst (arrow).

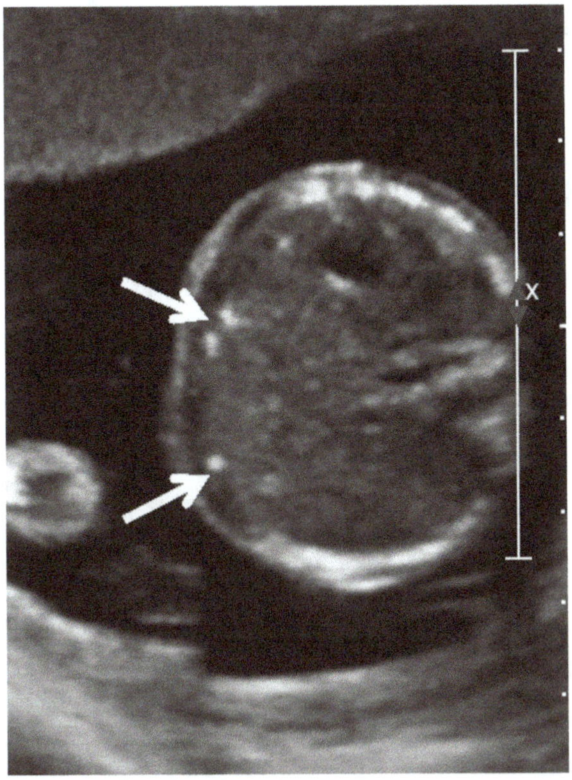


**FIGURE 9.1E** Cytomegalovirus. Hepatic calcifications (arrows).

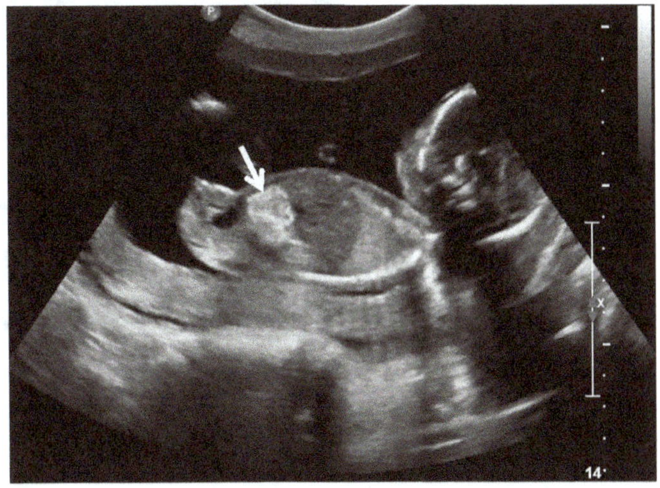


**FIGURE 9.1F** Cytomegalovirus. Echogenic small bowel (arrow).

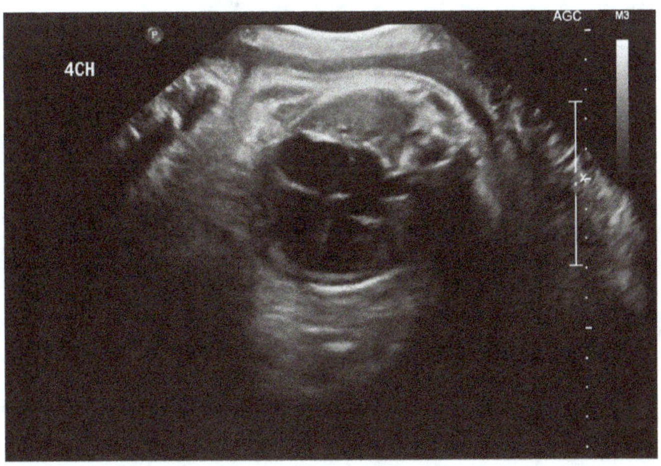


**FIGURE 9.1G** Cytomegalovirus cardiomegaly.

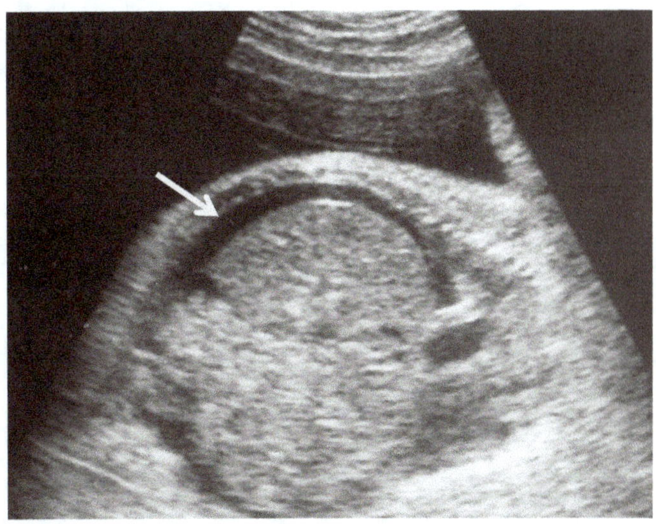

**FIGURE 9.1H** Cytomegalovirus ascites (arrow).

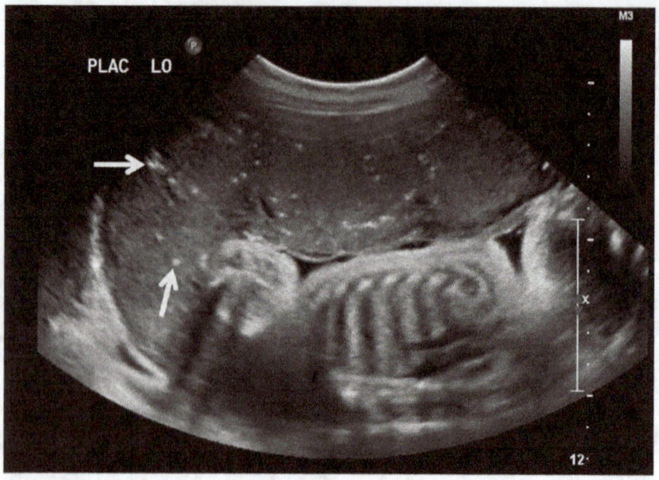


**FIGURE 9.1I** Cytomegalovirus. Placental microcalcifications (arrows).

# 9.2 PARVOVIRUS

## EPIDEMIOLOGY/GENETICS

**Definition** Parvovirus B19 is a small, nonenveloped DNA virus that exclusively infects humans. After infection, parvovirus B19 replication occurs primarily in erythrocytes and erythroblasts, which can lead to anemia in predisposed individuals. Children who are infected with parvovirus B19 typically develop erythema infectiosum (fifth disease) that is characterized by a "slapped-cheek" rash, low-grade fever, and mild influenza-like symptoms. Infected healthy adults generally have mild constitutional symptoms only. In contrast, immune-compromised individuals, including fetuses, can develop severe chronic anemia requiring directed therapies.

**Epidemiology** Transmission occurs via respiratory secretions. Although outbreaks may occur sporadically year-round, they are most prevalent in childcare facilities or schools in the spring. Infection transmitted in utero from a susceptible mother to the immune-incompetent fetus is recognized as an infrequent cause of fetal morbidity and mortality. Risk factors for maternal infection include large number of children in the household and occupational exposure (such as teacher or day-care worker). Fetal parvovirus B19 infection can cause spontaneous abortion in the early part of pregnancy and nonimmune hydrops fetalis secondary to aplastic anemia later in pregnancy.

**Prognosis** There is a 10% risk of fetal death due to hydrops secondary to severe fetal anemia. The risk of fetal death in utero is 17% before 20 weeks' gestation and 6% after 20 weeks. Most infected women give birth to normal neonates.

## SONOGRAPHY

### FREQUENT FINDINGS

- Hydrops
  - Pleural effusion
  - Pericardial effusion
  - Anasarca
  - Scalp edema
- Placentomegaly
- Polyhydramnios
- Cardiomegaly

### LESS FREQUENT

- Ventriculomegaly
- Microcephaly
- Hepatosplenomegaly
- Hepatic calcifications
- Echogenic small bowel

### KEY FINDINGS/PITFALLS

- The peak systolic velocity in the middle cerebral artery is elevated with severe anemia.
- The risk of hydrops decreases from 5% to 10% in the first trimester to 1% at 20 weeks' gestation.
- Hydrops develops between 3 and 12 weeks after maternal infection.
- Most cases of hydrops occur between 16 and 32 weeks' gestation.

## PREGNANCY MANAGEMENT

For women who report an exposure to an individual with parvovirus B19, we suggest following the screening and surveillance algorithm as outlined in the figure that follows.

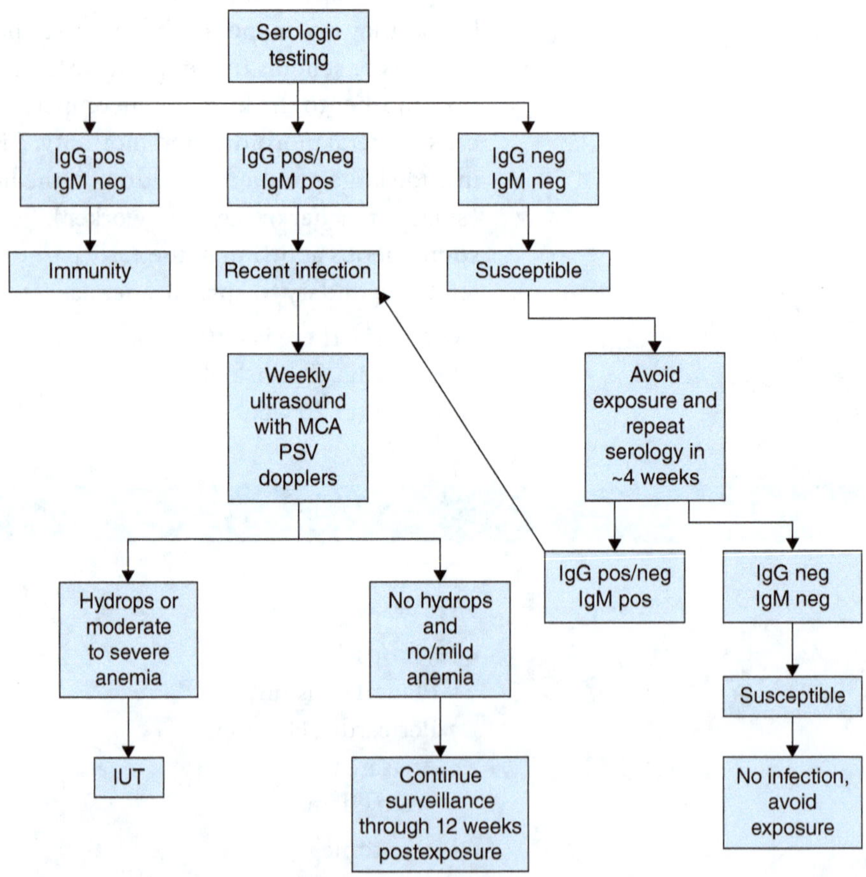


IUT: Intrauterine transfusion
MCA PSV: Middle cerebral artery peak systolic velocity

Pos: Positive
Neg: Negative

**Investigations and Consultations Required** Patients who are noted to have serologic confirmation of recent infection should be referred to a perinatal center that is equipped to perform sonographic surveillance for fetal anemia with middle cerebral artery peak systolic velocity.

**Maternal Treatment** There are no applicable antiviral therapies, vaccines, or immunological therapies during pregnancy or in the neonatal period.

**Monitoring** The serologic and sonographic surveillance strategy, as outlined in the figure, is recommended for monitoring.

**Fetal Intervention** Intrauterine transfusion is a successful treatment for fetal anemia secondary to parvovirus infection. Serial transfusions may be necessary, but as the infection is self-limited, they will not be necessary throughout the remainder of the pregnancy. Once the anemia has resolved with or without the need for transfusion, interval follow-up ultrasound examinations to monitor fetal growth and possible sequelae of the infection are warranted.

**Pregnancy Course** For women with maternal symptoms related to parvovirus infection, supportive care is reasonable, with antipyretics and analgesics for symptomatic relief. In pregnancies with an infected fetus, once the anemia is treated with transfusions, no other pregnancy complications are expected.

**Pregnancy Termination Issues** If pregnancy termination is undertaken, fetal and placental tissues should be tested for parvovirus B19 by PCR and histopathologic examination.

**Delivery** The mode of delivery should be based on obstetric indications and will vary depending on condition of the fetus.

## NEONATOLOGY

**Resuscitation** Respiratory depression and distress requiring mechanical ventilation are likely if hydrops or severe anemia is present. Resuscitative efforts, including drainage of pleural, pericardial, or peritoneal fluid, may be required at the time of delivery.

**Transport** Neonatal transport is indicated for treatment of respiratory distress, severe anemia, or hydrops. The infant may require ventilatory assistance in transit.

**Nursery Management** In the presence of hydrops or severe anemia, packed red blood cells or whole blood cross-matched with the mother's blood should be available for transfusion or partial exchange transfusion to correct severe anemia. Metabolic derangements, such as acidosis and hypoglycemia, should be anticipated and promptly corrected. Surfactant deficiency and hypoplastic lungs may be associated with hydrops and are managed with intubation and mechanical ventilation to provide respiratory support. Drainage of the pleural and abdominal cavities of pleural and ascitic fluid, respectively, may be necessary to adequately ventilate the infant. The infant may require prolonged respiratory assistance with mechanical ventilation. Umbilical arterial and venous catheters to monitor arterial pressure, blood gases, and venous pressure should be placed on delivery. Cranial imaging to assess for intracranial abnormalities, echocardiogram to assess for cardiac dysfunction, and abdominal ultrasound to detect the presence of intrahepatic calcifications are indicated.

## SUGGESTED READINGS

1. Cosmi E, Mari G, Delle Chiaie L, Detti L, et al: Non-invasive diagnosis by Doppler ultrasonography of fetal anemia resulting from parvovirus infection. Am J Obstet Gynecol 2002; 187:1290-1293.

2. Enders M, Weidner A, Zoellner I, et al: Fetal morbidity and mortality after acute human parvovirus B19 infection in pregnancy: prospective evaluation of 1018 cases. Prenat Diagn 2004; 24:513-518.
3. Harger JH, Adler SP, Koch WC, Harger GF: Prospective evaluation of 618 pregnant women exposed to parvovirus B19: risks and symptoms. Obstet Gynecol 1998: 91:413-420.
4. Kumar ML: Human parvovirus B19 and its associated diseases. Clin Perinatol 1991; 18:209-225.
5. Parovirus B19 infection in pregnancy. SOGC Clinical Practice Guidelines No. 199. J Obstet Gynaecol Can 2002; 24:727-734.
6. Prospective study of human parvovirus (B19) infection in pregnancy. Public Health Laboratory Service Working Party on Fifth Disease. BMJ 1990; 300:1166-1170.
7. Pryde PG, Nugent CE, Prijian G, et al: Spontaneous resolution of non-immune hydrops fetalis secondary to human parvovirus B19 infection. Obstet Gynecol 1992; 79:859-861.
8. Rodis JF, Quinn DL, Gary GW Jr, et al: Management and outcomes of pregnancies complicated by human B19 parvovirus infection: a prospective study. Am J Obstet Gynecol 1990; 163:1168-1171.
9. Schild R, Bald R, Plath H, et al: Intrauterine management of fetal parvovirus B19 infection. Ultrasound Obstet Gynecol 1999; 13:161-166.
10. Sheikh AU, Ernest JM, O'Shea M: Long-term outcome in fetal hydrops from parvovirus B19 infection. Am J Obstet Gynecol 1992; 167:337-341.
11. Von Kaiserburg CS, Jonat W: Fetal parvovirus infection. Ultrasound Obstet Gynecol 2001; 18:280-288.


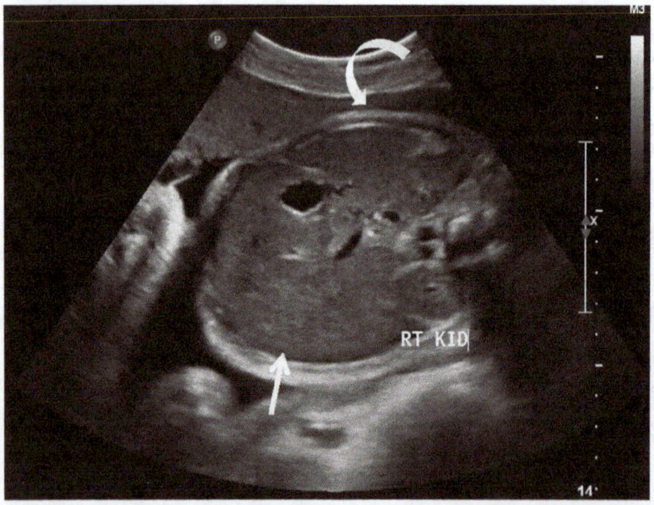


**FIGURE 9.2A** Parvovirus. Hepatomegaly (straight arrow) and splenomegaly (curved arrow).

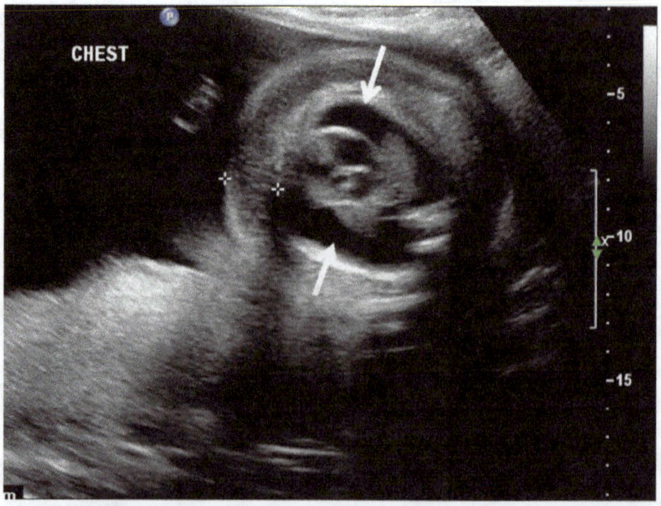


**FIGURE 9.2B** Parvovirus. Anasarca (+ … +) and bilateral pleural effusions (arrows).

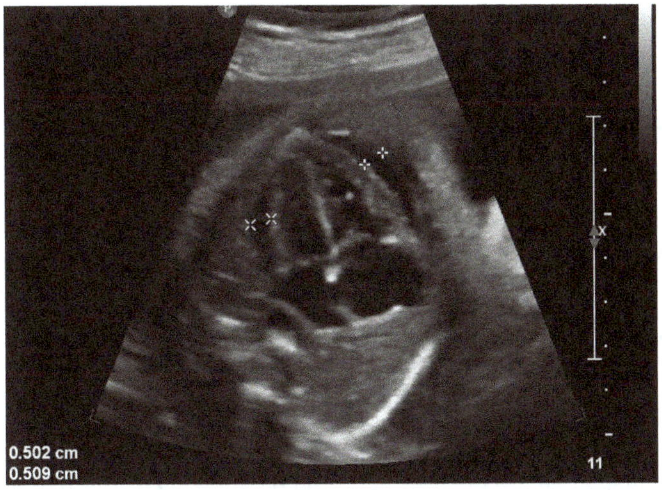


FIGURE 9.2C Parvovirus. Cardiomegaly with a pericardial effusion (+ … +).

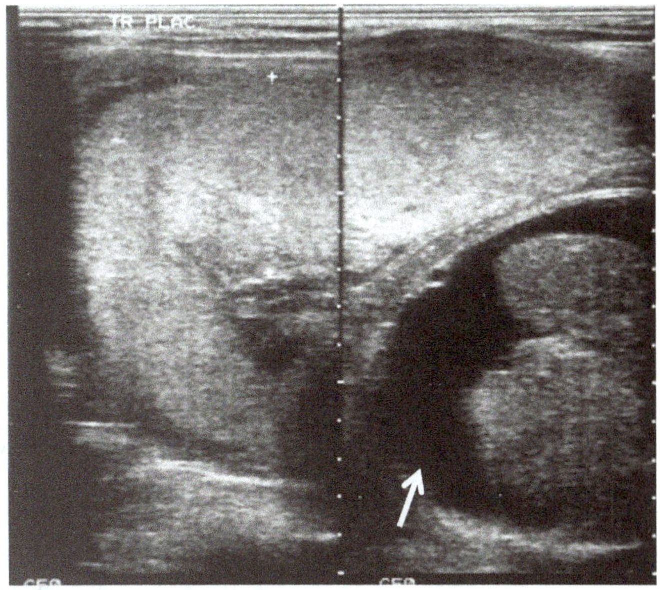


FIGURE 9.2D Parvovirus. Placentomegaly (+ … +). Fetal ascites (arrow).

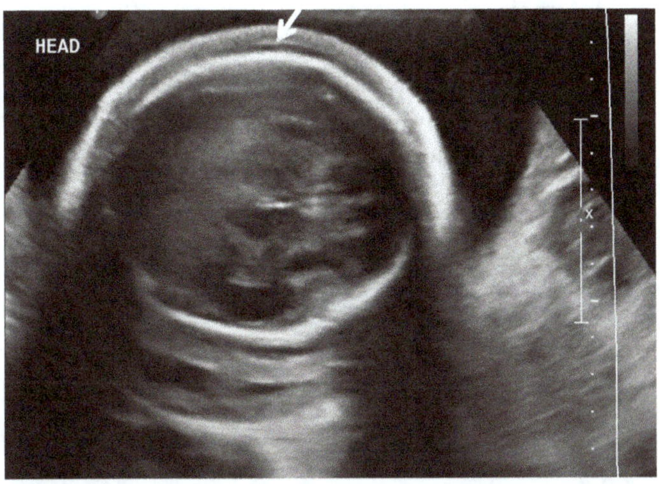


FIGURE 9.2E Parvovirus. Scalp edema (arrow).

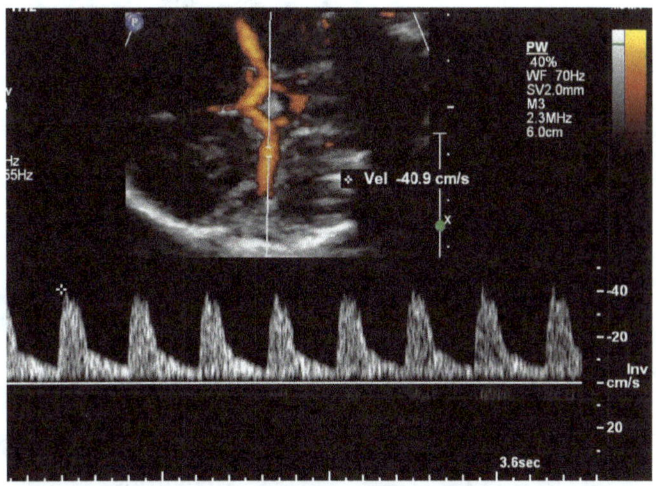


FIGURE 9.2F Parvovirus. Color Doppler of the middle cerebral artery indicating increased peak systolic velocity, consistent with severe anemia.

# 9.3 SYPHILIS, CONGENITAL

## EPIDEMIOLOGY/GENETICS

**Definition** Syphilis is a systemic disease caused by *Treponema pallidum*. The disease has been divided into stages based on clinical findings that help to guide treatment and follow-up.

**Epidemiology** Persons who have syphilis might seek treatment for signs or symptoms of primary syphilis infection (i.e., ulcers or chancre); secondary syphilis (i.e., manifestations that include, but are not limited to, skin rash, mucocutaneous lesions, and lymphadenopathy); or tertiary syphilis (i.e., cardiac, gummatous lesions, tabes dorsalis, and general paresis). Latent infections (i.e., those lacking clinical manifestations) are detected by serologic testing. Latent syphilis acquired within the preceding year is referred to as early latent syphilis; all other cases of latent syphilis are late latent syphilis or syphilis of unknown duration.

**Prognosis** In the absence of timely and effective penicillin treatment, congenital syphilis occurs in about 50% of babies of women with primary or secondary syphilis during pregnancy. Maternal early latent syphilis carries a ~40% risk of congenital syphilis, and late latent carries ~10% risk of congenital syphilis. Adequate maternal treatment during pregnancy reduces, but does not eradicate, the risk of congenital syphilis. The clinical spectrum in congenital syphilis includes stillbirth/neonatal death, clinically apparent congenital syphilis during the first few months of life, and late congenital syphilis.

## SONOGRAPHY

### FREQUENT FINDINGS

- Hepatosplenomegaly
- Hydrops
  - Pleural effusion
  - Pericardial effusion
  - Ascites
  - Anasarca

### LESS FREQUENT

- Intracerebral calcifications
- Echogenic bowel
- Bowel dilatation secondary to enterocolitis
- Hepatic calcifications
- Long-bone shortening
- Abnormal curvature of the long bones with focal bowing
- Placentomegaly
- Polyhydramnios

### KEY FINDINGS/PITFALLS

- The risk of fetal acquisition increases with gestational age.
- Ultrasound stigmata of fetal syphilis are only consistently identified after 18 to 20 weeks' gestation, that is, after the fetus can develop an inflammatory reaction to disease.
- A normal ultrasound does not rule out a congenitally infected neonate.

## PREGNANCY MANAGEMENT

**Investigations and Consultations Required** All women should be screened serologically for syphilis early in pregnancy. Pregnant women with reactive treponemal screening tests should have additional quantitative nontreponemal testing because titers are essential for monitoring treatment response. For communities and populations in which the prevalence of syphilis is high and for women at high risk for infection, serologic testing should also be performed twice during the third trimester: once at 28 to 32 weeks' gestation and again at delivery. Any woman who has a fetal death after 20 weeks' gestation should be tested for syphilis. When syphilis is confirmed with serologic testing, referral to maternal-fetal medicine or infectious disease specialist is advisable. An extended ultrasound examination should be performed.

**Fetal Intervention** There is no intervention suggested other than treatment of the mother with penicillin.

**Monitoring** Ultrasound will detect abnormalities in some, but not all, infected fetuses. Fetuses with this diagnosis should undergo an extended ultrasound examination in the second trimester and follow-up examinations at intervals thereafter, directed at the stigmata of congenital syphilis. Even if these were not present when therapy was initiated, these findings may develop later in gestation.

**Pregnancy Course** The course of pregnancy is largely driven by the course of syphilis. In the presence of timely and adequate treatment and improvement of titers, the probability of progression to neurosyphilis is low. Penicillin is the drug of choice for the treatment of syphilis in pregnant (and nonpregnant) women. No proven alternatives to penicillin are available for treatment of syphilis during pregnancy. Pregnant women who have a history of penicillin allergy should be desensitized and treated with penicillin. The recommended regimens are as follows:

- Early syphilis (primary, secondary, and latent syphilis of less than 1 year's duration)
  - Penicillin G benzathine 2.4 million units IM given once
- Syphilis of more than 1 year's duration
  - Penicillin G benzathine 2.4 million units IM weekly for 3 doses (total 7.2 million units)
- Neurosyphilis
  - Aqueous crystalline penicillin G 2-4 million units IV every 4 hours for 10-14 days, followed by penicillin G benzathine 2.4 million units IM one time

OR

- Aqueous penicillin G procaine 2.4 million units IM daily plus probenicid 500 mg orally four times a day, both for 10-14 days, followed by penicillin G benzathine 2.4 million units IM one time

Women treated for syphilis during the second half of pregnancy are at risk for premature labor or fetal distress if the treatment precipitates the Jarisch-Herxheimer reaction. It usually manifests within a few hours of the first dose of antibiotic as fever, chills, rigor, hypotension, headache, and tachycardia. These women should be advised to seek obstetric attention after treatment if they notice any fever, contractions, or decrease in fetal movements. Clinical and serologic evaluation should be performed at 6 and 12 months after treatment.

**Pregnancy Termination Issues** If pregnancy termination is undertaken, fetal and placental tissues should be tested for syphilis with molecular testing, and histopathologic examination.

**Delivery** The mode of delivery should be based on obstetric indications and will vary depending on the condition of the fetus. For symptomatic fetuses, delivery should be at a tertiary center.

## NEONATOLOGY

**Resuscitation** In the absence of other conditions, resuscitative efforts are not usually required.

**Transport** Care in a tertiary center, with expertise in diagnosing and treating congenital syphilis, is advisable in the event of untreated or incompletely treated maternal syphilis or with antenatally identified fetal features of congenital syphilis.

**Testing and Confirmation** All neonates born to mothers who have reactive nontreponemal and treponemal test results should be evaluated with a quantitative nontreponemal serologic test (RPR [rapid plasma reagin] or VDRL) performed on the neonate's serum. Conducting a treponemal test (i.e., TP-PA, [treponema pallidum particle agglutination], fluorescent treponemal antibody absorption [FTA-ABS] test, enzyme immunoassay [EIA], or chemiluminescence immunoassay [CIA]) on neonatal serum is not recommended because it is difficult to interpret. No commercially available immunoglobulin (IgM) test can be recommended.

**Nursery Management** The Centers for Disease Control and Prevention (CDC) continues to update the guidelines for treatment of congenital syphilis in neonates. Penicillin remains the drug of choice. The use of alternative antibiotics requires close serologic follow-up to assess the adequacy of therapy. All neonates with reactive nontreponemal tests should receive careful follow-up examinations and serologic testing (i.e., nontreponemal test) every 2-3 months until the test becomes nonreactive. If the nontreponemal test is still reactive at 6 months, the infant is likely to be infected and should be retreated.

## SUGGESTED READINGS


1. Barton JR, Thorpe EM Jr, Shaver DC, et al: Nonimmune hydrops fetalis associated with maternal infection with syphilis. Am J Obstet Gynecol 1992; 167:56-58.
2. Centers for Disease Control and Prevention: Congenital syphilis. MMWR Morb Mortal Wkly Rep 1989; 38:825-829.
3. Crino JP: Ultrasound and fetal diagnosis of perinatal infection. Clin Obstet Gynecol 1999; 42:71-80.
4. Hill LM, Maloney JB: An unusual constellation of sonographic findings associated with congenital syphilis. Obstet Gynecol 1991; 78:895-897.
5. Hollier LM, Harstad TW, Sanchez PJ: Fetal syphilis: clinical laboratory characteristics. Obstet Gynecol 2001; 97:447-453.
6. Minkoff HL: Preventing fetal damage from sexually transmitted diseases. Clin Obstet Gynecol 1991; 34:336-344.
7. Nathan L, Bohman VR, Sanchez PJ, et al: In utero infection with *Treponema pallidum* in early pregnancy. Prenat Diagn 1997; 17:119-123.
8. Nathan L, Twickler DM, Peters MT, et al: Fetal syphilis: correlation of sonographic findings and rabbit infectivity testing of amniotic fluid. J Ultrasound Med 1993; 12:97-101.
9. Raafat NA, Birch AA, Altieri LA, et al: Sonographic osseous manifestations of fetal syphilis: a case report. J Ultrasound Med 1993; 12:783-785.
10. Rac MNF, Bryant SN, McIntire DD, et al: Progression of ultrasound findings of fetal syphilis after maternal treatment. Am J Obstet Gynecol 2014; 211:426.e1-6.
11. Simchen MJ, Toi A, Bona M, et al: Fetal hepatic calcifications: prenatal diagnosis and outcome. Am J Obstet Gynecol 2002; 187:1617-1622.


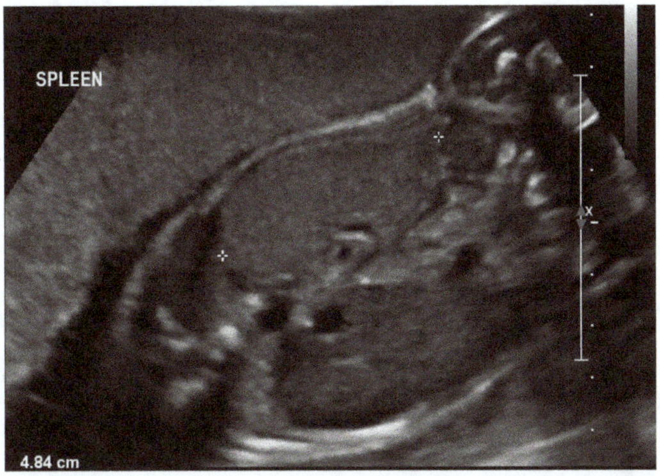


**FIGURE 9.3A** Syphilis. Splenomegaly (+ … +).

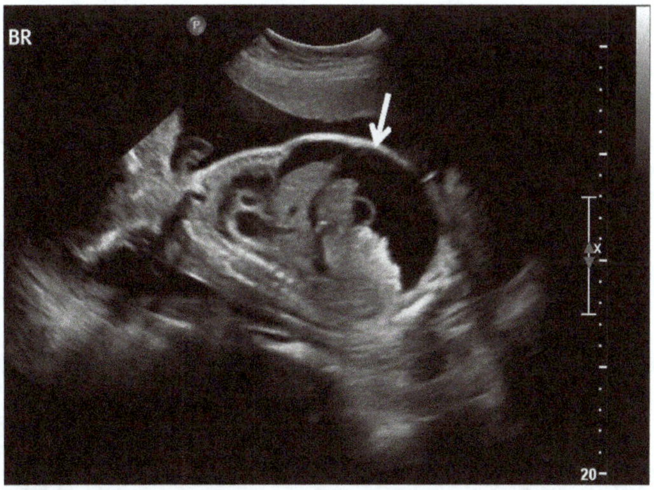


**FIGURE 9.3B** Syphilis. Ascites (arrow).

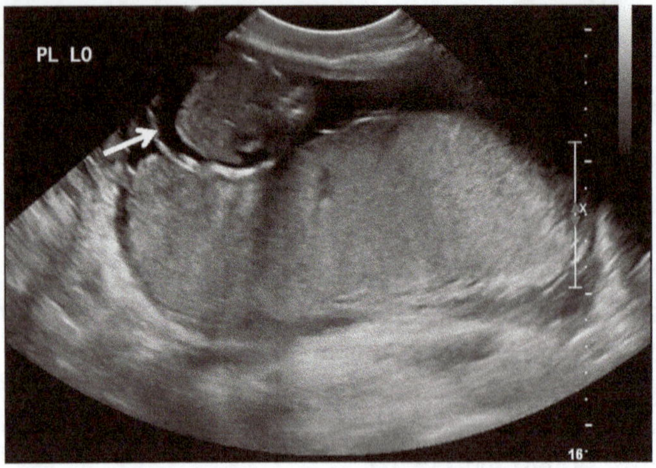


**FIGURE 9.3C** Syphilis. Fetal ascites (arrow) and placentomegaly.

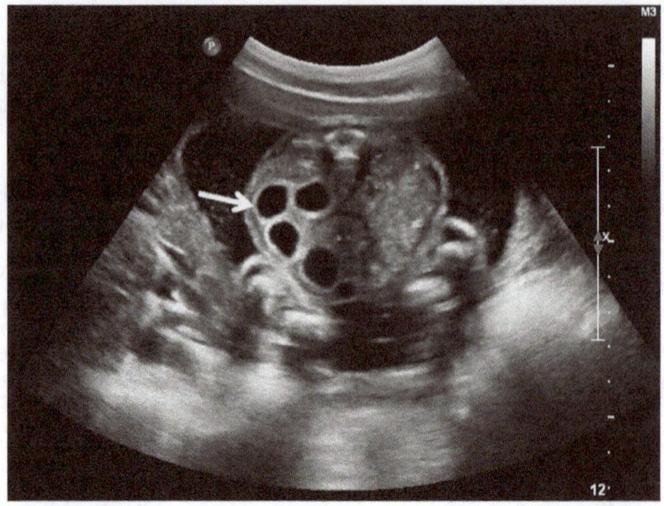


**FIGURE 9.3D** Syphilis. Dilated loops of small bowel (arrow).

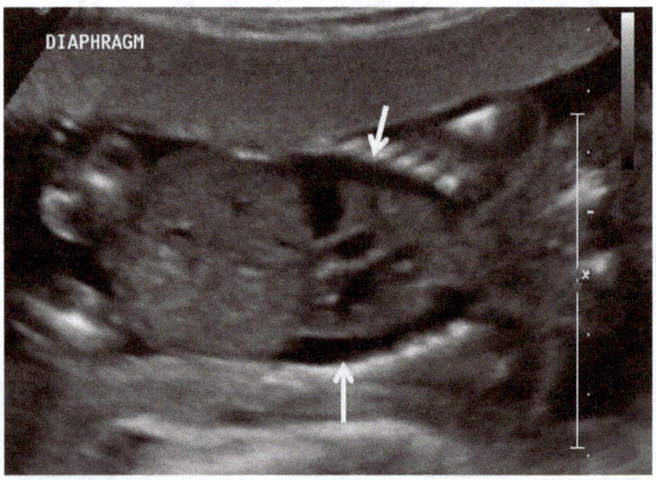


**FIGURE 9.3E** Syphilis. Bilateral pleural effusions (arrows).

# 9.4 TOXOPLASMOSIS

## EPIDEMIOLOGY/GENETICS

**Definition** Toxoplasmosis is an infection caused by the parasite *Toxoplasma gondii.*

**Epidemiology** The cat is the definitive host for *T. gondii.* Cats acquire toxoplasmosis by eating infected mice or other animals. In general, toxoplasmosis is thought to be most common in cats that go outdoors. Human infection may be acquired by consuming raw, or undercooked, meat of infected animals (particularly pork, beef, or lamb) or by contact with oocysts from the feces of an infected cat.

Seroprevalence of *Toxoplasma* varies across populations. In France, where consumption of raw or undercooked meat is common, seroprevalence is 55% to 65%. In the United States, however, seroprevalence is lower (~10% to 14%), with acute maternal infection in pregnancy occurring with a frequency of about 0.2% to 1%.

## SONOGRAPHY

### FREQUENT FINDINGS

- Central nervous system
  - Random intracerebral calcifications
  - Ventriculomegaly
- Hepatic calcifications

### LESS FREQUENT

- Microcephaly
- Microphthalmia
- Cataracts
- Hepatosplenomegaly
- Hydrops
  - Pleural effusions
  - Pericardial effusions
  - Ascites
  - Anasarca
  - Scalp edema

## PREGNANCY MANAGEMENT

**Investigations and Consultations Required** If the features on ultrasound are suspicious for toxoplasmosis and the patient's history is consistent with the diagnosis, an amniocentesis for polymerase chain reaction (PCR) *T. gondii* DNA should be performed at least 4 to 5 weeks after maternal exposure.

Real-time PCR is a rapid and more sensitive method for detecting *T. gondii* in amniotic fluid. If toxoplasmosis is suspected in a pregnant woman, serologic testing should be undertaken:

- A positive IgG titer indicates a prior toxoplasmosis infection with time of onset unknown.
- Serologic testing in the first trimester is preferred.
  - Serum samples obtained after the second trimester may not be able to exclude an infection early in the first trimester.
  - A positive IgG result and a negative IgM result essentially exclude a recent infection.
- A toxoplasmosis-specific IgM enzyme immunoassay (EIA) may be positive for 18 months after an acquired infection.
- Toxoplasmosis IgM testing lacks specificity.
  - An immunosorbent agglutination assay (ISAGA) is more sensitive and specific than the direct immunofluorescent test.
  - If a test for toxoplasmosis IgG is negative on two occasions with positive IgM results, the IgM result should be considered a false positive.
- Prior to the initiation of patient management for acute toxoplasmosis, all IgG/IgM positive tests should be submitted to a reference laboratory (Toxoplasmosis Serology Laboratory, Palo Alto, CA) for IgG avidity testing.
  - A high-avidity result in the first 12-16 weeks of pregnancy essentially rules out an infection acquired during gestation.
  - A low-avidity IgG is suspicious for a recent infection, but some patients have low-avidity IgG results for months after an acute infection.
- If serum testing is equivocal, a follow-up serum sample for parallel testing is usually obtained.

**Maternal Treatment** For women with acute *T. gondii* infection diagnosed at a reference laboratory during gestation, spiramycin is recommended (for the first and early second trimesters) or pyrimethamine/sulfadiazine and leucovorin (for late second and third trimesters). The effectiveness of maternal therapy on fetal outcome has not been adequately studied, but it is more likely to be effective in the absence of fetal manifestations on ultrasound.

**Fetal Intervention** No specific fetal interventions, except maternal medical treatment as noted previously, are advised in congenital toxoplasmosis.

**Monitoring** Sonographic surveillance for the development of fetal growth restriction or ventriculomegaly should be performed.

**Pregnancy Course** Pregnancy course is uncomplicated unless there is development of ventriculomegaly or growth restriction.

**Pregnancy Termination Issues** If pregnancy termination is undertaken, fetal and placental tissues should be tested for toxoplasmosis by PCR and histopathologic examination.

**Delivery** The mode of delivery should be based on obstetric indications and may vary depending on the condition of the fetus.

## NEONATOLOGY

**Resuscitation** Neonatal resuscitation and care should be anticipated based on the relevant findings that are identified prenatally.

**Transport** Delivery should take place in a tertiary center that is capable of the appropriate neonatal testing and treatment.

**Testing and Confirmation** Toxoplasma-specific laboratory tests for IgG, IgM (detected by enzyme-linked immunosorbent assay [ELISA] or ISAGA), Ig A, and IgE (detected by ELISA) should be obtained on both the mother and infant in suspected cases of congenital toxoplasmosis. The infant's peripheral blood white cells, cerebrospinal fluid, and amniotic fluid should be assayed for *T. gondii* by PCR assay in a reference laboratory. In the United States, the Toxoplasmosis Serology Laboratory at the Palo Alto Medical Foundation is suggested. Serial serologic testing during the first year of life is required for diagnosis when the initial results are equivocal.

**Nursery Management** Clinical findings associated with congenital toxoplasmosis include chorioretinitis, intracranial calcifications, fetal growth restriction, microcephaly, hepatosplenomegaly, ventriculomegaly, and hematologic abnormalities. Infants with suspected congenital toxoplasmosis require ophthalmologic evaluation and neurologic evaluation, consisting of cranial imaging, hearing screening, and a lumbar puncture to detect possible central nervous system involvement. Congenital toxoplasmosis should be treated with an antiparasitic regimen, consisting of sulfadiazine, pyrimethamine, and folinic acid supplementation. Referral to a pediatric infectious disease specialist is recommended for long-term follow-up and management.

## SUGGESTED READINGS

1. American Academy of Pediatrics: *Toxoplasma gondii* infections (Toxoplasmosis). In Kimberlin DW, ed. Red Book: 2015 Report of the Committee on Infectious Diseases. 30th ed. Elk Grove Village, IL: American Academy of Pediatrics; 2015: 787-796.
2. Bailao LA, Osborne NG, Rizzi MC, et al: Ultrasound markers of fetal infection. Part 2. Bacterial, parasitic, and fungal infections. Ultrasound Q 2006; 22:137-151.
3. Carter AO, Frank JW: Congenital toxoplasmosis: epidemiologic features and control. CMAJ 1986; 135:618-623.
4. Crino JP: Ultrasound and fetal diagnosis of perinatal infection. Clin Obstet Gynecol 1999; 42:71-80.
5. Daffos F, Forestier F, Capella-Pavlovsky M, et al: Prenatal management of 746 pregnancies at risk for congenital toxoplasmosis. N Engl J Med 1988; 318:271-275.
6. Desmonts G, Convreur J: Congenital toxoplasmosis: a prospective study of 378 pregnancies. N Engl J Med 1974; 290:1110-1116.

7. Friedman S, Ford-Jones LE, Toi A, et al: Congenital toxoplasmosis: prenatal diagnosis, treatment and postnatal outcome. Prenat Diagn 1999; 19:330-333.
8. Hohlfeld P, MacAleese J, Capella-Pavlovski M, et al: Fetal toxoplasmosis: ultrasonographic signs. Ultrasound Obstet Gynecol 1991; 1:241-244.
9. Pedreira DA, Diniz EM, Schultz R, et al: Fetal cataract in congenital toxoplasmosis. Ultrasound Obstet Gynecol 1999; 13:266-267.
10. Robert-Gangneux F, Gavinet MF, Ancelle T, et al: Value of prenatal diagnosis and early postnatal diagnosis of congenital toxoplasmosis: retrospective study of 110 cases. J Clin Microbiol 1999; 37:2893-2298.
11. Sever JL, Ellenberg JH, Ley AC, et al: Toxoplasmosis: maternal and pediatric findings in 23,000 pregnancies. Pediatrics 1988; 82:181-192.
12. Skinner FJ, Chatterton JM, Joss AW, et al: The use of an IgM immunosorbent agglutination assay to diagnose congenital toxoplasmosis. J Med Microbiol 1989; 28:125-128.
13. Wallon M, Franck J, Thulliez P, et al: Accuracy of real-time polymerase chain reaction for *Toxoplasmosis gondii* in amniotic fluid. Obstet Gynecol 2010; 115:727-733.

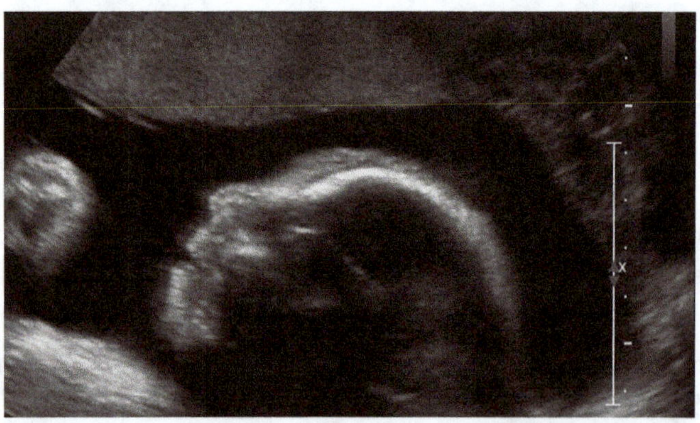

**FIGURE 9.4A** Toxoplasmosis. Sloping forehead indicative of microcephaly.

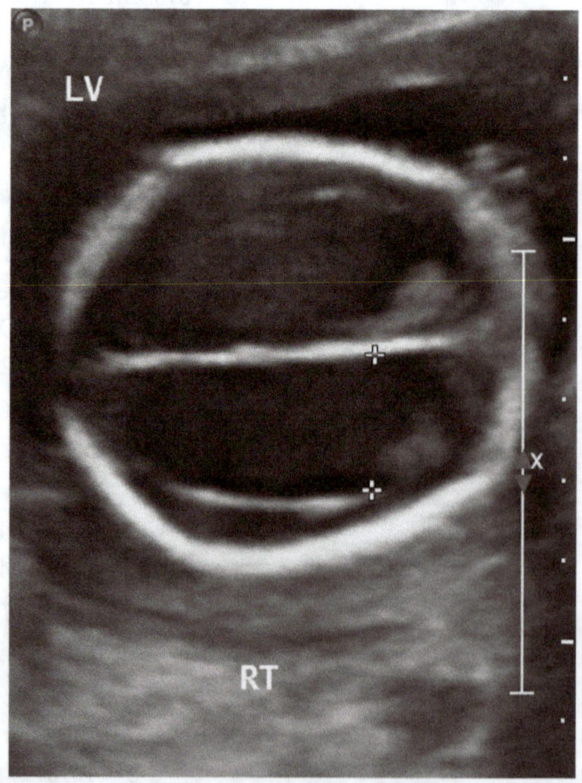


**FIGURE 9.4B** Toxoplasmosis. Ventriculomegaly (+ … +).

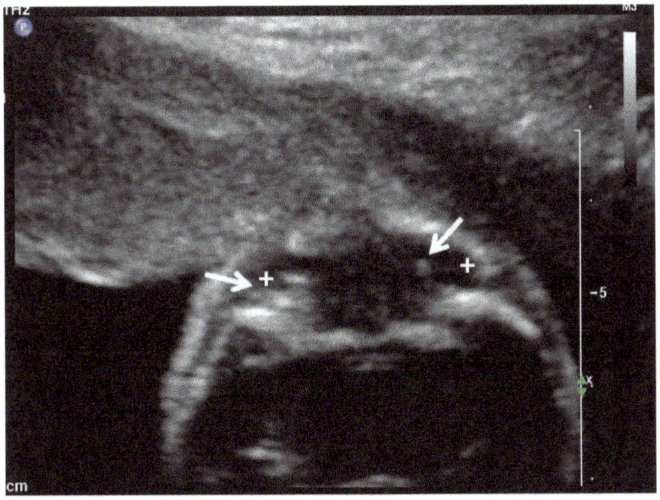


FIGURE 9.4C Toxoplasmosis. Cataracts (arrows).

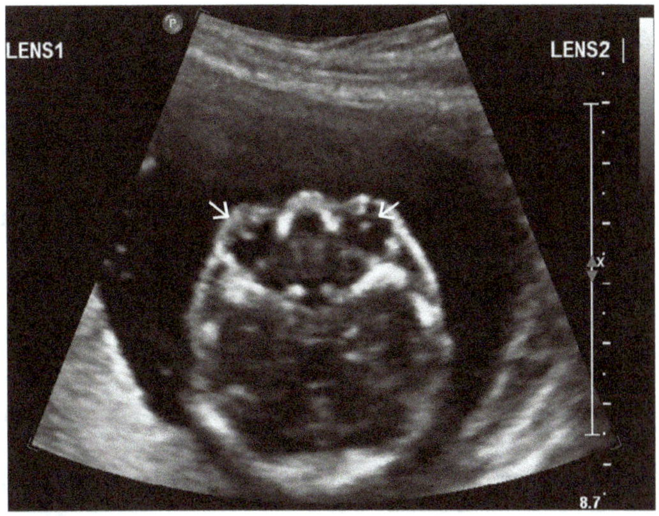


FIGURE 9.4D Toxoplasmosis. Normal lens (arrows).

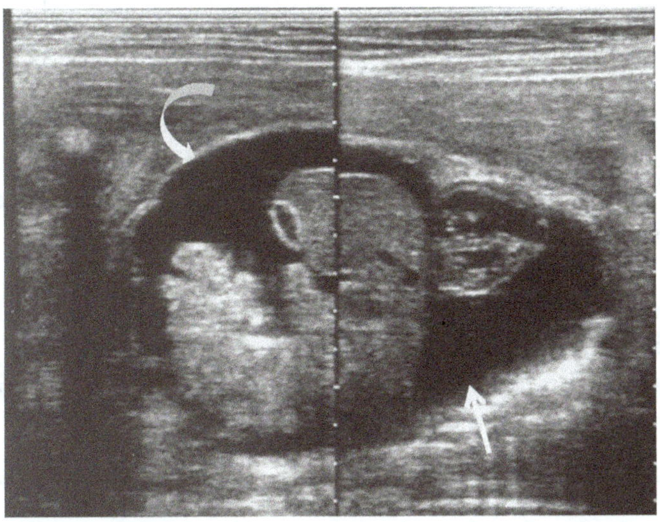

FIGURE 9.4E Toxoplasmosis. Plural effusion (straight arrow) and ascites (curved arrow).

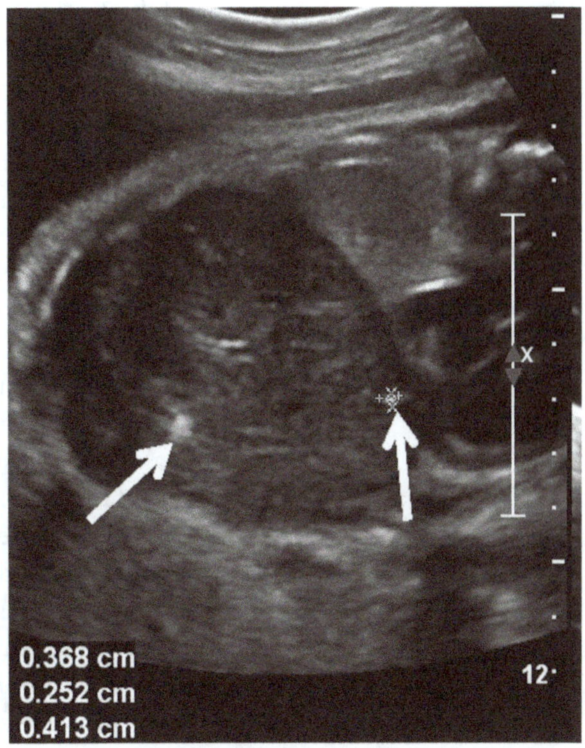


FIGURE 9.4F Toxoplasmosis. Hepatic calcifications (arrows).

# 9.5 VARICELLA

## EPIDEMIOLOGY/GENETICS

**Definition** Varicella zoster virus (VZV) is a member of the herpesvirus family and is a DNA virus.

**Epidemiology** Initial, or primary, infection with VZV results in varicella (chickenpox). Like other herpesviruses, VZV has the capacity to persist in the body after the primary infection as a latent infection. VZV persists in sensory nerve ganglia. Herpes zoster (shingles) is the result of reactivation of latent VZV infection.

Varicella is a human disease. No animal or insect source or vector is known to exist. In the United States, incidence is highest between March and May and lowest between September and November. Infection with VZV occurs through the respiratory tract. The most common mode of transmission of VZV is believed to be person to person from infected respiratory tract secretions. In adults, fever and generalized malaise typically precede the classic rash of chickenpox by several days. The rash typically begins on the face and scalp and spreads to the trunk, with generally minimal involvement of the extremities. The highly pruritic skin lesions vary in appearance based on their age, with progression from macules, to vesicles, then pustules, crusts, and scabs. Patients are contagious from 1 to 2 days prior to the onset of the rash until the lesions have become dried and crusted. The incubation period is 14 to 16 days after exposure, with a range of 10 to 21 days. Oral acyclovir or valacyclovir is recommended for mild maternal varicella in pregnancy. The most serious complication of varicella is pneumonia, occurring in 5% to 10% of adults with chickenpox. If unrecognized and untreated, varicella pneumonia carries significant morbidity and mortality risk to the mother. Hospitalization, respiratory evaluation and support, and intravenous acyclovir are recommended in the setting of respiratory symptoms in a pregnant woman with varicella.

Primary maternal varicella infection in the first 20 weeks of gestation is occasionally associated with abnormalities in the newborn, including low birth weight, hypoplasia of an extremity, skin scarring, localized muscular atrophy, encephalitis, cortical atrophy, chorioretinitis, and microcephaly. The risk of congenital abnormalities from primary maternal varicella infection appears to be very low (less than 2%).

## SONOGRAPHY

### FREQUENT FINDINGS

- Ventriculomegaly
- Cerebral calcifications
- Clubfeet
- Limb contractures
- Limb atrophy

- Decreased limb movement
- Polyhydramnios

### LESS FREQUENT

- Cataracts
- Microcephaly
- Microphthalmia
- Myocardial echogenicities
- Lung echogenicities
- Renal echogenicities
- Oligohydramnios

## PREGNANCY MANAGEMENT

**Investigations and Consultations Required** If the varicella syndrome is suspected, a history of recent chickenpox or exposure to someone with chickenpox or shingles should be ascertained. An infectious disease specialist should be consulted and IgG and IgM titers for varicella obtained. Amniotic fluid should be obtained and tested by PCR for varicella.

**Fetal intervention** No specific fetal interventions are indicated in congenital varicella.

**Monitoring** Serial sonography to assess for limb abnormalities, progressive ventriculomegaly, and fetal growth restriction should be performed. If these are found, the prognosis is poor. Antenatal consultations with neonatology and the appropriate pediatric subspecialty services may be helpful to the parents. Delivery should be planned at a tertiary center. In cases of intrauterine growth restriction, changes in obstetrical management, including antenatal testing, may be appropriate. There is no evidence that the initiation of antiviral medication to treat the fetus after these changes are found would affect outcome, and it is therefore not recommended.

**Pregnancy Termination Issues** If pregnancy termination is undertaken, fetal and placenta tissues should be tested for VZV by PCR and histopathology evaluation.

**Delivery** The mode of delivery should be based on obstetrical indications and will vary depending on the condition of the fetus.

## NEONATOLOGY

**Resuscitation** No specific issues are expected.

**Transport** Referral to a tertiary perinatal center is indicated if the infant is symptomatic or the diagnosis is uncertain.

**Testing and Confirmation** Anti–varicella zoster antibodies may persist after birth. VZV-specific IgM antibodies can be detected in cord blood, and VZV IgG may be detected in the newborn for up to 7 months after delivery. Evaluation for central nervous system, limb, and ophthalmic abnormalities is required.

**Nursery Management** Infants with congenital varicella syndrome require delineation of the extent of organ involvement and supportive care. Isolation of infants with structural defects secondary to varicella is not necessary as the virus is not shed. However, such infants may have episodic outbreaks of zoster skin lesions and become infectious while the lesions are acute. Treatment with acyclovir may be considered during such episodes.

## SUGGESTED READINGS

1. American Academy of Pediatrics: Varicella-zoster infections. In Kimberlin DW, ed. Red Book: 2015 Report of the Committee on Infectious Diseases. 30th ed. Elk Grove Village, IL: American Academy of Pediatrics; 2015: 846-860.
2. Bale J, Murphy J: Congenital infections and the nervous system. Pediatr Neurol 1992; 39:669-690.
3. Chapman SJ: Varicella in pregnancy. Semin Perinatol 1998; 22:339-346.
4. Hartung J, Enders G, Chaoui R, et al: Prenatal diagnosis of congenital varicella syndrome and detection of varicella-zoster virus in the fetus: a case report. Prenat Diagn 1999; 19:163-166.
5. Lamont RF, Sobel JD, Carrington D, et al: Varicella zoster virus (chickenpox) infection in pregnancy. Br J Obstet Gynaecol 2011; 118: 1155–1162.
6. Meyberg-Solomayer GC: Prenatal ultrasound diagnosis, follow-up, and outcome of congenital varicella syndrome. Fetal Diagn Ther 2006; 21:296-301.
7. Mouly F, Mirlesse V, Meritet JF, et al: Prenatal diagnosis of fetal varicella-zoster virus infection with polymerase chain reaction of amniotic fluid in 107 cases. Am J Obstet Gynecol 1997; 177:894-898.
8. Paryani SJ, Arvin AM: Intrauterine infection with varicella-zoster virus after maternal varicella. N Engl J Med 1986; 314:1542-1546.
9. Petignat P, Vial Y, Lavrini R, et al: Fetal varicella-herpes zoster syndrome in early pregnancy: ultrasonographic and morphological correlations. Prenat Diagn 2001; 21:121-124.
10. Pretorius DH, Hayward I, Jones KL, Stamm E: Sonographic evaluation of pregnancies with maternal varicella infection. J Ultrasound Med 1992; 11:459-463.
11. Sauerbrei A, Wutzler P: The congenital varicella syndrome. J Perinatol 2000; 20:548-554.
12. Sauerbrei A, Wutzler P: Herpes simplex and varicella-zoster virus infection during pregnancy: current concepts of prevention, diagnosis and therapy. Part II. Varicella-zoster virus infection. Med Microbiol Immunol 2007; 196:95-102.

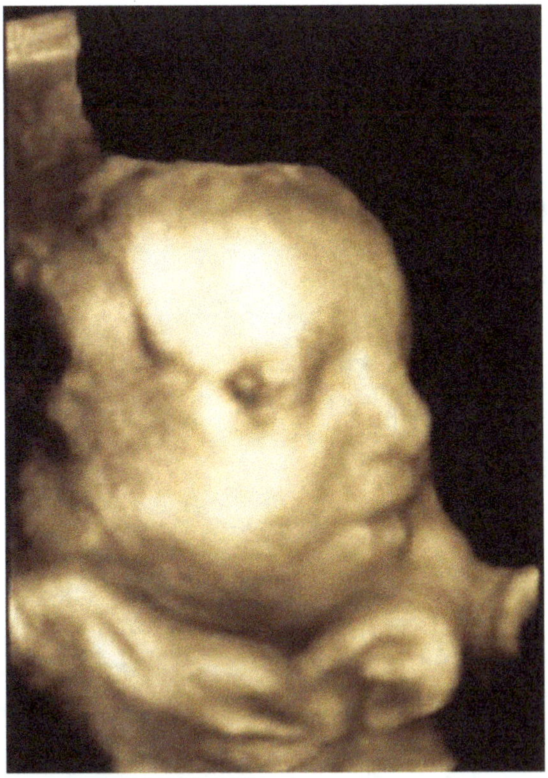

FIGURE 9.5A Varicella. Microcephaly.

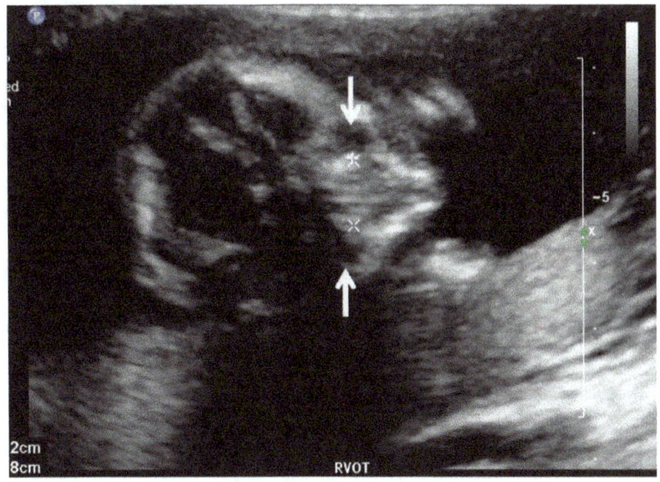


FIGURE 9.5B Varicella. Microphthalmia (arrows).

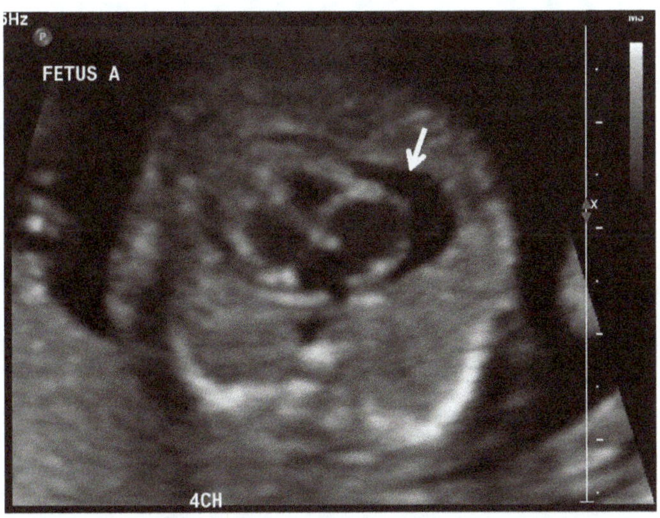


FIGURE 9.5C Varicella. Pericardial effusion (arrow).

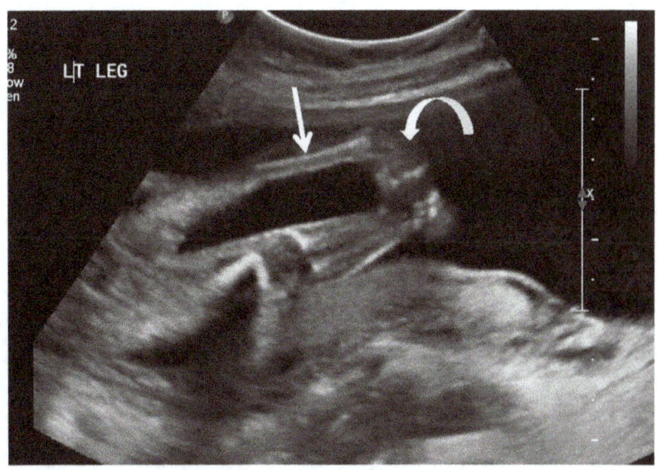


FIGURE 9.5D Varicella. Muscle atrophy (straight arrow) and clubfoot (curved arrow).

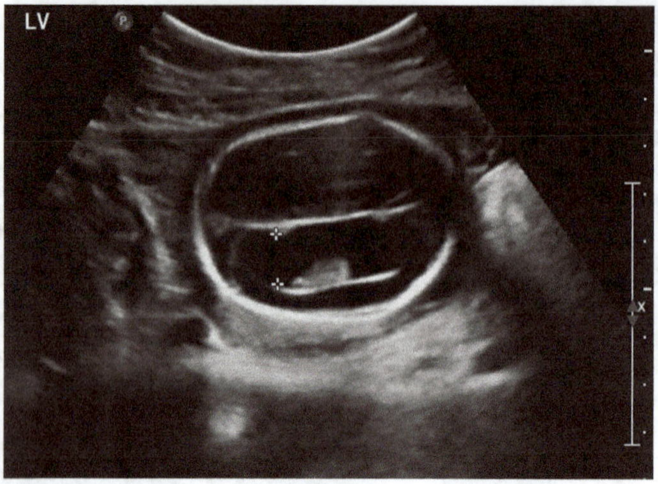


**FIGURE 9.5E** Varicella. Ventriculomegaly (+ … +).

# CHAPTER 10

# SYNDROMES

# 10.1 BECKWITH-WIEDEMANN SYNDROME

## EPIDEMIOLOGY/GENETICS

**Definition** Beckwith-Wiedemann syndrome (BWS) is a somatic overgrowth syndrome characterized by macrosomia, omphalocele, macroglossia, and ear creases.

**Epidemiology** Occurrence is 1 in 13,700 births (M1:F1).

**Embryology** BWS is caused by an imbalance of gene dosage involving a number of genes clustered at 11p15, a chromosomal region that is highly imprinted. Both genetic and epigenetic factors are implicated in the etiology of BWS. Microduplications and microdeletions on chromosome 11, as well as uniparental disomy, have been found in cases of BWS. Pregnancies conceived by assisted reproductive technologies have a higher incidence of BWS. Major malformations seen with BWS include ventral wall defects (omphalocele and umbilical hernia) and cleft palate. Congenital heart defects (20%) are common, with about 50% of the defects being cardiomegaly, which usually resolves spontaneously. Additional clinical findings include neonatal hypoglycemia, ear pits or creases, hemihypertrophy, Wilms tumor, neuroblastoma, and hepatoblastoma.

**Inheritance Patterns** Inheritance patterns are complex. Most cases are sporadic, but approximately 10% to 15% of families have shown autosomal dominant inheritance, with preferential maternal transmission. Careful examination of parents and genetic counseling are recommended to provide an accurate recurrence risk. Testing is available for approximately 80% of the mechanisms causing BWS, and consultation with a geneticist is recommended to discuss available testing options.

**Teratogens** None are known.

**Prognosis** Prognosis is good with successful surgical repair of omphaloceles and control of neonatal hypoglycemia. Some children require a tracheostomy, because of macroglossia, until surgical tongue reduction can be achieved. Intelligence is generally within the normal range. However, learning disabilities are increased, especially in children with 11p15 microduplications or infants with prematurity or refractory hypoglycemia. Hemihypertrophy and nephromegaly are risk factors for tumor development. The overall risk for tumor development is 8%, with most occurring by age 8.

## SONOGRAPHY

### FREQUENT FINDINGS

- Macrosomia
- Macroglossia
- Mild microcephaly
- Distended abdomen
- Omphalocele } 75%
- Umbilical hernia }

- Hepatomegaly
- Cardiomegaly
- Nephromegaly
- Placentomegaly
- Polyhydramnios (50%)

### LESS FREQUENT

- Hemihypertrophy
- Bilateral adrenal cysts
- Adrenal enlargement
- Prune belly
- Clitoromegaly
- Midface hypoplasia
- Cardiac defects (25%)
- Hyperplastic pancreas

### KEY FINDINGS/PITFALLS

- Fetuses with BWS may be larger than expected by 20 weeks' gestation.

## PREGNANCY MANAGEMENT

**Investigations and Consultations Required** The most likely feature to be detected by ultrasonography is omphalocele. Therefore, chromosome studies, including microarray, and fetal echocardiography should be performed to exclude other causes for the omphalocele. A pediatric surgeon and neonatologist should be consulted to discuss the immediate neonatal management of the infant.

**Fetal Intervention** None is available.

**Monitoring** Third-trimester sonographic evaluations should be performed to assess fetal weight and amniotic fluid volume. To prevent the complications of extreme macrosomia, assessment of lung maturity and induction of labor may be appropriate in some situations.

**Pregnancy Course** The third trimester may be complicated by polyhydramnios and preterm labor. Aggressive therapy for preterm labor is appropriate to allow time for fetal lung maturity.

**Pregnancy Termination Issues** The subtle features of the Beckwith-Wiedemann syndrome would require an intact fetus to establish a precise diagnosis.

**Delivery** The significant neonatal complications in this disorder require delivery in a tertiary center. The obstetrician should be prepared for the possible complications of macrosomia, especially shoulder dystocia.

## NEONATOLOGY

**Resuscitation** Most newborns with this disorder do not require intervention for the onset of breathing, although respiratory distress may be noted in association with preterm delivery as a consequence of polyhydramnios, which occurs frequently. On occasion, the macroglossia can be severe enough to compromise the airway. Oral intubation may be difficult. Use of a nasal trumpet airway is an alternative. The presence of associated major cardiothoracic anomalies may also complicate early adaptation. Management of an omphalocele, if present, consists of avoiding gastric distension and encasing the lower body in a sterile plastic bag. A bowel bag helps to prevent evaporative heat and water loss and to protect the omphalocele sac and its contents.

**Transport** Transfer to a tertiary center with pediatric surgery capability is necessary if there is an omphalocele or airway compromise. Transfer also is recommended to confirm the diagnosis, manage the almost-universal hypoglycemia, and establish the multidisciplinary follow-up usually required.

**Testing and Confirmation** Careful physical examination combined with diagnostic imaging form the primary methods of diagnosis. Molecular genetic studies, if not done prenatally, are indicated, as is careful assessment of the parents to facilitate further genetic counseling.

**Nursery Management** In addition to the unique management requirements for surgical repair of an omphalocele, two other major issues are management of hyperinsulinemic hypoglycemia, which can be severe and prolonged, and stabilization of the airway. Suckle feeding can be compromised by the macroglossia, in some cases necessitating alternative feeding methods. Because there is a significant association of embryonally derived neoplasia, a thorough search for such is essential. The most frequently reported site is renal, but hepatic and adrenal tumors have also been seen.

## SUGGESTED READINGS

1. Elliott M, Bayly R, Colet T, et al: Clinical features and natural history of Beckwith-Wiedemann syndrome: presentation of 74 new cases. Clin Genet 1994; 46:168-174.
2. Laje P, Palladino AA, Bhatti TR, et al: Pancreatic surgery in infants with Beckwith-Wiedemann syndrome and hyperinsulinism. J Pediatr Surg 2013; 48:2511-2516.
3. Lenke RR, Schmidt EK: Diagnosis of Beckwith-Wiedemann syndrome in the second trimester of pregnancy. J Reprod Med 1986; 31:514-516.
4. Pettenati MJ, Haines JL, Higgins RR, et al: Wiedemann-Beckwith syndrome: presentation of clinical and cytogenetics data on 22 new cases and review of the literature. Hum Genet 1986; 74:143-154.
5. Ranzini AC, Day-Salvatore D, Turner T, et al: Intrauterine growth and ultrasound findings in fetuses with Beckwith-Wiedemann syndrome. Obstet Gynecol 1997; 89:538-542.
6. Weinstein L, Anderson C: In utero diagnosis of Beckwith-Wiedemann syndrome by ultrasound. Radiology 1980; 134:474.
7. Weissman A, Mashiach S, Achiron R: Macroglossia: Prenatal ultrasonographic diagnosis and proposed management. Prenat Diagn 1995; 15:66-69.
8. Weksberg R, Chuman C, Beckwith JB: Beckwith-Wiedemann syndrome. Eur J Hum Genet 2010; 18:8-14.

9. Weng EY, Moeschler JB, Graham JM Jr: Longitudinal observations on 15 children with Wiedemann-Beckwith Syndrome. Am J Med Genet 1995; 56:366-373.

10. Williams DH, Gauthier DW, Maizels M: Prenatal diagnosis of Beckwith-Wiedemann syndrome. Prenat Diagn 2005; 25:879-884.

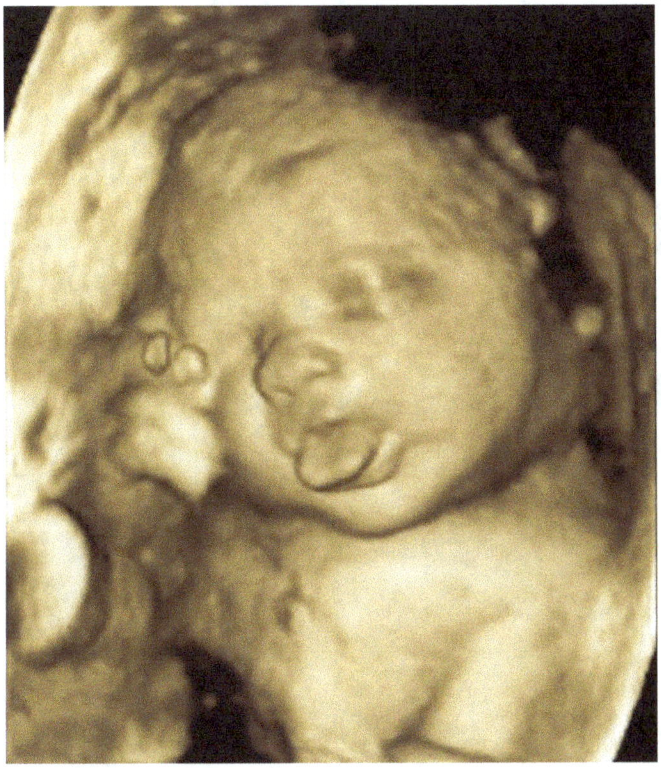

**FIGURE 10.1A** Three-dimensional view of macroglossia.

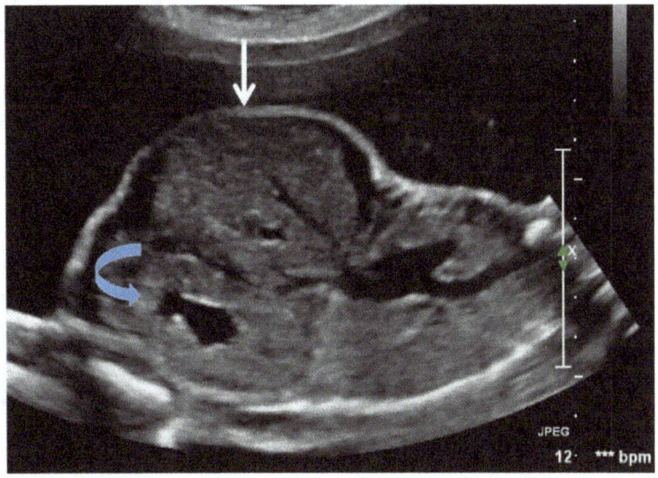


**FIGURE 10.1B** Distended abdomen with enlarged liver (straight arrow) and enlarged kidney (curved arrow). Polyhydramnios.

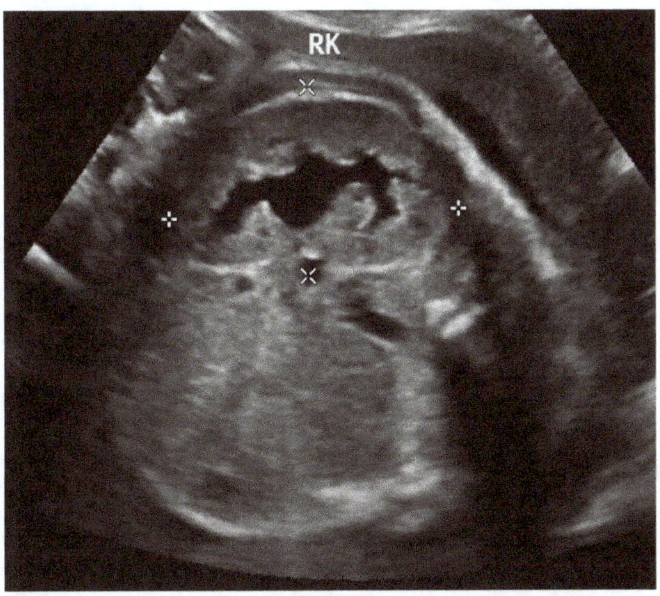


**FIGURE 10.1C** Renomegaly (+ … +).

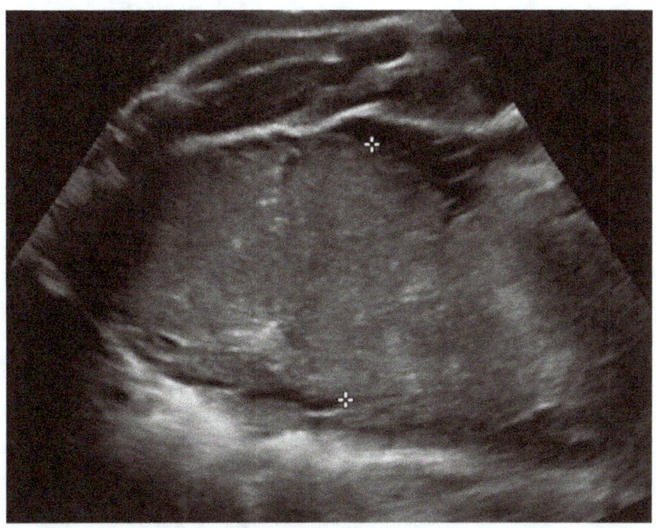

**FIGURE 10.1D** Placentomegaly (+ … +).

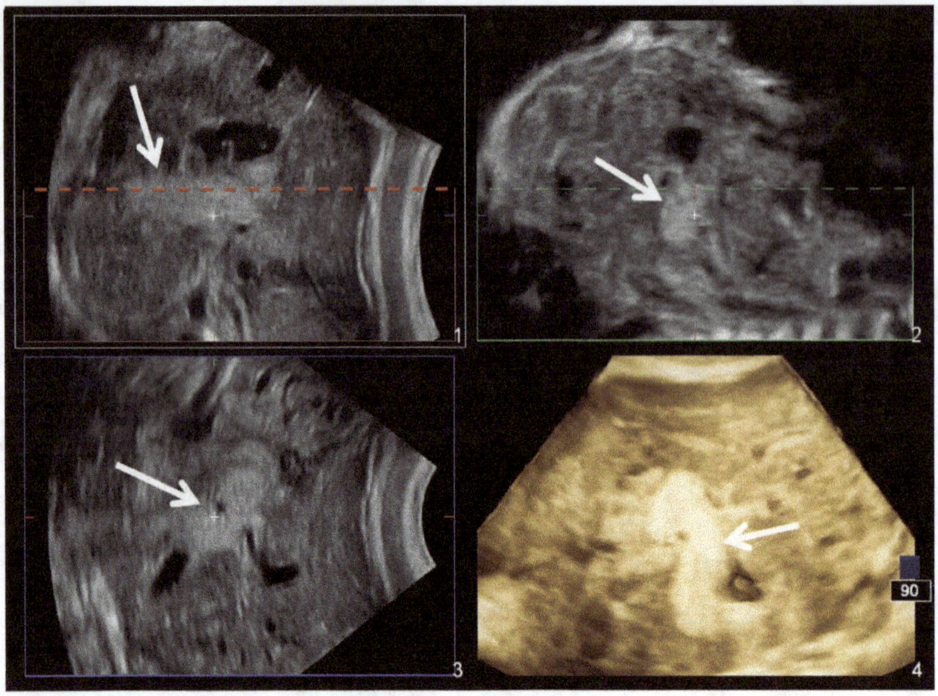


**FIGURE 10.1E** Three-dimensional view of hyperplastic pancreas (arrows).

# 10.2 CYSTIC FIBROSIS

## EPIDEMIOLOGY/GENETICS

**Definition** Cystic fibrosis is a hereditary disorder affecting the exocrine glands. It causes the production of abnormally thick mucus, leading to the blockage of the pancreatic ducts, intestines, and bronchi and often results in respiratory infection.

**Epidemiology** Incidence is 1 in 3,000 newborns.

**Embryology** Mutation in the *CFTR* gene causes abnormal fluid transport across cell membranes, resulting in thick secretions. These abnormal secretions block the bronchi, resulting in recurrent respiratory infections, and the pancreatic ducts, leading to a deficiency of pancreatic enzymes. The absence of pancreatic enzymes, with abnormal intestinal secretions, leads to meconium ileus. Meconium ileus is seen in 15% to 20% of newborns with cystic fibrosis.

**Inheritance Patterns** Cystic fibrosis is an autosomal recessive single-gene disorder with over 1000 mutations known to be causative. A 23-mutation panel can detect 30% to 97% of cystic fibrosis carriers, depending on ethnic background.

**Teratogens** None are known.

**Prognosis** Average life span is between 30 and 40 years, with most deaths secondary to respiratory complications. Survival is higher for males than females.

## SONOGRAPHY

### FREQUENT FINDINGS

- Second trimester: echogenic bowel, bright as bone
- Third trimester: dilated colon with meconium

### LESS FREQUENT

- Mildly dilated loops of bowel
- Dilated loops of bowel with diffuse meconium
- Nonvisualization of the gallbladder

### KEY FINDINGS/PITFALLS

- Prevalence of second-trimester echogenic bowel is 1%.
  - High inter- and intraobserver variability
  - Overdiagnosis with high-frequency (8-MHz) transducers
- Risk of cystic fibrosis with second-trimester echogenic bowel is 2.5%.
  - A 20-fold higher risk over the general population
- Risk of cystic fibrosis with the dilated loops of small bowel in the second trimester is 2.9%.
- Second-trimester echogenic small bowel will detect 11% of fetuses affected with cystic fibrosis.

- Nonvisualization of the fetal gallbladder has a sensitivity of 75% for detecting cystic fibrosis.
  - Risk of cystic fibrosis is 11.6-fold higher with nonvisualization of the gallbladder and echogenic small bowel, versus fetuses with just echogenic small bowel.

### DIFFERENTIAL DIAGNOSIS

The differential diagnosis for second-trimester echogenic bowel includes

- Physiologic variation of normal
- Aneuploidy
- Early-onset intrauterine growth restriction
- Intra-amniotic hemorrhage
- Congenital infection
- Bowel obstruction

## PREGNANCY MANAGEMENT

**Investigations and Consultations Required** Once the molecular diagnosis of cystic fibrosis is established, genetic counseling and referral of the family to a center with special expertise in the management of cystic fibrosis should be made. If any intra-abdominal abnormalities are noted, consultation with pediatric surgery is indicated.

**Fetal Intervention** None

**Monitoring** Periodic ultrasound examinations are indicated to assess for the development of bowel dilatation and meconium peritonitis. In the absence of intra-abdominal abnormalities, no special fetal assessment is necessary. Prenatal care should be coordinated in a tertiary center.

**Pregnancy Course** Polyhydramnios, secondary to intestinal obstructions, may result in preterm labor.

**Pregnancy Termination Issues** There are no special concerns if a molecular diagnosis has been established. Without a diagnosis, a complete autopsy and appropriate molecular studies on fetal tissue are essential.

**Delivery** Prenatal care and delivery should be at a tertiary center. In the absence of intra-abdominal abnormalities, routine obstetrical management is indicated.

## NEONATOLOGY

**Resuscitation** No special resuscitation measures are usually required. If meconium ileus has resulted in severe abdominal distension at birth, respiration may be hindered, necessitating endotracheal intubation at birth.

**Transport** Delivery at a tertiary center with neonatology, pediatric surgery, genetics, and pulmonary specialists is recommended if the diagnosis is known or suspected antenatally.

**Testing and Confirmation** A positive state newborn screen indicates a risk of CF and needs to be followed up with genetic testing for mutations in the *CFTR* gene and with a sweat test. The sweat test is the diagnostic gold standard for the diagnosis of cystic fibrosis and can be performed after 2 weeks of age in term infants.

**Nursery Management** In cases of meconium ileus or peritonitis, transfer to a tertiary center for management is indicated (see discussion of meconium ileus/peritonitis in section 6.6). Long-term follow-up at a tertiary center with an established cystic fibrosis clinic is recommended.

## SUGGESTED READINGS


1. Boue A, Muller F, Nezelop C, et al: Prenatal diagnosis in 200 pregnancies with a 1 in 4 risk of cystic fibrosis. Hum Genet 1986; 74:288-297.
2. Duchatel F, Muller F, Oury JF, et al: Prenatal diagnosis of cystic fibrosis: ultrasonography of the gall bladder at 17-19 weeks of gestation. Fetal Diagn Ther 1993; 8:28-36.
3. Duguépéroux I, Scotel V, Audrézet MP, et al: Non visualization of fetal gallbladder increases the risk of cystic fibrosis. Prenat Diagn 2012; 32:21-28.
4. Font GE, Solari M: Prenatal diagnosis of bowel obstruction initially manifested as isolated hyperechoic bowel. J Ultrasound Med 1998; 17:721-723.
5. Hill LM, Fries J, Hecker J, Grzybeck P: Second trimester echogenic small bowel: an increased risk for adverse perinatal outcome. Prenat Diagn 1994; 14:845-850.
6. Muller F, Dommengues M, Simon-Bouy B, et al: Cystic fibrosis screening: a fetus with hyperechogenic bowel may be the index case. J Med Genet 1998; 35:657-660.
7. Muller F, Simon-Bouy B, Girodon E, et al, French Collaborative Group: Predicting the risk of cystic fibrosis with abnormal ultrasound signs of fetal bowel: results of a French Molecular Collaborative Study based on 641 prospective cases. Am J Med Genet 2002; 110:109-115.
8. Scotet V, DeBraekeleer M, Audrézet MP, et al: Prenatal detection of cystic fibrosis by ultrasonography: a retrospective study of more than 346,000 pregnancies. J Med Genet 2002; 38:443-448.
9. Sepulveda W, Sebire NJ: Fetal echogenic bowel: a complex scenario (Opinion). Ultrasound Obstet Gynecol 2000; 16:510-514.
10. Watson MS, Cutting GR, Desnick RJ, et al: Cystic fibrosis population carrier screening: 2004 revision of American College of Medical Genetics mutation panel. Genet Med 2004; 6:387-391.

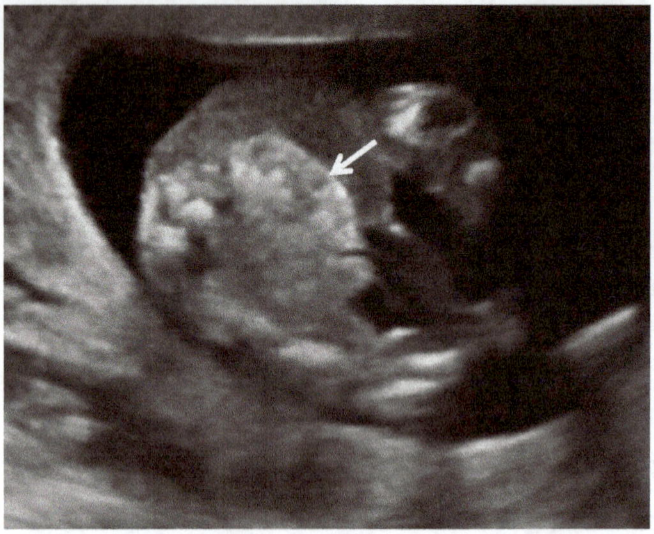

FIGURE 10.2A Echogenic small bowel (arrow).

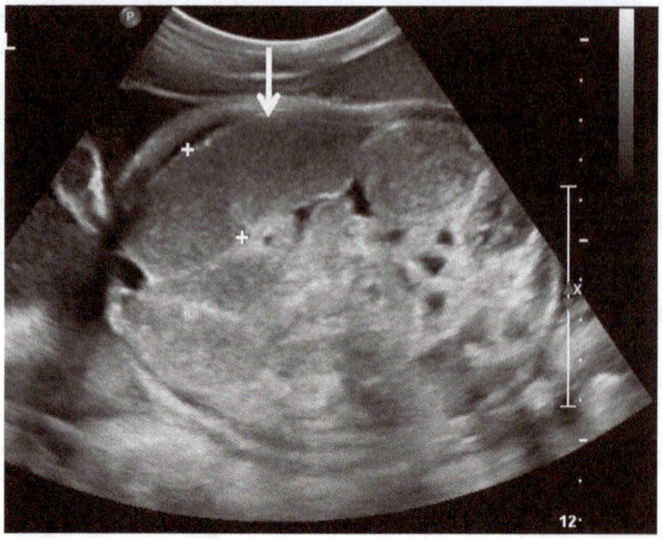

FIGURE 10.2B Meconium ileus (arrow; + … +).

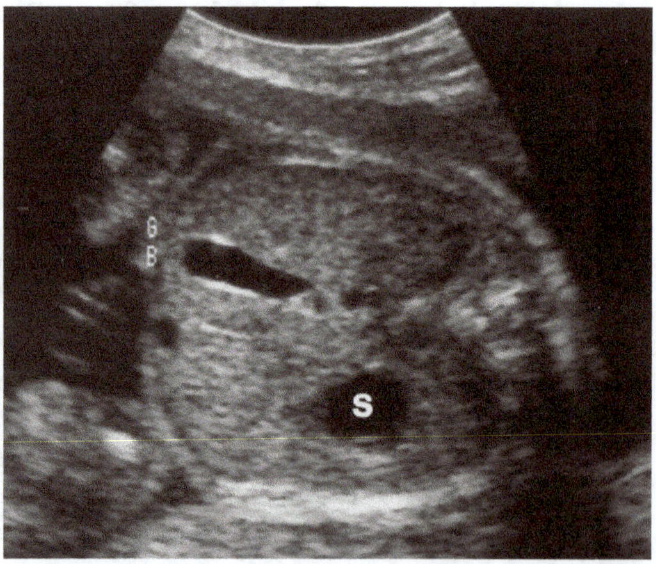


FIGURE 10.2C Normal gallbladder (GB) and stomach (S).

# 10.3 DIGEORGE SYNDROME (22Q11.2 SYNDROME)

## EPIDEMIOLOGY/GENETICS

**Definition** Deletion of chromosome 22q11.2 is now recognized as the cause for the DiGeorge syndrome (DGS) and velocardiofacial syndrome (Shprintzen syndrome). Common features include cardiac malformations (85%), cleft palate or velopharyngeal insufficiency (48%), neonatal hypocalcemia (63%), thymic hypoplasia (65%), dysmorphic face (95%), microcephaly (40%), and moderate-to-severe learning disabilities (20%).

**Epidemiology** Prevalence is 1 in 4000 live births (M1:F1).

**Embryology** DGS represents a developmental defect of the third and fourth pharyngeal pouches, resulting in conotruncal, thymus, and parathyroid effects. Deletion 22q11.2 has been found in 50% of children with interrupted aortic arch, 35% of children with truncus arteriosus, and 16% of children with tetralogy of Fallot. It is rarely found in cases of transposition of the great vessels. It is commonly detected in children with apparently isolated cleft palate (10%) or velopharyngeal insufficiency with developmental delays.

**Inheritance Patterns** It is a chromosome microdeletion that is inherited in an autosomal dominant fashion, with the majority (>90%) of cases being new mutations. Because of only mild-to-moderate developmental disabilities and significant intrafamilial phenotypic variability, affected parents are found in 10% to 15% of cases. These parents are at a 50% risk of having affected offspring. Parental studies should always be performed when a 22q11.2 deletion is found in the fetus.

**Teratogens** None are known.

**Prognosis** Significant neonatal morbidity and mortality exist related to the cardiac defects and sequelae of the immunodeficiency. Extensive cardiac and cleft palate surgery may be needed, depending on associated malformations. IQ generally ranges from 70 to 90, but both speech and language development are delayed/impaired. There is significant variability in clinical and cognitive presentation. Children with 22q11.22 have a high prevalence of autism spectrum, attention deficit, and anxiety disorders, as well as psychotic-like features. Up to 30% of adolescents and adults develop schizophrenia-like psychosis.

## SONOGRAPHY

### FREQUENT FINDINGS

- Thymic hypoplasia (90%)
- Congenital cardiac defects (80%)
  - Conotruncal abnormalities
    - Truncus arteriosus
    - Tetralogy of Fallot
    - Double-outlet right ventricle
    - Interrupted aortic arch
- Microcephaly (40%)

### LESS FREQUENT

- Unilateral renal agenesis
- Horseshoe kidney
- Multicystic dysplastic kidney
- Hypospadias
- First-trimester thickened nuchal translucency
- Intrauterine growth restriction
- Polyhydramnios

### KEY FINDINGS/PITFALLS

- The characteristic facial dysmorphology associated with DGS cannot be detected sonographically.
- Severe polyhydramnios may be a harbinger of neonatal feeding difficulties.
- The fetal thymus is best viewed on a three-vessel view. An absence of the thymus on this view is diagnostic for DGS.

## PREGNANCY MANAGEMENT

**Investigations and Consultations Required** The presence of any conotruncal abnormality or cleft palate detected in utero should prompt chromosome evaluation, including a karyotype, microarray, and fluorescent in situ hybridization study for the 22q11.2 deletion. Fetal blood sampling to assess fetal T-cell function can be performed to assess immune function. Because of the significant risk of neonatal complications, consultation with a neonatologist is essential. Other consultations will depend on what other structural malformations are present. When fetal DGS is diagnosed, maternal evaluation for DGS is appropriate to eliminate subclinical phenotypic features, particularly a maternal congenital heart defect that may have an impact on labor and delivery.

**Fetal Intervention** This multisystem disorder is not amenable to in utero therapy.

**Monitoring** Polyhydramnios is a frequent complication, and both clinical and sonographic assessment of amniotic fluid volume should be done regularly. Significant polyhydramnios may result in preterm labor.

**Pregnancy Course** Generally, pregnancy course is unremarkable unless complicated by polyhydramnios.

**Pregnancy Termination Issues** If a cytogenetic diagnosis has been established, there are no special autopsy requirements.

**Delivery** The site of delivery must be a tertiary center where the multiple neonatal complications can be managed.

## NEONATOLOGY

**Resuscitation** In general, management of the onset of respiration and the need for assistance is influenced by the nature of the associated cardiac defect. If a ductus-dependent lesion has been identified or is suspected, oxygen supplementation may be limited to 40% to 60%, while oxygen saturation is monitored to avoid hyperoxemia. Immediate infusion of prostaglandin $E_1$ should be instituted. Other abnormalities affecting onset of respiration include orofacial clefts, Pierre Robin variants, and diaphragmatic hernia, although these are infrequent in occurrence, except with the velocardiofacial syndrome.

**Transport** Immediate transport to a tertiary center with pediatric cardiac capabilities, both diagnostic and surgical, is essential. During transport, the infusion of prostaglandin $E_1$ should be maintained. Because apnea is a frequent side effect of prostaglandin infusion, intubation and assisted ventilation during transport may be necessary. Supplemental oxygen should be limited to that necessary to maintain acceptable oxygen saturation.

**Testing and Confirmation** The complete delineation of the cardiac defect is accomplished by echocardiography in the majority of cases. Additional laboratory testing should include serum calcium concentrations on a frequent basis, quantification of the T lymphocytes, and appropriate genetic studies, if not obtained prenatally.

**Nursery Management** The specific defects present will dictate the direction of care. The key issues are airway adequacy, hemodynamic stability, oxygen delivery, and the identification of concomitant problems, such as immunodeficiency and hypocalcemia. Seizures from the hypocalcemia may manifest in the absence of careful monitoring and maintenance of adequate serum calcium concentrations.

## SUGGESTED READINGS

1. Bassett AS, McDonald-McGinn DM, Devriendt K, et al, Internal 22q11.2 Deletion Syndrome Consortium: Practical guidelines for managing patients with 22q11.2 deletion syndrome. J Pediatr 2011; 159:332-339.
2. Botto LD, May K, Fernhoff PM, et al: A population-based study of the 22q11.2 deletion: phenotype, incidence, and contribution to major birth defects in the population. Pediatrics 2003; 112:101-107.
3. Chaoui R, Kalache KD, Heling KS, et al: Absent or hypoplastic thymus on ultrasound: a marker for deletion 22q11.2 in fetal cardiac defects. Ultrasound Obstet Gynecol 2002; 20:546-552.
4. Debrus S, Berger G, de Meeus A, et al: Familial non-syndromic conotruncal defects are not associated with a 22q11 microdeletion. Hum Genet 1996; 97:138-144.
5. DeVriendt K, Van Schoubroeck, Eyskens B, et al: Polyhydramnios as a prenatal symptom of the DiGeorge/velo-cardio-facial syndrome. Prenat Diagn 1998; 18:68-72.
6. Goodship J, Robson SC, Sturgiss S, et al: Renal abnormalities on obstetric ultrasound as a presentation of DiGeorge syndrome. Prenat Diagn 1997; 17:867-870.
7. Jonas RK, Montojo CA, Bearden CE: The 22q11.2 deletion syndrome as a window into complex neuropsychiatric disorders over the lifespan. Biol Psychiatry 2014; 75:351-360.
8. Markert ML, Sarzotti M, Ozaki DA, et al: Thymus transplantation in complete DiGeorge syndrome: immunologic and safety evaluations in 12 patients. Blood 2003; 102:1121-1130.

9. Thomas JA, Graham JM Jr: Chromosome 22q11 deletion syndrome: an update and review for the primary pediatrician. Clin Pediatr 1997; 36:253-266.

10. Wufsberg EA, Leana-Cox J, Neni G: What's in a name? Chromosome 22q abnormalities and the DiGeorge velocardiofacial, and conotruncal anomalies face syndromes. Am J Med Genet 1996; 65:317-319.

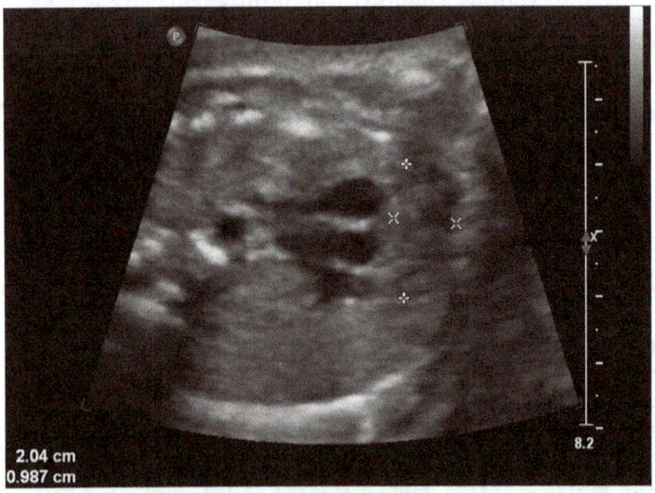


**FIGURE 10.3A** Three-vessel view and normal thymus (+ … +; x … x).

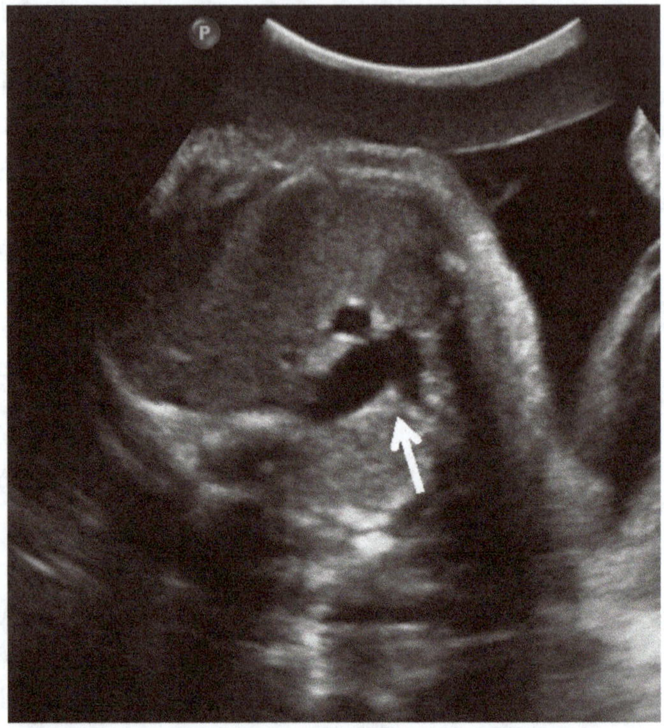

**FIGURE 10.3B** Truncus arteriosus results in two vessels at the level of a normal three-vessel view. The truncus is the larger vessel (arrow).

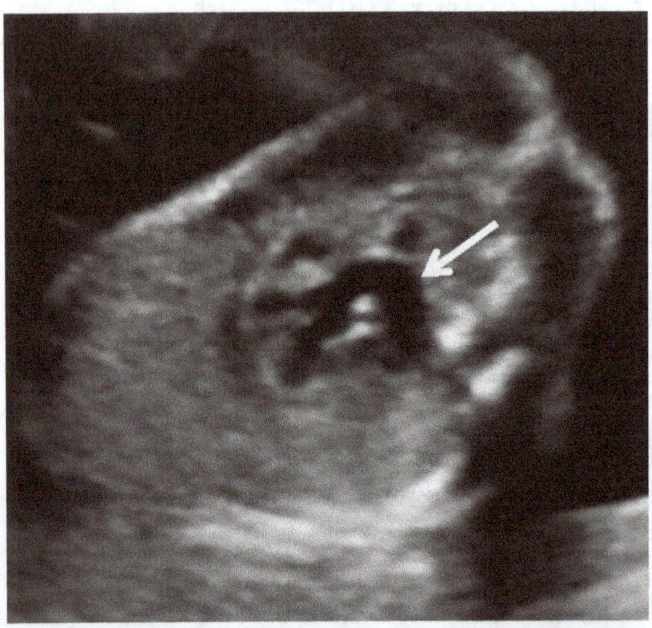

**FIGURE 10.3C** Truncus arteriosus (arrow).

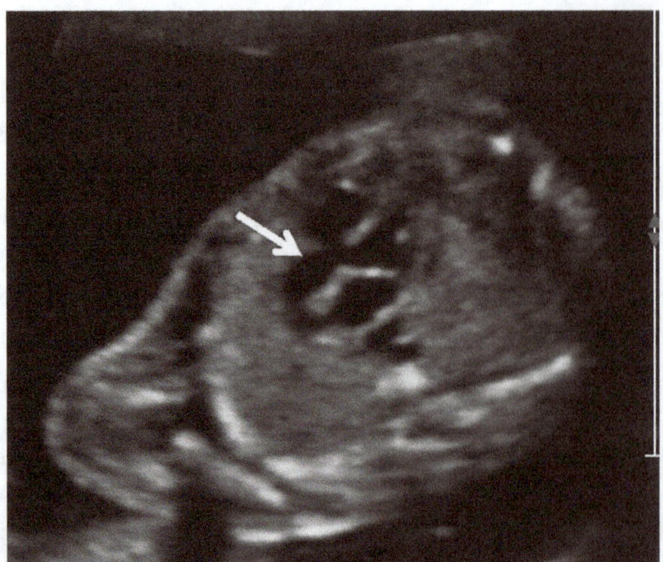

**FIGURE 10.3D** Tetralogy of Fallot with VSD and overriding aorta (arrow).

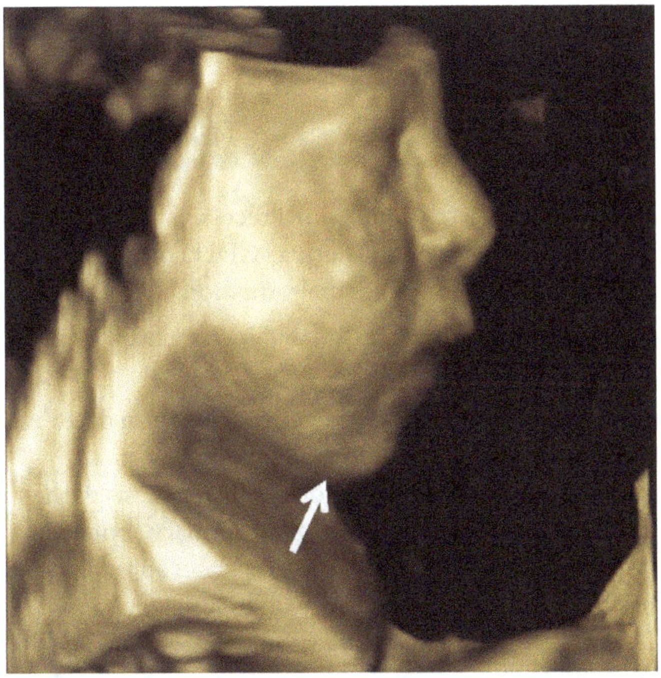

**FIGURE 10.3E** Mild micrognathia.

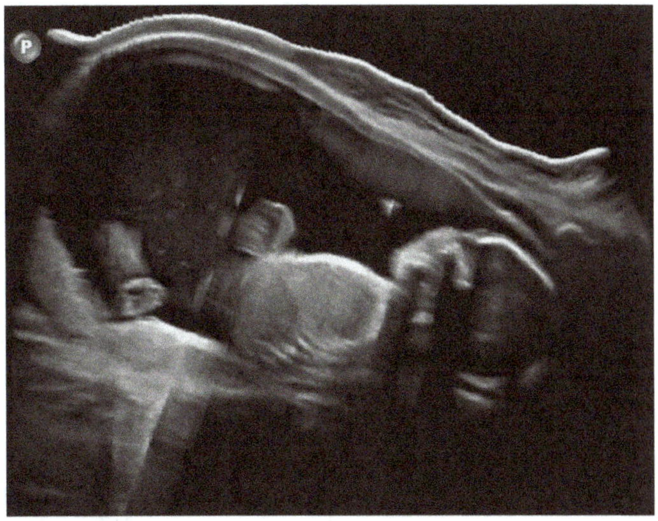

**FIGURE 10.3F** Severe polyhydramnios.

# 10.4 FRYNS SYNDROME

## EPIDEMIOLOGY/GENETICS

**Definition** Fryns syndrome is a highly lethal, autosomal recessive genetic condition characterized by congenital diaphragmatic hernia (CDH) or other defects of the diaphragm in association with other malformations.

**Epidemiology** Fryns syndrome is rare, with an estimated incidence of 0.7 in 10,000 births.

**Embryology** Diaphragmatic hernia or other defects in the diaphragm occur in 90% of cases. Other common abnormalities include the following: central nervous system malformations (Dandy-Walker malformation, agenesis of the corpus callosum); cystic kidneys; microretrognathia; genitourinary abnormalities; distal digital hypoplasia; cleft lip with or without cleft palate; and cystic hygroma. Fryns syndrome should be considered in the differential diagnosis with the detection of a CDH and any additional major congenital anomaly.

**Inheritance Patterns** Inheritance is autosomal recessive, with a 25% recurrence risk in future pregnancies. The gene responsible for the disorder has not yet been identified.

**Teratogens** None are known.

**Prognosis** Prognosis is poor, with most cases ending in stillbirth or early neonatal death due to pulmonary hypoplasia. In Fryns syndrome, the CDH-associated pulmonary hypoplasia is not due solely to mechanical compression. Intrinsic pulmonary arrest appears to account for a portion of CDH-associated pulmonary hypoplasia. Rare survivors without pulmonary hypoplasia had severe intellectual disability.

## SONOGRAPHY

### FREQUENT FINDINGS

- Congenital diaphragmatic hernia (90%)
- Pulmonary hypoplasia (65%)
- Dysmorphic facial features
  - Hypertelorism
  - Midface hypoplasia
  - Low-set/malformed ears
  - Micrognathia
  - Macrostomia
- Distal limb hypoplasia
  - Rudimentary development of the distal phalanges
- Congenital heart defects (50%)
  - Ventricular septal defect
  - Tetralogy of Fallot

    - Truncus arteriosis
    - Transposition of the great vessels
- Polyhydramnios (55%)

### LESS FREQUENT

- Ventriculomegaly (23%)
- Agenesis of the corpus callosum (13.5%)
- Dandy-Walker malformation
- Cystic hygroma
- Cleft lip and palate

### KEY FINDINGS/PITFALLS

- Polyhydramnios occurs in the late second and third trimesters.

## PREGNANCY MANAGEMENT

**Investigations and Consultations Required** Prenatal diagnosis of Fryns syndrome is unusual but may be suspected based on a previously affected child or when a CDH is associated with other anomalies. This syndrome will generally be a diagnosis of exclusion. Therefore, chromosome studies, microarray, and fetal echocardiography are essential to exclude other conditions. It is especially important that the chromosome studies be done on amniotic fluid, not fetal blood, and that fluorescent in situ hybridization be done on uncultured cells to exclude the Pallister-Killian syndrome (iso-12p). Fetal blood may be more prone to tissue-specific mosaicism and not demonstrate iso-12p found in amniocytes.

**Fetal Intervention** Because of the lethality of the condition, in utero repair should not be considered in cases of diaphragmatic hernia if there are limb or renal abnormalities suggestive of Fryns syndrome.

**Monitoring** No additional monitoring other than routine obstetric care is indicated.

**Pregnancy Course** Usually, pregnancy is uncomplicated unless polyhydramnios develops secondary to the diaphragmatic hernia.

**Pregnancy Termination Issues** To make an accurate diagnosis of Fryns syndrome, labor induction is the best alternative.

**Delivery** A precise prospective diagnosis is unlikely before birth. Therefore, standard obstetric care is indicated, including appropriate fetal surveillance.

## NEONATOLOGY

**Resuscitation** A full discussion with the parents about the limited prognosis for fetuses with this syndrome is essential prior to delivery. Because the majority of infants reported in the literature have not survived the neonatal period, the decision to attempt resuscitation should be based on the spectrum of organ malformations that are present. The absence of a diaphragmatic hernia or diaphragmatic abnormality seems to improve survival potential. However, significant neuroanatomic abnormalities have been reported in the survivors, with a high incidence of mental retardation. A decision for limited or no support following delivery is an option, particularly with evidence of a severe diaphragmatic abnormality and other serious organ system malformations.

**Transport** If there is uncertainty about the survivability of the infant, transport to a tertiary center with multiple pediatric and surgical subspecialists and neonatal intensive care capabilities is indicated.

**Testing and Confirmation** Careful physical examination will identify the characteristic facial features and limb abnormalities of Fryns syndrome. Diagnostic imaging (echocardiography and cranial ultrasonography) will delineate other significant organ system malformations. Magnetic resonance imaging is the preferred technique for evaluation of intracranial malformations.

**Nursery Management** Full ventilatory support from birth is required if diaphragmatic hernia is present. Often, the accompanying pulmonary hypoplasia is the predominant factor dictating clinical management (see Chapter 5.3). If a cardiac malformation is also present, the management is further modified as needed for the specific abnormality.

## SUGGESTED READINGS


1. Aymé S, Julian C, Gambarelli D, et al: Fryns syndrome: report on 8 new cases. Clin Genet 1989; 35:191-201.
2. Davis C, Samarakkody U: Fryns syndrome: a surviving case with associated Hirschsprung's disease and hemidiaphragmatic agenesis. J Paediatr Child Health 2002; 38:318-320.
3. Fryns JP: Fryns syndrome: a variable MCA syndrome with diaphragmatic defects, coarse face, and distal limb hypoplasia. J Med Genet 1987; 24:271-274.
4. Keijzer R: Dual-hit hypothesis explains pulmonary hypoplasia in the nitrofen model of congenital diaphragmatic hernia. Am J Pathol 2000; 156:1299-1306.
5. Keijzer R, Puri P: Congenital diaphragmatic hernia. Semin Pediatr Surg 2010; 19:180-185.
6. Lin AE, Pober BR, Mullen MP, Slavotinek AM: Cardiovascular malformations in Fryns syndrome: is there a pathogenic role for neural crest cells? Am J Med Genet A 2005; 139A:186-193.
7. Pellissier MC, Philip N, Potier A, et al: Prenatal diagnosis of Fryns' syndrome. Prenat Diagn 1992; 12:299-303.
8. Peron A, Bedeschi MF, Fabietti I, et al: Prenatal and postnatal findings in five cases of Fryns syndrome. Prenat Diagn. 2014; 34:1227-1230.
9. Sheffield JS, Twickler DM, Timmons C, et al: Fryns syndrome: prenatal diagnosis and pathologic correlation. J Ultrasound Med 1998; 17:585-589.
10. Slavotinek AM: Fryns syndrome: a review of the diagnostic guidelines. Am J Med Genet 2004; 124A:427-433.

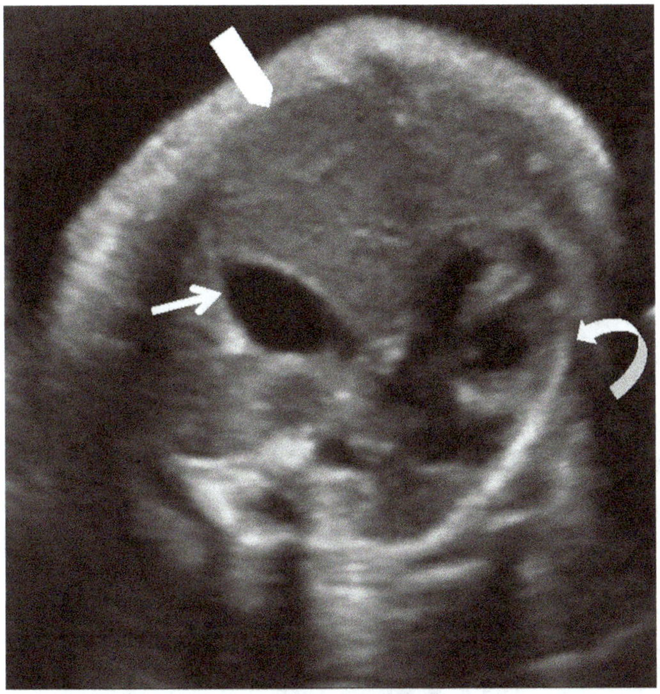

FIGURE 10.4A Fryns. Congenital diaphragmatic hernia with stomach (straight arrow) and liver (thick arrow) adjacent to the heart (curved arrow).

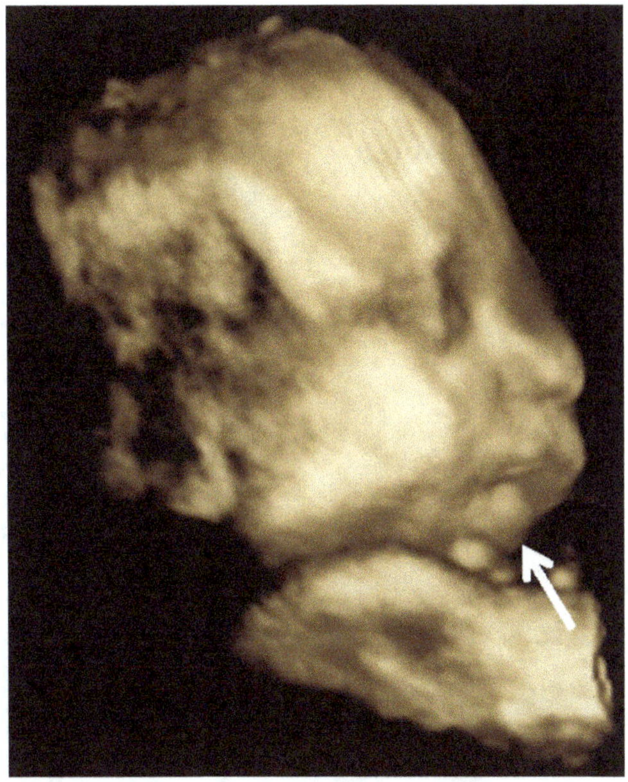

FIGURE 10.4B Fryns. Micrognathia (arrow).

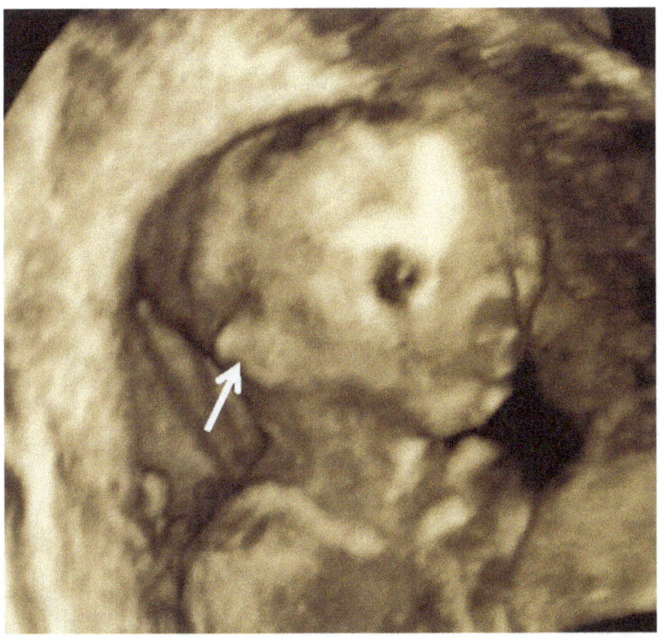

FIGURE 10.4C Fryns. Low-set abnormal ear (arrow).

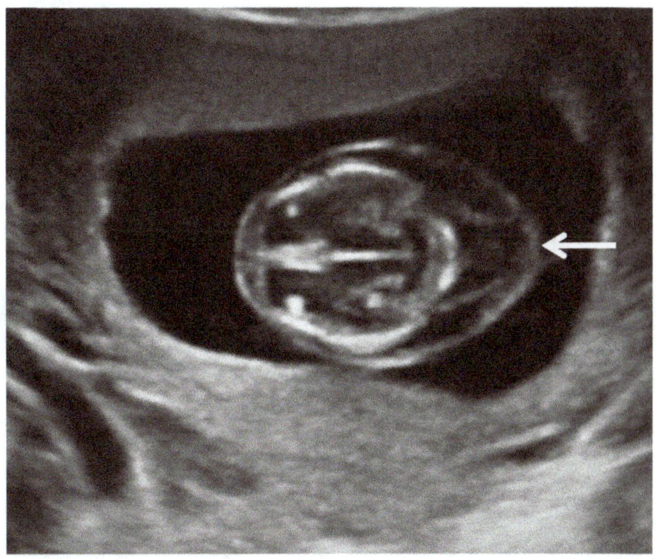

FIGURE 10.4D Fryns. Cystic hygroma (arrow).

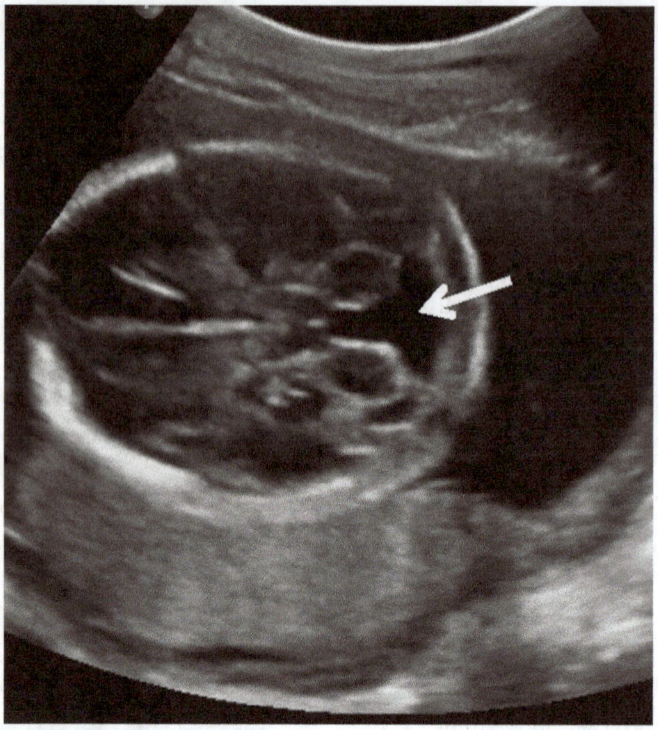

**FIGURE 10.4E** Fryns. Dandy-Walker malformation (arrow).

# 10.5 MECKEL-GRUBER SYNDROME

## EPIDEMIOLOGY/GENETICS

**Definition** Meckel-Gruber syndrome (MGS) is an autosomal recessive genetic syndrome characterized by an occipital encephalocele (63%), polydactyly (55%), and cystic dysplasia of the kidneys (100%). Of note, 18% have no brain abnormalities.

**Epidemiology** Incidence is 1 in 13,250 to 1 in 140,000 live births, with an increased incidence in the Finnish population (1 in 9000) (M1:F1).

**Embryology** MGS has been associated with a number of genes concerned with cilium function and is classified as one of the ciliopathies. Other abnormalities that may be seen include microcephaly, Dandy-Walker malformation, hydrocephalus, microphthalmia, cleft lip with or without cleft palate, and genital abnormalities.

**Inheritance Patterns** Inheritance is autosomal recessive with a 25% recurrence risk in future pregnancies. MGS has extreme genetic heterogeneity and displays allelism with other ciliopathies. Mutations in at least 12 genes have been reported to be causative, and consultation with a geneticist is appropriate to discuss testing options.

**Teratogens** None are known.

**Prognosis** MGS is lethal, with rare cases of survival of more than a few days or weeks.

## SONOGRAPHY

### FREQUENT FINDINGS

- Classic triad
  - Occipital encephalocele (90%)
  - Postaxial polydactyly (80%)
  - Renal dysplasia (100%)
- Microcephaly

### LESS FREQUENT

- Cerebellar hypoplasia
- Dandy-Walker malformation
- Micrognathia
- Cleft lip/palate
- Congenital heart defects
  - Ventricular septal defect
  - Atrioventricular septal defect
  - Coarctation of the aorta
- Bilateral clubbed feet
- Oligohydramnios

### KEY FINDINGS/PITFALLS

- The cephalocele is variable in size and may be difficult to detect.
- Both kidneys are enlarged and hyperechoic and contain multiple small cysts of varying sizes in both the medulla and cortex.
- Oligohydramnios is common in association with renal cystic dysplasia and may occur as early as 14 weeks' gestation.
- MGS has been diagnosed in the first trimester.
- Although MGS has been diagnosed in the first trimester, it should not be excluded until 20 weeks' gestation.

### DIFFERENTIAL DIAGNOSIS

- Trisomy 13
    - MGS has several stigmata of trisomy 13.
- Smith-Lemli-Opitz syndrome (SLOS): This is an autosomal recessive disorder with postaxial polydactyly and genitourinary and central nervous system malformations.
- Bardet-Biedl syndrome: This syndrome has postaxial polydactyly and renal dysplasia. The occipital encephalocele is absent.
- Joubert syndrome: This is an autosomal recessive disorder with microcephaly, meningoencephalocele, vermian hypoplasia, polydactyly, and renal abnormalities.

## PREGNANCY MANAGEMENT

**Investigations and Consultations Required** Chromosome studies should be done to exclude trisomy 13. As a number of genes and mutations have been implicated, molecular studies may only be informative in families with a previously affected individual with a known mutation. If continuation of the pregnancy is being considered, a consultation with a neonatologist is appropriate to develop a plan for management for the infant following delivery.

**Fetal Intervention** Intervention is not applicable to this lethal condition.

**Monitoring** Maternal status should be monitored in standard fashion. Fetal evaluation is not appropriate because emergency intervention is not indicated.

**Pregnancy Course** Renal malformations may result in oligohydramnios, and if monitoring is used in labor, severe fetal heart rate deceleration may be seen. Therefore, fetal monitoring in labor is not recommended.

**Pregnancy Termination Issues** Unless the features are classic for MGS, delivery of an intact fetus may be necessary to establish a precise anatomic diagnosis. Consideration should be given to DNA sequencing to allow molecular prenatal diagnosis in future pregnancies.

**Delivery** Electronic fetal monitoring and cesarean section should be avoided unless requested by the family after a thorough discussion of the prognosis for infants with MGS.

**Resuscitation** The reported prognosis is uniformly lethal, with the majority of perinatal deaths occurring before delivery. Neonatal resuscitation, with a known prenatal diagnosis, is not indicated. When the birth of an involved infant is unexpected and resuscitation is initiated, the result is minimal prolongation of survival. The accompanying pulmonary hypoplasia, associated with absent fetal renal function or central nervous system abnormalities, limits the response to resuscitation.

**Transport** Transport is indicated only if diagnostic confirmation and counseling are not available locally.

**Testing and Confirmation** The presence of an extracranial occipital mass, cystic dysplasia of the kidneys, and polydactyly are the classic findings of MGS. Other intracranial malformations may occur, and in a limited number of cases, polydactyly is absent. The concomitant occurrence of multiple organ system abnormalities is frequent. Diagnostic imaging (sonography, magnetic resonance imaging) will elucidate the characteristics of the major organ abnormalities.

**Nursery Management** Care is usually limited to provision of comfort measures once the diagnosis is confirmed. Support for parental grieving and genetic counseling for future pregnancies are essential.

## SUGGESTED READINGS

1. Alexiev BA, Lin X, Sun C-C, Brenner DS: Meckel-Gruber syndrome. Pathologic manifestations, minimal diagnostic criteria, and differential diagnosis. Arch Pathol Lab Med 2006; 130:1236-1238.
2. Ichowicz V, Eurin D, Maugey-Laulom B, et al: Meckel-Gruber syndrome: sonography and pathology. Ultrasound Obstet Gynecol 2006; 27:296-300.
3. Jones D, Fiozzo F, Waters B, et al: First-trimester diagnosis of Meckel-Gruber syndromes by fetal ultrasound with molecular identification of CCZDZA mutations by next generation sequencing. Ultrasound Obstet Gynecol 2014; 44:712-721.
4. Nyberg DA, Hallesy D, Mahony BS, et al: Meckel-Gruber syndrome. Importance of prenatal diagnosis. J Ultrasound Med 1990; 9:691-696.
5. Salonen R, Norio R: The Meckel syndrome in Finland: epidemiologic and genetic aspects. Am J Med Genet 1984; 18:691-698.
6. Szymanska K, Hartill VL, Johnson CA: Unraveling the genetics of Joubert and Meckel-Gruber syndromes. J Pediatr Genet. 2014; 3:65-78.
7. Wright C, Healicon R, English C, Burn J: Meckel syndrome: what are the minimum diagnostic criteria? J Med Genet 1994; 31:482-485.

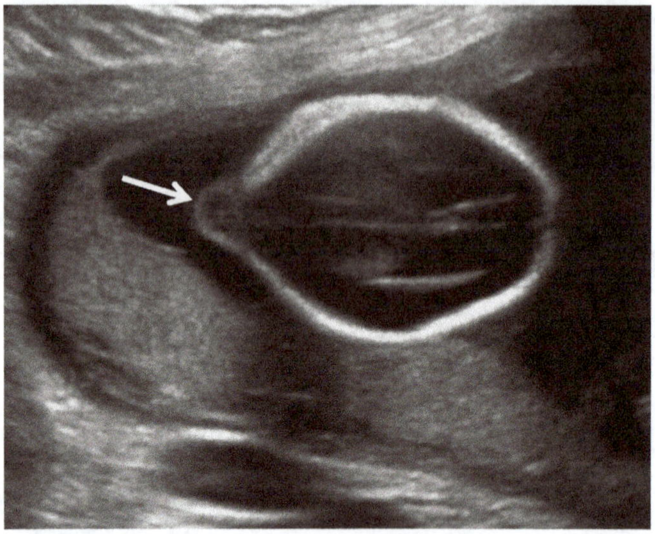

FIGURE 10.5A Cranial meningocele (arrow).

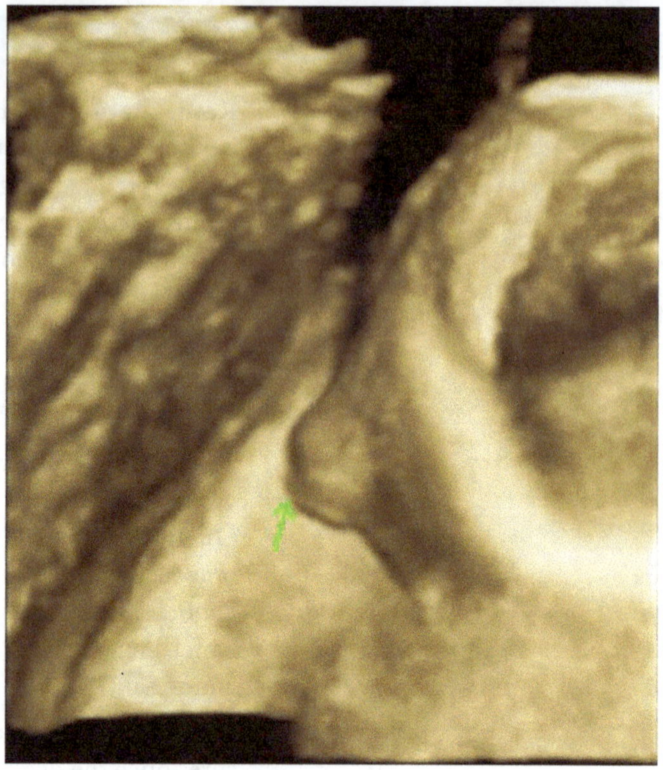

FIGURE 10.5B Three-dimensional image of cranial meningocele (arrow).

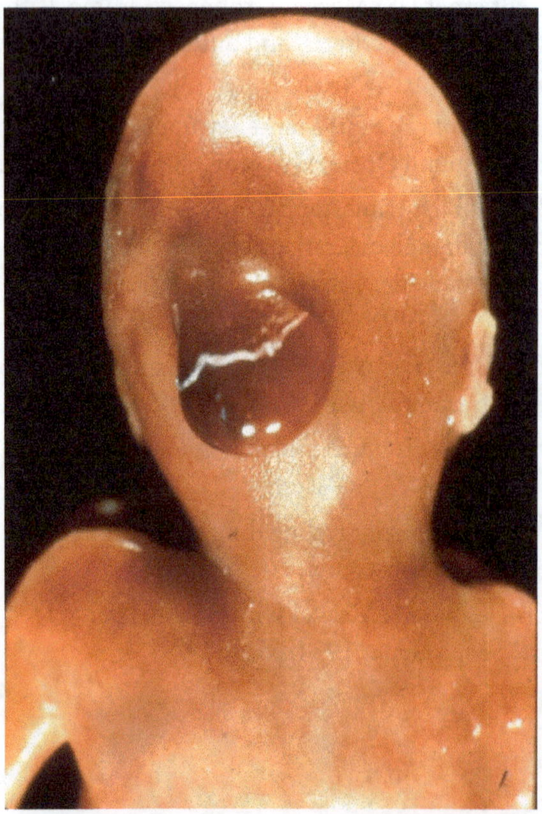

FIGURE 10.5C Fetus with a cranial meningocele.

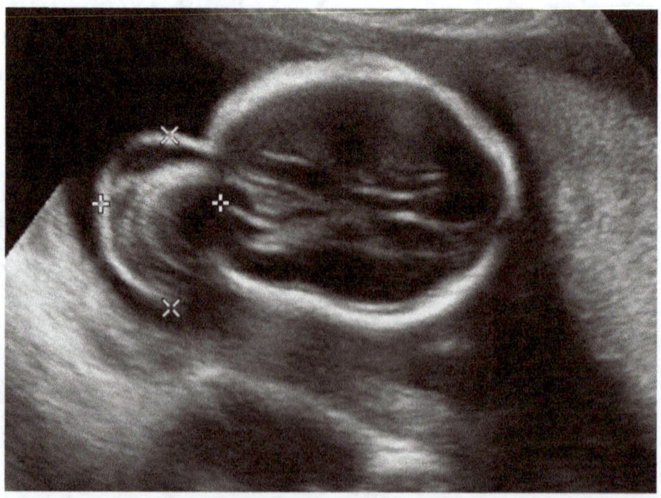

FIGURE 10.5D Encephalomeningocele (+ … +; x … x).

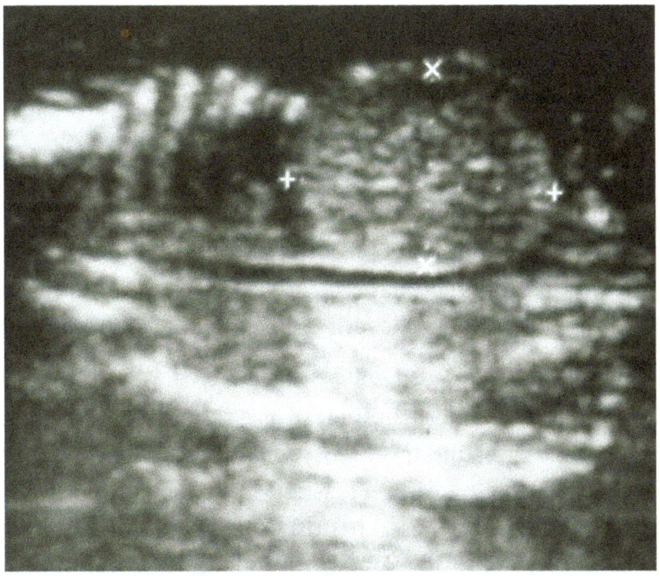

FIGURE 10.5E Renal dysplasia (+ … +; x … x).

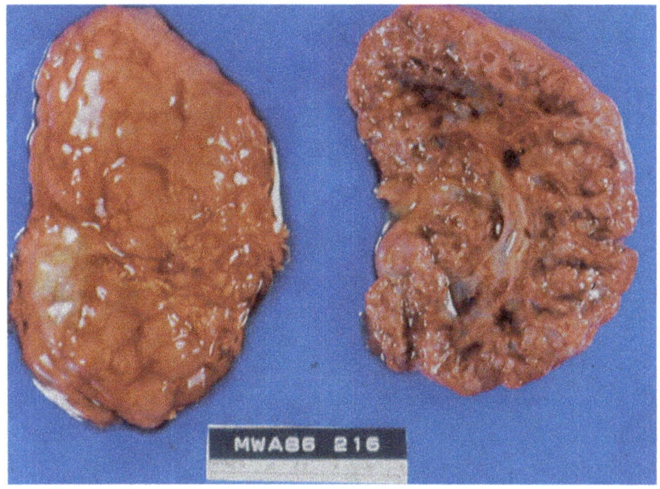


FIGURE 10.5F Pathologic specimen of renal dysplasia.

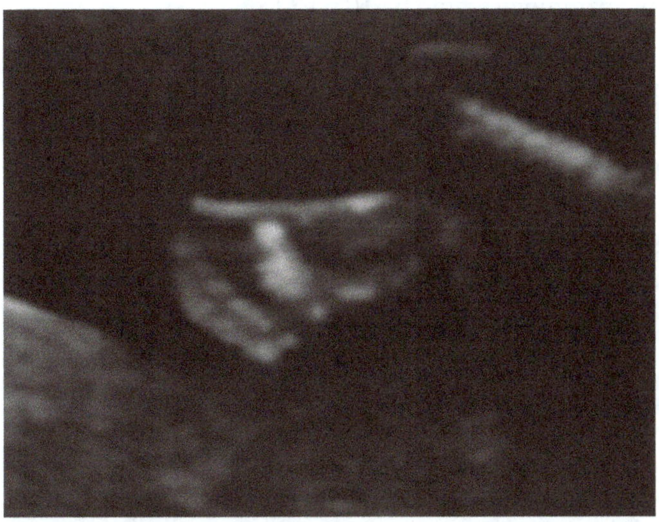

FIGURE 10.5G Polydactyly.

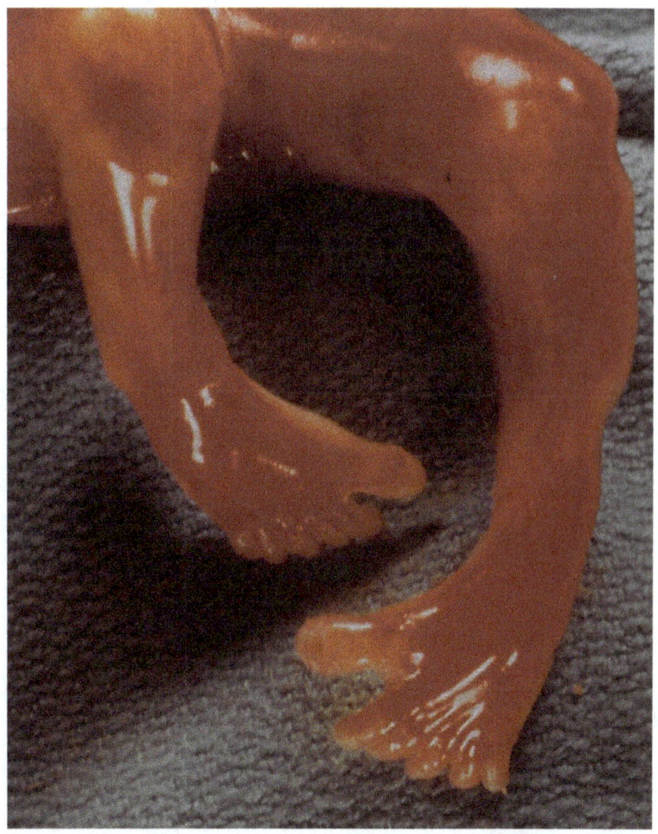

FIGURE 10.5H Polydactyly in a fetus with MGS.

# 10.6 PENA-SHOKEIR SYNDROME

## EPIDEMIOLOGY/GENETICS

**Definition** Pena-Shokeir syndrome is a heterogeneous group of disorders characterized by polyhydramnios, prenatal onset of growth restriction with head sparing, multiple joint contractures, characteristic facies, and pulmonary hypoplasia. The term *fetal akinesia* is preferable to describe this group of disorders.

**Epidemiology** Incidence is 1 in 3000 to 1 in 15,000 births (M1:F1).

**Embryology** Pena-Shokeir syndrome is best thought of as a number of separate neuromuscular disorders resulting in a similar phenotype. The phenotype consists of polyhydramnios, prenatal onset of growth restriction with head sparing, multiple joint contractures, webbed neck, closed hands, flexed wrists, absence of flexion creases, rocker-bottom feet, rigid and expressionless face, hypertelorism, prominent eyes, short umbilical cord, and pulmonary hypoplasia. The common pathophysiology of the phenotypic features is thought to be decreased, or absent, fetal movement in utero. Pathologic findings have been heterogeneous and include congenital myopathies, anterior horn cell abnormalities, in utero vascular accidents, and abnormalities of the brain. At least 20 specific familial types of Pena-Shokeir syndrome are recognizable.

**Inheritance Patterns** Autosomal recessive inheritance has been seen in approximately one-half of reported cases. Empiric recurrence risk for an isolated case with nonspecific pathology would be 10% to 15%.

**Teratogens** Maternal myasthenia gravis and any agent causing central nervous system damage, including infectious agents, fetal hypotension, or stroke are teratogenic.

**Prognosis** Cases with a classic phenotype are lethal and may be stillborn (30%) or die in the first few months of life due to respiratory complications. Because of the heterogeneous nature of this phenotype, the prognosis is dependent on the etiology of the causative disorder.

## SONOGRAPHY

### FREQUENT FINDINGS

- Reduced fetal movements
- Micrognathia
- Low-set ears
- Hypotelorism
- Fixed, open mouth
- Diffuse muscle atrophy
- Pulmonary hypoplasia/small chest
- Intrauterine growth restriction
- Polyhydramnios

### LESS FREQUENT

- Cleft palate
- Cerebellar hypoplasia
- Agenesis of the corpus callosum
- Congenital heart disease

### KEY FINDINGS/PITFALLS

- There is a variable time of onset, even within families.
  - An unaffected pregnancy cannot be ensured until the end of the second trimester.
- Pulmonary hypoplasia results from an absence of the appropriate development of the intercostal and diaphragmatic muscles.
  - Fetal breathing movements are not detected.
- A decrease in fetal swallowing results in polyhydramnios.
- The diagnosis of Pena-Shokeir syndrome has been made as early as 12 weeks' gestation.
- Three-dimensional imaging permits a better assessment of abnormal limb positions and micrognathia.

### DIFFERENTIAL DIAGNOSIS

- Trisomy 18: Micrognathia, arthrogryposis, and rocker-bottom feet occur in both trisomy 18 and Pena-Shokeir syndrome.
- Multiple pterygium syndrome is characterized by contractures, pterygia (webbing of the skin) at the joints, and cystic hygroma.

## PREGNANCY MANAGEMENT

**Investigations and Consultations Required** Chromosome studies with microarray should be performed to exclude chromosomal abnormalities. Amniotic fluid cultures for cytomegalovirus and maternal serum for TORCH (toxoplasmosis, other infections, rubella, cytomegalovirus infection, and herpes simplex) titers should be considered. Fetal echocardiography should be performed to detect the associated cardiac malformations.

**Fetal Intervention** Intervention is not appropriate for this usually lethal condition.

**Monitoring** Prenatal growth deficiency and polyhydramnios are commonly seen as components of the fetal akinesia sequence. Ultrasonography may be useful to document these findings, but fetal surveillance and assessment of placental function (including Doppler velocimetry) are inappropriate for this condition.

**Pregnancy Course** Polyhydramnios and preterm labor are common findings in this disorder. Therapeutic amniocentesis and tocolytic agents are contraindicated to prolong the pregnancy.

**Pregnancy Termination Issues** The multiple etiologies for the fetal akinesia syndromes almost always require a complete pathologic examination of an intact fetus to establish a precise diagnosis.

**Delivery** Fetuses with a small chest and polyhydramnios are likely to die of pulmonary hypoplasia. After an in-depth discussion of the implications of the diagnosis, most couples will concur with the recommendation that fetal monitoring and intervention for "nonreassuring fetal status" not be performed in labor.

## NEONATOLOGY

**Resuscitation** Pulmonary hypoplasia or the underlying central nervous system defect is most likely the dominant abnormalities affecting the survival potential for this group of infants. A full discussion with the parents about the limited prognosis for fetuses with this syndrome, and the decision not to attempt resuscitation is essential prior to delivery.

**Transport** Transfer to a tertiary center with pediatric subspecialty capabilities is appropriate to confirm the diagnosis. Once the diagnosis is confirmed, the parents should be provided with counseling regarding prolonged life support.

**Testing and Confirmation** There is no definitive diagnostic test antemortem, although magnetic resonance imaging or computed tomography may be helpful in delineating the underlying neurologic defects. Peripheral nerve and muscle biopsies may also be helpful.

**Nursery Management** At present, providing life support while proceeding with the diagnostic evaluation and facilitating the adjustment of the parents to the diagnosis and likely prognosis are the primary components of care. There are no reported cases of long-term survival that could inform a long-term management approach.

### SUGGESTED READINGS

1. Ajayi RA, Keen CE, Knott PD: Ultrasound diagnosis of the Pena-Shokeir phenotype at 14 weeks of pregnancy. Prenat Diagn 1995; 15:762-764.
2. Gerkins SM, Hertzberg BJ, Bovie JD, Beow O: Pena-Shokeir type I syndrome: in utero sonographic appearance. J Clin Ultrasound 1989; 17:56-61.
3. Gupta P, Sharma JB, Sharma R, et al: Antenatal ultrasound and MRI findings of Pena-Shokeir syndrome. Arch Gynecol Obstet 2011; 283:S27-S29.
4. Hall JG: Pena-Shokeir phenotype (fetal akinesia deformation sequence) revisited. Birth Defects Res A Clin Mol Teratol 2009; 85:677-694.
5. Ochi H, Kobeyashi E, Matsubara K, et al: Prenatal sonographic diagnosis of Pena-Shokeir syndrome type I. Ultrasound Obstet Gynecol 2001; 17:546-547.
6. Pena SK, Shokeir MH: Autosomal recessive cerebro-oculo-facial-skeletal (COFS) syndrome. Clin Genet 1974; 5:285-293.

7. Pena SDJ, Shokeir MH: Syndrome of camptodactyly, multiple ankyloses, facial anomalies, and pulmonary hypoplasia: a lethal condition. J Pediatr 1974; 85:373-375.
8. Senocak EU, Oguz KK, Halliloglu G, et al: Prenatal diagnosis of Pena-Shokeir syndrome phenotype by ultrasonography and MR imaging. Pediatr Radiol 2009; 39:377-380.
9. Tongsong T, Chanprapaph P, Khunamornpong S: Prenatal ultrasound of regional akinesia with Pena-Shokeir phenotype. Prenat Diagn 2000; 20:422-425.

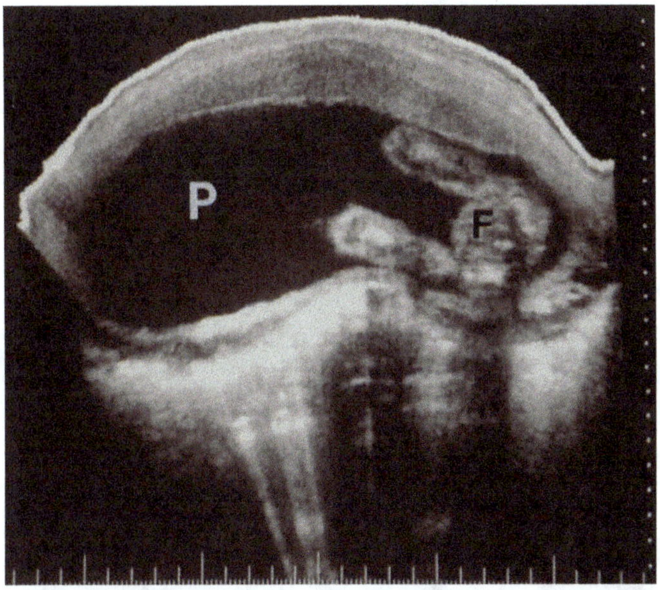


FIGURE 10.6A Polyhydramnios (P); fetus (F) with fetal akinesia.

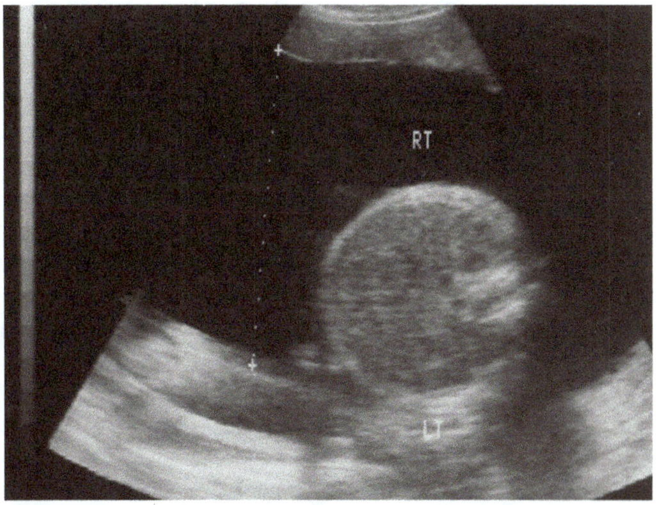


FIGURE 10.6B Polyhydramnios and absent fetal stomach. RT, right; LT, left.

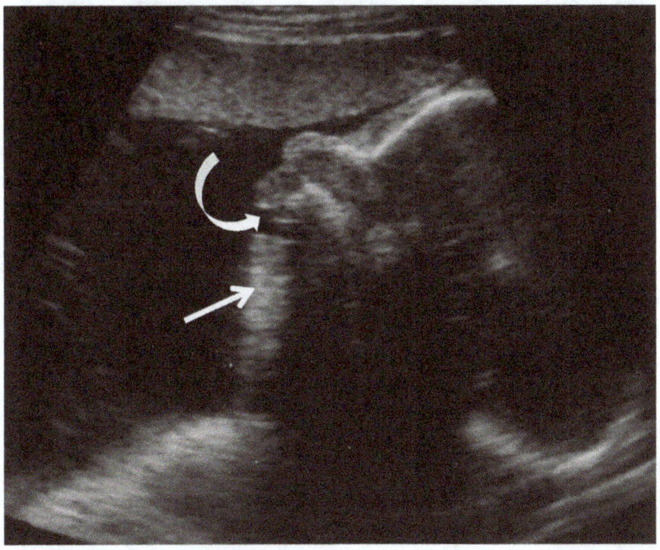

FIGURE 10.6C Micrognathia (straight arrow) with mouth fixed open (curved arrow).

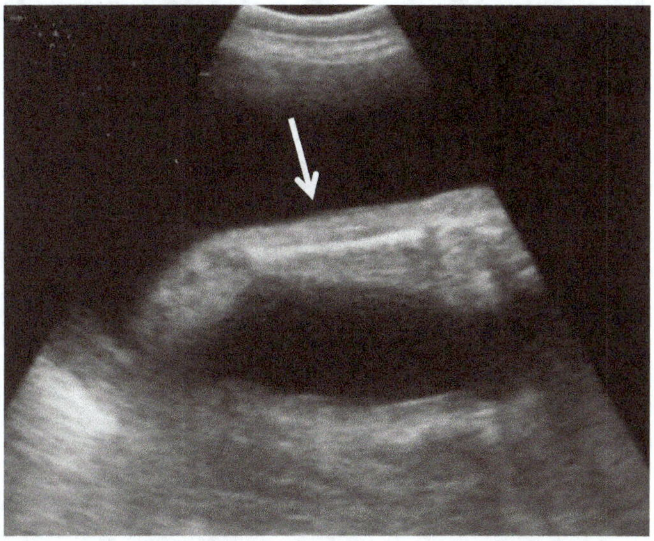

FIGURE 10.6D Rigidly fixed lower extremity; muscle atrophy (arrow).

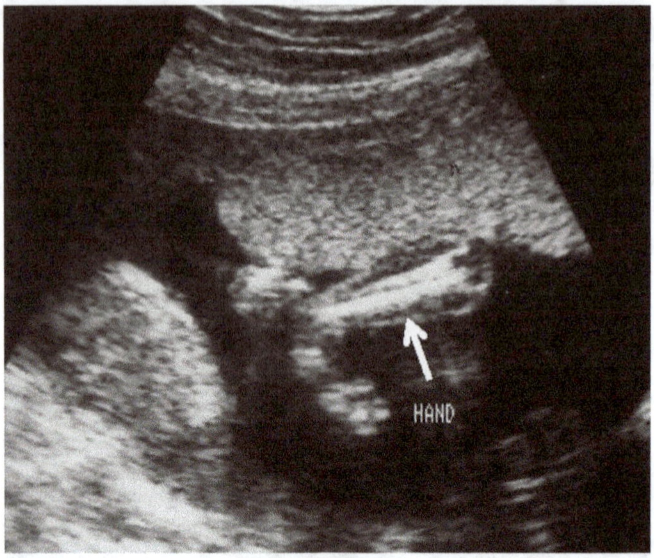


**FIGURE 10.6E** Fixed upper extremity with ulnar (arrow) deviation.

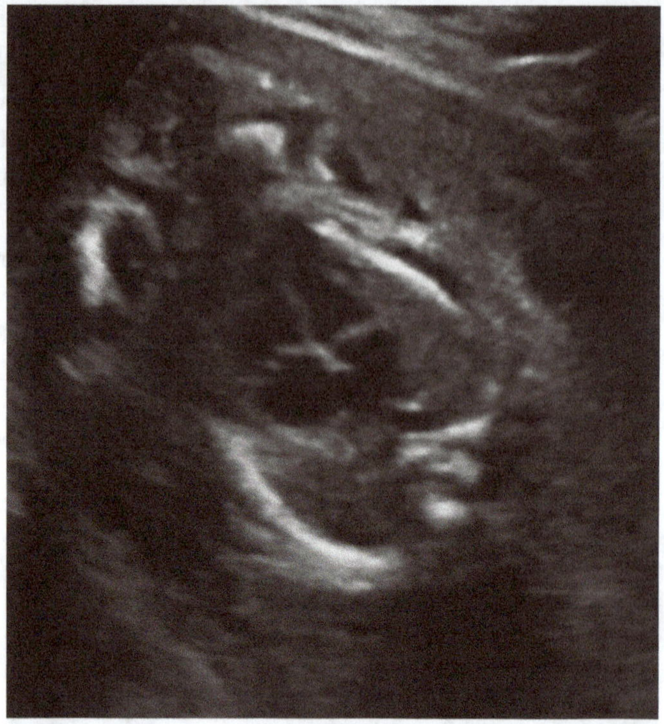

**FIGURE 10.6F** Normal heart circumference and small chest, suggestive of pulmonary hypoplasia.

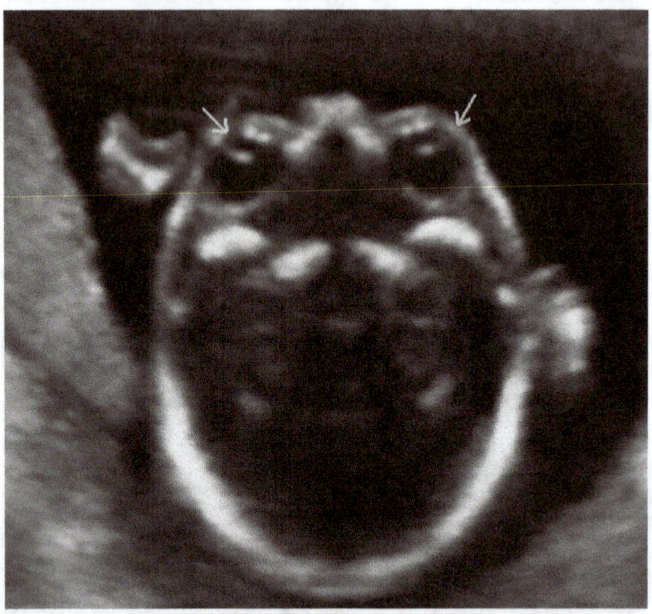

**FIGURE 10.6G** Normal lenses (arrows).

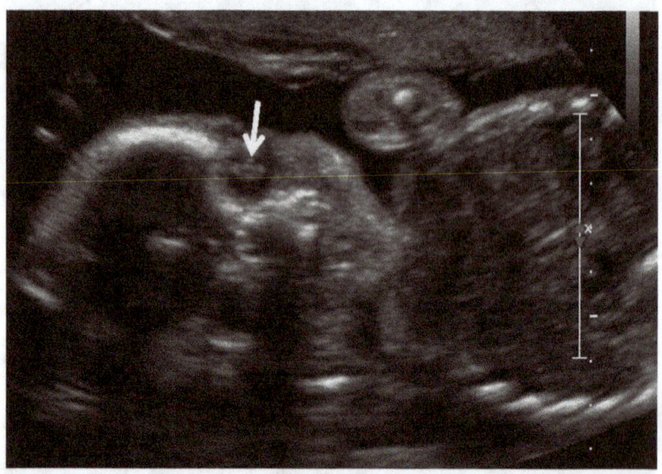

**FIGURE 10.6H** Type II Pena-Shokeir. Cataract (arrow).

# 10.7 SMITH-LEMLI-OPITZ SYNDROME

## EPIDEMIOLOGY/GENETICS

**Definition** Smith-Lemli-Opitz syndrome (SLOS) is a multiple congenital anomaly syndrome caused by a defect in cholesterol synthesis.

**Epidemiology** SLOS occurs in 1 in 20,000 to 1 in 60,000 births (M1:F1). The carrier frequency from population studies appears to be 1 in 25 to 1 in 33, suggesting that the incidence should be much higher. This discrepancy likely represents a very high in utero mortality in the form of spontaneous abortion and stillbirth. It is more common among northern Europeans, with a lower frequency in Africans and Asians.

**Embryology** This disorder is an inborn error of cholesterol metabolism due to mutations in the 7-dehydrocholesterol reductase gene. More than 100 mutations have been found to date. SLOS is characterized by prenatal onset of growth restriction, microcephaly (80%), and moderate-to-severe intellectual disability. Characteristic abnormalities include cleft palate (40% to 50%), cardiac defects (50%), postaxial polydactyly (50%), and two-to-three toe syndactyly (90% to 99%). Genitourinary malformations are seen in 90% of cases and include hypospadias, cryptorchidism, ambiguous genitalia, sex reversal, and upper tract abnormalities. Diagnosis is based on a consistent clinical phenotype with demonstration of elevated serum 7-dehydrocholesterol.

**Inheritance Patterns** Inheritance is autosomal recessive with a 25% recurrence risk in families with a previously affected child.

**Teratogens** None are known.

**Screening** 7-Dehydrocholesterol testing is recommended for families with a previously affected child. Elevated 7-dehydrocholesterol levels in amniotic fluid or in chorionic villi tissue samples are diagnostic. A markedly low unconjugated estriol, as part of a maternal serum screen, should prompt testing for SLOS.

**Prognosis** There is a continuum in SLOS that appears to be related to the specific mutations involved. Mildly affected children may survive into adulthood, but those with the more severe form often die in the newborn period from their lethal congenital anomalies. Of those who do survive, at least 20% will die in the first year of life. In those infants who survive, there is moderate-to-severe intellectual disability. Plasma cholesterol concentration correlates with the degree of severity. Dietary cholesterol supplementation has been used to treat these children, with some series showing benefit in growth and behavior. Randomized clinical trials have not shown a benefit.

## SONOGRAPHY

### FREQUENT FINDINGS

- First-trimester thick nuchal translucency
- Intrauterine growth restriction

- Microcephaly (84%)
- Agenesis of the corpus callosum
- Cardiac anomalies (54%)
  - Atrioventricular canal defect
  - Ventricular septal defect
  - Hypoplastic left heart
- Renal anomalies (25%)
  - Agenesis
  - Pyelectasis
- Ambiguous genitalia in males (70%)
  - Hypospadias
  - Bifid scrotum
- Syndactyly of the second and third toes (>95%)
- Postaxial polydactyly

### LESS FREQUENT

- Holoprosencephaly (5%)
- Ventriculomegaly
- Cerebellar hypoplasia
- Micrognathia
- Cleft palate
- Palmar simian crease
- Rhizomelic limb shortness
- Clubfeet

### KEY FINDINGS/PITFALLS

- Intrauterine growth restriction with polydactyly or a cardiac, renal, or genital malformation suggests a possible diagnosis of SLOS.

## PREGNANCY MANAGEMENT

**Investigations and Consultations Required** Because a precise diagnosis is not possible by ultrasonography, a complete evaluation of the fetus, including chromosome studies, microarray, and fetal echocardiography, is essential. A presumptive diagnosis can be made if maternal serum screening reveals a low serum unconjugated estriol value in conjunction with suggestive sonographic findings. Precise diagnostic testing is available using either chorionic villi or amniotic fluid cells and measuring 7-dehydrocholesterol.

**Fetal Intervention** At present, no fetal intervention is known to be effective. Current trials of dietary therapy in childhood may provide insights into possible fetal therapies.

**Monitoring** Prenatal growth deficiency and an increased incidence of stillbirth are found in this condition. Thorough discussion with the family and consultation with a pediatric geneticist should be undertaken before embarking on an intensive course of fetal surveillance.

**Pregnancy Course** Obstetric complications, such as intrauterine growth deficiency, stillbirth, and breech presentation, are not uncommon in fetuses affected with SLOS.

**Pregnancy Termination Issues** A precise biochemical diagnosis should be obtained before choosing the method of pregnancy termination. Following delivery, consideration could be given to molecular studies of the *DHCR7* gene (the only known causative gene) to allow molecular prenatal diagnosis in future pregnancies.

**Delivery** The significant incidence of neonatal complications makes delivery in a tertiary center the most appropriate option.

## NEONATOLOGY

**Resuscitation** When the prenatal diagnostic findings are suggestive of the severe form of the disorder, consideration of nonintervention in the event of respiratory depression at birth is appropriate. This recommendation is based on the severe prognosis for early infant death, moderate-to-severe intellectual disability in survivors, and, as yet, no effective treatment of the metabolic defect.

**Transport** Transfer of the newborn to a tertiary center with pediatric subspecialty diagnostic capabilities for confirmation of the diagnosis is appropriate.

**Testing and Confirmation** A defect in cholesterol biosynthesis has been identified. The characteristic plasma findings are abnormally low plasma cholesterol and elevated precursor, 7-dehydrocholesterol, concentrations. Ambiguous or female-appearing genitalia with a 46,XY karyotype occur frequently.

**Nursery Management** Cholesterol therapy may improve growth and development and currently is the recommended treatment. Other possible treatments, such as simvastatin and antioxidants, are currently being investigated in clinical trials. Surgery may be required to correct some of the anatomic abnormalities associated with the disorder. In general, management consists of supportive care, with attention to appropriate management of the associated renal and cardiac anomalies. Supporting the parents in long-term care planning for infants is essential.

### SUGGESTED READINGS


1. Bialer MG, Penshaszadeh VB, Kahn E, et al: Female external genitalia and mullerian duct derivatives in a 46,XY infant with Smith-Lemli-Opitz syndrome. Am J Med Genet 1987; 25:723-731.
2. Goldenberg A, Wolf C, Chevy F, et al: Antenatal manifestations of Smith-Lemli-Opitz (RSH) syndromes: a retrospective survey of 30 cases. Am J Med Genet 2004; 124A:423-426.
3. Hu H, Patel SB: Recent insights into the Smith-Lemli-Opitz syndrome. Clin Genet 2005; 68:383-391.
4. Hyatt JA, Clayton PT, Moscoso G, Nicolaides KH: Increased first trimester nuchal translucency as a prenatal manifestation of Smith-Lemli-Opitz syndrome. Am J Med Genet 1995; 58:374-376.

5. Irons MG, Nores J, Stewart TL, et al: Antenatal therapy of Smith-Lemli-Opitz syndrome. Fetal Diagn Ther 1999; 14:133-137.
6. Kelley RI, Hennekam RCM: The Smith-Lemli-Opitz syndrome. J Med Genet 2000; 37:321-335.
7. Ryan AK, Bartlett K, Clayton P, et al: Smith-Lemli-Opitz syndrome: a variable clinical and biochemical phenotype. J Med Genet 1998; 35:558-565.

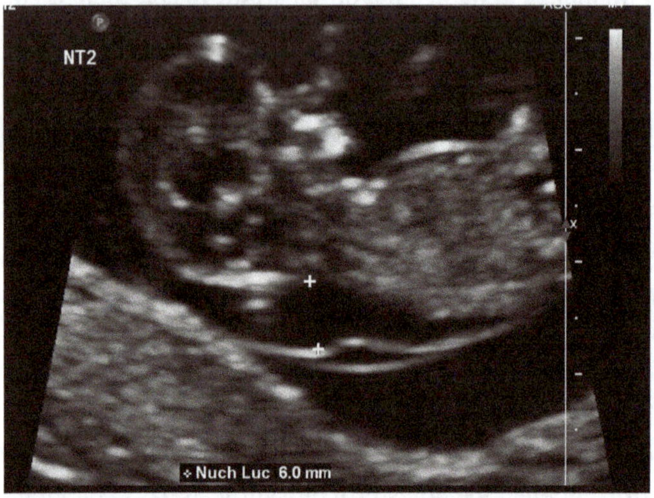


**FIGURE 10.7A** Enlarged nuchal translucency (+ … +).

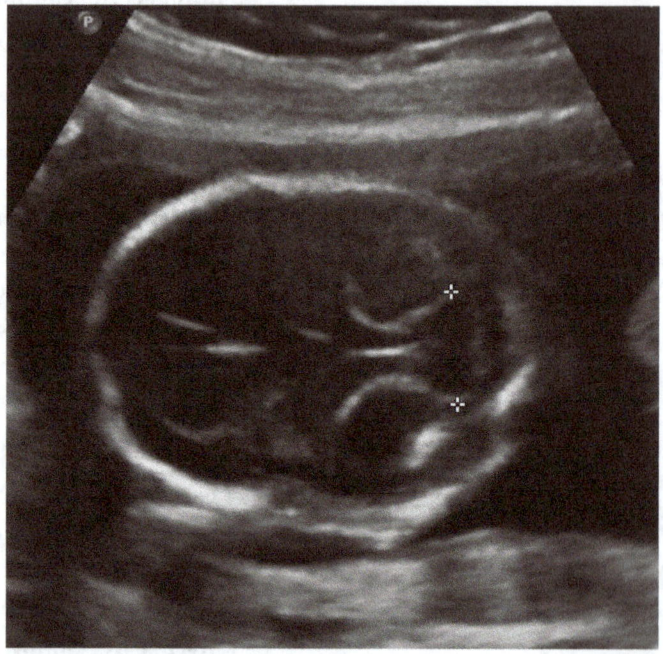

**FIGURE 10.7B** Cerebellar hypoplasia (+ … +).

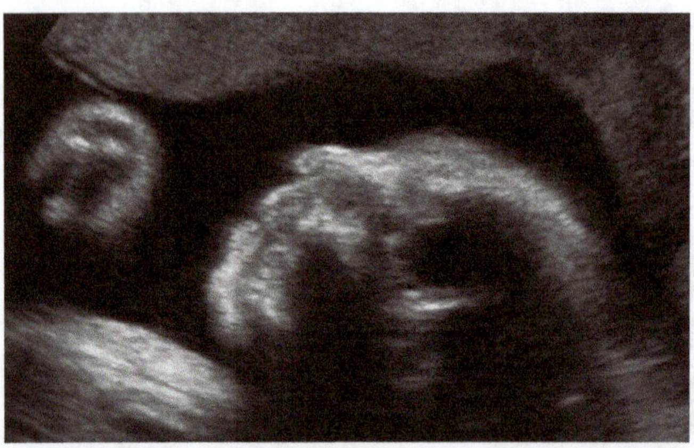

**FIGURE 10.7C** Microcephaly.

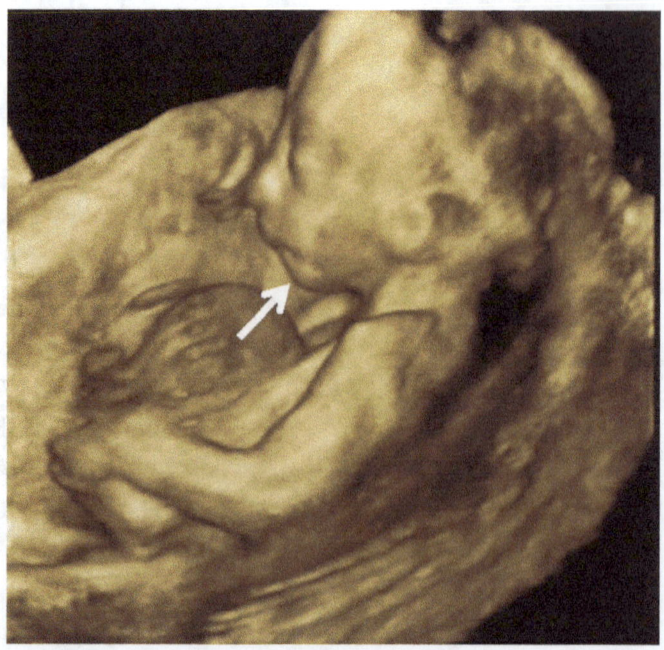

**FIGURE 10.7D** Micrognathia (arrow).

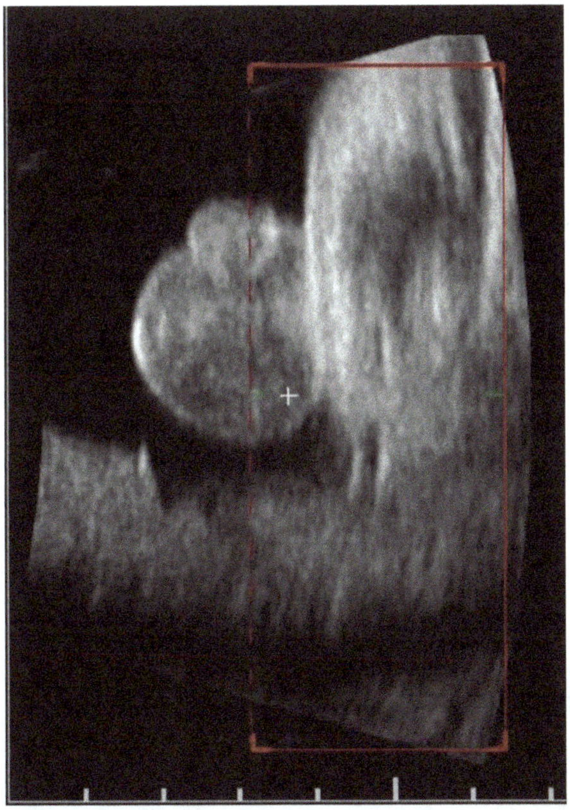

**FIGURE 10.7E** Severe hypospadias.

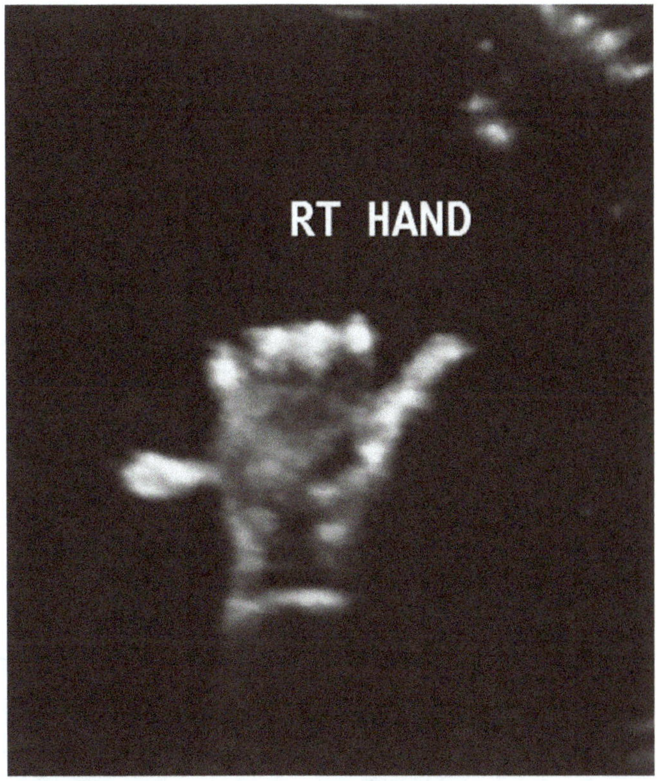


**FIGURE 10.7F** Postaxial polydactyly.

# 10.8 TUBEROUS SCLEROSIS COMPLEX

## EPIDEMIOLOGY/GENETICS

**Definition** Tuberous sclerosis complex (TSC) is an autosomal dominant, multisystem disorder characterized by the formation of hamartomas in multiple organ systems, most commonly the brain, skin, kidney, and eye.

**Epidemiology** TSC occurs in about 1 in 6000 births (M1:F1).

**Embryology** Postnatally, TSC is characterized by

- Facial angiofibromas (83%)
- Seizures (80%)
- Intellectual disability (50%)
- Renal angiomyolipomas and cysts (60%)
- Dental pitting (7%)
- Cardiac rhabdomyomas
- Intracranial calcification (50%)
- Brain, retina, optic nerve, and periungual hamartomas
- Hypopigmented macules (60%).

A definitive diagnosis of TSC requires two major features or one major plus two minor features. Antenatally, cardiac rhabdomyomas are the most common feature, and it is estimated that 30% to 50% of children with TSC have antenatal cardiac rhabdomyoma. The majority (50% to 80%) of children with cardiac rhabdomyomas have TSC.

**Inheritance Patterns** Inheritance is autosomal dominant with great variability. Approximately two-thirds of cases represent new mutations. Individuals with TSC have a 50% chance of passing the condition to each of their children. Gonadal mosaicism has been reported in some families. Two genetic loci, TSC1 located on chromosomes 9q34 and TSC2 located on 16p13, have been identified and account for 85% of the cases.

**Teratogens** None are known.

**Prognosis** Seizures and intellectual disability are the most important contributors to the morbidity associated with TSC. Childhood brain tumors and kidney failure are uncommon complications. Cardiac rhabdomyomas almost always regress spontaneously postnatally.

## SONOGRAPHY

### FREQUENT FINDINGS

- Cardiac tumor/tumors
  - Echogenic
  - Globular
  - Usually located within the ventricles or interventricular septum

### LESS FREQUENT

- Cardiac dysrhythmia
- Nonimmune hydrops
- Cerebral hamartomas

### KEY FINDINGS/PITFALLS

- Cardiac rhabdomyoma
  - Most common benign congenital tumor
  - May result in dysrhythmia (16% to 47%) and nonimmune hydrops
  - Single or multiple lesions
    - Usually, these are within the ventricle.
    - Fifty percent to 86% occur with TSC.
    - Most regress after birth.
      - Complete resolution of 80% in infancy
    - The detection of multiple cardiac tumors increases the likelihood of tuberous sclerosis over patients with a single tumor.
      - Of fetuses with multiple ventricular tumors, 95% have tuberous sclerosis.
    - Atrial tumors are only rarely associated with tuberous sclerosis.
- Cerebral periventricular nodules are rarely identified on antenatal sonography.
  - Nodule size is 1-4 mm.
  - A normal prenatal magnetic resonance image cannot exclude a diagnosis of cerebral tuberous sclerosis.
- A single cardiac tumor and the presence of one or more nodules on a fetal cerebral magnetic resonance image fulfill the criteria for a diagnosis of tuberous sclerosis.

## PREGNANCY MANAGEMENT

**Investigation and Consultation Required** Additional investigations depend on which structural malformations are present. Careful evaluation of the parents for signs of tuberous sclerosis is necessary if a presumptive diagnosis of fetal tuberous sclerosis is made. Additional consultations, such as with cardiology, will depend on the malformations seen.

**Fetal Intervention** None is indicated unless cardiac complications develop (hydrops or arrhythmia). Management would follow usual guidelines for these complications.

**Monitoring** As the rhabdomyomas can grow, possibly causing obstruction, serial sonographic examinations should be performed to detect signs of arrhythmia or hydrops. If these complications arise, consideration can be given to early delivery, but only after full discussion with the family regarding the significant complications associated with TSC.

**Pregnancy Course** No specific obstetric complications are to be expected unless fetal hydrops develops.

**Pregnancy Termination Issues** Unless the diagnosis has been made in one of the parents, an intact fetus is necessary for a complete autopsy.

**Delivery** Site of delivery will depend on the type of malformations seen and fetal status. In general, delivery is best accomplished in a tertiary center, particularly when rhabdomyomas are present.

## NEONATOLOGY

**Resuscitation** Management of the onset of respiration is determined by the spectrum of fetal abnormalities identified. Hydrops fetalis, either from cardiac arrhythmia or from intracavital obstruction of blood flow, may be present. If so, interventions must be directed at reducing the impingement of lung expansion by a pericardial fluid collection and pleural or peritoneal effusions. The specific arrhythmic type will determine the appropriate antiarrhythmic therapy. The presence of intracranial tubers rarely affects onset of respiration.

**Transport** Transfer to a tertiary center with the appropriate pediatric and surgical subspecialists and diagnostic capabilities is determined by the clinical presentation of the disorder. Immediate transfer is recommended with any evidence of hemodynamic instability or neurologic symptomatology. The neonate who has an uneventful adaptation and remains asymptomatic may be referred for outpatient evaluation within the first few weeks following birth.

**Testing and Confirmation** Appropriate evaluation of cardiac tumors includes electrocardiography, echocardiography, and, in selected cases, cardiac catheterization or cardiothoracic magnetic resonance imaging. Appropriately weighted magnetic resonance imaging is the modality of choice for demonstration of intracranial lesions, although both ultrasonography and computed tomography have been used.

**Nursery Management** Interventions should be directed at amelioration and correction of any hemodynamic abnormalities and cardiac arrhythmias. Most reports of fetal/neonatal rhabdomyomas indicate resolution of the tumors during the first several months, leading to the recommendation that surgical excision of the tumor in early infancy be limited to cases with persistent symptoms and the lack of evidence of tumor regression. The onset of seizures in early infancy from tuberous sclerosis has been reported and, if present, requires anticonvulsant therapy.

### SUGGESTED READINGS


1. Alkalay A, Ferry DA, Lin B, et al: Spontaneous regression of cardiac tumor rhabdomyoma in tuberous sclerosis. Clin Pediatr 1987; 26:532-535.
2. Bader RM, Chitayat D, Kelly E, et al: Fetal rhabdomyoma: prenatal diagnosis, clinical outcomes, and incidence of associated tuberous sclerosis complex. J Pediatr 2003; 143:620-624.
3. Calhoun BC, Watson PT, Hegge F: Ultrasound diagnosis of an obstructive cardiac rhabdomyoma with severe hydrops and hypoplastic lungs. A case report. J Reprod Med 1991; 36:317-319.
4. Fenoglio JJ, McAllister HA, Ferrans VJ: Cardiac rhabdomyoma: a clinicopathologic and electron microscopy study. Am J Cardiol 1976; 38:241-251.

5. Holley DG, Martin GR, Brenner JI, et al: Diagnosis and management of fetal cardiac tumors: a multicenter experience and review of published reports. J Am Coll Cardiol 1995; 26:516-520.
6. Roach ES, Gomez MR, Northrup H: Tuberous sclerosis complex consensus conference: revised clinical diagnostic criteria. J Child Neurol 1998; 13:624-628.
7. Sgro M, Garozzino T, Toi A, et al: Prenatal detection of cerebral lesions in a fetus with tuberous sclerosis. Ultrasound Obstet Gynecol 1999; 14:356-359.
8. Staley BA, Vail EA, Thiele EA: Tuberous sclerosis complex: diagnostic challenges, presenting symptoms, and commonly missed signs. Pediatrics 2011; 127:e117-e125.
9. Tworetzsky W, McElhinney DB, Margossian R, et al: Association between cardiac tumors and tuberous sclerosis in the fetus and neonate. Am J Cardiol 2003; 92:487-489.
10. Weiderholt WC, Gomez MR, Kurland LT: Incidence and prevalence of tuberous sclerosis in Rochester, Minnesota 1950 through 1982. Neurology 1985; 35:600-603.

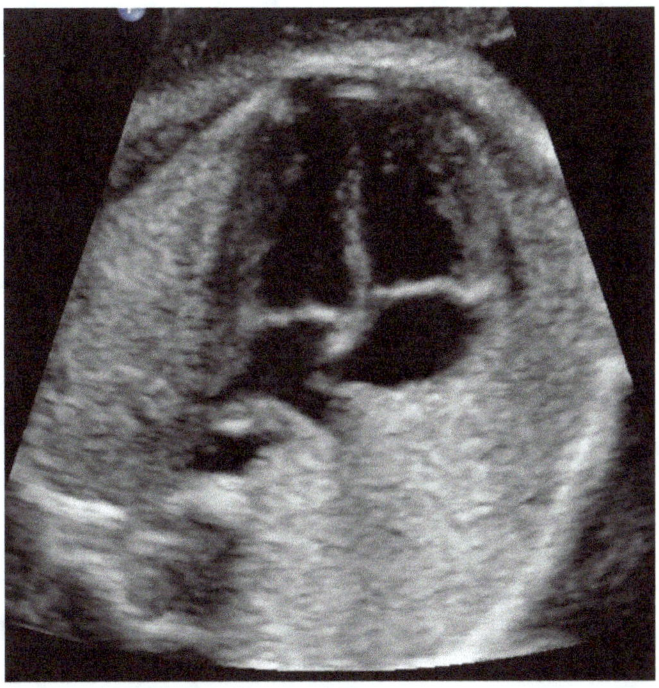

**FIGURE 10.8A** Normal four-chamber cardiac view.

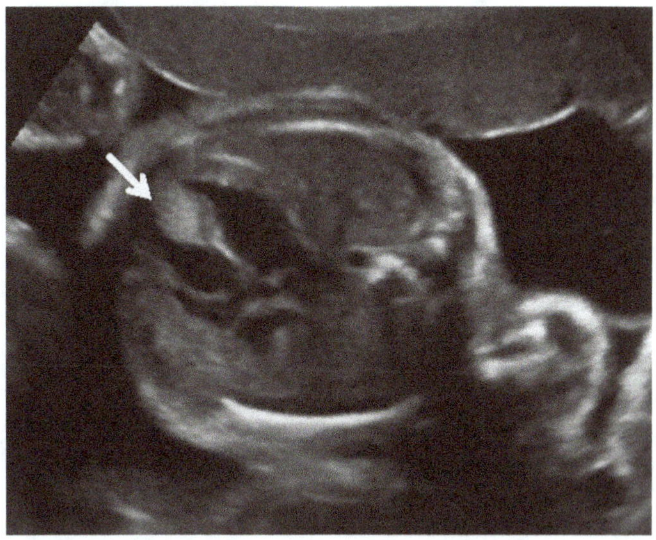

**FIGURE 10.8B** Single cardiac ventricle septal rhabdomyoma (arrow).

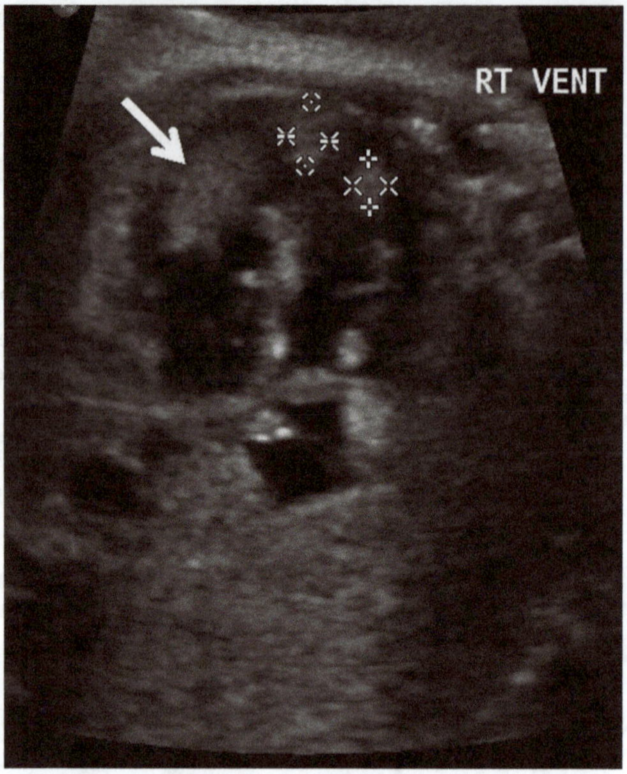


**FIGURE 10.8C** Large left ventricular rhabdomyoma (arrow); two smaller (markers) right ventricular (RT VENT) rhabdomyomas.

# 10.9 VACTERL SYNDROME

## EPIDEMIOLOGY/GENETICS

**Definition** VACTERL is an acronym for a nonrandom association of birth defects, including vertebral anomalies, anal atresia, cardiac defects, tracheo-esophageal fistula, renal anomalies, and radial limb abnormalities. Diagnosis is based on the presence of at least three of these defects.

**Epidemiology** Occurrence is 1 in 10,000 to 1 in 40,000 live births (M1:F1).

**Embryology** Etiology is unknown. To date, no unifying etiology has been found, and no specific genes have been implicated. Fanconi syndrome may present with similar clinical features and must be excluded. Trisomy 18 and del 13q can present with a VACTERL phenotype.

**Inheritance Pattern** Inheritance is sporadic. However, there have been reports of familial clustering. There is a VACTERL-like syndrome with hydrocephalus that has autosomal recessive or X-linked inheritance. Accurate recurrence risk depends on ruling out disorders with similar features that are inherited in a Mendelian fashion.

**Teratogens** Maternal diabetes mellitus is teratogenic.

**Prognosis** With modern surgical techniques, there is an excellent survival rate. Central nervous system abnormalities are rare, and most children have normal intelligence.

## SONOGRAPHY

### FINDINGS

- Vertebral (60% to 90%)
  - Hemivertebrae
  - Scoliosis
  - Spina bifida
- Anal (55% to 90%)
  - Imperforate anus
- Cardiac (40% to 80%)
  - Two-vessel umbilical cord
  - Ventricular septal defect
  - Tetralogy of Fallot
  - Transposition of the great vessels
  - Truncus arteriosis
  - Hypoplastic left heart
- Tracheoesophageal fistula (50% to 80%)
  - Esophageal atresia
- Renal (50% to 80%)
  - Pyelocaliectasis
  - Renal agenesis

- Cystic renal dysplasia
- Horseshoe kidney

- Limb (40% to 55%)
  - Polydactyly
  - Syndactyly
  - Radial ray defect
- Polyhydramnios
- Single umbilical artery (30%)

### KEY FINDINGS/PITFALLS

- The finding of one anomaly of the VACTERL association should prompt an extended fetal anatomic survey that looks for other potential anomalies.
- Sonographic clues to the diagnosis of VACTERL depend on the specific congenital anomalies in a given case.
  - Single umbilical artery (should prompt a thorough fetal anatomic survey)
  - Abnormal cardiac axis with tetralogy of Fallot, transposition of the great vessels, and truncus arteriosus
  - Abnormal spinal contour with hemivertebrae
  - Absent fetal stomach with esophageal atresia or tracheoesophageal fistula
  - Dilated colon due to anal atresia

### DIFFERENTIAL DIAGNOSIS

| SYNDROMES IN COMMON WITH VACTERL | | | |
|---|---|---|---|
| Syndrome | Cardiac | Renal | Other |
| CHARGE | √ | √ | |
| DiGeorge | √ | √ | |
| Fanconi syndrome | √ | √ | Radial array anomalies |
| Goldenhar | √ | √ | Limb anomalies, vertebral anomalies |
| Holt-Oram | √ | – | Limb anomalies |

## PREGNANCY MANAGEMENT

**Investigations and Consultations Required** As with all multiple-malformation cases, chromosome studies and microarray studies are essential, even though VACTERL itself is not associated with a chromosomal abnormality. Fetal echocardiography should be performed to delineate the severity of the cardiac defect. A pediatric surgeon should be consulted to discuss surgical management with the family.

**Monitoring** In the absence of polyhydramnios, no specific changes in obstetric care are required. Serial sonograms to detect increasing amniotic fluid volumes are appropriate.

**Pregnancy Course** Polyhydramnios may be a complicating factor and may result in preterm labor.

**Pregnancy Termination Issues** To establish a precise diagnosis, an intact fetus must be delivered and appropriate morphologic, radiologic, and pathologic examinations performed.

**Delivery** Once the diagnosis is made (based on three or more of the associated anomalies), the possibility of other associated anomalies that were not prenatally diagnosed must be anticipated. The site of delivery should be a tertiary center with appropriate medical and surgical specialists available to deal with the multiple malformations that are a part of this syndrome. The mode of delivery should be based on obstetric indications.

## NEONATOLOGY

**Resuscitation** The special management issues at birth are based on the specific organ defects known to be present. Among the ones included in the VACTERL association, tracheoesophageal fistula and cardiac defects have an impact on the onset of respiration and early adaptation. Resuscitation and stabilization of cardiorespiratory function measures to be instituted are discussed in the chapters concerned with those specific defects.

**Transport** Referral to a tertiary perinatal center with multiple pediatric and surgical subspecialists is always indicated. Care during transport should include the specific measures for each of the defects known or suspected to be present.

**Testing and Confirmation** A diagnosis can be made at birth. Radiographic studies are recommended to look for associated spinal abnormalities.

**Nursery Management** Priority in management is determined by the specific malformations known to be present. Thus, immediate diagnostic evaluation to identify the defects the infant manifests should be instituted. The next step is to coordinate the various surgical interventions to address the specific congenital anomalies: anal atresia, cardiac malformations, or tracheoesophageal fistula. In general, the vertebral, extremity, and renal defects are not associated with significant dysfunction in the neonatal period and therefore have less influence on the initial plan of care. If optimal surgical correction is achievable, the prognosis can be relatively positive. Patients with VACTERL syndrome do not tend to have neurocognitive deficits.

### SUGGESTED READINGS


1. Botto LD, Khoury MK, Mastroiacovo P, et al: The spectrum of congenital anomalies of the VATER association: an international study. Am J Med Genet 1997; 71:8-15.
2. Caston M, Rinaldi R, Capocaccia P, et al: VACTERL association and maternal diabetes: a possible causal relationship? Birth Defects Res A Clin Mol Teratol 2008; 82:169-172.
3. Khoury MJ, Cordero JF, Greenberg F, et al: A population study of the VACTERL association: evidence for its etiologic heterogeneity. Pediatrics 1983; 71:815-820.

4. Miller OF, Kolon TF: Prenatal diagnosis of VACTERL association. J Urol 2001; 166:2389-2391.
5. Ritter M, Paz JE, Castilla EE: VACTERL association, epidemiologic definition, and delineation. Am J Med Genet 1996; 63:529-536.
6. Solomon BD, Pineda-Alvarez DE, Raam MS, et al: Analysis of component findings in 79 patients diagnosed with VACTERL association. Am J Med Genet A. 2010; 152A:2236-2244.
7. Solomon BD, Baker LA, Bear KA, et al: An approach to the identification of anomalies and etiologies in neonates with identified or suspected VACTERL (vertebral defects, anal atresia, trachea-esophageal fistula with esophageal atresia, cardiac defects, renal and limb anomalies) association. J Pediatr 2014; 164:451-457.
8. Tongsong T, Wanapirak C, Piyamongkol W, Sudasana J: Prenatal sonographic diagnosis of VATER association. J Clin Ultarsound 1999; 27:378-384.

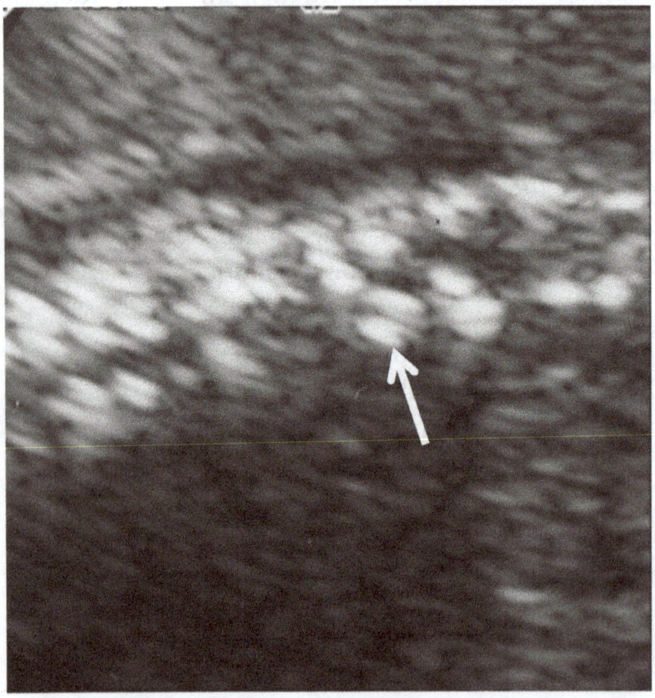

FIGURE 10.9A Hemivertebra (arrow).

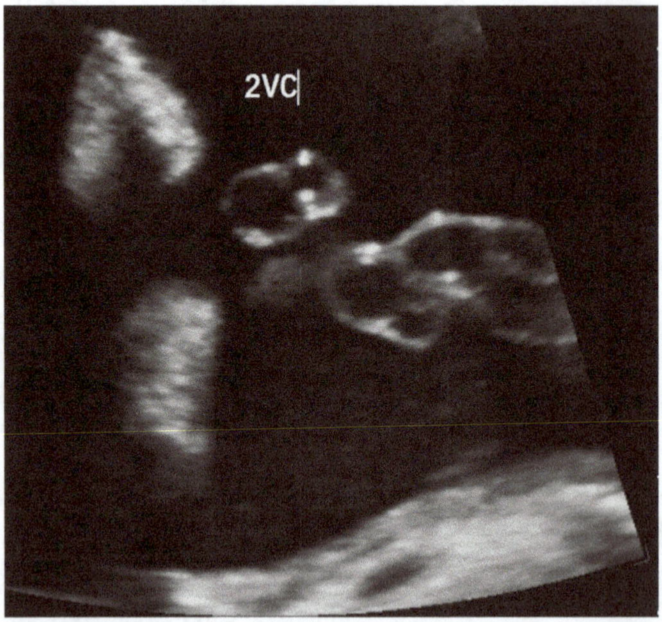


FIGURE 10.9B Two-vessel umbilical cord (2VC).

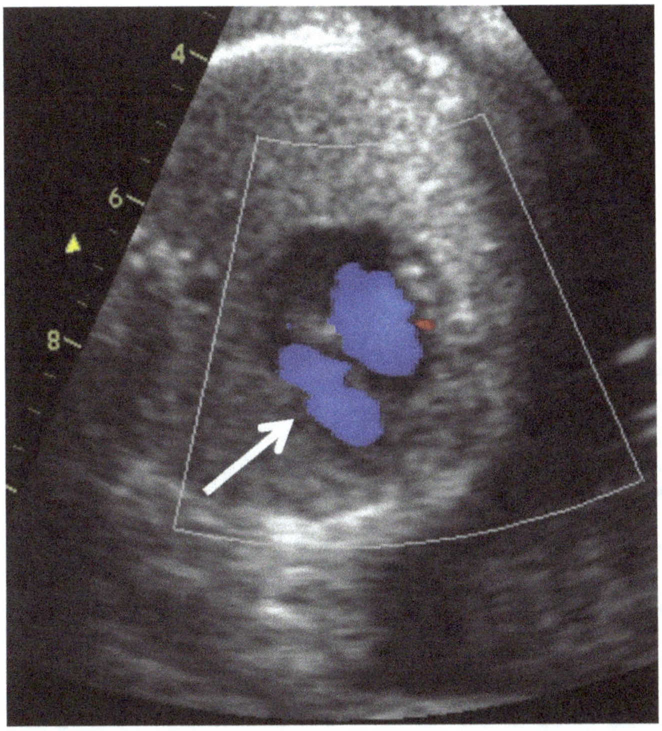

**FIGURE 10.9C** Small left ventricle (arrow) due to aortic coarctation.

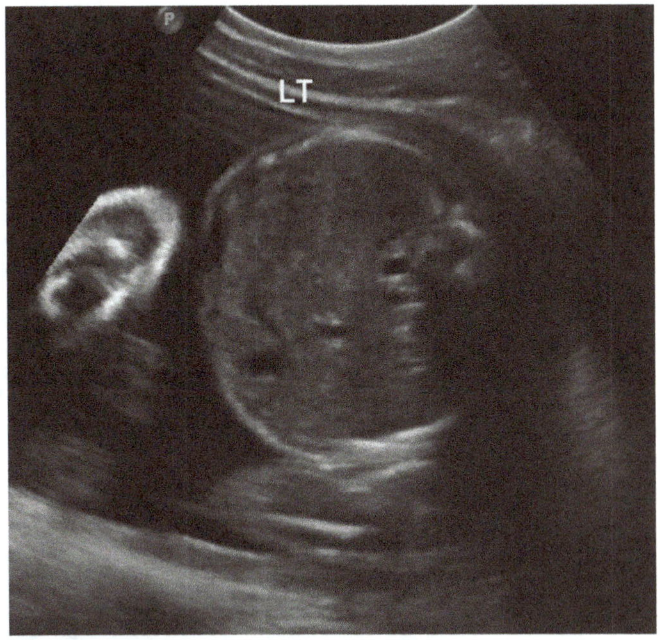


**FIGURE 10.9D** Absent fetal stomach (LT, left) due to esophageal atresia.

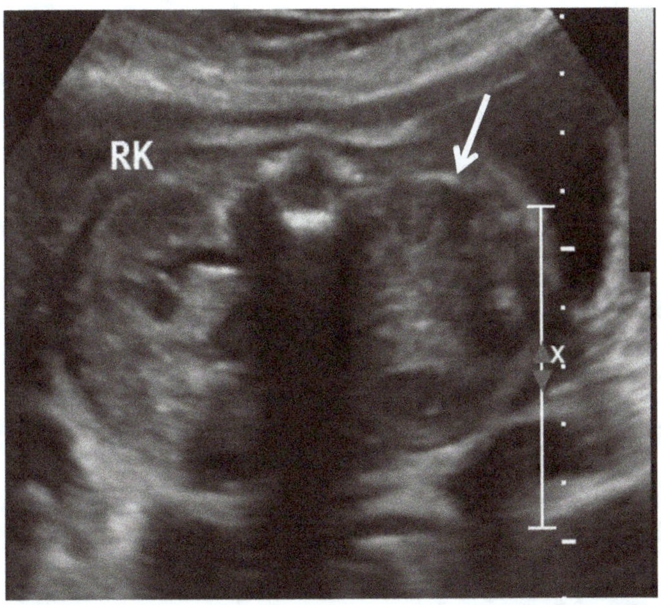


**FIGURE 10.9E** Left renal agenesis (arrow). RK, right kidney.

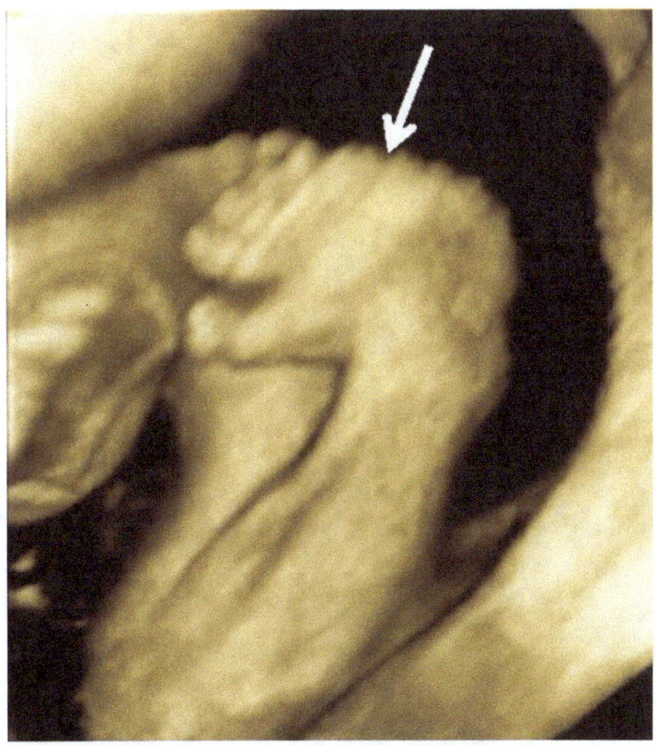

**FIGURE 10.9F** Three-dimensional image of clubfoot (arrow).

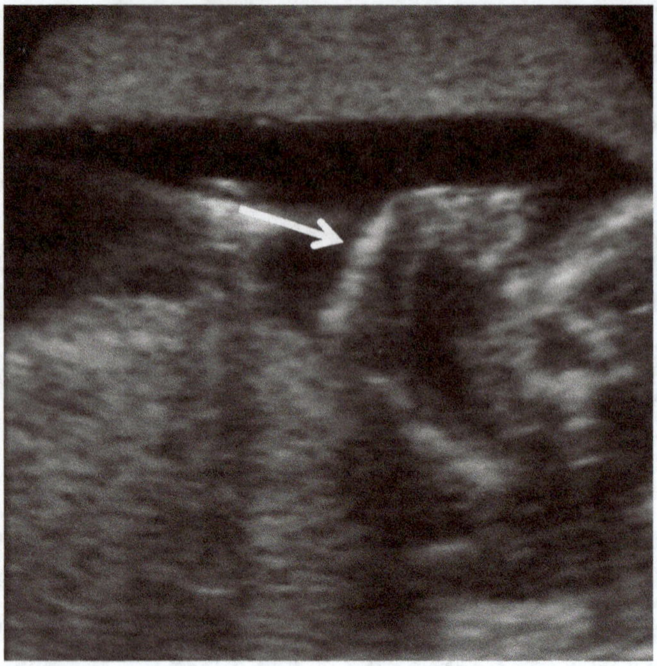

FIGURE 10.9G Absent radius (arrow).

# CHAPTER 11

# TWINS

# 11.1 MONOCHORIONIC/MONOAMNIOTIC TWINNING

## EPIDEMIOLOGY/GENETICS

**Definition** Monoamniotic (MA) twins share a common amniotic sac. Triplets and higher-order multifetal gestations also may contain a monochorionic (MC) twin pair. The most severe form of MA twins is conjoined (CJ) twins, which are defined by the shared body region ("pagus"), and can be dorsally (more common) or ventrally conjoined.

**Incidence** The reported incidence of MA twinning ranges from 1 in 1650 to 1 in 93,734 live births. Up to 20% of higher-order multifetal gestations can contain a MC pair. CJ twins are the rarest MC complication, occurring at an approximate rate of 10.25 per million births.

**Embryology** MA and CJ twins are at the last part of a spectrum of incomplete cleavage. Discordant anomalies occur more commonly in MC gestations (6% to 8%).

There are several proposed mechanisms for the increased incidence of structural anomalies in MC twins, including teratogenicity of zygotic splitting and vascular "accidents." Because of their unique angioarchitecture, MC twins have a higher incidence of morbidity and mortality than dichorionic (DC) twins. This is likely due to the sharing of a single placenta and the vascular communications that exist between twins. Loss of one twin can result in death (~15%) or significant neurologic injury (~30%) in the surviving twin. The suspected mechanism is pressure and volume shifts that occur at the time of death of one twin: the surviving twin exsanguinates into the demised twin.

**Inheritance Patterns** Inheritance is sporadic.

**Teratogenesis** None are known.

**Prognosis** The prognosis for MA twins is largely related to the presence of congenital malformations and the gestational age at delivery. Multifetal MC gestations are at a high risk for pregnancy complications and invariably result in preterm birth, either iatrogenic or spontaneous. Only 18% of prenatally diagnosed CJ twins survive.

## SONOGRAPHY

### FINDINGS

- MA twins are suspected when an intertwin membrane cannot be identified in association with other sonographic stigmata of an MC gestation.
  - Single placental mass
  - Concordant gender
- Documenting cord entanglement confirms the diagnosis.
- Other complications of MC gestations can occur within a MA gestation.
  - Twin-twin transfusion syndrome (TTTS)

- Selective fetal growth restriction (sFGR)
- Twin anemia-polycythemia sequence (TAPS)
- Discordant anomalies

### KEY FINDINGS/PITFALLS

- Some major structural anomalies, such as anencephaly and lower urinary tract obstruction, can be reliably detected in the late first trimester.
- Chorionicity in high-order multifetal gestations is best determined in the first trimester.
- The diagnosis of CJ twins is relatively straightforward.
  - No intervening amniotic fluid
  - Single umbilical cord with more than three vessels
  - Persistence of heads at the same body plane
  - Lack of separation of fetuses over time
- Defining the degree of conjoining can be challenging and may require high-resolution two-dimensional ultrasound, three-dimensional ultrasound, color Doppler mapping, magnetic resonance imaging (MRI), and fetal echocardiography.

### DIFFERENTIAL DIAGNOSIS

- Twin-twin transfusion syndrome
- Preterm premature rupture of one sac
- Selective fetal growth restriction
- Bilateral renal agenesis in one fetus

## PREGNANCY MANAGEMENT

**Investigations and Consults Required** Multidisciplinary collaboration and prenatal consultation are essential in developing a newborn management plan. The services involved will depend on the nature of the structural anomalies identified.

**Monitoring** MA twins typically undergo intensive antenatal surveillance beginning at the point of viability, as either inpatients or outpatients, until delivery, typically at 32 weeks. MC gestations discordant for anomalies and multifetal MC gestations that are not reduced should be monitored intensively, especially after the point of viability. Those that are reduced can be offered more routine surveillance, as the risk of acute twin-twin exsanguination is eliminated by cord coagulation.

**Fetal Intervention** MA twin gestations discordant for major anomalies may be candidates for selective termination of the anomalous fetus as a means of pregnancy prolongation for the healthy co-twin. Cord transection after occlusion is recommended to avoid cord accident. Consideration should be given to reduction of the MC pair of a high-order MC gestation as these pregnancies are at a high risk for complications and preterm birth. Unlike other circumstances of selective termination in MC gestations where cord occlusion is required, multifetal pregnancy reduction of the MC pair can be performed using standard techniques of injection of cardioplegic medications under ultrasound guidance and should be performed in the late first trimester.

**Pregnancy Termination Issues** Selective feticide in MC gestations must be performed by a cord occlusive technique, as cardioplegic medications can pass from one twin to the other through patent vascular channels.

**Delivery** Delivery should occur in a tertiary center because of the high risk of prematurity. Because of the risk of cord entanglement, MA twins are generally delivered by cesarean section. Gestational age, the patient's wishes regarding neonatal management, and the risk of maternal harm must be weighed when considering route of delivery for CJ twins.

## NEONATOLOGY

**Resuscitation** Anticipate difficulty with spontaneous onset of respiration, as well as problems associated with preterm delivery.

**Transport** Transfer to a tertiary center for neonatal intensive care is necessary in the majority of cases. Respiratory assistance, as well as support of myocardial function with continuous infusion of inotropic medication, may be required during transport.

**Nursery Management** Respiratory support, relief of myocardial stress, reduction of congestive heart failure, and correction of perinatal asphyxia are usually needed; thus, it is necessary to institute measures to accomplish these goals immediately following birth. Because most twin pregnancies are delivered prematurely, respiratory distress syndrome may also further complicate the clinical course. Early administration of surfactant replacement therapy may hasten the resolution of the latter.

### SUGGESTED READINGS


1. Bajoria R, Wee LY, Anwar S, Ward S: Outcome of twin pregnancies complicated by single intrauterine death in relation to vascular anatomy of the monochorionic placenta. Hum Reprod 1999; 14:2124-2130.
2. Bebbington M: Selective reduction in complex monochorionic gestations. Am J Perinatology 2014; 31:S51-S58.
3. Chervenak FA, McCullough LB: Ethical challenges in the management of multiple pregnancies: the professional responsibility model of perinatal ethics. J Perinatal Med 2013; 41:61-64.
4. Geipel A, Berg C, Katalinic A, et al: Prenatal diagnosis and obstetric outcomes in triplet pregnancies in relation to chorionicity. Br J Obset Gynaecol 2005; 112:554-558.
5. Lewi L, Jani J, Blickstein I, et al: The outcome of monochorionic diamniotic twin gestations in the era of invasive fetal therapy: a prospective cohort study. Am J Obstet Gynecol 2008; 199:514 e1-8.
6. Lewi L, Gratacos E, Ortibus E, et al: Pregnancy and infant outcome of 80 consecutive cord coagulations in complicated monochorionic multiple pregnancies. Am J Obstet Gynecol 2006; 194:782-789.

7. Mackenzie TC, Crombleholme TM, Johnson MP, et al: The natural history of prenatally diagnosed conjoined twins. J Pediatr Surg 2002; 37:303-309.
8. Van Mieghem T, De Heus R, Lewi L, et al: Prenatal management of monoamniotic twin pregnancies. Obstet Gynecol 2014; 124:498-506.

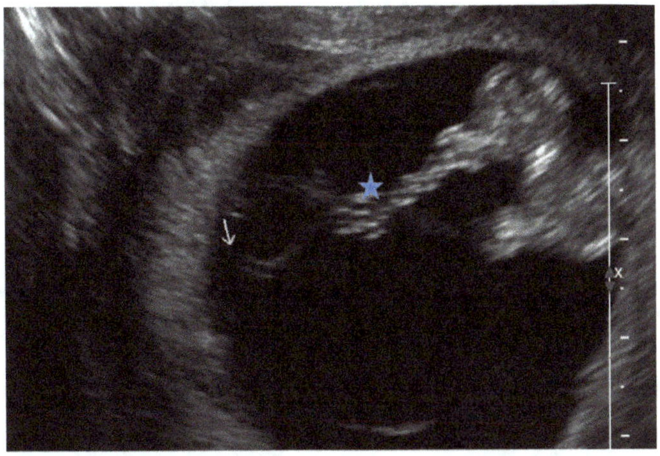

**FIGURE 11.1A** First trimester monoamniotic twins. Cord entanglement (star).

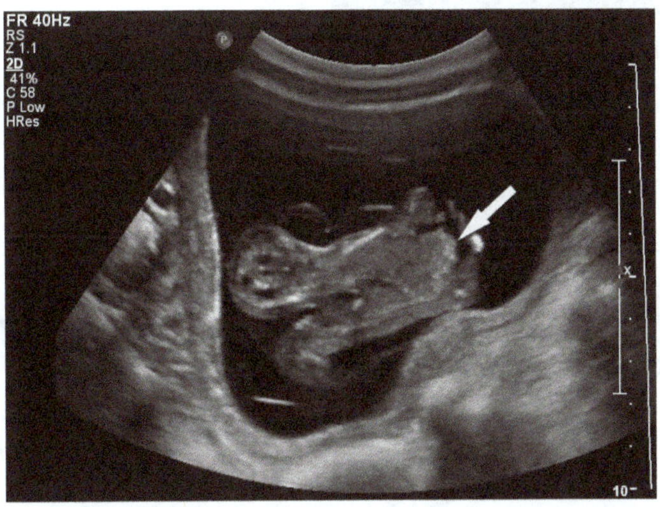


**FIGURE 11.1B** Omphalopagus conjoined twins (arrow).

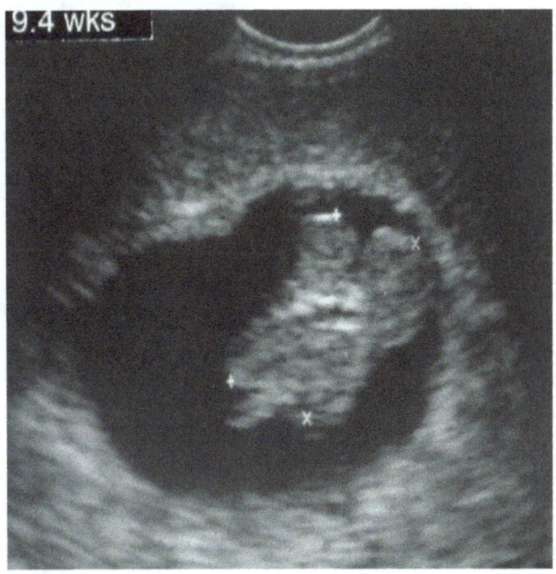


**FIGURE 11.1C** 9.3 week conjoined twins.

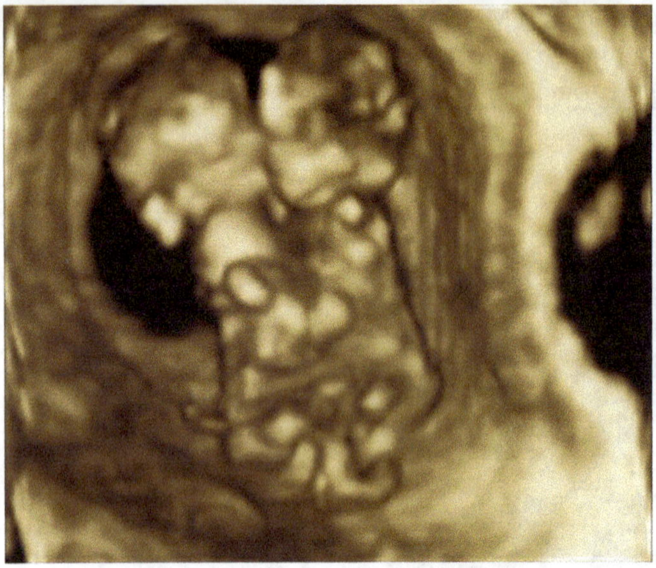

**FIGURE 11.1D** Three-dimensional image of conjoined (omphalopagus) first trimester twins.

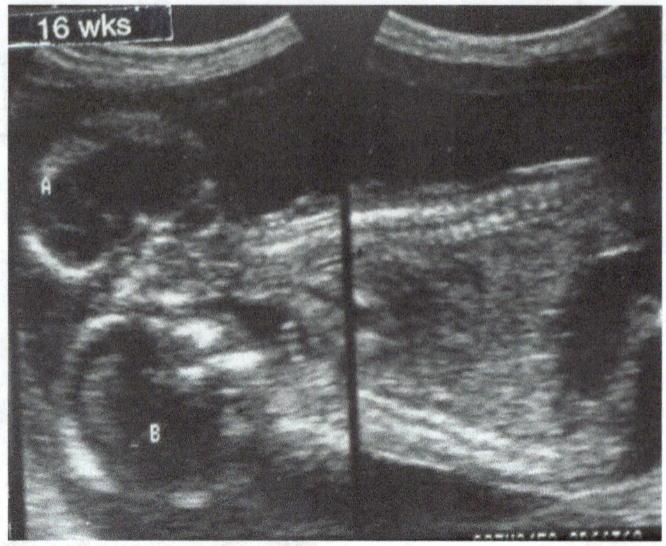


**FIGURE 11.1E** 16 week conjoined twins

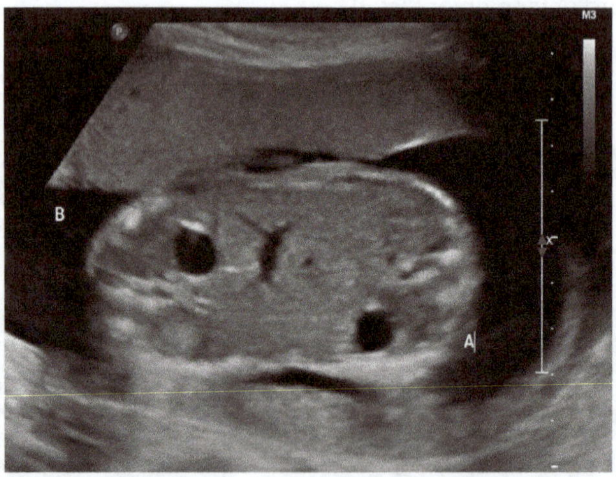


**FIGURE 11.1F** 30 week conjoined (omphalopagus) twins (A and B).

# 11.2 OTHER COMPLICATIONS OF MONOCHORIONIC PLACENTATION: TWIN ANEMIA-POLYCYTHEMIA SEQUENCE, TWIN REVERSED ARTERIAL PERFUSION, AND SELECTIVE FETAL GROWTH RESTRICTION

## EPIDEMIOLOGY/GENETICS

**Definition** Although twin to twin transfusion syndrome (TTTS) is the most widely recognized complication of MC gestations, other complications include twin anemia-polycythemia sequence (TAPS), twin reversed arterial perfusion (TRAP), and selective fetal growth restriction (sFGR). TAPS describes the condition of chronic and unreciprocated transfusion of red cells from one twin, the donor, to the other, the recipient, which results in chronic anemia and polycythemia, respectively, without the polyhydramnios/oligohydramnios associated with TTTS. TRAP describes chronic perfusion of an "acardiac" twin, or a twin with a rudimentary heart, by a "pump" twin through patent intertwin vascular channels, resulting in shunt physiology in the pump twin. sFGR describes growth discordance of 25% or more or an estimated fetal weight less than the 10th percentile in one nonanomalous twin. It can be further classified by characteristic Doppler waveforms.

**Epidemiology** TAPS occurs spontaneously in 3% to 5% of MC twins. It also can occur in up to 13% of laser-treated TTTS pregnancies. TRAP occurs in 1 in 35,000 births or 1 in 100 monozygotic twin pairs. Karyotypic abnormalities can occur in as many as 9% of pump twins. sFGR can complicate 10% to 15% of MC twins. TAPS and sFGR can occur independently or in association with TTTS.

**Embryology** TAPS, TRAP, and sFGR are all the consequence of the unique angioarchitecture of the MC placenta. Multiple vascular connections within the placenta allow for varying patterns of intertwin transfusion and placental partition or sharing or both. The forces responsible for abnormal sharing and partition are unknown. The cause of TRAP is unknown but may be the consequence of abnormal embryogenesis in one twin resulting in early demise. Ongoing perfusion of the acardiac, or amorphous, twin with deoxygenated blood from the pump twin allows for continued growth of the acardiac twin, although often in the presence of grotesquely abnormal morphological development.

**Inheritance Patterns** Inheritance is sporadic.

**Teratogens** None are known.

**Prognosis** The natural history of TAPS remains poorly defined. Case reports describe consequences of severe anemia in the donor (hydrops fetalis) and polycythemia in the recipient (sludging and thrombosis). Survival of the pump twin in TRAP is approximately 50%. Regarding sFGR, gestational age at delivery, rate of deterioration, loss of co-twin, and the risk of brain parenchymal lesions are associated with characteristic Doppler waveforms.

## SONOGRAPHY

### FINDINGS

- TAPS, TRAP, and sFGR all occur in MC gestations, the majority of which are diamniotic.
- TAPS can be suspected when hydrops is detected in one twin without the sonographic stigmata of TTTS.
- Discordant fetal hemoglobin in TAPS can be detected noninvasively by middle cerebral artery peak systolic velocity (MCA PSV) measurements. A staging system has been proposed based on MCA PSV findings.
- TRAP is diagnosed by the sonographic findings of a normally developed fetus, possibly in high-output heart failure, and an amorphous mass often with discernible fetal parts, such as long bones or ribs. Careful Doppler interrogation reveals blood flow toward the acardiac twin within the umbilical artery and away in the umbilical vein.
- sFGR demonstrates often-obvious growth discordance and frequent oligohydramnios and abnormal Doppler waveforms in the growth-restricted fetus.

### DIFFERENTIAL DIAGNOSIS

- The sonographic diagnosis of TRAP is relatively straightforward. Hydrops and polyhydramnios of the pump twin may be confused with stage IV TTTS initially.
- TAPS and sFGR can occur singularly or in association with each other and with TTTS. Only TTTS will reliably demonstrate the polyhydramnios/oligohydramnios sequence.
- TAPS generally has normal fluid in both sacs.
- sFGR may demonstrate oligohydramnios in the donor sac but normal fluid in the sac of the co-twin.

## PREGNANCY MANAGEMENT

**Investigations and Consultations Required** Referral to a regional treatment center is appropriate if the patient opts for intervention after consultation with maternal-fetal medicine. Consultation with neonatology is appropriate if delivery is anticipated. It is imperative that individual twin identities be maintained through the antepartum and intrapartum periods so that prenatally acquired data (TAPS donor vs. recipient, for example) can be assigned to the correct newborn.

**Fetal Intervention** Management options for TAPS include expectant management, selective feticide by cord occlusion, delivery, intrauterine transfusion (intravascular or intraperitoneal) of the anemic fetus with or without partial exchange transfusion of the polycythemic fetus, and laser photocoagulation of communicating intertwin vessels.

The goal for management of TRAP is the disruption of the vascular circuit between the pump twin and the acardiac twin. Intrafetal radio-frequency ablation is an effective, minimally invasive, ultrasound-guided technique with a low complication rate.

Management of sFGR largely depends on gestational age. Selective feticide can be offered if diagnosed before the legal limit for termination. Laser photocoagulation of communicating intertwin vessels is associated with a high risk of demise of the growth-restricted fetus but may be protective of the normally grown twin. Loss of one twin is associated with a 15% risk of loss of the co-twin and a 33% chance of neurologic injury in the survivor, likely secondary to acute intravascular pressure and volume shifts.

**Monitoring** Type and frequency of antenatal monitoring will depend on the diagnosis and stage. Monitoring strategies are usually tailored to the unique circumstances on a case-by-case basis. It should be noted that no amount of monitoring will guarantee a good outcome in these highly complex and often-volatile pregnancies.

**Pregnancy Termination Issues** Selective feticide in MC gestations must be performed by a cord occlusive technique, as cardioplegic medications can pass from one twin to the other through patent vascular channels. Selective feticide for TAPS and sFGR is limited by gestational age restrictions, while TRAP is generally not because the acardiac fetus is technically not "living."

**Delivery** Delivery should occur in a tertiary center because of the high risk of prematurity, as well as inherent complications from the underlying disease processes (anemia, polycythemia, growth restriction, hydrops).

## NEONATOLOGY

**Resuscitation** Anticipate difficulty with spontaneous onset of respiration, as well as problems associated with preterm delivery in the pump twin. The team must be prepared to deal with congestive heart failure early in the course.

**Transport** Transfer to a tertiary center for neonatal intensive care is necessary in the majority of cases. Respiratory assistance, as well as support of myocardial function, may be required during transport.

**Nursery Management** Respiratory support, relief of myocardial stress, reduction of congestive heart failure, and correction of perinatal asphyxia are usually needed, and it is necessary to institute measures to accomplish these goals immediately following birth. Because most TRAP sequence pregnancies are delivered prematurely, respiratory distress syndrome may also further complicate the clinical course. Early administration of surfactant replacement therapy may hasten the resolution the respiratory distress.

### SUGGESTED READINGS

1. Baschat AA, Oepkes D: Twin anemia-polycythemia sequence in monochorionic twins: implications for diagnosis and treatment. Am J Perinatol 2014; 31:S25-S30.
2. Borrell A, Pesarrodona A, Puerto B, et al: Ultrasound diagnostic features of twin reversed arterial perfusion sequence. Prenat Diagn 1990; 10:443-448.

3. Gratacos E, Lewi L, Munoz B, et al: A classification system for selective intrauterine growth restriction in monochorionic pregnancies according to umbilical artery Doppler flow in the smaller twin. Ultrasound Obstet Gynecol 2007; 30:28-34.
4. Ishii K, Murakoshi T, Hayashi S, et al: Ultrasound predictors of mortality in monochorionic twins with selective intrauterine growth restriction. Ultrasound Obstet Gynecol 2011; 37:22-26.
5. Lewi L, Deprest J, Hecher K: The vascular anastomoses in monochorionic twin pregnancies and their clinical consequences. Am J Obstet Gynecol 2013; 208:19-30.
6. Rossi AC, Prefumo F: Perinatal outcomes of twin anemia-polycythemia sequence: a systematic review. J Obstet Gynaecol Canada 2014; 36:701-707.
7. Sueters M, Oepkes D: Diagnosis of twin-to-twin transfusion syndrome, selective fetal growth restriction, twin anaemia-polycythaemia sequence, and twin reversed arterial perfusion sequence. Best Pract Clin Obstet Gynaecol. 2014; 28:215-226.
8. Valsky DV, Eixarch E, Martinez JM, Gratacos E: Selective intrauterine growth restriction in monochorionic diamniotic twin pregnancies. Prenat Diagn 2010; 30:719-726.
9. Veujoz M, Sananes N, Severac F, et al: Evaluation of prenatal and postnatal diagnostic criteria for twin anemia-polycythemia sequence. Prenat Diagn 2015; 35:281-288.

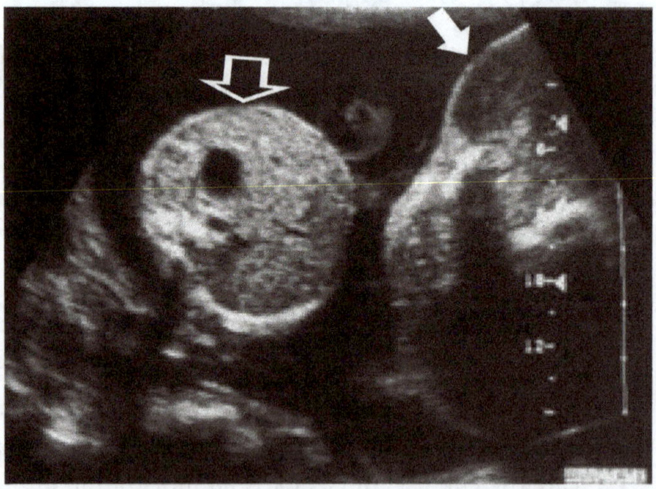

**FIGURE 11.2A** Normal "pump" twin (open arrow). Acardiac acephalic twin (closed arrow).

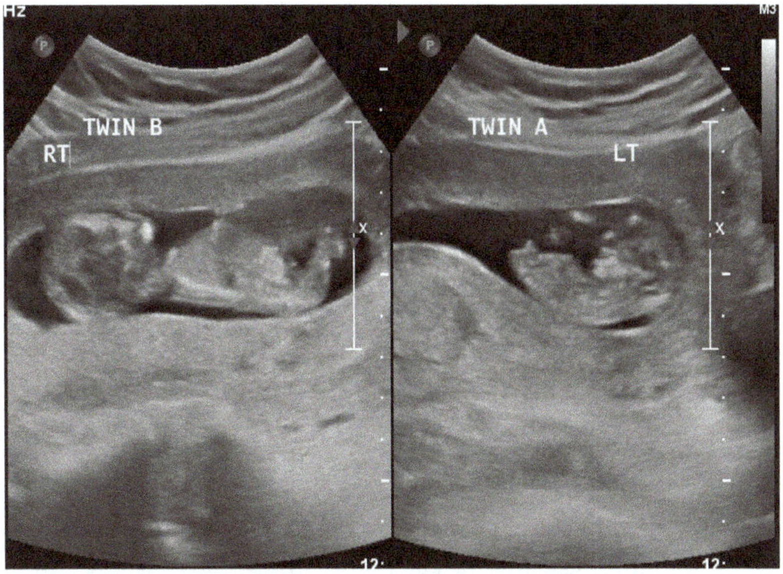


FIGURE 11.2B Monochorionic diamniotic twin discordancy. Crown rump lengths of 46 and 67 mm for fetuses A and B, respectively.

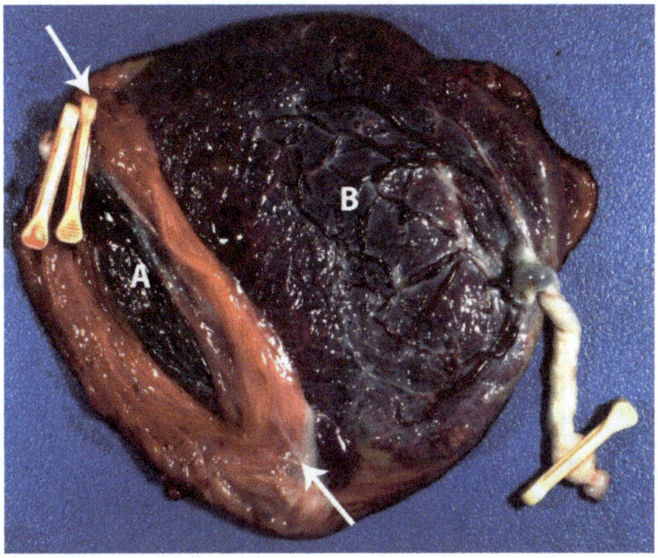


FIGURE 11.2C Monochorionic diamniotic placenta. Significant discordance in the placental distribution between fetuses A and B.

# 11.3 TWIN-TWIN TRANSFUSION SYNDROME

## EPIDEMIOLOGY/GENETICS

**Definition** Twin-twin transfusion syndrome (TTTS) describes a spectrum of fetal disorders involving hypovolemia and hypervolemia of donor and recipient MC twins, respectively, due to unreciprocated passage of blood and vasoactive substances through patent placental vascular channels.

**Epidemiology** TTTS affects approximately 10% of MC twins and accounts for the majority of morbidity and mortality in MC gestations. The peak incidence is approximately 20 weeks, but it can occur at any time in the second and third trimesters, including first appearing during labor.

**Embryology** Because of the unique angioarchitecture of the MC placenta, intraplacental vascular communications allow for unidirectional and unreciprocated passage of intravascular volume from one twin (the donor) to the other (the recipient). The donor becomes hypovolemic and oliguric. The recipient becomes hypervolemic and polyuric. In addition, vasoactive elements cause counterproductive cardiovascular signaling, resulting in exacerbation of the hemodynamic disequilibrium. The donor develops placental insufficiency, while the recipient develops hypertensive cardiomyopathy.

**Inheritance** The incidence of MC twinning is stable across all populations at approximately 3 to 5 per 1000 births and is increased with the use of in vitro fertilization. TTTS is a sporadic event unique to MC gestations.

**Prognosis** Left untreated, the mortality rate of TTTS is 70% to 100%. The recipient twin is at risk for demise due to hypertension, cardiac overload, and pump failure with consequent hydrops, whereas the donor is at risk of loss from hypovolemia and inadequate oxygen and nutrient supply. Loss of one twin can result in loss of the co-twin due to acute exsanguination of the surviving twin into the deceased twin. Survivors have a high incidence of neurologic morbidity (10% to 30%). Another mechanism of loss is preterm premature rupture of membranes (PPROM) and preterm delivery due to uterine overdistention from massive polyhydramnios.

## SONOGRAPHY

The most commonly used staging system is that of Quintero, for which progressive hypo- and hypervolemia are manifest sonographically. Stage I is oligohydramnios of the donor (maximum vertical pocket or MVP < 20 mm) and polyhydramnios of the recipient (MVP > 80 mm). Stage II adds a collapsed bladder in the donor. Stage III adds critically abnormal Doppler waveforms in either twin. Stage IV adds hydrops of either twin. Stage V is demise of one or both twins. Progression can be rapid and not necessarily in order (for example, donor bladder present, but critically abnormal Doppler waveforms in either twin). Other staging systems incorporate echocardiographic findings.

## FINDINGS

### Placenta

- TTTS occurs only in MC gestations.
- Sonographic markers of monochorionicity are
  - a single placental mass,
  - a thin intertwin membrane, and
  - the "T" sign, where the intertwin membrane meets the placenta at a right angle.
- Rarely, placental partitioning can occur, giving the appearance of a DC gestation.

### Amniotic Fluid

- Polyhydramnios/oligohydramnios sequence is pathognomonic for TTTS.
- Extreme cases are obvious with massive polyhydramnios of the recipient and anhydramnios of the donor, who is "stuck" to the uterine wall ("stuck twin syndrome").
- Membrane folding is common in less-severe forms, which can make an accurate assessment of fluid volumes in each sac difficult.

### Fetuses

- Although size discrepancy is not part of staging, an obvious size discrepancy between donor and recipient is common.
- The donor appears to be hypovolemic (collapsed bladder, abnormal umbilical artery Doppler waveforms).
- The recipient appears hypervolemic (distended bladder, cardiomyopathy, edematous umbilical cord).
- Color Doppler interrogation may reveal abnormal arterial (absent or reversed umbilical artery diastolic flow) or venous (absent or reversed ductus venosus a-wave, pulsatile umbilical vein) waveforms, indicating uteroplacental insufficiency and pump failure, respectively.

## KEY FINDINGS/PITFALLS

- Polyhydramnios/oligohydramnios sequence is the sine qua non of TTTS; the diagnosis cannot be made without it.
- Donor anhydramnios may mimic MA twins, as the intertwin membrane may be difficult to identify.
- Oligohydramnios in one twin may represent membrane rupture or renal agenesis.
- Hydrops of one or both twins may be unrelated to TTTS.
- Polyhydramnios of one twin may be due to discordant structural anomalies, such as esophageal atresia or a central nervous system lesion.
- Selective fetal growth restriction can present as oligohydramnios of the growth-restricted fetus but as normal fluid in the cotwin.

## PREGNANCY MANAGEMENT

**Investigations and Consultations Required** Early detection of TTTS is key as outcomes correlate with stage at diagnosis. A widely accepted strategy is to perform limited ultrasound screening evaluations every 2 weeks in all MC twins, from 16 weeks until delivery, to assess for amniotic fluid volume and bladder status. Increased surveillance and multivessel Doppler interrogation are performed for abnormal screening results. This is in addition to the usual anatomic survey and fetal echocardiography at 18-22 weeks and growth evaluations subsequently at regular intervals. Once TTTS is diagnosed, consultation with maternal-fetal medicine is warranted.

**Fetal Intervention** Management options depend on gestational age, disease severity, patient preference, and resource availability and include expectant management, pregnancy termination before viability, delivery, serial amnioreduction, selective feticide, and fetoscopic laser photocoagulation of communicating intertwin vessels. Fetoscopic laser photocoagulation has been shown to be superior to amnioreduction by a randomized controlled trial and is considered by many experts to be the treatment of choice for severe disease. Serial amnioreduction is widely available and may be the only option in certain circumstances, such as in low-resource areas. Selective feticide by cord occlusion is technically simple and can convert a complicated MC twin gestation to a relatively straightforward singleton gestation, but at the cost of sacrificing one fetus. Pregnancy termination may be preferable to some patients as all other strategies carry significant perinatal risk. Equipoise exists regarding the management of early-stage disease (stage I), with many centers offering expectant management with close ultrasound surveillance. Symptomatic polyhydramnios, a short cervix, and recipient cardiomyopathy may prompt early intervention. Finally, delivery may be the only available option when all other methods of safe pregnancy prolongation are exhausted. Pregnancy termination and selective feticide are limited by state laws, and fetoscopic laser is not available beyond 26 weeks due to Food and Drug Administration restrictions.

**Delivery** Vaginal delivery is preferred, reserving cesarean section for routine obstetric indications. Most centers deliver laser-treated TTTS twins at 36 weeks unless complications (PPROM, recurrent TTTS, sFGR, TAPS) arise. In general, delivery is indicated when the risks of an ongoing pregnancy exceed the risks of preterm birth of ill twin neonates.

## NEONATOLOGY

**Resuscitation** With chronic in utero twin-to-twin transfusion, both infants frequently are depressed at birth and require immediate attention to facilitate the onset of respiration and resolution of birth asphyxia. Two skilled resuscitation teams are required, and each must be prepared to deal with the resultant blood and red blood cell volume problem unique to the respective infant: severe anemia in the donor and severe polycythemia/hypervolemia in recipient. Either one or both twins could present with hydrops.

**Transport** Transfer of both infants to a tertiary perinatal center is indicated when there is preterm delivery, respiratory distress, or distress secondary to anemia or polycythemia. In utero transfer is the best transfer technique.

**Nursery Management** Issues of respiratory support, transfusion, cardiac failure, perinatal asphyxia, hypoglycemia, and prematurity are frequently encountered. Correction of anemia in the donor twin and partial exchange transfusion to correct polycythemia in the recipient twin may be indicated.

## SUGGESTED READINGS

1. Gratacos E, Lewi L, Munoz B, et al: A classification system for selective intrauterine growth restriction in monochorionic pregnancies according to umbilical artery Doppler flow in the smaller twin. Ultrasound Obstet Gynecol 2007; 30:28-34.
2. Lewi L, Jani J, Blickstein I, et al: The outcome of monochorionic diamniotic twin gestations in the era of invasive fetal therapy: a prospective cohort study. Am J Obstet Gynecol 2008; 199:514 e1-8.
3. Senat MV, Deprest J, Boulvain M, et al: Endoscopic laser surgery versus serial amnioreduction for severe twin-to-twin transfusion syndrome. N Engl Med 2004; 351:136-144.
4. Society for Maternal-Fetal Medicine (SMFM), Simpson LL: Twin-twin transfusion syndrome. Am J Obstet Gynecol 2013; 208:3-18.
5. Thorson HL, Ramaeker DM, Emery SP: Optimal interval for ultrasound surveillance in monochorionic twin gestations. Obstet Gynecol 2011; 117:131-135.
6. van Klink JM, Koopman HM, van Zwet EW, et al: Improvement in neurodevelopmental outcome in survivors of twin-twin transfusion syndrome treated with laser surgery. Am J Obstet Gynecol. 2014; 210:540 e1-7.

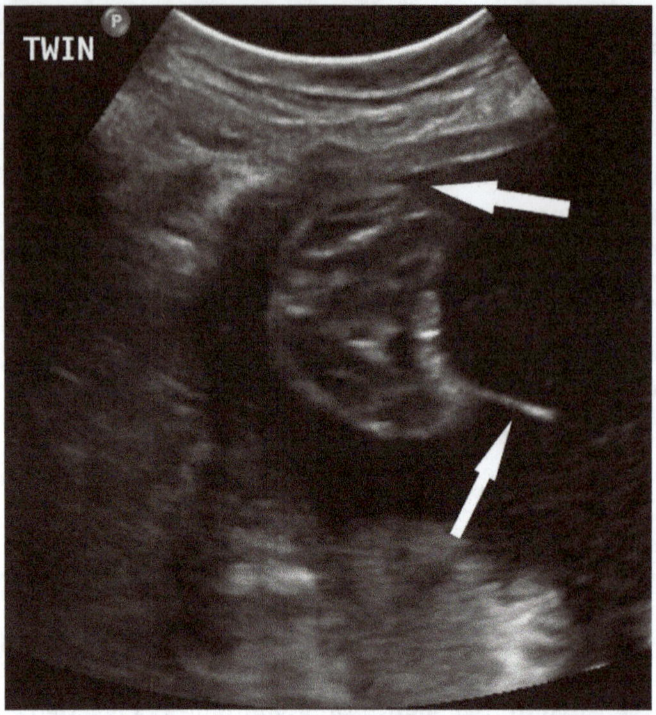


**FIGURE 11.3A** Twin-to-twin transfusion syndrome. The membrane (arrows) wraps around the stuck twin.

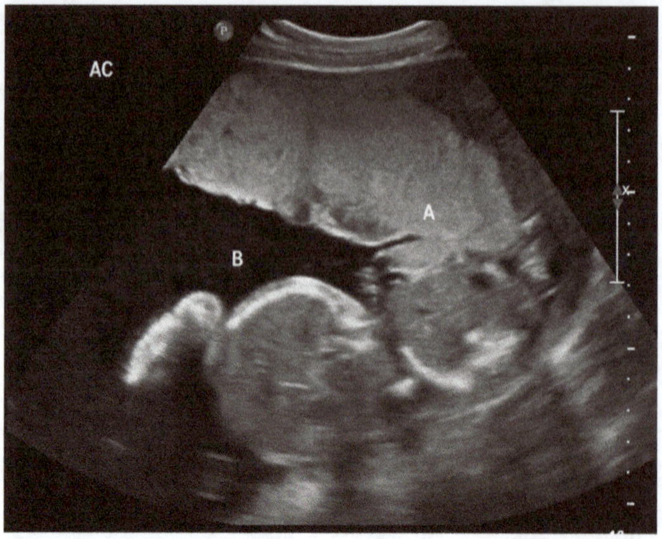


**FIGURE 11.3B** Twin-to-twin transfusion syndrome. Discordant growth fetus A is smaller than fetus B.

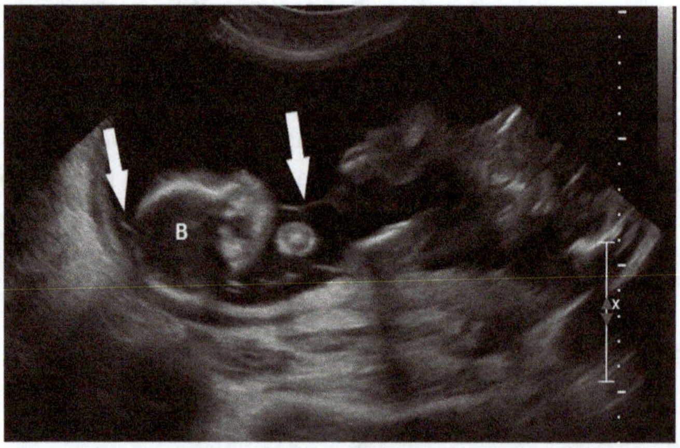


**FIGURE 11.3C** Stage II twin-to-twin transfusion syndrome. Infolding of the membrane (arrows) around the donor twin with oligohydramnios.

# CHAPTER 12

# MISCELLANEOUS ABNORMALITIES

# 12.1 AMNIOTIC BAND SYNDROME

## EPIDEMIOLOGY/GENETICS

**Definition** Amniotic band syndrome (ABS) is a rare spectrum of congenital anomalies caused by entanglement of fetal parts, or disruption of anatomic structures, by fibrous amniotic bands.

**Epidemiology** The exact incidence of ABS is uncertain but may be as high as 1 in 15,000 live births.

**Embryology** There are two theories proposed for ABS: (1) The bands are due to early amniotic rupture, leaving fibrous bands floating in the amniotic fluid to become entangled with the fetus; or (2) the bands are secondary to membrane malformations caused by ischemia. There are others who postulate that ABS is part of the limb–body wall spectrum. The timing of the insult determines the effect of the amniotic band on fetal development. An amniotic band can be: (1) **disruptive**, resulting in finger, toe, or extremity amputation; (2) an early insult may give rise to a **malformation** (i.e., an encephalocele); and (3) if a band constricts movement, a **deformation** (scoliosis) may result.

**Inheritance Pattern** ABS appears to be sporadic. ABS has been associated with maternal Ehlers-Danlos syndrome and epidermolysis bullosa.

**Teratogens** None are known.

**Prognosis** The prognosis depends on the resulting anomalies. Cranial and chest anomalies are more likely to be fatal, while limb involvement may have a better prognosis.

## SONOGRAPHY

### FINDINGS

- Atypical anomalies or an unusual constellation of abnormalities are frequently the presenting findings for ABS. Some anomalies that have been associated with ABS are as follows:
  - Isolated limb amputations or missing hands, feet, or digits in 80% of cases
  - Midline cleft lip, or transverse facial clefts
  - Asymmetric craniofacial defects
  - Acrania or encephalocele
  - Body wall defects (i.e., ectopia cordis, gastroschisis, omphalocele, and limb–body wall)

### KEY FINDINGS/PITFALLS

- If an isolated abnormality, or group of anomalies, seems asymmetric or atypical, ABS should be considered.
- The amniotic fluid volume may be decreased.
- ABS has been detected as early as the first trimester.
- ABS can be definitively identified when the following occur:

  - Bands can be visualized within the amniotic fluid and appear as single or multiple thin membranes that attach to, or limit the motion of, specific fetal parts.
    - They can be difficult to identify; only the sequelae of the amniotic bands may be apparent.
    - Extremity constriction can be the first sign and usually presents with edema of the distal extremity. This is frequently followed by limb amputation.
- Look for
  - Amnion in continuity with the fetal parts
  - Extremity edema/localized swelling with reduced distal vascular flow detected with Doppler
  - Fetal scoliosis
  - Echogenic debris within the amniotic fluid

### DIFFERENTIAL DIAGNOSIS

- Anomalies that can be isolated, can be related to aneuploidy or a syndrome, or can be ABS-related defects, including
  - Body stalk anomaly
  - Cephalocele
  - Acrania
  - Cleft lip
  - Omphalocele
  - Amniotic sheets
  - Chorioamniotic separation

## PREGNANCY MANAGEMENT

**Investigations and Consultations Required** Further consultation depends on the site(s) involved.

**Fetal Intervention** Fetoscopic intervention has been performed to lyse bands that show evidence of increasing vascular compromise of a limb; however, the diagnosis is frequently made after the damage has occurred.

**Monitoring** Frequent ultrasound examination of the extremities is critical to monitor for evidence of vascular compromise. Monitoring should be in a facility with the means for fetal intervention.

**Pregnancy Course** In most cases, the damage from the bands has preceded ultrasound diagnosis; further ultrasound examinations may be useful to monitor for further injury.

**Delivery** Most deliveries will need to occur in a tertiary center for newborn evaluation and treatment planning. The mode of delivery will depend on the location and extent of the defects.

## NEONATOLOGY

**Resuscitation** In general, most fetuses that have been affected by ABS do not experience distress in labor and thus do not require assistance with the onset of respiration. Only those with significant chest, face, or cranial defects are at risk for respiratory compromise and will need intervention.

**Transport** Indications for referral to a tertiary perinatal center immediately following birth include anomalies that will require specialist pediatric surgical correction, such as abdominal wall defects or partially compromised extremities.

**Testing and Confirmation** There are no specific tests for the evaluation of fetuses with suspected ABS. Pathological evaluation of the membranes and placenta is suggested.

**Nursery Management** Nursery management is supportive, depending on the location and extent of the associated defects.

## SUGGESTED READINGS

1. Barzilay E, Harel Y, Haas J, et al: Prenatal diagnosis of amniotic band syndrome—risk factors and ultrasonic signs. J Matern Fetal Neonatal Med 2015; 28:281-283.
2. Cignini P, Giorlandino C, Padula F, et al: Epidemiology and risk factors of amniotic band syndrome, or ADAM sequence. J Prenat Med 2012; 6:59-63.
3. Derderian SC, Iqbal CW, Goldstein R, et al: Fetoscopic approach to amniotic band syndrome. J Pediatr Surg 2014; 49:359-362.
4. Hata T, Tanaka H, Noguchi J: 3D/4D sonographic evaluation of amniotic band syndrome in early pregnancy: a supplement to 2D ultrasound. J Obstet Gynaecol Res 2011; 37:656-660.
5. Iqbal CW, Derderian SC, Cheng Y, et al: Amniotic band syndrome: a single-institutional experience. Fetal Diagn Ther 2015; 37:1-5.
6. Nishi T, Nakano R: Amniotic band syndrome: serial ultrasonographic observations in the first trimester. Clin Ultrasound 1994; 22:275-278.
7. Ross MG: Pathogenesis of amniotic band syndrome. Am J Obstet Gynecol 2007; 197:219-220.
8. van der Meulen JC: The amniotic band syndrome. Plast Reconstr Surg 1999; 103:1087-1090.
9. Walter JH Jr, Goss LR, Lazzara AT: Amniotic band syndrome. J Foot Ankle Surg 1998; 37:325-333.

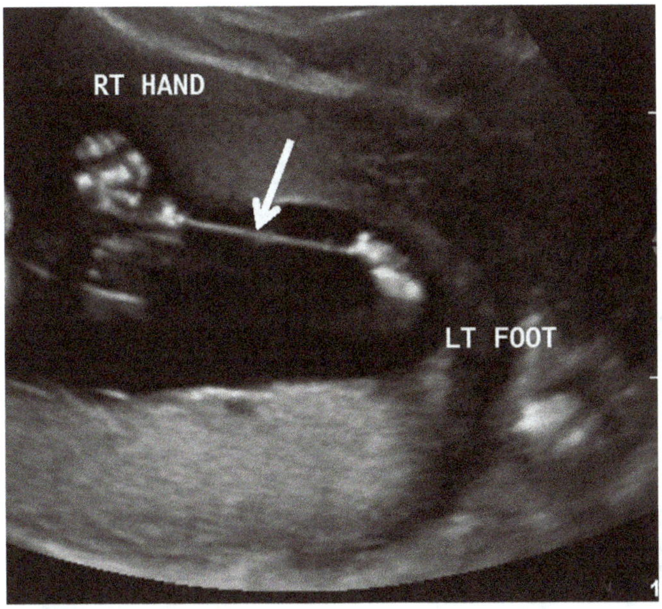


**FIGURE 12.1A** Amniotic band (arrow).

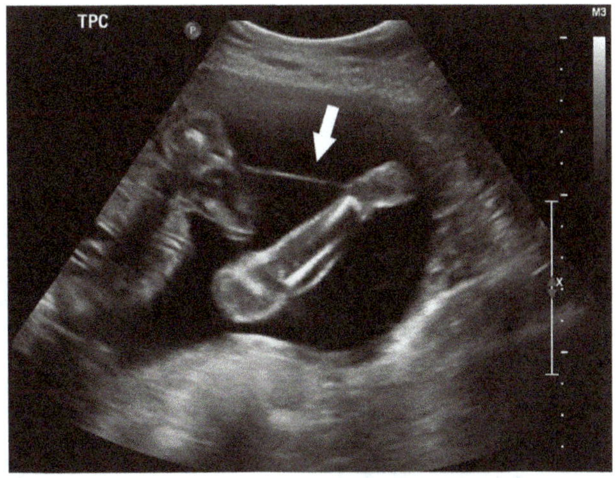


**FIGURE 12.1B** Amniotic band (white arrow) extending from the amnion to the left lower extremity, constricting the limb at the ankle.

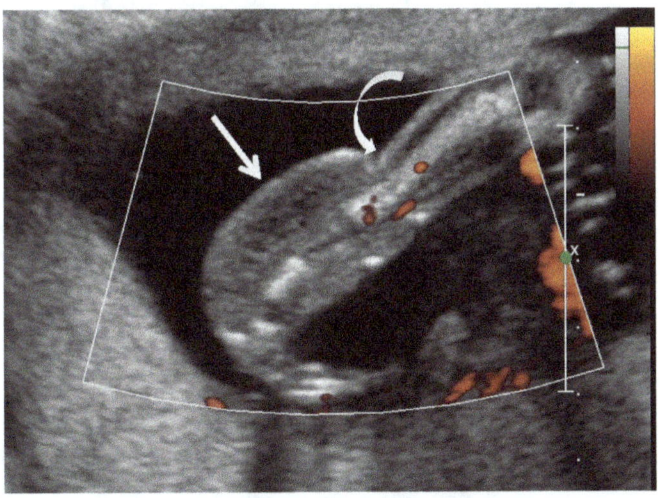

**FIGURE 12.1C** Distal limb edema (straight arrow). Amniotic band indentation (curved arrow).

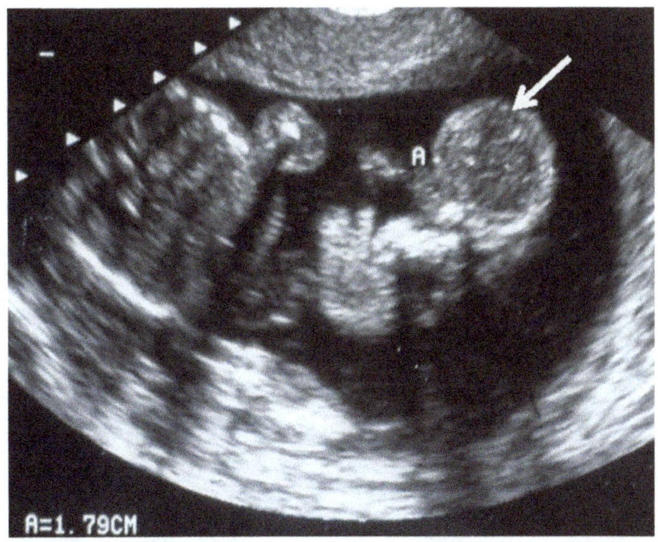


**FIGURE 12.1D** Amniotic band resulting in an anterior encephalocele (A; arrow).

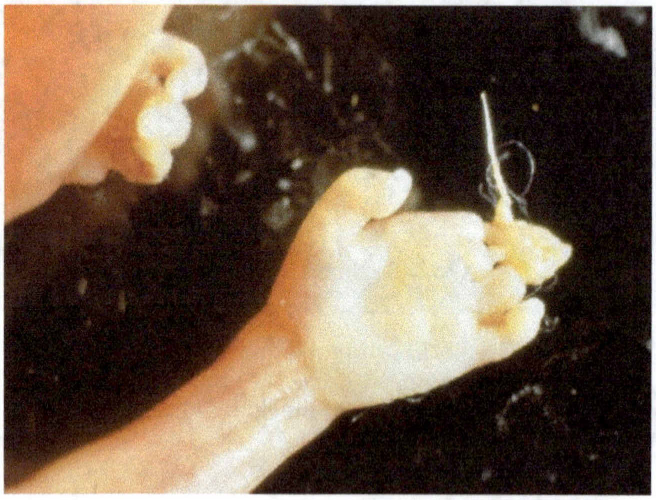

**FIGURE 12.1E** Fetus with an amniotic band around the second and third fingers.

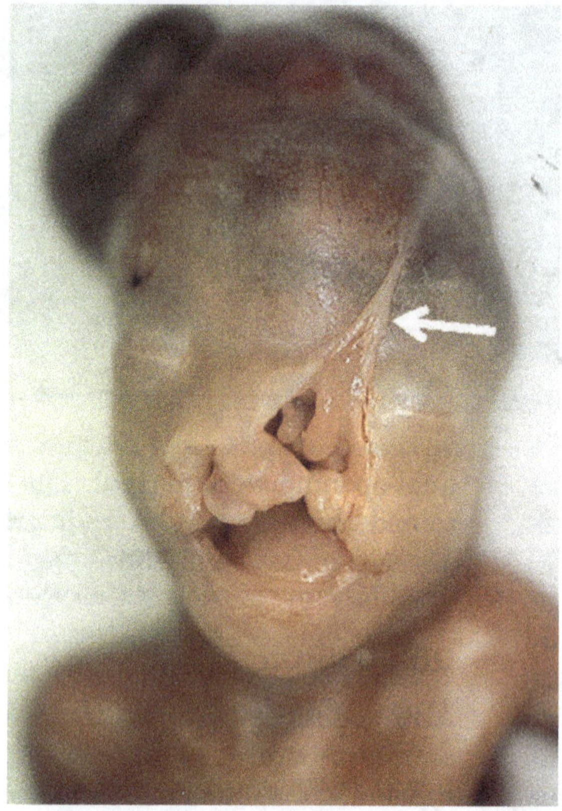

**FIGURE 12.1F** Fetus with an amniotic band (arrow) causing cleft lip and palate.

# 12.2 CHORIOANGIOMA

## EPIDEMIOLOGY/GENETICS

**Definition** Chorioangiomas are benign vascular tumors of the placenta that are most commonly encapsulated and intraplacental and found on the fetal side of the placenta.

**Epidemiology** Chorioangiomas are the most common primary tumors of the placenta and are found in approximately 1% of term placentas.

**Embryology** Chorioangiomas are either hamartomas derived from primitive chorionic mesenchyme or placental hemangiomas arising from the chorionic plate.

**Inheritance** These tumors are sporadic, with no increased risk in future pregnancies.

**Prognosis** Most chorioangiomas are incidental findings. Very rarely, secondary fetal hydrops can develop.

## SONOGRAPHY

### FINDINGS

**Fetus**

- The fetus is usually normal.
- On rare occasions, severe fetal anemia develops because the mass shunts blood and acts as an arteriovenous malformation.
- Hydrops may develop, with the earliest signs being hepatosplenomegaly and small pericardial effusions.

**Amniotic Fluid**

- If a large mass is present, the amniotic fluid volume is almost always increased.

**Placenta**

- A well-defined mass is present in the placenta that demonstrates arterial flow on color Doppler.
- The mass is usually solitary, but can be multiple, and usually protrudes into the amniotic cavity.
- It is often located near the cord insertion, and vascularity varies.
- Color Doppler mapping usually demonstrates arterial flow compatible with an arteriovenous malformation.
- Vascularity and size (≥5 cm) tend to correlate with polyhydramnios and hydrops.
- Chorioangiomas are usually not associated with any complications if they are less than 5 cm in diameter.

### KEY FINDING/PITFALLS

- Earliest detection reported is at 15 weeks' gestation, but chorioangiomas often develop in the second trimester of pregnancy.
- Venous lakes can be confused with chorioangiomas. Venous flow within a venous lake may not be visible with color flow or Doppler sonography. Observation with real-time imaging can reveal blood flow movement. Venous lakes often lie at the edge of the placenta and can protrude into the amniotic fluid.
- The chorioangioma may lie alongside the fetus and be mistaken for a fetal mass, such as a sacrococcygeal teratoma.

### DIFFERENTIAL DIAGNOSIS

- Placental hematoma: This is a mass with a similar appearance to a chorioangioma arising from the placental surface. No flow will be seen in real time or with Doppler imaging.
- Placental lake on placental surface: The apparent mass will show venous flow with real-time imaging and no flow with color flow or Doppler imaging.
- Placental cyst: Cysts arising from the placental surface often have a solid component at the base. A round, thin membrane outlining the echo-free component of the cyst will be seen. These cysts may represent a resolving hematoma.

## PREGNANCY MANAGEMENT

**Investigations and Consultations Required** No further investigations or consultations are required at diagnosis unless fetal growth restriction or hydrops is found.

**Monitoring** Serial sonographic examinations are needed to monitor the size of the mass and the amniotic fluid volume. Fetal growth should be assessed regularly. If the mass is large or grows rapidly, more frequent examinations should be performed to look for early signs of hydrops. In the absence of complications, aggressive intervention is unnecessary, as many of these masses will remain asymptomatic or spontaneously regress.

**Fetal Intervention** If hydrops develops, intervention should be considered. A thorough evaluation should be undertaken to ensure that the tumor is the cause of the hydrops. Early delivery should be weighed against aggressive in utero intervention and will depend largely on gestational age when the hydrops develops. Treatment options are directed at ablation or occlusion of the feeding vessel. Laser ablation is the most common intervention, although there is a small amount of evidence using intravascular glue for occlusion. In the case of large feeding vessels, interventional radiologic embolization with coils can be considered. However, this method should be considered with caution because there are no data on the risks. Prior to intervention, assessment of the middle cerebral artery peak systolic velocity should be performed to evaluate the fetus for anemia and prepare for an intrauterine transfusion, if necessary.

**Pregnancy Course** In the absence of hydrops or intrauterine growth restriction, no pregnancy complications are expected. In those rare cases when these develop, intervention to treat the hydrops or further evaluation for causes of intrauterine growth restriction should be undertaken. Similarly, antenatal testing should be performed in those complicated cases but is not indicated otherwise.

**Pregnancy Termination Issues** If pregnancy termination is chosen, delivery of an intact fetus and placenta is ideal to confirm the sonographic diagnosis and evaluate for any additional fetal findings.

**Delivery** In the absence of fetal complications, delivery at a tertiary center is not necessary. Pregnancies with polyhydramnios or fetal hydrops should deliver at a tertiary center.

## NEONATOLOGY

**Resuscitation** There are no specific measures required unless fetal anemia or hydrops fetalis is present.

**Transport** Unless there are concurrent fetal complications, transfer of the newborn is not indicated.

**Nursery Management** There are no special care requirements for the newborn except for the infant who has developed hydrops fetalis.

### SUGGESTED READINGS


1. Al Wattar BH, Hillman SC, Marton T, et al: Placenta chorioangioma: a rare case and systematic review of literature. J Maternal-Fetal Neonat Med 2014; 27:1055-1063.
2. Amer HZ, Heller DS: Chorangioma and related vascular lesions of the placenta—a review. Fetal Pediatr Pathol 2010; 29:199-206.
3. Garcia-Diaz L, Carreto P, Costa-Pereira S, Antinolo G: Prenatal management and perinatal outcome in giant placental chorioangioma complicated with hydrops fetalis, fetal anemia, and maternal mirror syndrome. BMC Pregnancy Childbirth 2012; 12:72.
4. Jauniaux E, Ogle R: Color Doppler imaging in the diagnosis and management of chorioangiomas. Ultrasound Obstet Gynecol 2000; 15:463-467.
5. Sepulveda W, Alcalde JL, Schnapp C, Bravo M: Perinatal outcome after prenatal diagnosis of placental chorioangioma. Obstet Gynecol 2003; 102:1028-1033.
6. Shih JC, Ko TL, Lin MC, et al: Quantitative three-dimensional power Doppler ultrasound predicts the outcome of placental chorioangioma. Ultrasound Obstet Gynecol 2004; 24:202-206.
7. Zalel Y, Weisz B, Gamzu R, et al: Chorioangiomas of the placenta: sonographic and Doppler flow characteristics. J Ultrasound Med 2002; 21:909-913.

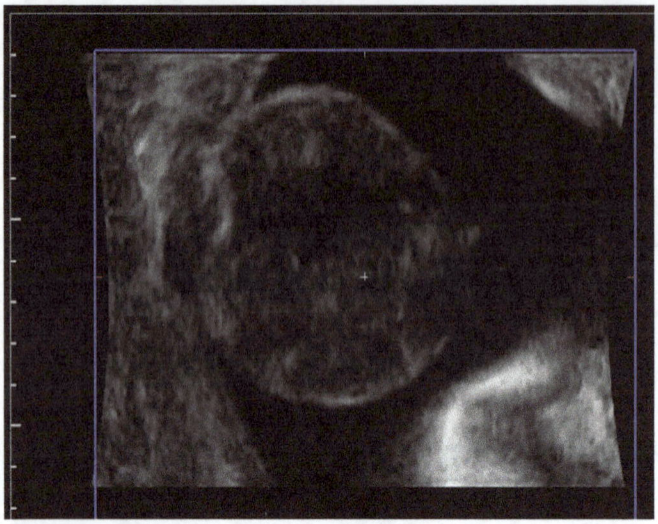

**FIGURE 12.2A** Mass arising from the placenta measuring 75 mm in maximal diameter at 23 weeks 5 days' gestation. Despite the large size, there was no evidence of fetal hydrops.

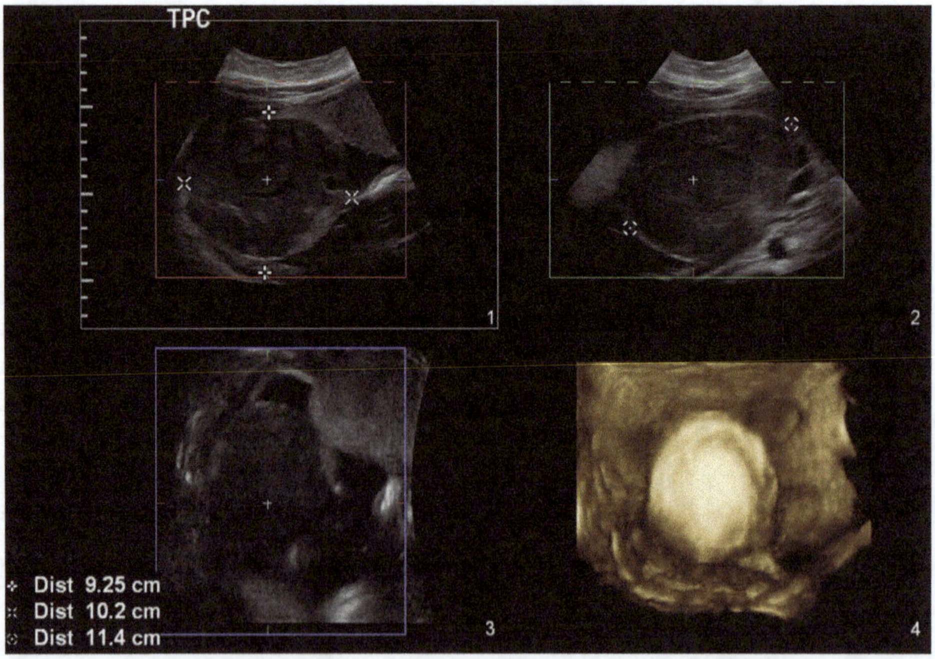


**FIGURE 12.2B** Multiplanar image of the same pregnancy as in Figure 12.2A at 25 weeks 6 days. The placental mass had increased to a maximal diameter of 114 mm, and hydrops was now present.

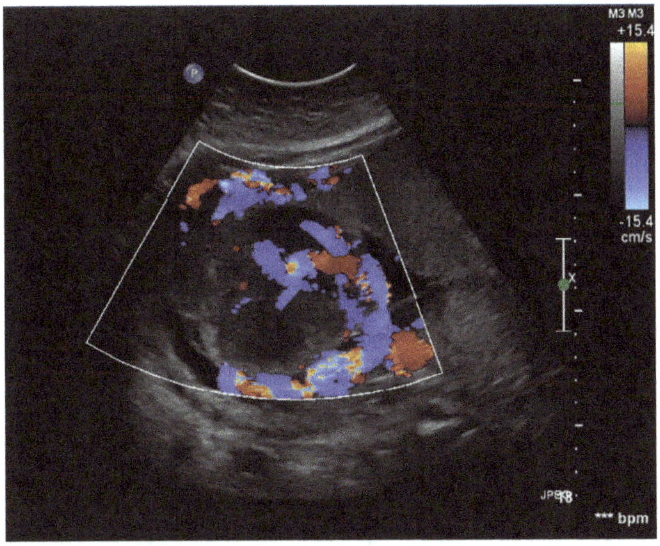


**FIGURE 12.2C** Color Doppler mapping of the chorioangioma in Figure 12.2A indicating significant vascular flow with large feeding vessels extending directly from the umbilical cord into the mass.

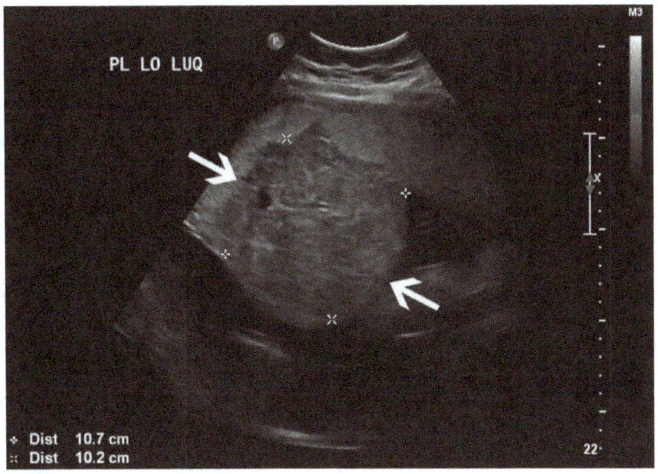


**FIGURE 12.2D** Mass (arrows) arising from the placenta at 29 weeks 1 day gestation. Despite the large (10.7 × 10.2 cm) size, no fetal hydrops developed.

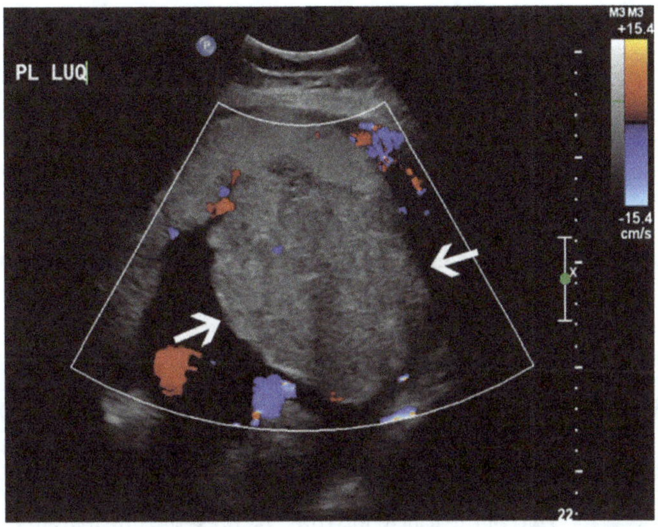


**FIGURE 12.2E** Color Doppler mapping of the chorioangioma in Figure 12.2D. This mass (between the arrows), arising from the placenta, shows minimal vascular flow.

# 12.3 NONIMMUNE HYDROPS FETALIS

## EPIDEMIOLOGY/GENETICS

**Definition** Hydrops fetalis is defined by abnormal fluid accumulation in serous cavities and soft tissues of the fetus. It is characterized as nonimmune if there is no indication of maternal red cell alloimmunization. To meet the criteria for hydrops, two of the following four must be present: pleural effusion, pericardial effusion, ascites, or skin edema. Some older series include cases with isolated skin edema or isolated ascites. These cases have a better prognosis than cases with more than one involved serous space.

**Epidemiology** The incidence of prenatally identified cases of hydrops fetalis is approximately 1 in 1700 to 1 in 3000.

**Embryology** Nonimmune hydrops fetalis (NIHF) may present in any trimester, but the underlying etiology differs by the gestational age at its onset. Hydrops can best be thought of as a final common pathway for a large number of fetal diseases and conditions. The causes are diverse and include numerous maternal, fetal, and placental disorders. Table 12.3-1 outlines some of the conditions that have been associated with NIHF.

**Inheritance** The heterogeneous nature of the etiologic conditions results in a wide range of inheritance patterns and therefore of recurrence risks. Many causes are not inherited conditions and have a sporadic recurrence. Some are due to recessive conditions with a 25% risk of recurrence. Families with no identified etiology but with recurrence of NIHF have been reported. In cases without an identified cause, an empiric risk of recurrence of 5% is appropriate for counseling purposes.

**Prognosis** Overall, the prognosis is poor, with a perinatal mortality of approximately 50% to 90%, depending on etiology and timing of onset.

## SONOGRAPHY

### FREQUENT FINDINGS

- Two of the following must be present, although in many cases more, or all, are noted:
  - Ascites
  - Skin edema
  - Pleural effusion
  - Pericardial effusion

### LESS FREQUENT

- Polyhydramnios
- Thickened placenta
- Cardiac arrhythmias, particularly tachyarrhythmias
- Structural cardiac defects
- Cystic hygroma
- Twins
- Other ultrasound findings may give clues of etiology.

### KEY FINDINGS/PITFALLS

- Once fluid is visualized in one space, a search should be made for accumulations in the other serous spaces.
- Skin edema is best detected over bony structures, such as chest wall or skull.
- Echo dropout in the abdomen may mimic ascites.
- A small amount of pericardial fluid is a normal finding in the third trimester and does not represent a pathologic effusion.
- Once a diagnosis of NIHF is made, a search for any congenital anomalies is warranted and may lead to identifying an etiology.
- If fetal anemia is considered a possible cause of NIHF, Doppler studies of the middle cerebral artery are indicated.

**TABLE 12.3-1** Causes of Nonimmune Hydrops (Partial List)

| |
|---|
| Cardiovascular |
| • Tachyarrythmia |
| • Bradyarrythmia |
| • Structural heart defect |
| Thoracic |
| • Pleural effusion |
| • Congenital pulmonary airway malformation |
| Fetal chromosome abnormalities |
| • Turner syndrome |
| • Trisomy 21 |
| Twinning |
| • Twin-to-twin transfusion syndrome |
| • Twin reversed arterial perfusion |
| Fetal anemia |
| • Fetomaternal hemorrhage |
| • α-Thalassemia |
| Fetal infection |
| • Cytomegalovirus |
| • Parvovirus B19 |
| • Syphilis |
| Lysosomal storage disease |
| • Mucopolysaccharidosis type VII |
| • Gaucher disease |
| • GM1-gangliosidosis |
| Placental chorioangioma |
| Sacrococcygeal teratoma |

## PREGNANCY MANAGEMENT

**Investigations and Consultations Required** Pregnancy management relies heavily on subsequent investigations to determine the underlying etiology. Successful antenatal detection of an etiology occurs in approximately 60% of cases. A family history and a review of pregnancy complications and maternal risk factors should be obtained. Maternal blood should be obtained for an indirect Coombs test to rule out immune hydrops. In addition, a maternal complete blood cell count (CBC), Kleihauer-Betke, cytomegalovirus (CMV) and parvovirus B19 serology and a serologic test for syphilis should be performed. A fetal echocardiogram with special emphasis on the cardiac rhythm and function should be obtained. Doppler of the middle cerebral artery for peak systolic velocity will help to exclude or suggest fetal anemia as an etiology of hydrops. Karyotyping and microarray should be performed, as well as polymerase chain reaction (PCR) for CMV and parvovirus. A listing of the diagnostic tests used in the evaluation of the pregnancy complicated by hydrops is outlined in Table 12.3-2. Other laboratory tests and consultations will vary. For example, if the mother has a very low mean corpuscular volume and mild anemia suggestive of the α-thalassemia carrier state, specialized DNA testing may be warranted. If fetal anemia is suspected, percutaneous umbilical blood sampling (PUBS) with availability of blood for a possible fetal transfusion should be performed.

Fetal hydrops may be diagnosed in the first trimester, most commonly in association with a cystic hygroma. In these cases, chromosomal studies can be obtained by chorionic villus sampling. If aneuploidy is not found and the maternal serologic evaluation is negative, a detailed ultrasonographic

**TABLE 12.3-2** Diagnostic Steps in the Prenatal Evaluation of Nonimmune Hydrops Fetalis

Maternal blood work
- Blood type and indirect Coombs
- Complete blood cell count
- Kleihauer-Betke
- Serology for syphilis, CMV, parvovirus B19

Imaging
- Extended ultrasound examination
- Middle cerebral artery Doppler
- Fetal echocardiogram

Invasive testing
- Karyotype
- Microarray
- PUBS, if anemia is suspected
- PCR studies for viral etiologies
- Genetic studies, as indicated

evaluation and fetal echocardiography at 18 weeks' gestation may help to determine the etiology of first-trimester hydrops.

**Fetal Intervention** Intervention should be reserved for those cases in which a precise diagnosis has been established. Intrauterine transfusion has been successful for anemia secondary to parvovirus infection and for fetomaternal hemorrhage. Resolution of fetal hydrops has been reported with a unilateral pleural effusion treated by shunt placement. Control of fetal cardiac tachyarrhythmias with maternally administered antiarrhythmic medications has been a successful intervention for associated fetal hydrops. Twins with hydrops from twin reversed arterial perfusion or twin-to-twin transfusion syndrome also may benefit from intervention.

**Monitoring** If a diagnosis and etiology are established, the management will be dictated by the treatment of that disorder. In cases with an unknown etiology, close monitoring for fetal decompensation is warranted. In general, outcome in stable cases is not improved by early delivery, most likely because of the underlying etiology of the hydrops.

**Pregnancy Course** There is a significant risk of polyhydramnios and preterm labor with NIHF. An uncommon, but important, maternal complication is a form of severe preeclampsia called mirror syndrome. This is an indication for delivery for maternal indications.

**Pregnancy Termination Issues** Unless a precise diagnosis has been made antenatally, an intact fetus must be delivered for a complete pathologic evaluation.

**Delivery** Because of the complicated neonatal resuscitation likely to be required, delivery must occur at a tertiary center. The mode of delivery should be based on obstetric indications and will vary depending on the condition of the fetus, underlying cause of the hydrops, and the gestational age.

## NEONATOLOGY

**Resuscitation** Fetuses with hydrops tolerate labor poorly. They develop asphyxia secondary to the accompanying placental pathologic lesions, as well as from the disorder causing the hydrops. Except in uncommon cases, extensive resuscitation with immediate respiratory support is required. Both thoracentesis and paracentesis may be needed following delivery to permit adequate ventilatory excursions.

**Transport** Referral to a tertiary perinatal center is mandatory because of both the very high mortality risk and the extensive technical support required for diagnostic evaluation and management.

**Nursery Management** The management approach is determined by two factors: the effects on cardiorespiratory function of the hydropic state and the underlying cause. If not established prenatally, determining the cause is imperative both to facilitate therapeutic intervention and to provide accurate counseling regarding prognosis and recurrence risk.

## SUGGESTED READINGS


1. Gimovsky AC, Luzi P, Berghella V: Lysosomal storage disease as an etiology of nonimmune hydrops. Am J Obstet Gynecol 2015; 212:281-290.
2. Heinonen S, Ryynanen M, Kirkinen P: Etiology and outcome of second trimester non-immunologic fetal hydrops. Acta Obstet Gynecol Scand 2000; 79:15-18.
3. Ismail KM, Martin WL, Ghosh S, et al: Etiology and outcome of hydrops fetalis. J Matern Fetal Med 2001; 10:175-181.
4. Machin GA: Hydrops revisited: literature review of 1,414 cases published in the 1980s. Am J Med Genet 1989; 34:366-390.
5. Mari G. The middle cerebral artery peak systolic velocity for the diagnosis of fetal anemia—the untold story (Opinion). Ultrasound Obstet Gynecol 2005; 25:323-330.
6. McCoy MC, Katz VL, Gould N, et al: Non-immune hydrops after 20 weeks' gestation: review of 10 years' experience with suggestions for management. Obstet Gynecol 1995; 85:578-582.
7. Santolaya J, Alley D, Jaffe R, Warsof SL: Antenatal classification of hydrops fetalis. Obstet Gynecol 1992; 79:256-259.
8. Schild Rl, Bald R, Plath H, et al: Intrauterine management of fetal parvovirus B19 infection. Ultrasound Obstet Gynecol 1999; 13:161-166.
9. Sohan K, Carroll SG, De La Fuente S, et al: Analysis of outcome in hydrops fetalis in relation to gestation age at diagnosis, cause, and treatment. Acta Obstet Gynecol Scand 2001; 80:726-730.
10. Uzun O, Babaoglu K, Sinha A, et al. Rapid control of foetal supraventricular tachycardia with digoxin and flecainide combination treatment. Cardiol Young 2012; 22:372-380.
11. Van Maldergem L, Jauniaux E, Fourneau C, Gillerot Y: Genetic causes of hydrops fetalis. Pediatrics 1992; 89:81-86.
12. Watson J, Campbell S: Antenatal evaluation and management of non- immune hydrops fetalis. Obstet Gynecol 1986; 67:589-593.

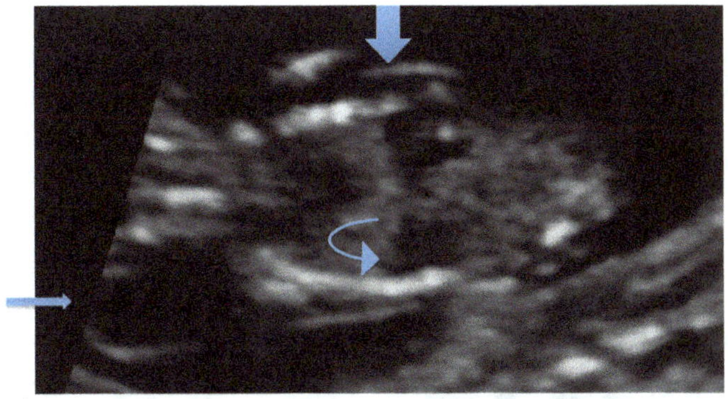

**FIGURE 12.3A** First-trimester fetus with cystic hygroma (narrow arrow), skin edema (broad arrow), and ascites (curved arrow).

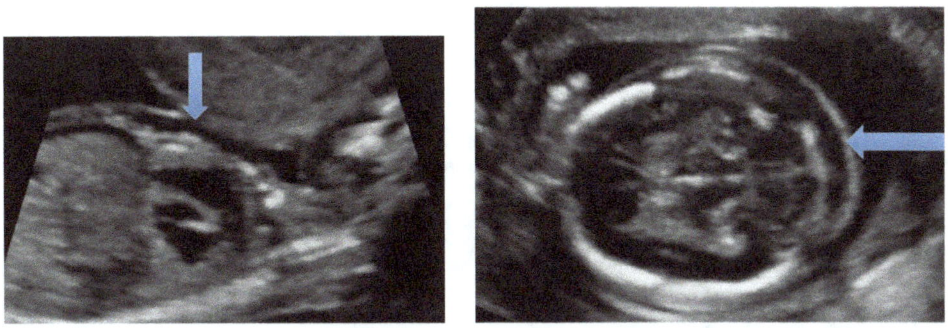

**FIGURE 12.3B,C** Fetus with edema demonstrated over chest wall (B, arrow) and scalp (C, arrow).

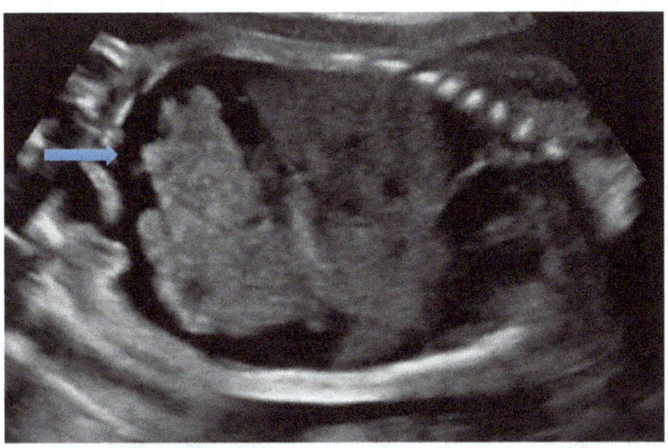

**FIGURE 12.3D** Fetal ascites (arrow).

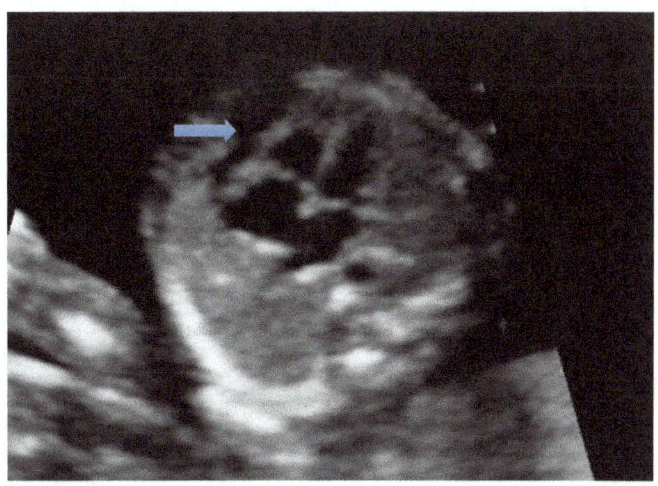

**FIGURE 12.3E** Pericardial effusion (arrow).

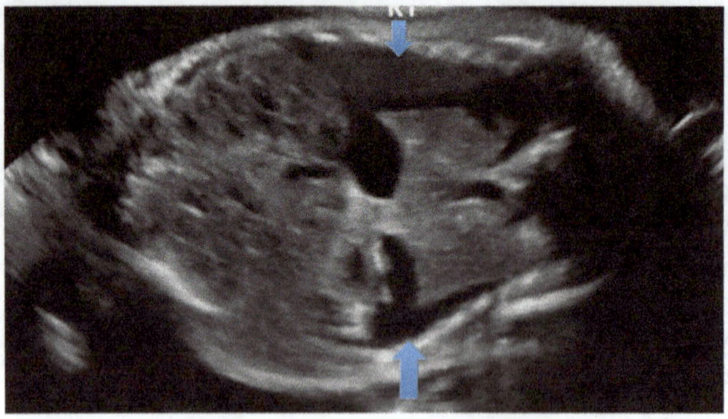

**FIGURE 12.3F** Bilateral pleural effusions (arrows).

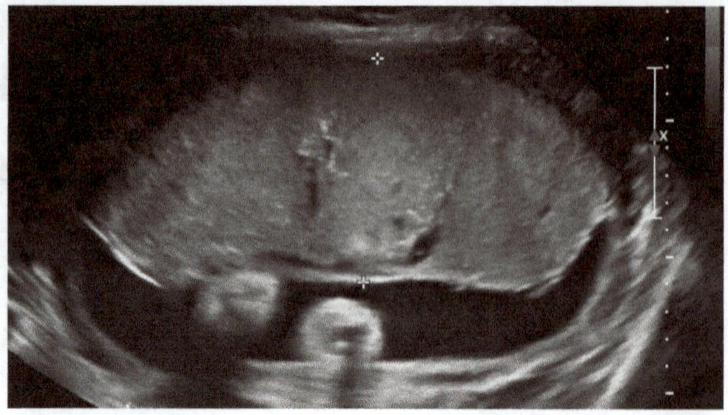

**FIGURE 12.3G** Placentomegaly. The placenta measures 82 mm.

# 12.4 UMBILICAL CORD CYSTS

## EPIDEMIOLOGY/GENETICS

**Definition** An umbilical cord cyst is a cyst arising from the cord.

**Epidemiology** The prevalence in the first trimester is 0.4% to 3.4%.

**Embryology** "True" cysts are derived from the allantois (i.e., urachus) or the omphalomesenteric duct. They are epithelial lined and usually found at the fetal end of the umbilical cord. These cysts have been associated with omphaloceles and a patent urachus. "False" cysts, or pseudocysts, are derived from edema of Wharton's jelly. Umbilical vessels may course through the cyst (i.e. Wharton's jelly). False cysts are likely formed by increased hydrostatic pressure associated with cord coiling.

**Inheritance Patterns** Inheritance is sporadic.

**Prognosis** If isolated, there are no clinical implications.

## SONOGRAPHY

### FREQUENT FINDINGS

- Anechoic 4- to 50-mm cyst, usually near the fetal end of the umbilical cord

### LESS FREQUENT

- Umbilical vessels appear to transect the cyst
- Notching of the umbilical artery waveform pattern due to cyst compression

### KEY FINDINGS/PITFALLS

- False cysts are more frequent than true cysts.
  - Generally, the sonographer cannot distinguish between a true cyst and a pseudocyst.
- Umbilical cord cysts are usually only several millimeters in diameter.
  - Cysts greater than 50 mm have been reported.
  - With sufficient size, an umbilical cord cyst may compress the umbilical vessels, resulting in fetal distress.
- First-trimester cysts that resolve by the second trimester are not associated with an increase in karyotypic abnormalities or poor outcome.
- Multiple first-trimester umbilical cord cysts are associated with aneuploidy and an increased risk of miscarriage.
- Umbilical cord cysts that persist into the second trimester are associated with an increased risk of karyotypic abnormalities (trisomy 18) and structural defects.
- The association of umbilical cord cysts with aneuploidy may be biased due to
  - The tendency to report adverse outcomes
  - Small sample size

- A second-trimester umbilical cord cyst should be considered an indication for an extended fetal anatomic survey.

## PREGNANCY MANAGEMENT

**Investigations and Consultations Required** An apparently isolated cyst seen in the first trimester may resolve by the time of the second-trimester anatomic survey. In these cases, no further investigation is needed. If the cyst persists, if there are multiple cysts, or if there are associated fetal anomalies, fetal chromosome studies should be performed.

**Monitoring** Follow-up sonograms may be useful to exclude progression and to assess for other abnormalities that may have been missed. Cord compression by an enlarging cord cyst, as evidenced by abnormal Doppler patterns (i.e., early diastolic notching), has been reported.

**Pregnancy Course** Pregnancy course is unremarkable in almost all cases.

**Delivery** Ensure that the cord is sent for pathologic analysis.

### SUGGESTED READINGS

1. Battaglic C, Artini PG, D'Ambrogio G, Genezzani AR: Cord vessel compression by an expanding allantoic cyst: case report. Ultrasound Obstet Gynecol 1992; 2:58-60.
2. Ghezzi F, Raio L, DiNaro E, et al: Single and multiple umbilical cord cysts in early gestation: two different entities. Ultrasound Obstet Gynecol 2003; 21:215-219.
3. Ross JA, Jurkovic D, Zosmer N, et al: Umbilical cord cysts in early pregnancy. Obstet Gynecol 1997; 89:442-445.
4. Sepulveda W: Beware of the umbilical cord "cyst." Ultrasound Obstet Gynecol 2003; 21:213-214.
5. Sepulveda W, Gutierrez J, Sanchez J, et al: Pseudocyst of the umbilical cord: prenatal sonographic appearance and clinical significance. Obstet Gynecol 1999; 93:377-381.
6. Skibo LK, Lyons EA, Levi CS: First-trimester umbilical cord cysts. Radiology 1992; 182:719-722.
7. Zanger R, Boldes R, Yaffe H, et al: Umbilical cord cysts in the second and third trimesters: significance and prenatal approach. Ultrasound Obstet Gynecol 2010; 36:296-301.

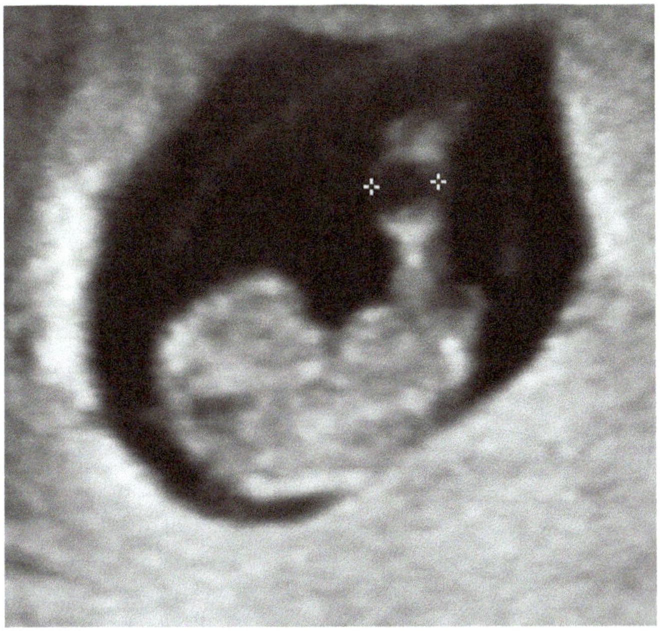

FIGURE 12.4A Umbilical cord cyst (+ … +).

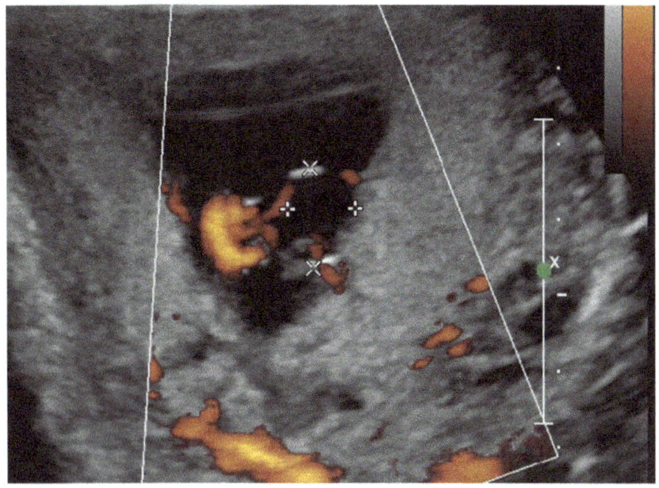

FIGURE 12.4B Umbilical cord cyst (+ … +; x … x).

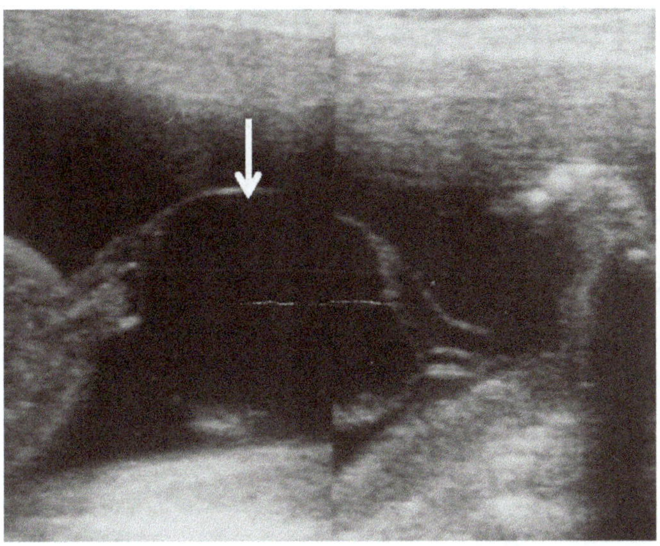

FIGURE 12.4C Large umbilical cord cyst (arrow).

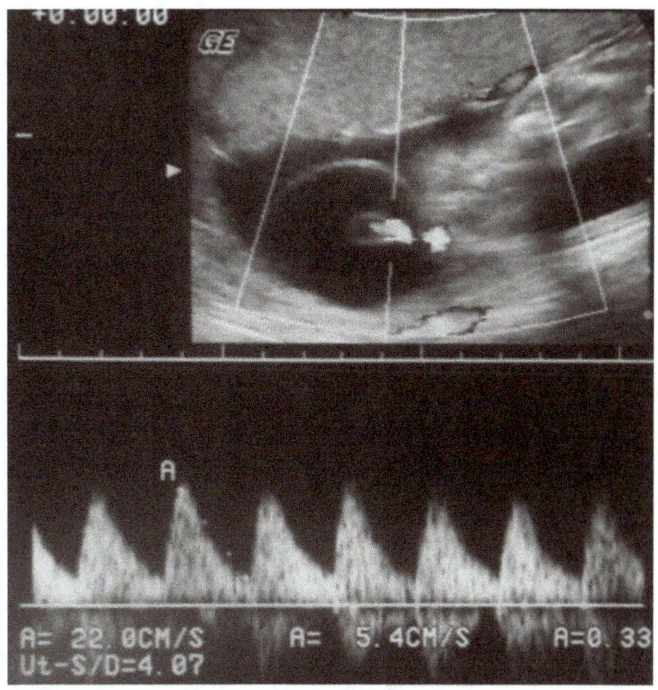


FIGURE 12.4D Umbilical cord cyst adjacent to umbilical artery (Doppler waveform).

# APPENDIX 1

# DIFFERENTIAL DIAGNOSES OF ABNORMAL IN UTERO SONOGRAPHIC FINDINGS

# ABDOMEN

Note: Items in bold represent most common diagnosis.

## ABDOMINAL CYST OR FLUID COLLECTION

**Dilated bladder**
**Dilated bowel**
**Hydroureter**
**Ovarian cyst (in females)**
**Renal cystic lesions, particularly ureteropelvic junction with anterior pelvis or pelvic dysplastic kidney**
Adrenal cyst or hemorrhage
Choledochal cyst
Duodenal atresia, anal atresia, gut atresia
Enteric duplication cyst
Hepatic arteriovenous malformation
Hepatic cyst
Hydrometrocolpos
Liver cyst
Lymphangioma
Meckel's diverticulum
Meconium pseudocyst
Mesenteric cyst
Rectal dilation
Sacrococcygeal (cystic) teratoma
Splenic cyst
Umbilical vein varix
Urachal cyst

## ABDOMINAL WALL PROCESS

**Omphalocele**
**Gastroschisis**
**Physiologic gut herniation (8 to 12 weeks' gestation)**
**Limb–body wall complex**
**Umbilical hernia**
Bladder exstrophy
Cloacal exstrophy (OEIS [omphalocele, exstrophy of the bladder, imperforate anus, and spinal defects] complex)
Pentalogy of Cantrell
Vesicoallantoic cyst
Urachal cyst

## STOMACH NONVISUALIZATION

**Diaphragmatic hernia (left sided)**
**Normal variant**
**Tracheoesophageal atresia or fistula/esophageal atresia**
Microgastria
Central nervous system problems that prevent swallowing
Hiatal hernia
Facial cleft
Micrognathia

## ASCITES (ISOLATED)

**Renal obstruction**
Trisomy 21
Meconium peritonitis
Fetal infections (especially parvovirus and cytomegalovirus)

## DILATED STOMACH AND DUODENUM

**Duodenal atresia**
**Normal variant**
Annular pancreas
Antral web
Diabetic embryopathy
Gut malrotation

## ECHOGENIC AREA IN ABDOMEN

### ECHOGENIC MASS

**Adrenal hemorrhage**
**Dysplastic second collecting system**
**Extralobar sequestration**
**Hepatic tumor**
Neuroblastoma
Ovarian cyst with hemorrhage
Sacrococcygeal teratoma
Fetus in fetu

### ECHOGENIC BOWEL

**Cystic fibrosis**

**Intragut or intra-abdominal bleed**

**Meconium in the third trimester**

**Normal variant at term**

**Trisomy 21**

**Intrauterine growth restriction**

**Fetal infections (cytomegalovirus)**

**Meconium peritonitis**

### CALCIFICATION

**Normal variant**

Fetal infections (cytomegalovirus infection, toxoplasmosis)

Gallstones

Idiopathic arterial calcification

Teratoma (intrapelvic or in adrenal region)

Intraluminal calcification—imperforate anus/anal atresia

## LARGE BOWEL DILATION

**Anorectal malformation or atresia**

**Meconium plug syndrome**

Hirschprung disease

## OMPHALOCELE

**Chromosome anomaly—trisomy 13, 18, or 21, triploidy**

**Isolated**

**Umbilical hernia**

Amniotic band syndrome

Beckwith-Wiedemann syndrome

Carpenter syndrome

CHARGE association

Meckel-Gruber syndrome

Pentalogy of Cantrell

Short-rib polydactyly syndromes, various types

## SMALL BOWEL DILATION

**Jejunoileal atresia**

**Volvulus**

**Meconium ileus**
**Meconium peritonitis**
**Enteric duplications**
**Gastroschisis**
**Massive bilateral ureteropelvic junction obstruction**
**Cystic fibrosis**

# GENITOURINARY

## ABSENT BLADDER

**Following voiding**
**Renal agenesis (bilateral)**
**Technical—obese patient and prone fetus**
Bilateral renal dysplasia
Bladder exstrophy
Caudal regression
Cloacal exstrophy
Infantile polycystic kidney disease
Severe intrauterine growth restriction
Sirenomelia
Meckel-Gruber syndrome

## CYSTS IN KIDNEYS

**Multicystic dysplastic kidney**
**Severe hydronephrosis in single or double systems**
**Meckel-Gruber syndrome**
**Chromosomal—trisomy 13**
Adult polycystic kidney
Ellis–van Creveld syndrome
Fryns syndrome
Infantile polycystic kidney disease
Jeune asphyxiating thoracic dystrophy
Joubert syndrome
Marden-Walker syndrome
McKusik-Kaufman syndrome
Orofacial-digital syndrome, various types (microcysts)
Roberts syndrome
Short-rib polydactyly syndromes, various types
Smith-Lemli-Opitz syndrome
Tuberous sclerosis
Zellweger syndrome

## ENLARGED KIDNEYS OR KIDNEY

**Autosomal recessive (infantile polycystic) kidney disease**
**Autosomal dominant (adult) polycystic kidney disease**
**Compensatory hypertrophy**
**Crossed renal ectopia**
**Double collecting system**
**Hydronephrosis**
**Multicystic dysplastic kidney disease**
Beckwith-Wiedemann syndrome
Meckel-Gruber syndrome
Trisomy 13
Mesoblastic nephroma

## GENITAL ABNORMALITIES

**Smith-Lemli-Opitz syndrome**
**Campomelic dysplasia**
**Cloacal exstrophy**
**Chromosomal abnormalities, various**
CHARGE association
Cornelia de Lange syndrome
Ectrodactyly-ectodermal-dysplasia-clefting (EEC) syndrome
Fanconi syndrome
Fraser syndrome
Noonan syndrome
Pallister-Killian syndrome
Pena-Shokeir syndrome
Short-rib polydactyly syndrome
Fryns syndrome
MURCS (müllerian duct aplasia, renal aplasia, cervicothoracic somite dysplasia)

## HYDRONEPHROSIS ASSOCIATIONS

**Ectopic ureter**
**Posterior urethral valves**
**Reflux**
**Ureterocele and ectopic ureter**
**Ureteropelvic junction obstruction**
**Ureterovesical junction obstruction**

Bladder exstrophy
Cloacal exstrophy
Ectrodactyly-ectodermal-dysplasia-clefting (EEC) syndrome
Hemifacial microsomia (Goldenhar syndrome)
McKusik-Kaufman syndrome
Megacystis megaureter
Megacystis microcolon
Sacrococcygeal teratoma

## POSSIBLE SUPRARENAL MASS

**Adrenal hematoma**
**Multicystic duplicated collecting system**
**Extrapulmonary sequestration (left side)**
**Neuroblastoma**
Hepatic mass
Liver cyst

## RENAL AGENESIS

**Isolated**
**VACTERL (vertebral defects, anal atresia, cardiac defects, tracheoesophageal fistula, renal anomalies, limb abnormalities) association**
Caudal regression/sirenomelia
Diabetic embryopathy
Fraser syndrome (cryptophthalmos)
Hemifacial microsomia (Goldenhar syndrome)
Limb–body wall complex
MURCS (müllerian duct aplasia, renal aplasia, cervicothoracic somite dysplasia)
Short rib polydactyly
Townes-Brock syndrome

# CARDIAC

## ENLARGED HEART

**Cardiomyopathy**
**Hydrops**
**Anemia**
**Small chest (normal size heart appears large—dwarfing syndromes)**
**Bilateral atrioventricular valve regurgitation**
**Pronounced bradycardia**
**Severe mitral valve regurgitation**
**Pericardial effusion**

## LEFT HEART ENLARGEMENT

**Aortic stenosis**
**Cardiomyopathy**

## RIGHT HEART ENLARGEMENT

**Coarctation of the aorta (particularly relative to left heart)**
**Hypoplastic left heart syndrome (particularly if tricuspid regurgitation)**
**Dysplastic pulmonary valve syndromes (with severe pulmonary regurgitation)**
**Premature closure of the ductus (e.g., nonsteroidal anti-inflammatory drugs such as indomethacin and aspirin)**
**Tetralogy of Fallot**

## RIGHT ATRIAL ENLARGEMENT

**Ebstein anomaly**
**Tricuspid regurgitation**
**Tricuspid stenosis**
**Total anomalous pulmonary venous return (left atrial hypoplasia so right atrium appears large)**

## BRIGHT ECHOES IN THE HEART

**Chordae tendineae (normal variant)**
**Papillary muscle (normal variant)**
**Rhabdomyoma (tuberous sclerosis)**

**Dystrophic calcification syndrome**

**Angioma**

**Endocardial fibroelastosis (linear echogenic border to left ventricle)**

Critical aortic stenosis and aortic atresia

Myocarditis (congenital infections—toxoplasmosis, cytomegalovirus)

## CARDIAC ABNORMALITY ASSOCIATIONS

**Chromosome abnormalities**

**Noonan syndrome**

**VACTERL (vertebral defects, anal atresia, cardiac defects, tracheoesophageal fistula, renal anomalies, limb abnormalities) association**

**Diabetic embryopathy**

**Deletion 22q syndrome (DiGeorge/velocardiofacial syndrome)**

Adams-Oliver syndrome

Campomelic dysplasia

Cornelia de Lange syndrome

Cri-du-chat syndrome

Ellis–van Creveld syndrome (chondroectodermal dysplasia)

Fanconi syndrome

Fetal alcohol syndrome

Fetal infections

Hemifacial microsoma (Goldenhar syndrome)

Holt-Oram syndrome

Heterotaxy syndrome—situs inversus

Hydrolethalis

McKusik-Kaufman syndrome

Maternal phenylketonuria

Meckel-Gruber syndrome

Neu-Laxova syndrome

Retinoic acid embryopathy

Rubenstein-Taybi syndrome

Roberts syndrome

Short-rib polydactyly syndromes

Smith-Lemli-Opitz syndrome

Thrombocytopenia–absent radius syndrome (TAR)

Tuberous sclerosis (rhabdomyoma)

Williams syndrome

Zellweger syndrome

## CARDIAC MASS

**Rhabdomyoma (tuberous sclerosis)**

**Hypertrophic cardiomyopathy**

**Pericardiac masses (e.g., thymus, teratoma)**

**Basal cell nevus syndrome**

## PERICARDIAL EFFUSION

**Infections**

- Cytomegalovirus
- Parvovirus
- Myocarditis

**Valvular aortic stenosis (especially if mitral regurgitation is present)**

**Cardiomyopathy**

**Pronounced bradycardia**

**Tachycardia**

**Early sign of anemia—Rh, parvovirus, and α-thalassemia**

**Early sign of hydrops**

**Pericardial cyst**

**Normal echopenic rim (pseudopericardial effusion)**

Cardiac tumor

Chromosomal—45X (Turner syndrome), trisomy 21

Confusion with pleural effusion

## REVERSED ATRIAL SHUNT (LEFT ATRIUM TO RIGHT ATRIUM)

**Critical mitral stenosis, mitral atresia**

**Severe left ventricular dysfunction**

**Severe left ventricular hypoplasia**

**Critical aortic stenosis/atresia**

**Hypoplastic left heart syndrome**

## REVERSED DUCTAL FLOW (AORTA-PULMONARY ARTERY)

**Tricuspid atresia**

**Tetralogy of Fallot with severe pulmonary stenosis or atresia**

**Critical pulmonary stenosis or atresia**

## RETROGRADE FLOW IN THE AORTIC ARCH

**Critical mitral stenosis, mitral atresia**
**Severe left ventricular dysfunction**
**Severe left ventricular hypoplasia**
**Critical aortic stenosis/atresia**
**Hypoplastic left heart syndrome**
**Interrupted aortic arch**

## ABSENT DUCTUS ARTERIOSUS

**Tetralogy of Fallot/pulmonary atresia**
**Tetralogy of Fallot with dysplastic pulmonary valve syndrome**

## ABSENT DUCTUS VENOSUS

**Underdevelopment or agenesis of the fetal portal system**

- **Intrahepatic drainage—good prognosis**
- **Extrahepatic drainage—potential for hydrops**

## BRADYCARDIA

**Sinus node dysfunction**
**Atrioventricular node block (secondary or tertiary) (complete heart block)**
**Blocked premature atrial contractions**
**Structural heart abnormality**
**Maternal autoimmune disease**

## TACHYCARDIA

**Sinus tachycardia**
**Supraventricular tachycardia**
**Atrial flutter**
**Atrial fibrillation with rapid ventricular response**
**Ventricular tachycardia**
**Sepsis**
**Anemia**
**Thyrotoxicosis**

# CHEST

## FLUID COLLECTION IN CHEST

**Pleural effusion**
**Bronchogenic cyst**
**Congenital pulmonary adenomatoid malformation**
**Diaphragmatic hernia (stomach)**
Bronchial atresia
Cystic hygroma
Duplication cyst
Enlarged cardiac chamber
Hiatal hernia (stomach)
Pericardial cyst
Mediastinal teratoma
Neuroenteric cyst

## SOLID MASS IN CHEST

**Congenital pulmonary adenomatoid malformation**
**Pulmonary sequestration**
Cardiac tumor—rhabdomyoma
Chest wall hematoma
Mediastinal teratoma
Neuroblastoma metastases
Normal thymus

## DIAPHRAGMATIC HERNIA ASSOCIATIONS

**Fryns syndrome**
**Trisomy 18 and other chromosomal abnormalities**
**Pallister-Killian (tetrasomy 12p)**
Jarcho-Levin syndrome
Deletion 4p (Wolf-Hirschhorn syndrome)

## PLEURAL EFFUSION

**Chylothorax**
**Early sign of hydrops**

**Trisomy 21**

Hemothorax

Secondary to pulmonary sequestration, congenital pulmonary adenomatoid malformation, tracheal atresia

Lung agenesis

## SMALL CHEST

**Osteogenesis imperfecta type II**

**Thanatophoric dysplasia**

Achondrogenesis, all types

Atelosteogenesis, all types

Campomelic dysplasia

Chondrodyoplasia punctata

Ellis–van Creveld syndrome (chondroectodermal dysplasia)

Fibrochondrogenesis

Hypophosphatasia

Jeune asphyxiating thoracic dystrophy

Multiple pterygium syndrome

Short-rib polydactyly syndromes, all types

Spondyloepiphyseal dysplasia congenita

# CENTRAL NERVOUS SYSTEM

## AGENESIS OF THE CORPUS CALLOSUM ASSOCIATIONS

**Dandy-Walker malformation, isolated**
Aicardi syndrome
Acrocallosal syndrome
Apert syndrome
Chromosomal—trisomy 13
Chromosomal—trisomy 18
Encephalocele
Fetal alcohol syndrome
Fetal infections
Fryns syndrome
Hydrolethalus
Meckel-Gruber syndrome
Neu-Laxova syndrome
Smith-Lemli-Opitz syndrome
Walker-Warburg syndrome
Zellweger syndrome

## BRAIN TOO EASILY VISUALIZED (UNDEROSSIFICATION OF BONE)

**Osteogenesis imperfecta, type II**
Achondrogenesis, some types
Acrania
Atelosteogenesis
Hypophosphatasia
Short-rib polydactyly syndrome

## CEREBELLAR HYPOPLASIA

**Dandy-Walker malformation**
**Spinal dysraphism**
Chromosomal—trisomy 13
Chromosomal—trisomy 18
Cri-du-chat syndrome
Fetal infections
Joubert syndrome
Meckel-Gruber syndrome

Neu-Laxova syndrome
Smith-Lemli-Opitz syndrome
Walker-Warburg syndrome

## DANDY-WALKER MALFORMATION

**Cornelia de Lange syndrome**
**Chromosomal—triploidy**
**Chromosomal—trisomy 13**
**Chromosomal—trisomy 18**
Joubert syndrome
Aicardi syndrome
Fetal alcohol syndrome
CHARGE syndrome
Maternal diabetic embryopathy
Fryns syndrome
Meckel-Gruber syndrome
Neu-Laxova syndrome
Neural tube defect
Fetal infections
Smith-Lemli-Opitz syndrome
Walker-Warburg syndrome

## ECHOGENIC BRAIN FOCUS OR FOCI

**Cerebellar vermis (normal)**
**Choroid plexus (normal)**
Fetal infections (cytomegalovirus infection [wall of lateral ventricles] and toxoplasmosis)
Gyri in third trimester
Intrabrain hemorrhage when fresh
Intracranial tumor (teratoma and lipoma of the corpus callosum)
Tuberous sclerosis

## ENCEPHALOCELE

**Amniotic band syndrome—asymmetrical top of the head lesions**
**Isolated**
Adams-Oliver syndrome
Chromosomal—trisomy 13
Chromosomal—trisomy 18

Dandy-Walker malformation
Dysegmental dysplasia
Meckel-Gruber syndrome
Roberts syndrome (pseudothalidomide)
Walker-Warburg syndrome

## FLUID COLLECTION IN THE HEAD

### BILATERAL

**Choroid plexus cyst**
**Ventriculomegaly**

### SINGLE

**Cavum septum pellucidum or vergae (normal)**
**Quadrageminal cistern (normal)**
**Choroid plexus cyst**
**Third-ventricular enlargement**
Arachnoid cyst
Bleed
Porencephalic cyst
Schizencephaly
Tumor (cystic teratoma)
Dandy-Walker malformation
Mega cisterna magna
Aneurysm of vein of Galen
Holoprosencephaly
Intrahemispheric cyst with agenesis of the corpus callosum
Cystic encephalomalacia and periventricular encephalomalacia
Posterior fossa extra-axial cyst
Subdural hygroma
Unilateral ventriculomegaly

## HOLOPROSENCEPHALY

**Chromosomal—trisomy 13**
**Isolated**
Aicardi syndrome
Campomelic dysplasia
CHARGE association
Chromosomal—triploidy
Chromosomal—trisomy 18

Chromosomal—18p-
Diabetic embryopathy
DiGeorge syndrome
Frontonasal dysplasia
Fryns syndrome
Short-rib polydactyly syndrome
Smith-Lemli-Opitz syndrome

## HYDRANENCEPHALY CAUSES

**Isolated**
Fetal infections
Stuck twin (death of co-twin)
Cocaine embryopathy
Familial hydranencephaly (autosomal recessive)

## KLEEBLATTSCHÄDEL DEFORMITY OF SKULL (CLOVERLEAF SKULL)

**Apert syndrome**
**Pfeiffer syndrome**
**Thanatophoric dysplasia**
Amniotic band syndrome
Campomelic dysplasia
Crouzon syndrome

## MACROCEPHALY

**Familial macrocephaly**
**Ventriculomegaly**
Achondrogenesis, all types
Achondroplasia
Basal cell nevus syndrome
Beckwith-Wiedemann syndrome
Chromosomal—triploidy (relative enlargement)
Greig cephalopolysyndactyly syndrome
Intracranial tumor
Sotos syndrome
Thanatophoric dysplasia

## MICROCEPHALY

**Drugs (alcohol, hydantoin, aminopterin)**
**Fetal infections (cytomegalovirus infection, toxoplasmosis, rubella, Zika)**
**Isolated (including autosomal and X-linked recessive forms)**
**Spinal dysraphism**
**Cerebral atrophy**
**Chromosome abnormalities (especially trisomy 18)**
Adams-Oliver syndrome
Cornelia de Lange syndrome
Craniosynostosis
Cri-du-chat syndrome
Encephalocele
Freeman-Sheldon syndrome
Holoprosencephaly
Lenz syndrome
Lissencephaly (including Miller-Diecker syndrome)
Maternal phenylketonuria
Meckel-Gruber syndrome
Neu-Laxova syndrome
Roberts syndrome
Rubenstein-Taybi syndrome
Seckel syndrome
Smith-Lemli-Opitz syndrome
Teratogens
Walker-Warburg syndrome

## POSTERIOR FOSSA CYST

**Arachnoid cyst (extra-axial cyst)**
**Dandy-Walker malformation**
**Dilated cisterna magna**
Porencephalic cyst
Quadrageminal cyst
Vein of Galen aneurysm

## VENTRICULOMEGALY

**Aqueduct stenosis**
**Arnold-Chiari malformation (neural tube defect)**

**Dandy-Walker malformation**
**Encephalocele**
**Hydrocephalus ex vacuo (atrophy)**
**Normal variant (mild)**
Achondroplasia (third trimester)
Agenesis of the corpus callosum (colpocephaly)
Amniotic band syndrome
Arachnoid cyst
Baller-Gerold syndrome
Campomelic dysplasia
CHARGE association
Chromosomal abnormalities
Craniosynostosis
Fetal alcohol syndrome
Fetal infections (cytomegalovirus infection and toxoplasmosis)
Fryns syndrome
Holoprosencephaly
Hydrolethalis
Intracranial bleed
Meckel-Gruber syndrome
Lissencephaly, including Miller-Diecker syndrome
Neoplasms
Neu-Laxova syndrome
Roberts syndrome (pseudothalidomide)
Short-rib polydactyly syndromes
Smith-Lemli-Opitz syndrome
Thanatophoric dysplasia
Vein of Galen aneurysm
Walker-Warburg syndrome
Zellweger syndrome

# SPINE

## SHORT SPINE

**Iniencephaly**
**Caudal regression/sirenomelia**
Jarcho-Levin syndrome
Klippel-Feil syndrome

## SPINAL DYSRAPHISM ASSOCIATIONS

**Chromosome abnormalities (triploidy and trisomy 18)**
**Maternal diabetic embryopathy**
Aminopterin
Amniotic band syndrome
Anencephaly
Cataract
Caudal regression
Cloacal exstrophy (OEIS [omphalocele, exstrophy of the bladder, imperforate anus, and spinal defects] syndrome)
Diastematomyelia
Encephalocele
Valproic acid embryopathy
Retinoic acid embryopathy
Iniencephaly
Limb–body wall complex
Rachischisis
Roberts syndrome (pseudothalidomide)
Sacrococcygeal teratoma

## VERTEBRAL ABNORMALITIES

**Maternal diabetic embryopathy**
**Neural tube defect**
**VACTERL (vertebral defects, anal atresia, cardiac defects, tracheoesophageal fistula, renal anomalies, limb abnormalities) association**
Cloacal exstrophy (OEIS [omphalocele, exstrophy of the bladder, imperforate anus, and spinal defects] syndrome)
Diastomatomyelia
Hemifacial microsomia (Goldenhar syndrome)
Jarcho-Levin syndrome

Klippel-Feil syndrome

Kniest syndrome

Larsen syndrome

MURCS (müllerian duct aplasia, renal aplasia, cervicothoracic somite dysplasia)

Noonan syndrome

Skeletal dysplasia, many types

# EYES

## EXOPHTHALMOS/PROPTOSIS/PROMINENT EYES

**Craniosynostosis**

Apert syndrome (acrocephalosyndactyly, type I)

Carpenter syndrome

Crouzon syndrome

Jackson-Weiss syndrome

Melnick-Needles syndrome

Neu-Laxova syndrome

Pfeiffer syndrome

## CATARACT

**Fetal infections**

Neu-Laxova syndrome

Walker-Warburg syndrome

Zellweger syndrome

## HYPERTELORISM

Aarskog syndrome

Acrocallosal syndrome

Atelosteogenesis

Craniosynostosis syndromes

Chromosomal—4p- (Wolf-Hirschhorn syndrome)

Frontal encephalocele

Frontonasal dysplasia

Larsen syndrome

Marden-Walker syndrome

Melnick-Needles syndrome

Noonan syndrome

Neu-Laxova syndrome

Pena-Shokeir syndrome

Otopalatodigital syndrome

Opitz hypertelorism hypospadias syndrome

Robinow syndrome (fetal face syndrome)

## HYPOTELORISM

**Holoprosencephaly**

**Chromosomal abnormalities, particularly trisomy 13**

**Trigonocephaly**

**Baller-Gerald syndrome**

## MICROPHTHALMIA OR ANOPHTHALMIA

**Chromosomal abnormalities, especially trisomy 13**

**Isolated**

CHARGE association

Fetal infections (rubella, varicella, toxoplasmosis)

Fraser syndrome—cryptophthalmos

Goldenhar syndrome (hemifacial microsomia)

Hydrolethalis

Lenz syndrome

Neu-Laxova syndrome

Oculodentodigital syndrome

Walker-Warburg syndrome

# FACE

## ASYMMETRY

**Goldenhar syndrome (hemifacial microsomia)**
**Amniotic band syndrome with facial cleft**
Craniosynostosis and associated syndromes
CHARGE association
Greig cephalopolysyndactyly syndrome
Jackson-Weiss syndrome
Saethre-Chotzen syndrome
Townes-Brock syndrome

## CLEFT LIP AND PALATE (M = MIDLINE CLEFT LIP OR PALATE, L = LATERAL CLEFT OR PALATE, P = CLEFT PALATE ONLY)

**Isolated**
**Amniotic band syndrome (L)**
**Chromosome abnormalities, especially trisomy 13 (M, L, P)**
**Holoprosencephaly (M, L)**
**Stickler syndrome (P)**
Atelosteogenesis (P)
Campomelic dysplasia (P)
CHARGE association (P)
Cri-du-chat syndrome
Diastrophic dysplasia (P)
Ectrodactyly-ectodermal-dysplasia-clefting syndrome (L, P)
Fetal anticonvulsant syndrome (L)
Hydrolethalus
Maternal phenylketonuria (P)
Meckel-Gruber syndrome (M, L, P)
Mohr syndrome (M)
Multiple pterygium syndrome, lethal (P)
Orofacial-digital syndrome, various types (M, L, P)
Otopalatodigital syndrome
Retinoic acid embryopathy (L, P)
Roberts syndrome (L, P)
Robinow syndrome (L, P)
Short-rib polydactyly syndromes, various types (L, P)
Spondyloepiphyseal dysplasia congenita (P)

Stickler syndrome
Treacher-Collins syndrome (P)
Velocardiofacial syndrome/DiGeorge sequence (P)
Smith-Lemli-Opitz syndrome
Gorlin syndrome
Pierre Robin sequence

## MACROGLOSSIA

**Beckwith-Wiedemann syndrome**
**Chromosomal—trisomy 21 (Down syndrome)**
**Oral teratoma**

## MALFORMED EARS

**Chromosome abnormalities, especially trisomy 18**
Acrofacial dysostoses (microtia)
Branchio-otorenal syndrome
CHARGE association
Hemifacial microsomia (Goldenhar syndrome) (tags, microtia)
Retinoic acid embryopathy
Townes-Brock syndrome (tags)
Treacher-Collins syndrome (tags) (microtia)

## MICROGNATHIA

**Chromosomal abnormalities, especially trisomy 18**
**Pierre Robin sequence**
**Short-rib polydactyly syndrome**
**Stickler syndrome**
Acrofacial dysostoses, various types
Atelosteogenesis
Campomelic dysplasia
CHARGE association
Cri-du-chat syndrome
Fetal teratogens (alcohol, valproic acid, retinoic acid)
Freeman-Sheldon syndrome (whistling facies)
Hemifacial microsomia (Goldenhar syndrome)
Hypoglossia, hypodactyly
Joubert syndrome

Larsen syndrome
Melnick-Needles syndrome
Multiple pterygium syndrome
Marden-Walker syndrome
Neu-Laxova syndrome
Nager syndrome
Orofacial-digital syndrome, various types
Otocephaly
Seckel syndrome
Skeletal dysplasias, various types
Smith-Lemli-Opitz syndrome
Sotos syndrome
Treacher-Collins syndrome

## MIDFACE HYPOPLASIA/DEPRESSED NASAL BRIDGE/MAXILLARY HYPOPLASIA

**Achondroplasia (third trimester)**
**Atelosteogenesis**
**Campomelic dysplasia**
**Chondrodysplasia punctata (third trimester)**
**Cleidocranial dysostosis**
**Thanatophoric dysplasia**
**Apert syndrome**
**Carpenter syndrome**
**Fetal alcohol syndrome**
**Fetal warfarin syndrome**
**Larsen syndrome**
**Osteogenesis imperfecta, type II**
**Pfeiffer syndrome**
**Holoprosencephaly sequence**
**Pena-Shokeir syndrome**
**Smith-Lemli-Opitz syndrome**
**Stickler syndrome**

# LIMBS

## ABNORMAL THUMB

**Diabetic embryopathy**

**Holt-Oram syndrome**

**VACTERL (vertebral defects, anal atresia, cardiac defects, tracheoesophageal fistula, renal anomalies, limb abnormalities) association**

Acrofacial dysostoses, various types

Apert syndrome (acrocephalosyndactyly, type I)

Baller-Gerold syndrome

Carpenter syndrome (acrocephalopolysyndactyly, type II)

Chromosomal—trisomy 18

Cornelia de Lange syndrome

Diastrophic dysplasia

Ectrodactyly-tibial aplasia syndrome

Fanconi syndrome

Greig cephalopolysyndactyly syndrome

Hemifacial microsomia (Goldenhar syndrome)

Orofacial-digital syndrome, various types

Pfeiffer syndrome (acrocephalosyndactyly, type V)

Poland anomaly

Rubinstein-Taybi syndrome

Townes-Brock syndrome

## ABSENT DIGITS

**Amniotic band syndrome**

**Poland anomaly**

**Terminal transverse limb defect**

Acrofacial dysostoses, various types

Atelosteogenesis

Adams-Oliver syndrome

Baller-Gerold syndrome

Various chromosomal abnormalities

Cornelia de Lange syndrome

Ectrodactyly-ectodermal-dysplasia-clefting syndrome

Ectrodactyly-tibial aplasia syndrome

Fanconi syndrome

Fryns syndrome

Holt-Oram syndrome
Nager acrofacial dystosis
Oromandibular limb hypogenesis
Pfeiffer syndrome (acrocephalosyndactyly, type V)
Roberts syndrome (pseudothalidomide)
Townes-Brock syndrome
VACTERL (vertebral defects, anal atresia, cardiac defects, tracheoesophageal fistula, renal anomalies, limb abnormalities) association

## ASYMETRIC LIMBS

**Amniotic band syndrome**
**Osteogenesis imperfecta**
**Femoral hypoplasia**
**Terminal transverse limb deficiency**
**Femur-fibula-ulna syndrome**
**Proteus syndrome**
Klippel-Trenaunay-Weber syndrome
Rubenstein-Taybi syndrome

## ABSENT LIMBS

**Amniotic band syndrome**
**Diabetic embryopathy**
**Limb–body wall complex**
**Terminal transverse limb deficiency**
Acrofacial dysostoses, various types
Atelosteogenesis
Cornelia de Lange syndrome
Ectrodactyly-ectodermal-dysplasia-clefting syndrome
Grebe syndrome
Holt-Oram syndrome
Oromandibular limb hypogenesis
Poland anomaly
Retinoic acid embryopathy
Roberts syndrome (pseudothalidomide)
Sirenomelia
Thalidomide embryopathy
Thrombocytopenia–absent radius syndrome

## BONE HYPOMINERALIZATION

**Achondrogenesis**
**Hypophosphatasia**
**Osteogenesis imperfecta**

## BOWING

**Campomelic dysplasia—particularly tibia and femur**
**Osteogenesis imperfecta, type II—particularly tibia and femur**
**Thanatophoric dysplasia**
Achondrogenesis
Boomerang dysplasia
Diabetic embryopathy
Dyssegmental dysplasia
Fibrochondrogenesis
Focal femoral deficiency—only involves tibia and femur
Hypophosphatasia
Melnick-Needles syndrome
Normal (if femur scanned from medial aspect)
Oligohydramnios sequence
Roberts syndrome

## CLENCHED HANDS

**Arthrogryposis, various types**
**Chromosomal abnormalities, especially trisomy 18**
Amniotic band syndrome
Apert syndrome
Congenital muscular dystrophy, various types
Freeman-Sheldon syndrome
Harlequin icthyosis
Multiple pterygium syndrome
Neu-Laxova syndrome
Pena-Shokeir syndrome
Smith-Lemli-Opitz syndrome
X-linked hydrocephalus (fixed thumb in palm of hand)

## CLINODACTYLY

**Chromosomal abnormalities, especially trisomy 18 and trisomy 21**
**Normal variant**
Acrocephalosyndactyly syndromes
Amniotic band syndrome
Campomelic dysplasia
Cornelia de Lange syndrome
Ectrodactyly-ectodermal-dysplasia-clefting syndrome
Aarskog syndrome
Holt-Oram syndrome
Miller-Dieker syndrome
Orofacial-digital syndrome, various types
Poland anomaly
Roberts syndrome
Russell-Silver syndrome
Seckel syndrome
Saetre-Chotzen syndrome
Townes-Brock syndrome

## CLUBFOOT

**Arthrogryposis, various types**
**Chromosomal abnormalities, especially trisomy 18**
**Isolated**
**Neural tube defect**
Adam-Oliver syndrome
Amniotic band syndrome
Amyloplasia congenita
Atelosteogenesis
Campomelic dysplasia
Caudal regression, especially diabetic embryopathy
Chondrodysplasia punctata (rhizomelic type), lethal
Diabetic embryopathy
Ellis–van Creveld syndrome
Diastrophic dysplasia
Freeman-Sheldon syndrome (whistling face)
Fryns syndrome
Hydrolethalus
Larsen syndrome

Meckel-Gruber syndrome
Multiple pterygium syndrome
Pena-Shokeir syndrome
Seckel syndrome
Short-rib polydactyly syndromes, various types
Smith-Lemli-Opitz syndrome
Thrombocytopenia–absent radius syndrome (TAR)
Zellweger syndrome

## FRACTURES

**Osteogenesis imperfecta, all types**
Achondrogenesis
Hypophosphatasia

## JOINT CONTRACTURES—CONTRACTURES OF THE EXTREMITIES

**Arthrogryposis, various types**
**Caudal dysplasia sequence (diabetic embryopathy)**
**Chromosomal abnormalities, especially trisomy 18**
**Neural tube defect (lower limbs)**
Amniotic band syndrome
Amyloplasia congenita
Apert syndrome (acrocephalosyndactyly, type I)
Beals syndrome (contractual arachnodactyly)
Cornelia de Lange syndrome
Diastrophic dysplasia
Focal femoral deficiency
Freeman-Sheldon syndrome
Larsen syndrome
Multiple pterygium syndrome, various types
Neu-Laxova syndrome
Oligohydramnios sequence
Pena-Shokeir syndrome
Roberts syndrome
Seckel syndrome
Zellweger syndrome

# LIMB SHORTENING

**Achondrogenesis**
**Osteogenesis imperfecta, types II, III**
**Thanatophoric dysplasia**
Achondroplasia
Campomelic dysplasia
Diastrophic dysplasia
Early intrauterine growth restriction
Ellis–van Creveld syndrome
Hypophosphatasia
Kniest syndrome
Roberts syndrome
Short-rib polydactyly syndrome
Spondyloepiphyseal dysplasia congenita
Other rare dysplasias

## RHIZOMELIC SHORTENING

**Asphyxiating thoracic dysplasia (Jeune's syndrome)**
**Achondroplasia**
**Early intrauterine growth restriction**
**Thanatophoric dysplasia**
Atelosteogenesis
Chondrodysplasia punctata, rhizomelic type
Diabetic embryopathy
Familial
Fetal warfarin syndrome
Fibrochondrogenesis
Focal femoral deficiency
Neu-Laxova syndrome
Short-rib polydactyly syndromes

## SELECTED LIMBS

**Amniotic band syndrome**
**Caudal regression (diabetic embryopathy)**
**Focal femoral deficiency**
**Osteogenesis imperfecta**
**Campomelic dysplasia**
**Cornelia de Lange syndrome**
**Fanconi syndrome**
**Femur-fibula-ulna syndrome**
**Holt-Oram syndrome**

**Roberts syndrome**

**Thrombocytopenia–absent radius syndrome**

**VACTERL (vertebral defects, anal atresia, cardiac defects, tracheoesophageal fistula, renal anomalies, limb abnormalities) association**

## MUSCLE WASTING

**Arthrogryposis, various types**

**Congenital muscular dystrophy, various types**

**Amyoplasia congenita**

**Freeman-Sheldon syndrome**

**Neural tube defect, various types (lower limbs only)**

**Multiple pterygium syndrome (lethal)**

**Pena-Shokeir syndrome**

## POLYDACTYLY

### PREAXIAL

Carpenter syndrome

Greig cephalopolysyndactyly syndrome (feet)

Townes-Brock syndrome

Fanconi anemia

### POSTAXIAL

Chromosome abnormalities, especially trisomy 13

Familial, especially African American

Acrocallosal syndrome

Atelosteogenesis

Carpenter syndrome

Ellis–van Creveld syndrome (chondroectodermal dysplasia)

Grebe syndrome

Greig cephalopolysyndactyly syndrome (hands)

Hydrolethalis

Joubert syndrome

McKusik-Kaufman syndrome

Meckel-Gruber syndrome

Mohr syndrome

Orofacial-digital syndrome

Pallister-Hall syndrome

Short-rib polydactyly syndromes

Smith-Lemli-Opitz syndrome

## RADIAL HYPOPLASIA/SHORT RADIAL RAY

**Chromosomal abnormalities, especially trisomy 18**

**Cornelia de Lange syndrome**

**Holt-Oram syndrome**

**VACTERL (vertebral defects, anal atresia, cardiac defects, tracheoesophageal fistula, renal anomalies, limb abnormalities) association**

Aase syndrome

Acrofacial dysostoses, various types

Amniotic band

Baller-Gerold syndrome

Fanconi syndrome

Hemifacial microsomia (Goldenhar syndrome)

Roberts syndrome (pseudothalidomide)

Thrombocytopenia–absent radius syndrome (TAR)

Townes-Brock syndrome

## ROCKER-BOTTOM FEET

**Arthrogryposis, various types**

**Chromosomal abnormalities, especially trisomy 18**

Syndromes with severe neurologic impairment, including Fryns syndrome, multiple pterygium syndromes, Neu-Laxova syndrome

## SOFT TISSUE MASS

**Fibrosarcoma**

**Hemangioma**

**Infantile myofibromatosis**

**Klippel-Trenaunay-Weber syndrome**

**Mafucci syndrome**

**Proteus syndrome**

**Teratoma, including sacrococcygeal teratoma**

**Turner syndrome**

## STIPPLED EPIPHYSES

**Chondrodysplasia punctata**

**Chromosome anomalies, especially trisomy 18**

**Vitamin K deficiency**

**Warfarin syndrome**
**Zellweger syndrome**

## SYNDACTYLY

Neu-Laxova syndrome
Ectrodactyly-ectodermal-dysplasia-clefting syndrome
Apert syndrome
Cephalopolysyndactyly syndrome
Fraser syndrome
Mohr syndrome
Smith-Lemli-Opitz syndrome (second and third toes)
Chromosomal syndromes, especially triploidy

# NECK

## CYSTIC HYGROMA

**Chromosomal abnormalities, especially Turner syndrome, trisomy 21**
Acardiac, acephalic twin
Achondrogenesis
Multiple pterygium syndrome
Neu-Luxova syndrome
Noonan syndrome
Pena-Shokeir syndrome
Roberts syndrome

## HYPEREXTENDED NECK

**Anterior lymphangioma**
**Cervical neural tube defect (iniencephaly)**
**Cervical teratoma**
**Goiter**
**Neuromuscular disorder**
**Normal variant**
**Neu-Laxova syndrome**

## NUCHAL THICKENING OR INCREASED NUCHAL TRANSLUCENCY (MEMBRANE)

**Chromosomal abnormalities**
**Cardiac anomalies**
**Normal variant**
Achondrogenesis
Apert syndrome
Cri-du-chat syndrome
Jacobson syndrome
Joubert syndrome
Multiple pterygium syndrome
Noonan syndrome
Roberts syndrome
Spinal muscular atrophy
Smith-Lemli-Opitz syndrome
Zellweger syndrome

## NECK MASS

**Amniotic band syndrome**
**Anterior lymphangioma**
**Branchial cleft cyst**
**Cervical neural tube defect (iniencephaly)**
**Cystic hygroma (bilateral)**
**Cystic hygroma (unilateral)**
**Encephalocele**
**Goiter**
**Hemangioma**
**Nuchal thickening**
**Teratoma of neck**
**Thyroglossal duct cyst**

# OTHER

## AMNIOTIC MEMBRANE

**Amniotic band syndrome**
**Amniotic sheet**
**Subamniotic or subchorionic bleed**
**Twin membrane**
**Unfused amnion/chorion membranes**
Amniotic membrane displacement following amniocentesis
Limb–body wall complex (amniotic disruption sequence)
Placental cyst

## CHROMOSOMAL ANOMALY SONOGRAPHIC FINDINGS

**Central nervous system anomalies**
- **Holoprosencephaly**
- **Dandy-Walker malformation, cerebellar hypoplasia**
- **Ventriculomegaly**
- **Spina bifida**
- **Agenesis of the corpus callosum**

**Hypotelorism, cleft lip and palate, single nostril, absent nose**
**Cystic hygroma**
**Nuchal thickening/translucency**
**Cardiac malformations**
**Choroid plexus cysts (trisomy 18)**
**Duodenal atresia**
**Gastrointestinal atresias**
**Omphalocele**
**Genitourinary anomalies**
**Hydrothorax**
**Clubfoot, rocker-bottom foot**
**Club hand or clenched hand**
**Severe early intrauterine growth restriction**
**Polyhydramnios or oligohydramnios**
**Second-trimester cord cysts**

## CORD MASS

**Allantoic cyst**
**Wharton's jelly**

Aneurysm
Angiomyxoma cord cyst
Cord knot
Hemangioma
Hematoma
Mucoid degeneration of the cord
Omphalomesenteric cyst
Teratoma
Thrombosis of umbilical vessels
Umbilical vein varix
Urachal cyst

## HYDROPS

**Anemia, including Rh disease and α-thalassemia**
**Cardiac malformation (congenital heart disease)**
**Chromosomal abnormalities, especially Turner syndrome and trisomy 21**
**Chest masses, including congenital pulmonary adenomatoid malformation**
**Cystic hygroma**
**Fetal infections (cytomegalovirus infection, parvovirus infection, syphilis, toxoplasmosis)**
**Twin-to-twin transfusion syndrome**
Achondrogenesis
Cardiac tumor–rhabdomyoma–tuberous sclerosis
Chondrodysplasia punctata
Chorioangioma
Congenital nephrotic syndrome, Finnish type
Cornelia de Lange syndrome
Meconium peritonitis
Diaphragmatic hernia
Dysrhythmia
Extralobar pulmonary sequestration
Fetomaternal transfusion
Fibrochondrogenesis
Glycogen storage disease
Hepatic tumor
Hypophosphatasia
Lymphangioma
Multiple pterygium syndrome, lethal
Neu-Laxova syndrome

Noonan syndrome
Osteogenesis imperfecta, various types
Pena-Shokeir syndrome
Teratomas, including sacrococcygeal teratoma
Short-rib polydactyly syndromes, various types
Tracheal atresia

## INTRAUTERINE GROWTH RESTRICTION

**Chromosomal abnormalities, especially triploidy and trisomy 18**
**Poor-quality measurements**
**Small normal fetus**
Skeletal dysplasias, various types
CHARGE association
Cornelia de Lange syndrome
Fetal infections (cytomegalovirus, varicella, rubella)
Fetal alcohol syndrome
Fetal aminopterin/methotrexate syndrome
Fetal warfarin syndrome
Fibrochondrogenesis
Fryns syndrome
Harlequin syndrome (asymmetric)
Hypophosphatasia
Neu-Laxova syndrome
Osteogenesis imperfecta, various types
Pena-Shokeir syndrome
Roberts syndrome (pseudothalidomide)
Russell-Silver syndrome
Seckel syndrome
Short-rib polydactyly syndromes, various types
Smith-Lemli-Opitz syndrome
Spondyloepiphyseal dysplasia congenita

## MACROSOMIA

**Diabetic embryopathy**
**Familial**
**Poor-quality measurements**
**Wrong dates**
Beckwith-Wiedemann syndrome

Simpson-Golabi-Behmel syndrome
Sotos syndrome
Weaver syndrome

## OLIGOHYDRAMNIOS

**Bilateral dysplastic kidneys**
**Bilateral renal agenesis**
**Bilateral ureteral obstruction**
**Infantile polycystic kidney disease**
**Intrauterine growth restriction**
**Posterior urethral valves**
**Postmaturity**
**Premature rupture of membranes**
**Stuck twin**
Congenital infections
Sirenomelia and caudal regression
Chromosomal—various, especially triploidy

## PLACENTAL MASS

**Chorioangioma**
**Venous lake**
Fetal lobulation
Partial molar changes
Mole and normal fetus
Placental cyst
Placental infarct

## PLACENTAL THICKENING

**Normal variant**
Chorioangioma
Chromosome various, especially triploidy
Diabetic embryopathy
Fetal infections (cytomegalovirus, rubella, syphilis, toxoplasmosis)
Hydrops, especially Rh incompatibility
Beckwith-Wiedemann syndrome

## POLYHYDRAMNIOS

**Associated with fetal hydrops**
**Fetal infections—parvovirus**
**Duodenal atresia**
**Maternal diabetes**
**Gastrointestinal atresias**
**Macrosomia**
**Congenital myotonic dystrophy**
**Tracheoesophageal fistula (esophageal atresia)**
**Twins**
Anemias (thalassemia)
Cardiac malformation—heart failure, various types
Severe/lethal skeletal dysplasias, various types
Obstructing rhabdomyoma (tuberous sclerosis)
Chorioangioma
Congenital nephrotic syndrome, Finnish type
Congenital pulmonary adenomatoid malformation
Diaphragmatic hernia
Epignathus
Fetal goiter
Fryns syndrome
Hydrolethalus
Idiopathic
Intra-abdominal mass (e.g., mesoblastic nephroma)
Large ovarian cysts
Megacystis microcolon
Micrognathia—severe (e.g., otocephaly)
Multiple pterygium syndromes
Neck teratoma
Osteogenesis imperfecta, various types
Otocephaly
Sacrococcygeal teratoma
Short-rib polydactyly
Twin-to-twin transfusion syndrome

# APPENDIX 2

# SONOGRAPHIC FEATURES OF LESS-COMMON FETAL SYNDROMES/ ASSOCIATIONS

*Aarskog syndrome (X-linked recessive)*
- **Hypertelorism**
- **Short nose**
- **Clinodactyly**
- **Brachydactyly**

*Aase syndrome (autosomal dominant)*
- **Radial hypoplasia**
- **Cleft palate**
- **Ventricular septal defect**
- **Urogenital anomalies**

*Acrocallosal syndrome (autosomal recessive)*
- **Agenesis of corpus callosum**
- **Intracranial cysts**
- **Hypertelorism**
- **Macrocephaly**
- **Polydactyly—postaxial**

*Acrofacial dysostosis, Miller syndrome (autosomal recessive)*
- **Malformed ears**
- **Micrognathia**
- **Cleft lip/palate**
- **Absent digits, usually the fifth digits**
- **Radial hypoplasia**

*Acromesomelic dysplasia (autosomal recessive)*
- **Mesomelic (forearm/lower leg) shortness**
- **Bowed radius**

*Adams-Oliver syndrome (autosomal dominant)*
- **Absent digits**
- **Encephalocele**
- **Microcephaly**
- **Cardiac defects**
- **Clubfoot**
- **Intrauterine growth restriction**

*Aicardi syndrome (X-linked dominant)*
- **Agenesis of corpus callosum**
- **Arachnoid cyst**
- **Dandy-Walker malformation**
- **Ventriculomegaly**
- **Microcephaly**
- **Microphthalmia**

*Amyloplasia congenita (sporadic)*
- **Gastroschisis**
- **Micrognathia**
- **Clubfoot**
- **Joint contractures**
- **Decreased fetal movement**

*Atelosteogenesis (autosomal dominant)*
- **Small chest**
- **Eleven pairs of ribs**

Hypertelorism
Cleft lip and palate
Micrognathia
Absent humeri
Absent fibula
Bowed tibia
Clubfoot
Rhizomelic (proximal) shortening
Intrauterine growth restriction
Polyhydramnios

*Baller-Gerold syndrome (autosomal recessive)*
Malformed kidney
Mild ventriculomegaly
Hypotelorism
Micrognathia
Absent digits
Abnormal or absent thumb
Radial hypoplasia
Intrauterine growth restriction
Renal abnormalities

*Basal cell nevus (Gorlin) syndrome (autosomal dominant)*
Macrocephaly
Calcifications in falx cerebri
Ventriculomegaly—mild

*Beals syndrome (autosomal dominant)*
Joint contractures
Cardiac defects

*Boomerang dysplasia (autosomal dominant)*
Bowing
Severe micromelia
Hypertelorism
Clubfeet
Polyhydramnios

*Branchio-oto-renal (Melnick-Fraser) syndrome (autosomal dominant)*
Malformed ears
Renal abnormalities

*CHARGE association (autosomal dominant)*
Esophageal atresia
Cardiac abnormality
Anophthalmia
Holoprosencephaly
Cleft palate
Micrognathia
Genital hypoplasia

*Chondrodysplasia punctata (X-linked dominant, X-linked recessive, autosomal recessive)*
Small chest
Joint contractures

**Rhizomelic shortening**
**Hydrops**
**Stippled epiphyses**

*Chromosome: 18p-*
**Holoprosencephaly**
**Hypotelorism**
**Clubfoot**
**Cardiac abnormalities**

*Chromosome: 18q-*
**Microphthalmia/anophthalmia**
**Microcephaly**

*Chromosome: 47,XXY*
**Increased nuchal translucency**

*Chromosome: 4p- (Wolf-Hirschhorn)*
**Hypertelorism**
**Cardiac abnormality**
**Cleft lip/palate**
**Micrognathia**
**Malformed ears (tags)**
**Intrauterine growth restriction**
**Microcephaly**

*Cleidocranial dysplasia (autosomal dominant)*
**Partial or total aplasia of the clavicles**
**Brachycephaly**
**Hypertelorism**

*Congenital muscular dystrophy (autosomal recessive)*
**Clenched hands**
**Muscle wasting**

*Congenital nephrotic syndrome (autosomal recessive)*
**Polyhydramnios**
**Hydrops**
**Placentomegaly**

*Cornelia de Lange syndrome (autosomal dominant)*
**Cardiac abnormality**
**Dandy-Walker malformation**
**Microcephaly**
**Short nose**
**Midface hypoplasia**
**Abnormal thumb**
**Absent digits**
**Absent limbs**
**Clinodactyly**
**Radial hypoplasia**
**Short limbs**
**Hydrops**
**Intrauterine growth restriction**

*Cri-du-chat (5p deletion) syndrome*
- Microcephaly
- Micrognathia
- Cardiac malformation
- Facial abnormalities, such as cleft lip and palate
- Hypoplastic cerebellum
- Increased nuchal translucency
- Intrauterine growth restriction

*Diabetic embryopathy*
- Duodenal atresia
- Malformed kidney
- Renal agenesis
- Cardiac abnormality
- Holoprosencephaly
- Spinal dysraphism
- Vertebral defects
- Cleft lip/palate
- Macrosomia
- Polyhydramnios

*Dyssegmental dysplasia (autosomal recessive)*
- Bowing
- Severe shortening of all limbs
- Vertebral abnormalities
- Cleft palate

*Ectrodactyly-ectodermal-dysplasia-clefting syndrome (autosomal dominant)*
- Hydronephrosis
- Cleft lip with or without cleft palate
- Absent digits
- Absent limbs
- Clinodactyly
- Renal anomalies
- Holoprosencephaly

*Ectrodactyly–tibial aplasia syndrome (autosomal dominant)*
- Abnormal thumbs
- Absent digits
- Tibial aplasia
- Bifurcation of femora
- Ulna hypoplasia

*Ellis–Van Creveld syndrome (autosomal recessive)*
- Renal agenesis
- Cardiac abnormalities
- Small chest
- Clubfoot
- Polydactyly—postaxial
- Dandy Walker malformation
- Short limbs
- Intrauterine growth restriction

*Fanconi syndrome (autosomal recessive)*
**Cardiac abnormality**
**Thumb hypoplasia/aplasia**
**Microcephaly**
**Radial hypoplasia**
**Renal abnormalities**
**Absent cavum septum pellucidum**
**Cardiac defects**

*Fetal infections*
**Echogenic bowel**
**Echogenic brain foci**
**Hepatic calcifications**
**Microcephaly**
**Limb abnormalities (varicella)**
**Mild ventriculomegaly**
**Cataracts**
**Microphthalmia**
**Hydrops**
**Intrauterine growth restriction**
**Thick placenta**

*Fetal methotrexate embryopathy*
**Mesomelic shortness**
**Micrognathia**
**Intrauterine growth restriction**
**Clubfeet**
**Cleft palate**
**Neural tube defects**

*Fetal warfarin syndrome*
**Nasal hypoplasia**
**Rhizomelic shortening**
**Intrauterine growth restriction**
**Stippled epiphyses**

*Fibrochondrogenesis (autosomal dominant and autosomal recessive)*
**Small chest**
**Rhizomelic shortening**
**Cleft palate**
**Hydrops**
**Intrauterine growth restriction**
**Omphalocele**

*Fraser syndrome (autosomal recessive)*
**Microphthalmia or anophthalmia**
**Syndactyly**
**Genital abnormalities**
**Laryngeal atresia**
**Malformations of the nose and ear**
**Renal agenesis**

*Freeman-Sheldon syndrome (autosomal dominant)*
- Micrognathia
- Ulnar deviation of hands
- Clenched hands
- Clubfoot
- Joint contractures
- Microcephaly

*Frontonasal dysplasia sequence (autosomal recessive in some forms)*
- Frontal bone defect
- Median cleft lip
- Hypertelorism

*Grebe syndrome (autosomal recessive)*
- Acromesomelia
- Absent limbs
- Polydactyly—preaxial

*Greig cephalopolysyndactyly syndrome (autosomal dominant)*
- Macrocephaly
- Hypertelorism
- Abnormal thumb
- Hands: polydactyly—postaxial
- Feet: polydactyly—preaxial
- Absence of the corpus callosum
- Ventriculomegaly

*Harlequin icthyosis (autosomal recessive)*
- Open mouth with large tongue
- Clenched or fixed hands
- Limbs in fixed positions

*Holt-Oram syndrome (autosomal dominant)*
- Cardiac abnormality
- Abnormal thumb
- Absent digits
- Absent limbs
- Clinodactyly
- Radial hypoplasia

*Hydrolethalus (autosomal recessive)*
- Agenesis of the corpus callosum
- Microphthalmia or anophthalmia
- Polydactyly—postaxial
- Ventriculomegaly
- Polyhydramnios
- Micrognathia
- Cleft palate
- Heart defect
- Clubfoot

*Hypophosphatasia (autosomal recessive)*
- Small chest
- Easily visualized brain structures

**Bowed limbs**
**Moderate-to-severe bone shortening**
**Diffuse hypomineralization**
**Polyhydramnios**

***Ivemark syndrome (usually sporadic)***
**Situs inversus**
**Complex heart defect**
**Polysplenia**
**Renal abnormalities**

***Jackson-Weiss syndrome (autosomal dominant)***
**Exophthalmos/proptosis/prominent eyes**
**Facial asymmetry**

***Jacobsen syndrome (sporadic unless a parent has a balanced translocation)***
**Trigonocephaly**
**Microcephaly**
**Hypertelorism**
**Micrognathia**
**Cardiac defects**

***Jarcho-Levin syndrome, spondylocostal dysostosis (autosomal recessive)***
**Malaligned and malformed vertebra**
**Fan-shaped ribs**
**Severe shortening of the spine**

***Joubert syndrome (autosomal recessive)***
**Cerebellar hypoplasia**
**Dandy-Walker malformation**
**Renal abnormalities**
**Micrognathia**
**Polydactyly**

***Klippel-Feil sequence (sporadic)***
**Vertebral defects**
**Congenital heart defects**
**Cleft palate**

***Kniest syndrome (autosomal dominant)***
**Short limbs**
**Kyphoscoliosis**
**Platyspondyly**
**Hypoplastic pelvic bones**
**Cleft palate**

***Larsen syndrome (autosomal dominant and recessive)***
**Clubfoot**
**Abnormal vertebral segmentation with kyphoscoliosis**
**Hypertelorism**
**Micrognathia**
**Joint dislocation**
**Cleft palate (autosomal dominant form)**

*Lenz syndrome (X-linked recessive)*
- Microcephaly
- Renal aplasia/hypoplasia
- Microphthalmia

*Marden-Walker syndrome (autosomal recessive)*
- Microcephaly
- Micrognathia
- Cleft palate
- Clubfeet
- Joint contractures
- Renal cysts
- Intrauterine growth restriction

*Maternal phenylketonuria*
- Cardiac abnormality
- Microcephaly
- Intrauterine growth restriction

*McKusick-Kaufman syndrome (autosomal recessive)*
- Hydronephrosis
- Cardiac abnormality
- Polydactyly—postaxial
- Hydrometrocolpos (midline lower abdominal mass containing echogenic debris that is due to vaginal atresia/stenosis)
- Other genitourinary anomalies
- Anorectal atresia

*Megacystis megaureter (sporadic)*
- Hydronephrosis
- Large thick-walled bladder
- Dilated ureters
- Mostly male

*Megacystis microcolon intestinal hypoperistalsis syndrome (possibly autosomal recessive)*
- Large bladder without wall thickening
- Polyhydramnios
- Dilated small bowel
- Mostly female

*Melnick-Needles syndrome (X-linked dominant)*
- Exophthalmos
- Micrognathia
- Bowing of humerus, radius, ulna, tibia
- Small chest

*Miller-Dieker syndrome (17p13.3 deletion may be de novo or inherited from a parent with a balanced translocation)*
- Micrognathia
- Clinodactyly
- Absent parieto-occipital fissure
- Abnormal sylvian fissure

**Lissencephaly-only complete agyria can be diagnosed in utero (should not be considered until after 20 weeks' gestation)**
**Ventriculomegaly**
**Microcephaly**
**Intrauterine growth restriction**
**Polyhydramnios**
**Absence of the corpus callosum**

*MURCS (müllerian duct aplasia, renal aplasia, cervicothoracic somite dysplasia) association (sporadic)*
**Upper spine vertebral deformities**
**Absence or hypoplasia of uterus**
**Enlarged fetal bladder**
**Renal agenesis/ectopy**
**Cystic umbilical cord due to patent urachus**
**Oligohydramnios**
**Female fetus**

*Nager acrofacial dysostosis (autosomal dominant)*
**Micrognathia**
**Cleft palate**
**Deformed ears**
**Absent or hypoplastic thumb**

*Neu-Laxova syndrome (autosomal recessive)*
**Intrauterine growth restriction**
**Agenesis of the corpus callosum**
**Cerebellar hypoplasia**
**Lissencephaly**
**Microcephaly with sloping forehead**
**Cataract**
**Exophthalmos/proptosis/prominent eyes with hypertelorism**
**Extreme puffiness of hands and feet**
**Clenched hands**
**Joint contractures**
**Rocker-bottom feet**
**Micrognathia with flat nose**
**Malformed ears**
**Congenial heart disease**

*Noonan syndrome (autosomal dominant)*
**Cardiac abnormality—pulmonary stenosis**
**Other cardiac defects**
**Cystic hygroma**
**Hypertelorism**
**Hemivertebrae**

*Oculodentodigital syndrome (autosomal dominant)*
**Microphthalmia or anophthalmia**
**Aplasia of one or more fingers or toes**

*Opitz G/BBB syndrome (autosomal dominant, X-linked recessive)*
**Hypertelorism**
**Hypospadias**

Cleft lip with or without cleft palate
Micrognathia
Tracheoesophageal fistula
Genital abnormality

*Oral-facial-digital syndrome type I (X-linked dominant)*
Renal cystic disease
Median cleft lip and palate
Abnormal digits
Clinodactyly
Polydactyly—preaxial of feet

*Oromandibular limb hypogenesis spectrum (sporadic)*
Absent digits
Absent limbs
Micrognathia
Cleft palate
Syndactyly

*Otocephaly (likely sporadic)*
Hypoplasia or absence of the mandible and tongue
Agnathia
Cleft palate
Polyhydramnios

*Otopalatodigital syndrome (X-linked with intermediate expression in females)*
Hypertelorism
Cleft palate
Small thorax
Bowed tibia

*Pallister-Hall syndrome (autosomal dominant)*
Intracranial tumor—hypothalamic hamartoblastoma
Polydactyly—postaxial
Imperforate anus

*Poland sequence (sporadic)*
Absent digits
Absent or hypoplastic upper limb
Syndactyly

*Proteus syndrome (sporadic)*
Macrodactyly
Soft tissue masses
Variable-size limbs
Macrocephaly
Nephromegaly

*Retinoic acid embryopathy*
Cardiac abnormalities
Cerebellar hypoplasia
Microcephaly
Ventriculomegaly
Microtia

Micrognathia
Hypertelorism

*Roberts syndrome (autosomal recessive)*
Hypomelia, more severe in upper extremities
Phocomelia
Absent digits
Absent limbs
Cleft lip with or without cleft palate
Hypertelorism
Cardiac abnormality
Encephalocele
Cataract
Clinodactyly
Severe intrauterine growth restriction
Genitourinary anomaly

*Robinow syndrome (autosomal recessive and autosomal dominant)*
Hypertelorism
Cleft lip with or without cleft palate
Micrognathia
Midface hypoplasia
Macrocephaly
Hemivertebrae
Fused/missing ribs
Genital abnormalities
Shortened long bones
Cardiac defects

*Rubinstein-Taybi syndrome (sporadic)*
Broad thumbs with radial angulation
Microcephaly
Renal abnormalities
Cardiac defects

*Russell-Silver syndrome (sporadic)*
Asymmetrical intrauterine growth restriction with normal-size head
Asymmetric short long bones
Micrognathia
Clinodactyly

*Saethre-Chotzen syndrome (autosomal dominant)*
Exophthalmos/proptosis/prominent eyes
Hypertelorism
Facial asymmetry
Craniosynostosis
Frontal bossing
Small ears
Syndactyly
Broad/duplicated large toe

*Seckel syndrome (autosomal recessive)*
Microcephaly
Micrognathia

**Clinodactyly**
**Intrauterine growth restriction**

***Simpson-Golabi-Behnel syndrome (X-linked recessive)***
**Macrosomia**
**Polyhydramnios**
**Macrocephaly**
**Macroglossia**
**Polydactyly—postaxial**

***Sotos syndrome (autosomal dominant)***
**Dolichocephaly**
**Macrocephaly**
**Frontal bossing**
**Macrosomia**
**Ventriculomegaly**
**Absence of the corpus callosum**

***Spondyloepiphyseal dysplasia congenita (autosomal dominant)***
**Small chest**
**Cleft palate**
**Short limbs**
**Short spine with vertebral abnormalities**
**Kyphoscoliosis**
**Platyspondyly**
**Clubfeet**
**Intrauterine growth restriction**

***Stickler syndrome (autosomal dominant)***
**Cleft palate**
**Micrognathia**
**Cataracts**
**Scoliosis**
**Clubfoot**

***Thalidomide embryopathy***
**Absent limbs**
**Phocomelia**
**Cardiac defects**
**Microtia**
**Renal abnormalities**
**Gastrointestinal atresias**

***a-Thalassemia***
**Hydrops**

***Thrombocytopenia—absent radius (TAR) syndrome (autosomal recessive)***
**Absent radius bilaterally**
**Ulnar abnormalities**
**Cardiac abnormality**
**Absent limbs**
**Clubfoot**
**Renal abnormalities**

*Townes-Brock syndrome (autosomal dominant)*
**Facial asymmetry**
**Malformed ears**
**Abnormal thumb**
**Absent digits**
**Polydactyly—preaxial**
**Renal agenesis**
**Multicystic dysplastic kidneys**
**Duodenal atresia**

*Walker-Warburg syndrome (autosomal recessive)*
**Agenesis of the corpus callosum**
**Absent cavum septum pellucidum**
**Dandy-Walker malformation**
**Encephalocele**
**Lissencephaly**
**Mild ventriculomegaly**
**Cataracts**
**Microphthalmia or anophthalmia**

*Weaver syndrome (autosomal dominant)*
**Macrosomia**
**Micrognathia**
**Camptodactyly**
**Clubfoot**
**Cardiac defects**

*Williams syndrome (usually sporadic but transmitted from parent to child)*
**Cardiac defects—supravalvular aortic stenosis**
**Other cardiac defects**
**Renal abnormalities**
**Mild intrauterine growth restriction**

*Zellweger syndrome (autosomal recessive)*
**Renal cystic disease**
**Cataracts**
**Clubfoot**
**Joint contractures**
**Agenesis of the corpus callosum**
**Cardiac defects-septal defects**
**Decreased fetal movement**
**Stippled epiphyses**

Note: In this index, the letters "*f*" and "*t*" denote figures and tables, respectively.

www.ingramcontent.com/pod-product-compliance
Lightning Source LLC
LaVergne TN
LVHW080524210926
848481LV00022B/2823